ONCOLOGY NUTRITION FOR CLINICAL PRACTICE

Oncology Nutrition

a dietetic practice group of the

eat right. Academy of Nutrition and Dietetics

Maureen Leser, MS, RDN, CSO, LD

Natalie Ledesma, MS, RDN, CSO

Sara Bergerson, MS, RDN

Elaine Trujillo, MS, RDN

Editors

eat right. Academy of Nutrition and Dietetics

eat right. Academy of Nutrition and Dietetics

Academy of Nutrition and Dietetics
120 S. Riverside Plaza, Suite 2190
Chicago, IL 60606-6995

Oncology Nutrition for Clinical Practice

ISBN 978-0-88091-527-4
Catalog Number 527419

First published by Oncology Nutrition, a dietetic practice group of the Academy of Nutrition and Dietetics, 2013.

The views expressed in this publication are those of the authors and do not necessarily reflect policies and/or official positions of the Academy of Nutrition and Dietetics. Mention of product names in this publication does not constitute endorsement by the authors or the Academy of Nutrition and Dietetics. The Academy of Nutrition and Dietetics disclaims responsibility for the application of the information contained herein.

10   9   8   7   6   5   4   3

For more information on the Academy of Nutrition and Dietetics, visit www.eatright.org.

Maureen Leser, MS, RDN, CSO, LD
CAPT (retired) USPHS
Consultant
Nutrition, Food and Health Connections
Berlin, MD

Natalie Ledesma, MS, RDN, CSO
Oncology Dietitian
UCSF Helen Diller Family Comprehensive Cancer Center
University of California, San Francisco
Clinical Nutrition Specialist
Smith Integrative Oncology
San Francisco, CA

Sara Bergerson, MS, RDN, CNSC
Clinical Research Dietitian
National Institutes of Health
Clinical Research Center
Bethesda, MD

Elaine Trujillo, MS, RDN
Nutritional Science Research Group
Division of Cancer Prevention
National Cancer Institute
National Institutes of Health
Bethesda, MD

About the Editors

Maureen Leser has 30 years of clinical nutrition experience and is a board-certified specialist in oncology nutrition. After retiring from a career with the US Public Health Service, where she was stationed at the NIH Clinical Research Center in Bethesda, MD, Maureen and her husband Steve retired to the Eastern Shore of Maryland. She worked in the fields of cardiology, weight management, medical-surgical care and critical care before specializing in oncology, and served as the Director of the NIH Dietetic Internship prior to her retirement. Maureen has numerous publications and presentations and over the past several years has served as the editor of *Oncology Nutrition Connection,* the newsletter of the Oncology Nutrition Dietetic Practice Group of the Academy of Nutrition and Dietetics.

A board-certified specialist in oncology nutrition, **Natalie Ledesma** is a senior dietitian for the University of California, San Francisco Helen Diller Family Comprehensive Cancer Center as well as a clinical nutrition specialist at Smith Integrative Oncology in San Francisco. Natalie provides nutritional counseling to oncology patients and develops patient education materials specific to diet and cancer. She has taught college courses and classes, and gives frequent presentations about diet, nutrition, and cancer. Natalie has been interviewed by the *New York Times, NBC, Fortune* magazine, *Runner's World,* and the *San Francisco Chronicle.* Recent publications include nutrition chapters in *Clinical Nutrition for Oncology Patients, Everyone's Guide to Cancer Therapy, Everyone's Guide to Cancer Survivorship, Nutritional Issues in Cancer Care*, and *Supportive Cancer Care: The Complete Guide for Patients and their Families*.

Sara Bergerson has 30 years of clinical nutrition experience, most of it spent in the fields of oncology, critical care and nutrition support. Sara is employed at the NIH Clinical Research Center (CRC) in Bethesda, MD. After retiring from a 30-year career with the US Public Health Service, Sara remained at the NIH as a civil service dietitian. She has numerous publications and presentations and has received many awards for her dedication to patient care. Sara is the critical care and nutrition support preceptor for the NIH Dietetic Internship, and conducts seminars on nutrition support for medical fellows and RNs as well as other RDs at the NIH Clinical Research Center. She works closely with CRC pharmacists, with whom she has jointly developed the NIH Nutrition Support Manual.

Elaine Trujillo is a Nutritionist at the National Cancer Institute (NCI) where she promotes the translation of information about bioactive food components as modifiers of cancer. She collaborates with other federal agencies, and is serving on the management team for the *2015 Dietary Guidelines for Americans.* She currently is the Chair of the Oncology Nutrition Dietetic Practice Group and is former Chair of the Education and Research Division for the Maryland Academy of Nutrition and Dietetics. Prior to joining the NCI, Ms. Trujillo was a Senior Clinical and Research Dietitian at Brigham and Women's Hospital, Harvard Medical School in Boston. Elaine has numerous publications, including scientific journal articles, book chapters and textbooks. Along with Catherine Jones, she has authored the book, *Eating for Lower Cholesterol,* Da Capo Press, and is working on a second book, *The Calories In Calories Out Cookbook,* The Experiment Publishing, which is due out Spring 2014.

ONCOLOGY NUTRITION
FOR CLINICAL PRACTICE

Donald I. Abrams, MD
Chief, Hematology-Oncology
San Francisco General Hospital
Integrative Oncologist
UCSF Osher Center for Integrative Medicine
Professor of Clinical Medicine
University of California, San Francisco
San Francisco, CA

Alice Bender, MS, RDN
Associate Director, Nutrition Programs
American Institute for Cancer Research
Washington, DC

Shanna Bernstein, MPH, RD
Clinical Research Dietitian
National Institutes of Health
Clinical Research Center
Bethesda, MD

Karen Collins, MS, RDN, CDN
Nutrition Advisor
American Institute for Cancer Research
Washington, DC

Tricia Cox, RD, CSO, LD, CNSC
Oncology Dietitian
Baylor University Medical Center
Dallas, TX

Laura Elliott, MPH, RD, CSO, LD
Clinical Dietitian
Mary Greely Medical Center
Ames, IA

Danielle Fatemi, MS, RD, LD
Clinical Research Dietitian
National Institutes of Health
Clinical Research Center
Bethesda, MD

Colleen Gill, MS, RD, CSO
Oncology Dietitian
University of Colorado Cancer Center
Aurora, CO

Elizabeth M. Grainger, PhD, RD
Research Dietitian
Laboratory of Nutrition and Chemoprevention
Division of Hematology and Oncology
The Ohio State University Comprehensive Cancer Center
Columbus, OH

Barbara L. Grant, MS, RDN, CSO, LD
Oncology Dietitian
Saint Alphonsus Cancer Care Center
Boise, ID

Kathryn K Hamilton, MA, RD, CSO, CDN
Outpatient Oncology Dietitian
Carol G Simon Cancer Center
Morristown Medical Center
Morristown, NJ

Susan Higginbotham, PhD, RDN
Director of Research
American Institute for Cancer Research
Washington, DC

Maureen B Huhmann DCN, RD, CSO
Adjunct Assistant Professor
Department of Nutritional Sciences, School of Health Related Professions
Rutgers, The State University
Newark, NJ

Maki Inoue-Choi, PhD, MS, RD
Research Associate
Division of Epidemiology and Community Health
School of Public Health
University of Minnesota
Minneapolis, MN

Natalie Ledesma, MS, RDN, CSO
Oncology Dietitian
UCSF Helen Diller Family Comprehensive Cancer Center
University of California, San Francisco
Clinical Nutrition Specialist
Smith Integrative Oncology
San Francisco, CA

Maureen Leser, MS, RDN, CSO, LD
CAPT (retired) USPHS
Consultant
Nutrition, Food and Health Connections
Berlin, MD

Rhone Levin, MEd, RD, CSO, LD
St. Luke's Meridian Medical Center
Mountain States Tumor Institute
Meridian, ID

Greta Macaire, MA, RD, CSO
Oncology Dietitian
UCSF Helen Diller Family Comprehensive Cancer Center
University of California
Cancer Resource Center
San Francisco, CA

Paula Charuhas Macris, MS, RD, CSO, FADA
Nutrition Education Coordinator
Pediatric Nutrition Specialist
Seattle Cancer Care Alliance
Seattle, WA

Contributors

Mary Marian, MS, RD, CSO
Instructor & Clinical Dietitian
University of Arizona
Colleges of Medicine & Agriculture-Life Sciences
Consultant, AZ Oncology Associates
Tucson, AZ

Jeannine Mills, MS, RD, CSO, LD
Oncology Dietitian
Norris Cotton Cancer Center
Dartmouth Hitchcock Medical Center
Lebanon, NH

Eric Nadler, MD, MPP
Medical Oncologist
Charles A. Sammons Cancer Center
Baylor University Medical Center
Dallas, TX

Vicky A. Newman, MS, RD
Director, Nutrition Services
Cancer Prevention & Control Program
Moores UCSD Cancer Center
La Jolla, CA

Andreea Nguyen, MS, RD, CSO, LD, CNSC
Clinical Dietitian
Charles A. Sammons Cancer Center
Baylor University Medical Center
Dallas, TX

Sarah O'Brien, MS, RD, CSO
Clinical Dietitian
Denver, CO

Maria Q. B. Petzel, RD, CSO, LD, CNSC
Senior Clinical Dietitian
The University of Texas MD Anderson Cancer Center
Houston, TX

Kimberly Robien, PhD, RD, CSO, FAND
Associate Professor
Department of Epidemiology and Biostatistics
George Washington University School of Public Health
and Health Services
Washington, DC

Alison N. Ryan, MS, RDN, CSO, CNSC
Clinical Dietitian-Oncology/Hematology/Radiation
Stanford Hospital and Clinics
Palo Alto, CA

Shari Oakland Schulze, RD, CSO
Board Certified as a Specialist in Oncology Nutrition
ESJH Comprehensive Cancer Center
Denver, CO

Pamela Sheridan-Neumann, MPH, RD, LD
Pediatric Clinical Dietitian
Texas Children's Hospital
Houston, TX

Colleen Spees, PhD, MEd, RD, LD
Assistant Professor
Medical Dietetics & Health Sciences
Comprehensive Cancer Center
The Ohio State University Medical Center
Columbus, OH

Cynthia A Thomson, PhD, RD, FAND
Professor - Public Health, Division of Health Promotion Sciences
Member University of Arizona Cancer Center
University of Arizona
Tucson, AZ

Kelay Trentham, MS, RDN, CSO, CD
MultiCare Regional Cancer Center
Tacoma, WA

Ashley J. Vargas, PhD, RD, CSG
Post-doctoral Fellow, Cancer Prevention Fellowship Program
National Cancer Institute
Graduate student, Harvard School of Public Health
Harvard University
Boston, MA

Reviewers
Katrina Claghorn, MS, RD, LDN
Cynthia Clark, MS, RD, CSO
Mridul Datta, PhD, RD
Marnie Dobbin, MS, RD, CNSC
Rachael Drabot-Lopez, MPH, RD, CSO
Laura Elliott, MPH, RD, CSO, LD
Nicole Fox, RD, LMNT, CNSC
Jody Gilman, MS, RD, CNSC
Karen Huntzinger, MS, RD
Melissa Kingery, MS, RD
Dianne Kiyomoto, RD, CSO
Jeannine Mills, MS, RD CSO, LD
Laure Newton, MAEd, RD, LD
Lee Renda, RD
Nancy Sebring, MEd, RD
Karen Smith, MS, RDN
Leslie Shaw, RD, LD, CNSC
Paige Mller. PhD, MPH, RD
Holly Nicastro, PhD, MPH
Alice Shapiro, PhD, RD, LN
Kelly Verdin, RD

The editors would also like to thank Sara Bergerson, MS, RD and
Barbara Grant, MS, RD, CSO for expert technical consultation.

Cancer and Nutrition: Significance and Background

Maki Inoue-Choi, PhD, MS, RD
Kim Robien, PhD, RD, CSO, FAND

Introduction

The term *cancer* refers to a group of neoplastic diseases characterized by the uncontrollable growth and spread of abnormal cells, which if left untreated may result in death. There are more than 100 different types of cancer, each with different etiology, progression, recommended treatment, and prognosis. This chapter reviews cancer statistics in the United States (U.S.) adult population, cancer screening, classification methods, and health care expenditures for cancer care. This chapter also provides a general overview of the role of nutrition in carcinogenesis.

Cancer Statistics

Using data from the Surveillance, Epidemiology and End Results program of the National Cancer institute (NCI), a premier source for cancer statistics in the U.S., the American Cancer Society (ACS) estimates that approximately 1.6 million new cancer cases will be diagnosed in 2013 (1-2). The lifetime risk of developing cancer for men is 1 in 2; the risk for women is a little more than 1 in 3. In the U.S., whites and African Americans have the highest cancer incidence rates among all racial/ethnicity groups (3). The five most common cancer types in the U.S. are prostate, lung, colorectal, urinary bladder and melanoma skin cancers for men, and breast, lung, colorectal, uterine and thyroid cancers for women (1). Overall, cancer incidence rates increased from 1975 to 1989, were stable from 1989 to 1999, and have significantly declined since 1999 (2,4).

Cancer is the second most common cause of death in the U.S., accounting for nearly 1 of every 4 deaths, with heart disease as the leading cause of death. Approximately 580,350 Americans are expected to die of cancer in 2013 (1). Survival varies significantly by cancer types and staging. The five-year survival rate for all cancers improved from 49% for cancers diagnosed between 1975 and 1977 to 67% in 2007.

Cancer Screening

Regular screening examinations can result in the early detection of precancerous lesions and the diagnosis of cancers at an early stage, when they are most treatable. Early cancer detection refers to identifying tumors before they become palpable, and is an active area of cancer research with the potential to significantly decrease cancer morbidity, mortality and health care costs (5). Significant decreases in death rates from certain cancers such as breast and colorectal cancers over the last decade are attributed largely to the increase in the use of screening tests as well as improvement in treatment (1).

There are several different kinds of screening tests including physical examination, blood tests, imaging procedures, and molecular tests. Physical examination or palpation is the most common screening test. Examples include breast or testicle self-exams, or examination of the skin to look for pigmentation changes that may signal the development of skin cancer. However, once cancer is able to be detected by these techniques, it is often fairly advanced. Blood tests to determine levels of circulating tumor cell metabolites, such as prostate specific antigen testing, have been developed as early detection methods. Imaging procedures such as mammograms and colonoscopies are able to detect cancers that are too small to feel by physical exam. Molecular techniques, such as genotyping or gene expression assays, which look for certain genetic mutations that are linked to some types of cancer, are also being explored for possible use in early cancer detection, as are many radiographic techniques. False screening test results can occur. Test results may appear to be abnormal even though there is no cancer. A false-positive result may cause anxiety and is usually followed by more invasive tests and procedures. Conversely, screening test results may appear to be normal even though a cancer is present. A false-negative test result may delay appropriate medical care. The ACS publishes annual cancer screening and detection guidelines that are available on the ACS web site www.cancer.org (6).

Cancer Staging

Staging of cancer is essential to determine the appropriate treatment plan and to estimate prognosis at the time of diagnosis. Staging describes the severity of a cancer based on the extent of disease and whether the primary tumor has spread to other areas of the body. The Tumor, lymph Nodes, and Metastasis (TNM) classification system (7-8) is one of the most widely used tumor staging tools, especially for solid tumors. Each tumor is assigned grades for each initial: a T grade reflects the size and/or extent of the tumor; an N grade is for the extent of spread to local lymph nodes; and an M grade indicates the presence of distant metastasis. A number added to each letter indicates the size or extent of the primary cancer and the extent of cancer spread (Table 1). Additionally, tumor grading systems are used to classify cancer cells in terms of their appearance. Histologic grade describes how "differentiated" the tumor cells appear, in other words, how different the tumor cells appear from normal cells in the same tissue (Table 2). Each type of cancer has a unique grading system. Tumors are also described according to their nuclear grade, which refers to the size and shape of the nucleus in tumor cells, and the percentage of tumor cells that are actively dividing (8).

Cost of Cancer Care

The financial costs of cancer care are a burden to cancer patients, their families, and society. The NCI estimates that the direct medical cost of cancer care in 2010 was $125 billion, and is expected to reach $158 billion by 2020 given the growth and aging of the U.S. population (9-10). This represents a 27% increase in the national cancer financial burden over the next 10 years. The largest projected increase in costs for 2020 is expected to result from long-term continuing care for female breast and male prostate cancer survivors, the most common cancers in women and men, respectively (9). Additional costs will occur with the rise in cancer incidence expected with increased longevity (11). Individually, cancer survivors also face not only direct costs related to health care expenses, but lost income due to illness, decreased productivity, and premature mortality (10).

Carcinogenesis

The term carcinogenesis refers to the process by which normal cells transform into cancer cells, usually as a result of accumulating genetic damage. Figure 1 depicts the steps of the carcinogenesis process. Normal cells may develop genetic damage as a result of exposure to environmental factors such as radiation, chemicals, or viruses. Under normal conditions, cellular processes, such as DNA repair enzymes, allow cells to repair individual instances of DNA damage. If the damage cannot be repaired, it may trigger cell cycle arrest that results in a process called apoptosis, or programmed-cell death. However, genetic damage that occurs within the DNA repair genes, proto-oncogenes and/or tumor suppressor genes can lead to alterations in these normal repair processes and uncontrolled growth of the tumor.

Both hereditary and acquired factors influence the carcinogenic process. Although genetic susceptibility influences the risk of cancer, most cancers are caused by acquired factors, including internal factors such as hormones and the immune system, and external factors including infection, environmental toxins, and behaviors such as smoking, sunlight exposure, and an unhealthy diet (12-13). These factors may act together to initiate or promote the carcinogenic process. Many cancers take ten or more years to develop; therefore, nutrition may be crucial to prevention. According to the ACS and the World Cancer Research Fund / American Institute for Cancer Research report, one-third of cancer deaths are smoking-related, and another one-third are related to obesity or overweight, physical inactivity, and poor nutrition (1,14).

Nutrition and Carcinogenesis
There is evidence, primarily from *in vitro* studies, suggesting that nutrients may play a protective role in these early carcinogenesis processes (Figure 1). Food components may have protective effects

Table 1: Summary of the TNM Classification System (8)

Grade	Definition
Primary Tumor (T)	
Tx	Tumor cannot be evaluated
T0	No evidence of tumor
Tis	*Carcinoma in situ* (CIS): abnormal cells are present but have not spread to neighboring tissues. Although CIS is not cancer, it may become cancer.
T1	Tumor not palpable or visible by imaging
T2	Tumor confined to the primary cancer site
T3	Tumor extends to the neighboring tissue
T4	Metastatic disease
Lymph Nodes (N)	
Nx	Regional lymph nodes cannot be evaluated
N0	No regional lymph node involvement
N1, 2, 3	Involvement of regional lymph nodes (number of lymph nodes and/or extent of spread)
Distant Metastasis (M)	
Mx	Distant metastasis cannot be evaluated
M0	No distant metastasis
M1	Distant metastasis is present

Table 2: American Joint Committee on Cancer tumor grading system (8)

Grade	Description
GX	Grade cannot be assessed (Undetermined grade)
G1	Well-differentiated (low grade)
G2	Moderately differentiated (intermediate grade)
G3	Poorly differentiated (high grade)
G4	Undifferentiated (high grade)

in carcinogenesis through multiple mechanisms including cell growth cycle, apoptosis, DNA repair, cell differentiation, hormone regulation, carcinogen metabolism, and inflammatory response (Figure 2) (15). Antioxidants, such as vitamins C and E, may protect DNA from oxidative damage (16). Folate plays an important role in both DNA synthesis and DNA repair, and individuals who are folate deficient may be at increased risk of DNA damage and inefficient DNA repair (17). Adequate folate intake has been shown to be associated with lower risk of cancer in large, prospective cohort studies (18). Selenium has also been shown to play a number of roles in DNA protection and repair, including protection from DNA damage, support of DNA repair, and induction of cell cycle arrest (19). Soy isoflavones are known as phytoestrogens, which have hormonal effects and alter hormonal regulation (20-21). Curcumin, a polyphenol in turmeric, has been shown to induce apoptosis and inhibit angiogenesis, which is the formation of blood supply to the growing tumor (22). Indole-3-carbinol, a bioactive compound found in cruciferous vegetables, has been shown to influence estrogen regulation, induce cell cycle arrest and apoptosis, inhibit

Figure 1: Effect of nutrients during the various stages of carcinogenesis

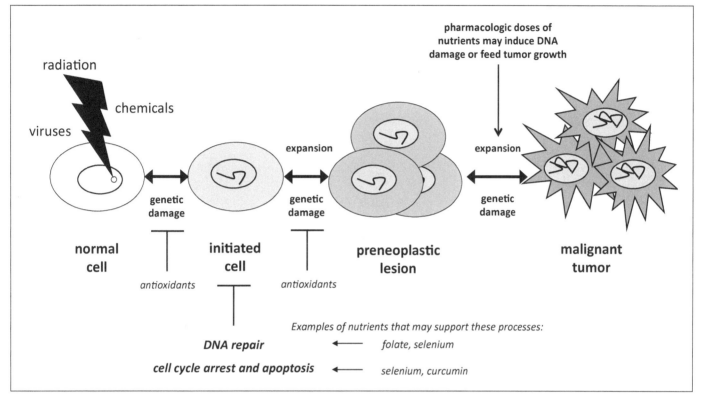

Legend. Normal healthy cells may develop genetic damage as a result of exposure to environmental factors such as radiation, chemicals or viruses. Nutrients may play a protective role in these early carcinogenesis processes. Antioxidants may protect DNA from oxidative damage. Folate provides methyl groups that are vital for both DNA synthesis and repair. Selenium has also been shown to provide protection from DNA damage, support of DNA repair, and induce cell cycle arrest. Curcumin has been shown to induce apoptosis. However, at pharmacologic doses, some nutrients have the potential to increase cancer risk. For example, extremely high folate may promote the growth of undetected cancers.

angiogenesis, and suppress inflammatory responses (23-24). Sulforaphane, another bioactive compound found in cruciferous vegetables, may inhibit carcinogen formation and induce apoptosis (25). Allyl sulfur compounds in garlic may block the formation and activation of carcinogens, enhance DNA repair, reduce cell proliferation, and/or induce apoptosis (26).

Nutrition recommendations and interventions may vary by cancer type, stage of the carcinogenesis, and/or planned treatment. Nutrients may play different roles in different stages of carcinogenesis (Figure 1) via a variety of mechanisms (Figure 2). For example, once carcinogenesis is initiated, folate provides substrates for DNA synthesis and accelerates cancer cell proliferation and tumor expansion (27). The anti-folate chemotherapeutic agent methotrexate actually targets this metabolic process, and inhibits folate-mediated DNA synthesis, thus stopping cancer cell proliferation. Folate in the form of calcium leucovorin may be used to "rescue" patients from methotrexate toxicity (28-29), or alternatively, to enhance the effectiveness of drugs such as 5-fluorouracil that target enzymes that use folate as a cofactor (30).

Pharmacologic doses of nutrients from dietary supplementation, especially in addition to adequate dietary intake, may enhance progression of clinically undetectable cancers. For example, Mason et al. hypothesized that the increased rates of colorectal cancers

observed around the time of mandatory folate fortification of enriched grain products in the U.S. in the late 1990s may be due to increased folate exposure promoting the growth of undetected cancers (31). Potential nutrition-related issues and outcomes by stages of the cancer continuum are outlined in Figure 3.

Cancer Treatment

Cancer is primarily treated with surgery, radiation, chemotherapy, hormone therapy, immunotherapy, biological therapy, targeted therapy, transplantation, or a combination of these modalities (1,32). Treatment selection depends on the cancer type, stage of disease and other factors such as a patient's age and comorbid conditions. Supportive care with nutrition and physical activity interventions, as well as complementary and alternative medicine approaches, are increasingly being used (1,32).

Chemotherapy agents are designed to kill cancer cells, which often grow and divide more rapidly than normal cells. However, most chemotherapy drugs are indiscriminate, and may also damage normal cells such as blood cells in the bone marrow; cells in the digestive tract, including the mouth, esophagus, stomach, and intestines; cells in the reproductive system; and hair follicles. Common side effects of chemotherapy, such as loss of appetite, nausea, mucositis, and diarrhea, are the result of this damage. Nutrition and pharmacologic intervention may help prevent

Figure 2: Mechanisms through which bioactive food components influence carcinogenesis

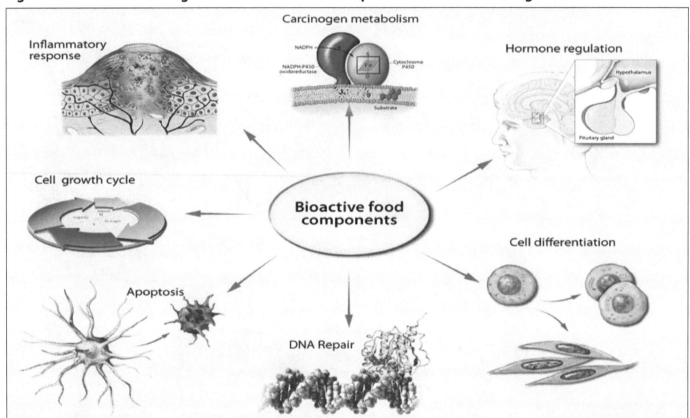

Legend. Food components may have protective effects on carcinogenesis through multiple mechanisms. For example, epigallocatechin-3-gallate (ECGC) found in green tea has been shown to modulate rates of cell differentiation. Antioxidants, such as vitamins C and E, may protect DNA from oxidative damage, while folate and selenium are necessary for DNA repair. Indole-3-carbinol (found in cruciferous vegetables) and selenium have been shown to alter cell cycle regulation by inducing cell cycle arrest, thus limiting growth of cancers. Curcumin, a polyphenol in turmeric, may induce apoptosis and inhibit the formation of the blood supply to a growing tumor (angiogenesis). Indole-3-carbinol and EGCG have been found to suppress inflammatory responses. Sulforaphane (a bioactive found in cruciferous vegetables) and allyl sulfur compounds in garlic may inhibit carcinogen formation. Soy isoflavones, which are phytoestrogens, have been shown to alter hormonal regulation.

Reprinted from *J Am Diet Assoc*, 2006, 106(3), Trujillo E, Davis C, Milner J. Nutrigenomics, Proteomics, Metabolomics, and Dietetic Practice, 103-113, 2006, with permission from Elsevier.

significant weight loss and malnutrition caused by these side effects. Radiation therapy can also cause side effects by damaging normal, healthy cells near the treatment site (32). Studies suggest that nutrition intervention during cancer treatment is associated with fewer side effects (33-37), fewer hospitalizations (34,36,38), and better quality of life (33,35,37). The role of nutrition interventions during cancer treatment is discussed in further detail in Chapters 12 and 16-26.

Conclusion

Nutrition plays a significant role throughout the carcinogenic process. Successful nutrition interventions to decrease cancer risk and improve cancer outcomes require understanding of cancer biology, treatment regimens, and management of side effects of cancer treatment.

References

1. American Cancer Society. *Cancer Facts & Figures 2013*. Atlanta, Georgia. Accessed National Cancer Institute. SEER Cancer Statistics Review, 1975-2009 (Vintage 2009 Populations). Bethesda, MD. http://www.cancer.org/research/cancerfactsfigures/cancerfactsfigures/cancer-facts-figures-2013. Accessed March 10, 2013.

2. Howlader N, Noone AM, Krapcho M, et al., eds. SEER Cancer Statistics Review, 1975-2009 (Vintage 2009 Populations), National Cancer Institute. Bethesda, MD, http://seer.cancer.gov/csr/1975_2009_pops09/, based on November 2011 SEER data submission, posted to the SEER web site April 2012. Accessed June 2012.

3. North American Association of Central Cancer Registries 2011. Available at: http://faststats.naaccr.org/selections.php?#Output. Accessed June 2012.

4. National Cancer Institute. Cancer Trends Progress Report - 2009/2010 Update. National Cancer Institute. Bethesda, MD. Available at: http://progressreport.cancer.gov/doc_detail.asp?pid=1&did=2009&chid=93&coid=920&mid#trends. Updated 4/15/10. Accessed June 2012.

5. Etzioni R, Urban N, Ramsey S, et al. The case for early detection. *Nat Rev Cancer.* 2003;3(4):243-252.

6. American Cancer Society. Guidelines for the Early Detection of Cancer. web site. Available at: http://www.cancer.org/Healthy/FindCancerEarly/CancerScreeningGuidelines/american-cancer-society-guidelines-for-the-early-detection-of-cancer. Last Medical Review 3/5/12. Accessed June 2012.

7. Sobin LH, Wittekind C, editors. *TNM: classification of malignant tumors.* 6th ed. New York, NY: Wiley-Liss; 2002.

8. American Joint Committee on Cancer. *AJCC Cancer Staging Manual.* 6th ed. New York, NY: Springer; 2002.

9. Mariotto AB, Yabroff KR, Shao Y, Feuer EJ, Brown ML. Projections of the cost of cancer care in the United States: 2010-2020. *J Natl Cancer Inst.* 2011;103(2):117-128.

Figure 3: Potential nutrition-related issues and outcomes across the cancer continuum

	Diagnosis		≥ 5 years after diagnosis	
	Cancer prevention	**Initial treatment**	**Early post-treatment**	**Long-term cancer survivorship**
Potential nutrition issues	Obesity, body fatness Energy-dense food intake Excessive micronutrient intake from dietary supplements Food contaminants (toxins, chemicals)	Side effects of treatment (e.g., nausea, vomiting, diarrhea, mucositits, taste changes) Fatigue Pain Anorexia Treatment-related cachexia Immunosuppression Weight/body composition changes Drug-nutrition interactions	Fatigue Pain Endocrine disorders Weight / body composition changes Cognitive deficits Dental caries/complications	Weight changes Osteoporosis Endocrine disorders Cardiovascular complications Cognitive deficits Dental caries/complications
Potential outcomes of nutrition interventions	Weight/body composition management Better blood sugar control Improved immune surveillance	Ability to adhere to scheduled treatment Fewer infectious complications Weight/body composition management Delay/prevent disease progression Improved survival Improved quality of life	Less fatigue Improved functional status More rapid recovery from treatment Weight/body composition management Decreased risk of cancer recurrence, subsequent primary cancers Improved survival Improved quality of life	Fewer late-effects of treatment Improved functional status Weight/body composition management Decreased risk of cancer recurrence, subsequent primary cancers Improved survival Improved quality of life Lower health care costs

10. National Cancer Institute. The Cost of Cancer. Available at: http://cancer.gov/aboutnci/servingpeople/cancer-statistics/costofcancer. Updated 2/18/11. Accessed June 2012.
11. Yabroff KR, Lamont EB, Mariotto A, et al. Cost of care for elderly cancer patients in the United States. *J Natl Cancer Inst.* 2008;100(9):630-641.
12. Willett WC. Balancing life-style and genomics research for disease prevention. *Science.* 2002;296(5568):695-698.
13. Czene K, Lichtenstein P, Hemminki K. Environmental and heritable causes of cancer among 9.6 million individuals in the Swedish Family-Cancer Database. *Int J Cancer.* 2002;99(2):260-266.
14. World Cancer Research Fund / American Institute for Cancer Research. *Food, Nutrition, Physical Activity and the Prevention of Cancer: a Global Perspective.* Washington DC: AICR; 2007.
15. Trujillo E, Davis C, Milner J. Nutrigenomics, proteomics, metabolomics, and the practice of dietetics. *J Am Diet Assoc.* 2006;106(3):403-413.
16. Loft S, Moller P, Cooke MS, Rozalski R, Olinski R. Antioxidant vitamins and cancer risk: is oxidative damage to DNA a relevant biomarker? *Eur J Nutr.* 2008;47 Suppl 2:19-28.
17. Duthie SJ, Hawdon A. DNA instability (strand breakage, uracil misincorporation, and defective repair) is increased by folic acid depletion in human lymphocytes in vitro. *FASEB J.* 1998;12(14):1491-1497.
18. Kim DH, Smith-Warner SA, Spiegelman D, et al. Pooled analyses of 13 prospective cohort studies on folate intake and colon cancer. *Cancer Causes Control.* 2010;21(11):1919-1930.
19. Valdiglesias V, Pasaro E, Mendez J, Laffon B. In vitro evaluation of selenium genotoxic, cytotoxic, and protective effects: a review. *Arch Toxicol.* 2010;84(5):337-351.
20. Duncan AM, Underhill KE, Xu X, Lavalleur J, Phipps WR, Kurzer MS. Modest hormonal effects of soy isoflavones in postmenopausal women. *J Clin Endocrinol Metab.*1999;84(10):3479-3484.
21. Cassidy A, Bingham S, Setchell KD. Biological effects of a diet of soy protein rich in isoflavones on the menstrual cycle of premenopausal women. *Am J Clin Nutr.* 1994;60(3):333-340.
22. Agrawal DK, Mishra PK. Curcumin and its analogues: potential anticancer agents. *Med Res Rev.* 2010;30(5):818-860.
23. Higdon JV, Delage B, Williams DE, Dashwood RH. Cruciferous vegetables and human cancer risk: epidemiologic evidence and mechanistic basis. *Pharmacol Res.* 2007;55(3):224-236.
24. Chinni SR, Li Y, Upadhyay S, Koppolu PK, Sarkar FH. Indole-3-carbinol (I3C) induced cell growth inhibition, G1 cell cycle arrest and apoptosis in prostate cancer cells. *Oncogene.* 2001;20(23):2927-2936.
25. Sarkar R, Mukherjee S, Biswas J, Roy M. Sulphoraphane, a naturally occurring isothiocyanate induces apoptosis in breast cancer cells by targeting heat shock proteins. *Biochem Biophys Res Commun.* 2012;427(1):80-85.
26. Milner JA. A historical perspective on garlic and cancer. *J Nutr.* 2001;131(3s):1027S-1031S.
27. Choi SW, Mason JB. Folate status: effects on pathways of colorectal carcinogenesis. *J Nutr.* 2002;132(8 Suppl):2413S-2418S.
28. Sullivan RD, Miller E, Sikes MP. Antimetabolite metabolite combination cancer chemotherapy. Effects of intraarterial methotrexate-intramuscular Citrovorum factor therapy in human cancer. *Cancer.* 1959;12:1248-1262.
29. Kamen BA. High-dose methotrexate and asparaginase for the treatment of children with acute lymphoblastic leukemia: why and how? *J Pediatr Hematol Oncol.* 2004;26(6):333-335.
30. Grem J. 5-Fluoropyrimidines. In: Chabner BA, Longo DL, eds. *Cancer Chemotherapy and Biotherapy.* 2nd ed. Philadelphia: Lippincott-Raven; 1996.
31. Mason JB, Dickstein A, Jacques PF, et al. A temporal association between folic acid fortification and an increase in colorectal cancer rates may be illuminating important biological principles: a hypothesis. *Cancer Epidemiol Biomarkers Prev.* 2007;16(7):1325-1329.

32. American Cancer Society. Treatments and Side Effects. Available at: http://www.cancer.org/Treatment/TreatmentsandSideEffects/index. Accessed June 2012.
33. Ravasco P, Monteiro-Grillo I, Vidal PM, Camilo ME. Dietary counseling improves patient outcomes: a prospective, randomized, controlled trial in colorectal cancer patients undergoing radiotherapy. *J Clin Oncol.* 2005;23(7):1431-1438.
34. Odelli C, Burgess D, Bateman L, et al. Nutrition support improves patient outcomes, treatment tolerance and admission characteristics in oesophageal cancer. *Clin Oncol* (R Coll Radiol). 2005;17(8):639-645.
35. Ravasco P, Monteiro-Grillo I, Marques Vidal P, Camilo ME. Impact of nutrition on outcome: a prospective randomized controlled trial in patients with head and neck cancer undergoing radiotherapy. *Head Neck.* 2005;27(8):659-668.
36. Paccagnella A, Morello M, Da Mosto MC, et al. Early nutritional intervention improves treatment tolerance and outcomes in head and neck cancer patients undergoing concurrent chemoradiotherapy. *Support Care Cancer.* 2010;18(7):837-845.
37. Ollenschlager G, Thomas W, Konkol K, Diehl V, Roth E. Nutritional behaviour and quality of life during oncological polychemotherapy: results of a prospective study on the efficacy of oral nutrition therapy in patients with acute leukaemia. *Eur J Clin Invest.* 1992;22(8):546-553.
38. Hill A, Kiss N, Hodgson B, Crowe TC, Walsh AD. Associations between nutritional status, weight loss, radiotherapy treatment toxicity and treatment outcomes in gastrointestinal cancer patients. *Clin Nutr.* 2011;30(1):92-98.

Nutrition and Cancer Prevention

Alice Bender, MS, RDN
Karen Collins, MS, RDN, CDN
Susan Higginbotham, PhD, RDN

A substantial proportion of cancer cases in the United States do not have to happen. An estimated one-third of some of the most common cancers and one-quarter of cancer overall could be prevented by healthy patterns of diet and physical activity (1). The American Institute for Cancer Research and the World Cancer Research Fund (AICR/WCRF) developed recommendations for cancer prevention that were based on systematic reviews of the literature on food, nutrition, physical activity and cancer. These recommendations and the science behind them are outlined in this chapter (2). The chapter also includes a section on "emerging topics" that focuses on selected foods and nutrients of special interest. These foods and nutrients are being actively studied but there is currently limited or inconsistent evidence regarding their effects on cancer risk.

Recommendations for Cancer Prevention

The AICR/WCRF recommendations were developed by an expert panel that reviewed and synthesized the large body of relevant peer-reviewed literature on diet, physical activity, and cancer. The recommendations are aimed at the prevention of cancer as a whole but they take the prevention of other diseases into account as well. The recommendations are compatible with the 2010 Dietary Guidelines for Americans, which were designed to promote health, reduce the risk of chronic diseases, and reduce the prevalence of overweight and obesity (3) as well as with the American Cancer Society guidelines on nutrition and physical activity for cancer prevention (4). Table 1 summarizes AICR/WCRF recommendations for cancer prevention. In addition, Appendix 1 compares cancer prevention nutrition and lifestyle recommendations from AICR, the World Health Organization, the American Cancer Society, and the National Comprehensive Cancer Network.

Body Fatness (Overweight and Obesity)

Second only to not using tobacco products, maintaining a healthy body weight throughout life may be the most important lifestyle factor to reduce cancer risk. There is convincing evidence that body fatness is a cause of cancer of the esophagus (adenocarcinoma), pancreas, colorectum, breast (postmenopause), endometrium, and kidney and evidence that body fatness probably is a cause of cancer of the gall bladder (2,5-7). Approximately 20 percent of these cancers in the United States are attributed to overweight and obesity (1).

There are several plausible mechanisms through which body fatness could influence cancer risk:

- Excess body fat is associated with insulin resistance, resulting in elevated levels of insulin and increased bioavailable insulin-like growth factor 1 (IGF-1) (8). This increase in IGF-1 can stimulate a mitogen-activated protein kinase pathway, promoting growth and reproduction of cancer cells and inhibiting apoptosis (i.e., programmed cell death).
- Adipose tissue is the primary site of estrogen production in postmenopausal women. Obese women tend to have higher levels of bioavailable estrogen, which is associated with endometrial cancer and postmenopausal breast cancer.
- Fat cells also produce other hormones, including leptin. Increased leptin levels associated with obesity may promote cell proliferation and angiogenesis while inhibiting apoptosis.
- Excess body fat is linked with decreased levels of the adipose hormone adiponectin. Adiponectin is a protective hormone that decreases insulin resistance and inflammation and promotes apoptosis (9).
- Overweight and obesity are associated with a state of low-grade chronic inflammation that can promote cancer development through elevations in DNA-damaging free radicals and cell-to-cell signaling proteins (2).
- Other possible mechanisms include altered immune responses and various organ-specific effects.

Abdominal fatness

Waist circumference is a measure of abdominal fatness that includes both subcutaneous and the more metabolically active visceral fat stores. The evidence that abdominal fatness is a cause of colorectal cancer is convincing. It is associated with increased risk of cancers of the endometrium, breast (postmenopause), and pancreas as well (2,5,7,10-11). Visceral fat stores are associated with hyperinsulinemia and influence the body's response to inflammation. AICR recommends that waist circumference be no larger than 37 inches in men, and 31.5 inches in women. Research is underway to develop standards that reflect ethnic differences in body fat deposition.

Key Practice Points

- Body fatness probably protects against premenopausal breast cancer but increases the risk of postmenopausal breast cancer, which is more common. Thus, any potential benefit of overweight and obesity decreasing risk for premenopausal breast cancer is outweighed by the increased risk for postmenopausal breast cancer as well as for other chronic diseases.

- For people already overweight or obese, there are benefits from even a modest reduction in weight. Data are limited but current studies suggest that intentional weight loss is associated with decreased cancer risk (12).
- Even within the normal range of body mass index (BMI), both large waist size and excessive adult weight gain are associated with unhealthy metabolic changes and increased risk of some cancers. Steps are warranted to change the balance of calories consumed and used in physical activity to achieve a more optimum metabolic environment and improved body composition.

Physical Activity

All forms of physical activity protect against cancers of the colon, breast (postmenopause), and endometrium (2,6-7). Physical activity also prevents many cancers indirectly through protection against weight gain, overweight, and obesity. The American Cancer Society recommends that adults get 150 minutes of moderate activity or 75 minutes of vigorous activity each week and that children and adolescents be physically active for a minimum of one hour each day, to include at least three days each week of vigorous activity (4). AICR/WCRF recommends at least 30 minutes of moderate physical activity every day. As fitness improves and for even more protection, aim for 60 minutes or more of moderate, or for 30 minutes or more of vigorous, physical activity every day.

An emerging body of research points to sedentary behavior, independent from physical activity, as a risk factor for cancer, possibly because of its effects on waist size, insulin levels, and inflammation (13-14). Both AICR/WCRF and the American Cancer Society recommend limiting sedentary behavior such as sitting, lying down, and watching television (2,4).

Mechanisms through which physical activity could influence cancer risk include:
- Reduced weight gain and easier maintenance of a healthy level of body fat;
- Improved insulin sensitivity and reduced insulin levels;
- Decreased levels of bioavailable sex steroid hormones;
- More rapid gut transit time, which reduces exposure of colon cells to carcinogens;
- Improved immune function.

Key Practice Points
- Increasing physical activity generally produces a modest and slow weight loss without changes in calorie consumption. People expecting rapid weight loss from exercise may become frustrated and stop exercising, so it is important to emphasize that regular physical activity is not aimed only at weight management, and provides cancer protective benefits regardless of body weight.

Foods and Drinks that Promote Weight Gain

Research indicates that diets rich in low energy-dense foods protect against weight gain, overweight, and obesity (2,15-16). By supporting a healthy body weight, low energy-dense diets help protect against cancer. They provide filling amounts of food that make it possible to limit calorie consumption without being hungry. Many foods low in energy density, including vegetables, fruits, and foods containing dietary fiber, are also associated with reduced cancer risk.

Box 1: What Is Energy Density?

Energy density (also called calorie density) describes how concentrated foods are in calories, and is defined as the calories per gram or per 100 grams of food. Foods high in energy density, including oils, fats, chips, crackers, and most cookies, tend to contain high amounts of fat and/or added sugar. Foods low in energy density, such as vegetables, fruits, legumes, whole grains, and broth-based soups, generally have higher water and fiber content.

Steps for promoting low energy-dense diets in weight management include substituting foods low in energy density such as vegetables, fruits, and relatively unprocessed grains for high energy-dense foods – particularly those with added fats and sugars (15,17).

Although sugar-sweetened beverages such as carbonated sodas, sweetened iced tea, and juice drinks are high in sugar, they are considered to be low in energy density because of their high water content. Nevertheless, research supports limiting sugar-sweetened beverages to reduce calorie consumption and promote weight loss (2,18). Recent studies suggest that the body is less able to recognize or compensate for calories from beverages than from solid foods, and this can contribute to long-term energy surplus and weight gain (19).

Key Practice Points
When discussing the concept of energy density with the public, it may be helpful to use the term calorie density, as the meaning of "energy" is often misunderstood by consumers.
- Not all energy-dense foods should be avoided. Some oils, nuts, and seeds provide important nutrients. Small servings fit within an overall low calorie-dense diet and are not associated with weight gain (20).
- Low energy-dense foods help people feel full on fewer calories. However, large portions of any food can promote overconsumption without regard to hunger, so portion control is still important (21). In order to decrease overall caloric intake, lower energy-dense foods should be chosen to replace higher energy-dense foods on the plate, not simply added as an addition to one's usual diet.

A Predominantly Plant-based Diet

High consumption of a variety of plant foods protects against cancers at various sites. Non-starchy vegetables and fruits protect against cancers of the mouth, pharynx, larynx, esophagus, stomach, and lung. Allium vegetables such as garlic, onions, and leeks protect against stomach cancer; garlic and foods that contain dietary fiber protect against colorectal cancer (2,6). Whole grain consumption protects against colorectal cancer as well (22).

Plant foods are rich in phytochemicals, vitamins, and minerals that, as part of the whole food, also protect against cancer. Foods containing selenium and foods containing lycopene protect against prostate cancer. Foods containing vitamin C and foods containing beta-carotene protect against esophageal cancer. Foods that supply carotenoids, such as dark green and orange vegetables and fruits, help protect against cancer of the mouth, pharynx, larynx, and lung (2).

Throughout the cancer process nutrients and phytochemicals from plant foods seem to work independently as well as synergistically to decrease risk. For example, a recent mouse study of prostate cancer showed that a combination tomato and broccoli diet was more effective at slowing tumor growth than either tomato or broccoli alone (23).

Many nutrients and phytochemicals, such as those highlighted below, show ability to inhibit phase I carcinogen-activating enzymes (such as cytochrome p450) and promote activity of phase II carcinogen-detoxifying enzymes (such as glutathione-S-transferase) in laboratory studies. In cell and animal studies, nutrients and phytochemicals found in plant foods show effects on cell cycle regulation, processes of angiogenesis, apoptosis, DNA repair, and inflammation (2). These effects may be accomplished through several mechanisms:

- Epigenetic effects refer to changes in gene expression that occur without mutations that change the genetic sequence itself. In laboratory studies, constituents in plant foods and their metabolites, including isothiocyanates and indole-3-carbinol formed from glucosinolates in cruciferous vegetables, allyl sulfides from garlic and onion family vegetables, genistein from soybeans and other legumes, folate from dark green vegetables, and stilbenes such as resveratrol from grapes and berries, can change histone acetylation, DNA methylation, and microRNAs that directly and indirectly regulate cancer progression. These epigenetic changes in essence may either silence or promote expression of genes such as tumor suppressor genes (24-27).
- Consumption of plant foods also may affect hormones influential in the cancer process. For example, the association of high dietary fiber intake and reduced risk of breast cancer may result from reduced levels of circulating insulin and related growth factors (such as IGF-1) that promote cell proliferation, and also from decreased circulating estrogen levels due to its decreased reabsorption from the digestive tract (28).
- Many vitamins and phytochemicals, such as carotenoids, flavonoids and other polyphenols, and allyl sulfur compounds act as antioxidants, and are important for protecting DNA. Alpha-carotene and beta-carotene promote gap junctional intercellular communication (cell-to-cell communication) that helps control cell growth (29).
- The intestinal microbiota, trillions of bacteria that live in the

Table 1: AICR/WCRF Personal Recommendations

BODY FATNESS
Be as lean as possible within the normal range of body weight
- Ensure that body weight through childhood and adolescent growth projects towards the lower end of normal BMI range at age 21
- Maintain body weight within the normal range from age 21
- Avoid weight gain and increases in waist circumference throughout adulthood

PHYSICAL ACTIVITY
Be physically active as part of everyday life
- Be moderately physically active, equivalent to brisk walking, for at least 30 minutes every day
- As fitness improves, aim for 60 minutes or more of moderate, or 30 minutes or more of vigorous, physical activity every day
- Limit sedentary habits such as watching television

FOODS AND DRINKS THAT PROMOTE WEIGHT GAIN
Limit consumption of energy-dense foods; avoid sugary drinks
- Consume energy-dense foods sparingly
- Avoid sugary drinks
- Consume "fast foods" sparingly, if at all

PLANT FOODS
Eat mostly foods of plant origin
- Eat at least five portions/servings (at least 400 g or 14 oz) of a variety of non-starchy vegetables and of fruits every day
- Eat relatively unprocessed cereals (grains) and/or pulses (legumes) with every meal
- Limit refined starchy foods

ANIMAL FOODS
Limit intake of red meat and avoid processed meat
- People who eat red meat to consume less than 500 g (18 oz) a week, very little if any to be processed

ALCOHOLIC DRINKS
Limit alcoholic drinks
- If alcoholic drinks are consumed, limit consumption to no more than two drinks a day for men and one drink a day for women

PRESERVATION, PROCESSING, PREPARATION
Limit consumption of salt; avoid moldy cereals (grains) or pulses (legumes)
- Avoid salt-preserved, salted, or salty foods; preserve foods without using salt
- Limit consumption of processed foods with added salt to ensure an intake of less than 2,400 mg of sodium a day

DIETARY SUPPLEMENTS
Aim to meet nutritional needs through diet alone
- Dietary supplements are not recommended for cancer prevention

BREASTFEEDING
Mothers to breastfeed; children to be breastfed
- Aim to breastfeed infants exclusively up to six months

CANCER SURVIVORS
Follow the recommendations for cancer prevention
- All cancer survivors to receive nutritional care from an appropriately trained professional
- If able to do so, and unless otherwise advised, aim to follow the recommendations for diet, healthy weight, and physical activity

colon, act on fermentable fiber and resistant starch to produce butyrate, a short-chain fatty acid that promotes normal colon cell development and may reduce inflammation. The microbiota also converts some phytochemicals to bioavailable active forms (30-31).

Emerging evidence suggests that a predominantly plant-based dietary pattern, which can be implemented in a variety of ways, may provide greater protective effects than consumption of any particular nutrients, compounds, or individual foods (2,32).

Key Practice Points

- Five or more standard servings of non-starchy vegetables and fruits daily (a total of 2.5 cups, though more when this includes raw leafy greens) meet recommendations to reduce cancer risk in addition to being linked with cardiovascular health benefits (2,4).
- Selecting a variety of vegetables and fruits is important to ensure a broad spectrum of protective compounds and the apparent additive and synergistic effects between them (23,33-34).
- The role of whole grains in protecting against cancer likely extends beyond dietary fiber to differences in nutrient and phytochemical content (35). Although the fiber content of whole grains and refined grains with added fiber may be comparable, it is unlikely that their benefits are equivalent.

Red and Processed Meats

AICR/WCRF recommendations for cancer prevention include limiting consumption of red meat (beef, lamb, and pork) and avoiding consumption of processed meats. People who eat red meat should consume less than 18 ounces per week and very little if any processed meat (2).

The term "processed meat" refers to meats (usually red meats) preserved by smoking, curing, or salting, or by the addition of chemical preservatives. Processed meat includes ham, bacon, frankfurters, hot dogs, pastrami, salami, and other sausages prepared by these methods. There is convincing evidence that red meat and processed meat are causes of colorectal cancer. The risk of colorectal cancer increases by an estimated 17 percent for every 100 grams of red meat consumed daily and by 18 percent for every 50 grams of processed meat consumed daily (6,36).

There are several plausible mechanisms to explain the association between consumption of red meat or processed meat and colorectal cancer (2,36-37).

- Red meat contains heme iron, which can lead to the production of free radicals, resulting in oxidative damage to DNA, protein, and cell membranes. Heme iron promotes formation of carcinogenic N-nitroso compounds (NOCs) within the gut.
- NOCs also form when nitrites used to preserve meat combine with amines from amino acids; they also can be created during the curing process as well as in the stomach.
- Cooking meat at high temperatures or over open flames causes production of heterocyclic amines and polycyclic aromatic hydrocarbons, both of which are carcinogenic in animals.

Vegan and other vegetarian diets have been associated with reduced incidence of cancer in many, but not all studies. Although observational studies adjust for known risk factors and lifestyle choices, vegetarians may differ from meat-eaters in unknown and unmeasured ways that could influence cancer risk. Also, various vegetarian eating patterns may differ in their overall effect on cancer risk. Thus a predominantly, but not exclusively, plant-based diet might provide similar reductions in cancer risk.

Other Animal Foods

Not all animal foods are associated with cancer. There is a lack of substantial evidence that poultry, fish, or eggs are associated with either an increase or decrease in cancer risk. Available evidence on milk, cheese, and other dairy products is difficult to interpret and appears to be in conflict regarding colorectal cancer (decreased risk) and prostate cancer (possible increased risk) (6). The AICR/WCRF Expert Panel did not make a recommendation regarding dairy products.

Key Practice Points

- Since red meat provides heme iron, which seems to underlie its association with cancer risk, the message to limit consumption is distinct from messages aimed at blood lipids, which focus on fat content of meat to define its healthfulness.
- Processed meat is produced by a variety of methods, yet because studies often classify all processed meat together it is not clear whether some pose more risk than others, or whether antioxidant or other additives, or changes in smoking or other procedures might lead to a lower-risk processed meat. That is why, for now, it is recommended that consumption of all forms of processed meat be minimized.

Alcoholic Drinks

There is convincing evidence that alcoholic drinks are a cause of cancers of the mouth, pharynx and larynx, esophagus, colorectum (men), and breast (both premenopause and postmenopause) and are probably a cause of cancers of the colorectum (women) and liver. The effect of alcoholic drinks is from ethanol, regardless of the type of drink. The extent to which alcohol increases cancer risk depends on the amount of alcohol consumed and the type of cancer being studied (2,6-7).

Alcohol increases cancer risk through several mechanisms:
- Ethanol in alcoholic beverages is classified as a human carcinogen, and when it is metabolized it forms acetaldehyde, another human carcinogen (38-39). Ethanol also acts as a solvent, enhancing penetration of carcinogens into cells.
- Alcohol metabolism also generates reactive oxygen species that can damage DNA.
- Alcohol acts synergistically with tobacco, multiplying risk of mouth and throat cancers for people exposed to both (2).
- Tissue-specific alcohol-related cancer risk may also reflect direct tissue damage and resulting inflammation, interactions with folate, and interference with estrogen pathways (40).

Key Practice Points
- A modest increase in breast cancer risk occurs even at intakes of the recommended maximum of one standard drink per day (2,7,41).
- Although small or moderate amounts of alcohol may protect against coronary heart disease, alcohol consumption is not recommended as a heart health strategy (42).
- Resveratrol is a phytochemical found in red wine that laboratory studies link with anti-carcinogenic effects. However, the overall body of research does not support considering red wine separately from other alcoholic beverages in relationship to cancer risk.

Foods Processed with Salt or Sodium
AICR/WCRF recommends that individuals limit consumption of salt and processed foods with added salt, aiming for an intake of less than 2,400 mg of sodium daily. Salt and salt-preserved foods are probably a cause of stomach cancer (2).

Excessive salt intake may lead to stomach cancer through several potential mechanisms (2,43):
- Excessive salt intake may damage the protective mucous lining of the stomach, leading to cell hyperplasia that increases inflammation and potential for mutations.
- Salt has been shown to increase formation of endogenous N-nitroso compounds.
- A high-salt diet may enhance *H. pylori* colonization and interact synergistically with these bacteria and with carcinogens.

Key Practice Points
- Using herbs, spices, and other flavor enhancers reduces the need for added salt while providing small amounts of potentially beneficial phytochemicals (44). However, laboratory studies showing health benefits from herbs, spices, and flavor enhancers generally involve larger amounts than are used in cooking, usually pharmaceutical doses or supplements.
- Regardless of sodium restrictions recommended for cardiovascular health, reducing intake substantially below 2,400 mg is not associated with further protection from cancer.

Dietary Supplements
Evidence indicates that dietary supplements can be protective or can cause cancer. Calcium supplements probably protect against colorectal cancer, but at levels above 1,500 mg calcium daily, risk for prostate cancer increases (2,6). The AICR/WCRF Expert Panel concluded that the overall body of evidence does not support the use of dietary supplements as an effective strategy to reduce cancer risk. However, the Panel recognized that dietary supplements may at times be beneficial for specific population groups, for reasons not related to cancer.

As research moves forward regarding the role of supplements in ensuring optimum nutrient levels, multiple factors need to be addressed, including the effects of differences in dietary intake, other lifestyle factors, and the environment. In addition, genetic

polymorphisms that affect nutrient metabolism need to be better understood, as does the impact of timing (both in the life cycle and within the stage of cancer development), dose, and duration of exposure.

Examples of dietary supplements associated with increased risk for cancer include beta-carotene and vitamin E. In early epidemiologic studies, evidence pointed to lower risk of lung cancer in people who consumed foods high in beta-carotene. However, two randomized controlled trials showed that smokers who took high-dose beta-carotene supplements developed lung cancer at higher rates than those taking a placebo (45-46). Also, the Selenium and Vitamin E Cancer Prevention Trial (SELECT) suggests that high-dose vitamin E supplements may promote a modest increase in the risk of prostate cancer (47).

Selenium from food and supplements may play a role in reducing the risk of prostate cancer, especially in its aggressive form (48). However, prostate cancer risk was not reduced by selenium supplements in the SELECT study (49). The benefit of selenium supplementation may be greater in populations in which the food supply is low in selenium resulting in low serum selenium levels than in people who already have adequate serum levels (50).

Vitamin D may act throughout the cancer process to reduce cancer risk (51), and a large randomized controlled trial, the VITamin D and Omega-3 TriaL (VITAL), is currently underway to examine effects of vitamin D and omega-3 fats on cancer risk (52). Some observational studies suggest benefit of higher blood levels of vitamin D, but results are inconsistent, especially regarding target blood levels and the level of intake different people need to reach any given target (53-56).

Key Practice Points
- Obtaining nutrients and other compounds from food rather than from dietary supplements provides the potential for beneficial and synergistic effects against carcinogenesis.
- The concept of a U-shaped curve refers to research showing supplementation with a particular nutrient in people with low dietary intake or low body levels of a nutrient may be beneficial, whereas supplements may have no effect or even be harmful in people who already have adequate amounts or if given to achieve super-physiologic levels (57). This stands in contrast to common beliefs among the public regarding antioxidants and nutrients that if some is good, more is better.

Breastfeeding
There is convincing evidence that breastfeeding reduces a mother's risk of both pre- and postmenopausal breast cancer. It is also well established that breastfeeding offers immune and other health benefits to babies, and as an additional benefit, babies who are breastfed are less likely to become overweight or obese in later childhood. Greater lifetime duration of breastfeeding is associated with greater reduction in breast cancer risk.

Mechanisms by which breastfeeding may protect against breast cancer include:

- Breastfeeding contributes to elimination of cells with potential DNA damage through exfoliation of breast tissue during lactation and a major apoptosis of epithelial cells at the end of breastfeeding (2).
- Breastfeeding leads to amenorrhea, reducing lifetime exposure to estrogen.

Key Practice Points

- Exclusive breastfeeding for the first six months means giving babies no other nourishment, including water, except for vitamin drops where needed. After that, solid foods and other liquids are to be added at age-appropriate times.
- Few mothers in the United States breastfeed exclusively for even three months, and less than half of babies are breastfed at all by age six months. Changing breastfeeding practices will require support and changes in current practice from many sources, including hospitals and birthing centers, employers, communities, and families.

Cancer Survivors

The term "cancer survivor" refers to people who have been diagnosed with cancer, including those who have recovered, from the time of diagnosis onward. During cancer treatment, and in cases in which ability to consume or metabolize food has been altered by treatment, people may have special nutritional needs. Especially in these cases, AICR/WCRF emphasizes the need for nutritional counseling from an appropriately trained health professional. Registered dietitians (RDs) and registered dietitian nutritionists (RDNs) who are Board Certified Specialists in Oncology (CSOs) have special expertise in oncology nutrition. AICR/WCRF advises that if possible, and unless otherwise advised by a qualified professional, that the recommendations for cancer prevention be followed by cancer survivors. As cancer survivors live increasingly longer they are at risk of developing new primary cancers as well as other chronic diseases and are likely to benefit from this guidance. The American Cancer Society has published a comprehensive set of nutrition and physical activity guidelines specifically for cancer survivors (58).

Since the publication of the AICR/WCRF Expert Report, the research evidence base regarding nutrition, physical activity, and cancer continues to expand. The AICR/WCRF Continuous Update Project (CUP) systematically identifies this evidence as it is published. A section on cancer survivorship has been added to the CUP and relevant papers on breast cancer survivors are being added to the CUP database. More information is available at the AICR/WCRF Expert Report website (www.dietandcancerreport.org).

Emerging Topics
Omega-3 Fatty Acids

Laboratory studies suggest that omega-3 fatty acids from both marine and plant sources may protect against cancer by acting to decrease inflammation, cell proliferation, and angiogenesis while increasing apoptosis. EPA (eicosapentaenoic acid) and DHA (docosahexaenoic acid) from fish and ALA (alpha-linolenic acid) from plants accomplish this by acting to suppress biosynthesis of tumorigenic, pro-inflammatory eicosanoids; altering cell membrane structure and receptor function; and influencing transcription factor activity, gene expression, signaling pathways, and production of reactive oxygen species (59). Recent human studies suggest that omega-3 fatty acids might also protect against the shortening of the telomeres at the ends of chromosomes, a process that has been identified as a marker of cell aging and associated with cancer risk (60-61).

Observational studies of omega-3 fatty acids face challenges in separating the effects of total omega-3 intake from those of long-chain omega-3s, ALA, fish intake, and supplemental forms of omega-3s. Although some observational studies in humans show an association of high fish consumption or omega-3 fatty acid intake with reduced risk of colorectal and other cancers (62-63), the overall body of research is inconsistent (64-65). The VITAL study now underway is testing the effect of daily supplements of 1,000 mg of omega-3 fatty acids (EPA and DHA) on cancer risk, but results will not be available for several years (52).

Soy Foods

Isoflavones in soy foods are often studied in relation to cancer risk. However, many soy foods are also good sources of dietary fiber and selenium, and some are fortified with calcium. Research suggests that soy foods do not increase cancer risk, and in some cases may lower it. The role of soy in an overall cancer-protective diet needs more study, as do individual differences that may modify its effects.

The soy isoflavones genistein and daidzein are classified as phytoestrogens and can bind to estrogen receptors. In cell and animal studies, these compounds have slowed growth of cancer cells. Some early studies in rodents suggested that genistein increased growth of estrogen receptor-positive (ER+) breast cancer cells and promoted breast cancer growth (66). However, later research showed that rats and mice metabolize phytoestrogens such as genistein differently than humans (67). The preferential binding of soy isoflavones to beta- rather than alpha- forms of estrogen receptors may be cancer-protective, but needs further study (68).

Observational studies in humans suggest that soy may protect against some forms of cancer. Soy consumption is associated with lower breast cancer risk in Asia, where throughout their lives women consume moderate amounts of soy. Protective effects of soy probably stem from consumption in childhood and adolescence (69-71). Soy may affect cancer risk in some people more than others due to individual differences in genetics and gut bacteria that ferment soy compounds into their active form (69,72).

Beyond breast cancer, only limited research in humans links soy or total isoflavone consumption to lower risk of cancers of the prostate, stomach, lung, and colon (2,73-75). Five population studies of breast cancer survivors and one pooled analysis concluded that moderate consumption of soy foods does not increase risk of recurrence of breast cancer, including estrogen receptor-positive types. In the pooled analysis of survivors in the United States and Asia, soy isoflavone consumption was associated with decreased recurrence. Further, these studies do not show any harmful interactions with tamoxifen, an anti-estrogen medication (76-81).

Moderate soy consumption is considered one to two standard servings daily of whole soy foods, such as tofu, soy milk, edamame, or soy nuts. (One serving averages about 7 grams of protein and 25 mg, isoflavones.) Up to 100 mg/day of isoflavones have been consumed in Asian populations long-term without link to increased breast cancer risk (79). The health effects of consuming more than 100 mg/day of isoflavones from high dose supplements or isolated soy protein are not known.

Flaxseed
Most research on flaxseed and cancer has focused on breast cancer. Emerging research also examines the effect of flaxseed on prostate and colon cancers. Studies have primarily focused on ALA and lignans present in flaxseed. Evidence suggests that consuming one to four tablespoons of ground flaxseed daily appears to be safe, and may contribute to lower risk of breast or other cancers (82). However, research is currently too limited to be conclusive or to support a recommendation.

When plant lignans are consumed, they are converted by intestinal bacteria into enterolignans, which can be absorbed from the colon and circulate in the blood. The amount of these enterolignans produced and absorbed varies substantially from person to person. Observational studies in humans show mixed results regarding an association between lignan intake and breast cancer risk, though some suggest a reduced risk of postmenopausal breast cancer (83-84). To avoid measurement error related to assessment of dietary lignan consumption, studies now can use serum or urinary levels of enterolactone (the main circulating enterolignan) as a biomarker of lignan consumption. Studies of serum enterolignans and breast cancer risk show mixed results, but a meta-analysis of 13 epidemiologic studies found that compared with women with the lowest serum enterolactone levels, women with the highest serum enterolactone levels had a lower breast cancer risk (85).

In some, but not all, studies, lignan consumption seems to promote a shift in women's serum estrogen to a form less likely to promote cancer (82,86-87). Some animal and human studies suggest that lignans may decrease IGF-1 and other growth factors to decrease cell proliferation and the angiogenesis that enables tumors to grow. Flaxseed is also a source of ALA, which can be converted in the body to the long-chain omega-3 fats EPA and DHA. This conversion is very inefficient, however, and research is investigating the role of ALA itself.

There has been concern whether, as phytoestrogens, the lignans in flaxseed could increase the incidence or recurrence of breast cancer, or interfere with tamoxifen. Studies do not support an association,

and according to animal studies, flaxseed may enhance tamoxifen's effectiveness (88-91). However, with no results from randomized controlled trials of flaxseed use during tamoxifen, aromatase inhibitor, or trastuzumab treatment, decisions about flaxseed use should be discussed carefully with a patient's physician.

In cell and animal studies, flaxseed or enterolactone has been shown to inhibit the growth and metastasis of prostate cancer (92-93). In men with prostate cancer, flaxseed has lowered tumor biomarkers and pre-surgery rates of cell proliferation (94).

Many questions about flaxseed's potential role in a diet to reduce cancer risk remain, including its safety throughout all life stages, its potential interactions with various forms of cancer treatment, and the differences in flaxseed's effects due to individual dietary, genetic, and hormonal differences.

Green Tea
Interest in green tea and cancer primarily relates to its epigallocatechin gallate (EGCG) content. In laboratory tests, EGCG, a catechin polyphenol, shows even more powerful antioxidant effects than vitamins C or E. In addition, cell and animal studies show tea polyphenols may directly inhibit development of various types of cancer. The epigenetic effects of tea polyphenols have been found to stimulate enzymes that deactivate carcinogens, decrease tumor growth, increase apoptosis, and restrain the ability of cancer cells to spread (95-96). The amounts of EGCG provided in some lab studies, however, when considered as human-equivalent doses, are higher than commonly consumed in tea beverages.

Small studies in humans show that drinking tea can raise antioxidant capacity (97). Some observational studies examine green and black tea separately, since they differ in particular polyphenol content, but others look at total tea consumption. Results are inconsistent, but show potential for reducing risk of several cancers, including cancer of the breast, ovary, and endometrium (96,98-100). Several small randomized controlled trials of green tea catechins show promise for decreasing development of prostate cancer but more studies are needed to clarify amounts needed, long-term effects, and individual differences (101-102).

If green tea can play a role in reducing cancer risk, research is needed to clarify the optimal amount; laboratory studies and intervention studies using green tea extract often involve doses of EGCG unlikely to be reached in typical dietary consumption of green tea, so the impact of moderate consumption needs clarification.

References
1. World Cancer Research Fund/American Institute for Cancer Research, *Policy and Action for Cancer Prevention. Food, Nutrition, and Physical Activity: a Global Perspective*, 2009, Washington, DC: AICR.
2. World Cancer Research Fund/American Institute for Cancer Research, *Food, Nutrition, Physical Activity, and the Prevention of Cancer: a Global Perspective*, 2007, Washington, DC: AICR.
3. U.S. Department of Agriculture and U.S. Department of Health and Human Services, *Dietary Guidelines for Americans, 2010, 7th Edition*: Washington, DC: U.S. Government Printing Office.

4. Kushi LH, Doyle C, McCullough M, et al. American Cancer Society Guidelines on nutrition and physical activity for cancer prevention: reducing the risk of cancer with healthy food choices and physical activity. *CA Cancer J Clin* 2012;62(1):30-67.

5. World Cancer Research Fund/American Institute for Cancer Research, *Continuous Update Project Report. Food, Nutrition, Physical Activity, and the Prevention of Pancreatic Cancer*, 2012.

6. World Cancer Research Fund/American Institute for Cancer Research, *Continuous Update Project Report. Food, Nutrition, Physical Activity, and the Prevention of Colorectal Cancer*, 2011.

7. World Cancer Research Fund/American Institute for Cancer Research, *Continuous Update Project Report. Food, Nutrition, Physical Activity, and the Prevention of Breast Cancer*, 2010.

8. Arcidiacono B, Iritano S, Nocera A, et al. Insulin resistance and cancer risk: an overview of the pathogenetic mechanisms. *Exp Diabetes Res.* 2012;2012:789174. doi: 10.1155/2012/789174.

9. Dalamaga M, Diakopoulos KN, Mantzoros CS. The role of adiponectin in cancer: a review of current evidence. *Endocr Rev.* 2012;33(4):547-594.

10. Perera, PS, Thompson RL, Wiseman MJ. Recent evidence for colorectal cancer prevention through healthy food, nutriton, and physical activity: implications for recommendations. *Curr Nutr Reports.* 2012;1(1):44-54.

11. Aune D, Greenwood DC, Chan DS, et al. Body mass index, abdominal fatness and pancreatic cancer risk: a systematic review and non-linear dose-response meta-analysis of prospective studies. *Ann Oncol.* 2012;23(4):843-852.

12. Byers T, Sedjo RL. Does intentional weight loss reduce cancer risk? *Diabetes Obes Metab.* 2011;13(12):1063-1072.

13. Lynch BM. Sedentary behavior and cancer: a systematic review of the literature and proposed biological mechanisms. *Cancer Epidemiol Biomarkers Prev.* 2010;19(11):2691-2709.

14. Healy GN, Matthews CE, Dunstan DW, Winkler EA, Owen N. Sedentary time and cardio-metabolic biomarkers in US adults: NHANES 2003-06. *Eur Heart J.* 2011;32(5):590-597.

15. Rolls BJ, Drewnowski A, Ledikwe JH. Changing the energy density of the diet as a strategy for weight management. *J Am Diet Assoc.* 2005;105(5 Suppl 1):S98-103.

16. Pérez-Escamilla R, Obbagy JE, Altman JM, et al. Dietary energy density and body weight in adults and children: a systematic review. *J Acad Nutr Diet.* 2012;112(5):671-684.

17. Blatt AD, Roe LS, Rolls BJ. Hidden vegetables: an effective strategy to reduce energy intake and increase vegetable intake in adults. *Am J Clin Nutr.* 2011;93(4):756-763.

18. Flood JE, Roe LS, Rolls BJ. The effect of increased beverage portion size on energy intake at a meal. *J Am Diet Assoc.* 2006;106(12):1984-1990; discussion 1990-1991.

19. Pan A, Hu FB. Effects of carbohydrates on satiety: differences between liquid and solid food. *Curr Opin Clin Nutr Metab Care.* 2011;14(4):385-390.

20. Mozaffarian D, Hao T, Rimm EB, Willett WC, Hu FB. Changes in diet and lifestyle and long-term weight gain in women and men. *N Engl J Med.* 2011;364(25):2392-2404.

21. Saquib N, Natarajan L, Rock CL, et al. The impact of a long-term reduction in dietary energy density on body weight within a randomized diet trial. *Nutr Cancer.* 2008;60(1):31-38.

22. Aune D, Chan DS, Lau R, et al. Dietary fibre, whole grains, and risk of colorectal cancer: systematic review and dose-response meta-analysis of prospective studies. *BMJ.* 2011 Nov 10;343:d6617. doi: 10.1136/bmj.d6617.

23. Canene-Adams K, Lindshield BL, Wang S, Jeffery EII, Clinton SK, Erdman JW Jr. Combinations of tomato and broccoli enhance antitumor activity in dunning r3327-h prostate adenocarcinomas. *Cancer Res.* 2007;67(2):836-843.

24. Meeran SM, Ahmed A, Tollefsbol TO. Epigenetic targets of bioactive dietary components for cancer prevention and therapy. *Clin Epigenetics.* 2010;1(3-4):101-116.

25. Navarro SL, Li F, Lampe JW. Mechanisms of action of isothiocyanates in cancer chemoprevention: an update. *Food Funct.* 2011;2(10):579-587.

26. Nian H, Delage B, Ho E, Dashwood RH. Modulation of histone deacetylase activity by dietary isothiocyanates and allyl sulfides: studies with sulforaphane and garlic organosulfur compounds. *Environ Mol Mutagen.* 2009;50(3):213-221.

27. Duthie SJ. Folate and cancer: how DNA damage, repair and methylation impact on colon carcinogenesis. *J Inherit Metab Dis.* 2011;34(1):101-109.

28. Aune D, Chan DS, Greenwood DC, et al. Dietary fiber and breast cancer risk: a systematic review and meta-analysis of prospective studies. *Ann Oncol.* 2012;23(6):1394-1402.

29. Tanaka T, Shnimizu M, Moriwaki H. Cancer chemoprevention by carotenoids. *Molecules.* 2012;17(3):3202-3242.

30. Bosscher D, Breynaert A, Pieters L, Hermans N. Food-based strategies to modulate the composition of the intestinal microbiota and their associated health effects. *J Physiol Pharmacol.* 2009;60Suppl6:5-11.

31. Tuohy KM, Conterno L, Gasperotti M, Viola R. Up-regulating the human intestinal microbiome using whole plant foods, polyphenols, and/or fiber. *J Agric Food Chem.* 2012;60(36):8776-8782.

32. Miller PE, Lesko SM, Muscat JE, Lazarus P, Hartman TJ. Dietary patterns and colorectal adenoma and cancer risk: a review of the epidemiological evidence. *Nutr Cancer.* 2010;62(4):413-424.

33. Jeurnink SM, Büchner FL, Bueno-de-Mesquita HB, et al. Variety in vegetable and fruit consumption and the risk of gastric and esophageal cancer in the European prospective investigation into cancer and nutrition. *Int J Cancer.* 2012 Sep 15;131(6):E963-973. doi: 10.1002/ijc.27517.

34. Liu RH. Potential synergy of phytochemicals in cancer prevention: mechanism of action. J Nutr. 2004;134(12 Suppl):3479S-3485S.

35. Adom KK, Liu RH. Antioxidant activity of grains. *J Agric Food Chem.* 2002;50(21):6182-6187.

36. Chan DS, Lau R, Aune D, et al. Red and processed meat and colorectal cancer incidence: meta-analysis of prospective studies. *PLoS One.* 2011;6(6):e20456. doi: 10.1371/journal.pone.0020456.

37. Cross AJ, Ferrucci LM, Risch A, et al. A large prospective study of meat consumption and colorectal cancer risk: an investigation of potential mechanisms underlying this association. *Cancer Res.* 2010;70(6):2406-2414.

38. Cogliano VJ, Baan RM, Straif K, et al. Preventable exposures associated with human cancers. *J Natl Cancer Inst.* 2011;103(24):1827-1839.

39. Secretan B, Straif K, Baan R, et al. A review of human carcinogens—Part E: tobacco, areca nut, alcohol, coal smoke, and salted fish. *Lancet Oncol.* 2009;10(11):1033-1034.

40. Oyesanmi O, Snyder D, Sullivan N, Reston J, Treadwell J, Schoelles KM. Alcohol consumption and cancer risk: understanding possible causal mechanisms for breast and colorectal cancers. *Evid Rep Technol Assess (Full Rep).* 2010;(197):1-151.

41. Allen NE, Beral V, Casabonne D, et al. Moderate alcohol intake and cancer incidence in women. *J Natl Cancer Inst.* 2009;101(5):296-305.

42. Lichtenstein AH, Appel LJ, Brands M, et al. Diet and lifestyle recommendations revision 2006: a scientific statement from the American Heart Association Nutrition Committee. *Circulation.* 2006;114(1):82-96.

43. Wang XQ, Terry PD, Yan H. Review of salt consumption and stomach cancer risk: epidemiological and biological evidence. *World J Gastroenterol.* 2009;15(18):2204-2213.

44. Kaefer CM, Milner JA. Herbs and Spices in Cancer Prevention and Treatment In: Benzie IFF, Wachtel-Galor S, eds. *Herbal Medicine: Biomolecular and Clinical Aspects,* 2nd edition. Boca Raton (FL): CRC Press; 2011: Chapter 17.

45. The Alpha-Tocopherol, Beta Carotene Cancer Prevention Study Group. The effect of vitamin E and beta carotene on the incidence of lung cancer and other cancers in male smokers. *N Engl J Med.* 1994;330(15):1029-1035.

46. Omenn GS, Goodman GE, Thornquist MD, et al. Effects of a combination of beta carotene and vitamin A on lung cancer and cardiovascular disease. *N Engl J Med.* 1996;334(18):1150-1155.

47. Klein EA, Thompson IM Jr, Tangen CM, et al. Vitamin E and the risk of prostate cancer: the Selenium and Vitamin E Cancer Prevention Trial (SELECT). *JAMA.* 2011;306(14):1549-1556.

48. Hurst R, Hooper L, Norat T, et al. Selenium and prostate cancer: systematic review and meta-analysis. *Am J Clin Nutr.* 2012;96(1):111-122.

49. Lippman SM, Klein EA, Goodman PJ, et al. Effect of selenium and vitamin E on risk of prostate cancer and other cancers: the Selenium and Vitamin E Cancer Prevention Trial (SELECT). *JAMA.* 2009;301(1):39-51.

50. Rayman MP. Selenium and human health. *Lancet*. 2012;379(9822):1256-1268.

51. Lazzeroni M, Serrano D, Pilz S, Gandini S. Vitamin d supplementation and cancer: review of randomized controlled trials. *Anticancer Agents Med Chem*. 2013;13(1):118-125.

52. Manson JE, Bassuk SS, Lee IM, et al. The VITamin D and OmegA-3 TriaL (VITAL): rationale and design of a large randomized controlled trial of vitamin D and marine omega-3 fatty acid supplements for the primary prevention of cancer and cardiovascular disease. *Contemp Clin Trials*. 2012;33(1):159-171.

53. Pilz S, Kienreich K, Tomaschitz A, et al. Vitamin D and cancer mortality: systematic review of prospective epidemiological studies. *Anticancer Agents Med Chem*. 2013;13(1):107-117.

54. Touvier M, Chan DS, Lau R, et al. Meta-analyses of vitamin D intake, 25-hydroxyvitamin D status, vitamin D receptor polymorphisms, and colorectal cancer risk. *Cancer Epidemiol Biomarkers Prev*. 2011;20(5):1003-1016.

55. Gandini S, Boniol M, Haukka J, et al. Meta-analysis of observational studies of serum 25-hydroxyvitamin D levels and colorectal, breast and prostate cancer and colorectal adenoma. *Int J Cancer*. 2011;128(6):1414-1424.

56. Chung M, Lee J, Terasawa T, Lau J, Trikalinos TA. Vitamin D with or without calcium supplementation for prevention of cancer and fractures: an updated meta-analysis for the U.S. Preventive Services Task Force. *Ann Intern Med*. 2011;155(12):827-838.

57. Mayne ST, Ferrucci LM, Cartmel B. Lessons learned from randomized clinical trials of micronutrient supplementation for cancer prevention. *Annu Rev Nutr*. 2012 Aug 21;32:369-390. doi: 10.1146/annurev-nutr-071811-150659.

58. Rock CL, Doyle C, Demark-Wahnefried W, et al. Nutrition and physical activity guidelines for cancer survivors. *CA Cancer J Clin*. 2012;62(4):243-274.

59. Cockbain AJ, Toogood GJ, Hull MA. Omega-3 polyunsaturated fatty acids for the treatment and prevention of colorectal cancer. *Gut*. 2012;61(1):135-149.

60. Kiecolt-Glaser JK, Epel ES, Belury MA, et al. Omega-3 fatty acids, oxidative stress, and leukocyte telomere length: A randomized controlled trial. *Brain Behav Immun*. 2013 28:16-24 doi: 10.1016/j.bbi.2012.09.004.

61. Farzaneh-Far R, Lin J, Epel ES, Harris WS, Blackburn EH, Whooley MA. Association of marine omega-3 fatty acid levels with telomeric aging in patients with coronary heart disease. *JAMA*. 2010;303(3):250-257.

62. Hall MN, Chavarro JE, Lee IM, Willett WC, Ma J. A 22-year prospective study of fish, n-3 fatty acid intake, and colorectal cancer risk in men. *Cancer Epidemiol Biomarkers Prev*. 2008;17(5):1136-1143.

63. Norat T, Bingham S, Ferrari P, et al. Meat, fish, and colorectal cancer risk: the European Prospective Investigation into cancer and nutrition. *J Natl Cancer Inst*. 2005;97(12):906-916.

64. MacLean CH, Newberry SJ, Mojica WA, et al. Effects of omega-3 fatty acids on cancer risk: a systematic review. *JAMA*. 2006;295(4):403-415.

65. Hooper L, Thompson RL, Harrison RA, et al. Risks and benefits of omega 3 fats for mortality, cardiovascular disease, and cancer: systematic review. *BMJ*. 2006;332(7544):752-760.

66. Ju YH, Allred CD, Allred KF, Karko KL, Doerge DR, Helferich WG. Physiological concentrations of dietary genistein dose-dependently stimulate growth of estrogen-dependent human breast cancer (MCF-7) tumors implanted in athymic nude mice. *J Nutr*. 2001;131(11):2957-2962.

67. Setchell KD, Brown NM, Zhao X, et al. Soy isoflavone phase II metabolism differs between rodents and humans: implications for the effect on breast cancer risk. *Am J Clin Nutr*. 2011;94(5):1284-1294.

68. Shanle EK, Xu W. Selectively targeting estrogen receptors for cancer treatment. *Adv Drug Deliv Rev*. 2010;62(13):1265-1276.

69. Nagata C. Factors to consider in the association between soy isoflavone intake and breast cancer risk. *J Epidemiol*. 2010;20(2):83-89.

70. Trock BJ, Hilakivi-Clarke L, Clarke R. Meta-analysis of soy intake and breast cancer risk. *J Natl Cancer Inst*. 2006;98(7):459-471.

71. Korde LA, Wu AG, Fears T, et al. Childhood soy intake and breast cancer risk in Asian American women. *Cancer Epidemiol Biomarkers Prev*. 2009;18(4):1050-1059.

72. Lampe JW. Emerging research on equol and cancer. *J Nutr*. 2010;140(7):1369S-1372S.

73. Hwang YW, Kim SY, Jee SH, Kim YN, Nam CM. Soy food consumption and risk of prostate cancer: a meta-analysis of observational studies. *Nutr Cancer*. 2009;61(5):598-606.

74. Shimazu T, Inoue M, Sasazuki S, et al. Isoflavone intake and risk of lung cancer: a prospective cohort study in Japan. *Am J Clin Nutr*. 2010;91(3):722-728.

75. Yan L, Spitznagel EL, Bosland MC. Soy consumption and colorectal cancer risk in humans: a meta-analysis. *Cancer Epidemiol Biomarkers Prev*. 2010;19(1):148-158.

76. Caan BJ, Natarajan L, Parker B, et al. Soy food consumption and breast cancer prognosis. *Cancer Epidemiol Biomarkers Prev*. 2011;20(5):854-858.

77. Kang X, Zhang Q, Wang S, Huang X, Jin S. Effect of soy isoflavones on breast cancer recurrence and death for patients receiving adjuvant endocrine therapy. *CMAJ*. 2010;182(17):1857-1862.

78. Guha N, Kwan ML, Quesenberry CP Jr, Weltzien EK, Castillo AL, Caan BJ. Soy isoflavones and risk of cancer recurrence in a cohort of breast cancer survivors: the Life After Cancer Epidemiology study. *Breast Cancer Res Treat*. 2009;118(2):395-405.

79. Shu XO, Zheng Y, Cai H, et al. Soy food intake and breast cancer survival. *JAMA*. 2009;302(22):2437-2443.

80. Nechuta SJ, Caan BJ, Chen WY, et al. Soy food intake after diagnosis of breast cancer and survival: an in-depth analysis of combined evidence from cohort studies of US and Chinese women. *Am J Clin Nutr*. 2012;96(1):123-132.

81. Zhang YF, Kang HB, Li BL, Zhang RM. Positive effects of soy isoflavone food on survival of breast cancer patients in China. *Asian Pac J Cancer Prev*. 2012;13(2):479-482.

82. Brooks JD, Ward WE, Lewis JE, et al. Supplementation with flaxseed alters estrogen metabolism in postmenopausal women to a greater extent than does supplementation with an equal amount of soy. *Am J Clin Nutr*. 2004;79(2):318-325.

83. Velentzis LS, Cantwell MM, Cardwell C, Keshtgar MR, Leathem AJ, Woodside JW. Lignans and breast cancer risk in pre- and post-menopausal women: meta-analyses of observational studies. *Br J Cancer*. 2009;100(9):1492-1498.

84. Ward HA, Kuhnle GG, Mulligan AA, Lentjes MA, Luben RN, Khaw KT. Breast, colorectal, and prostate cancer risk in the European Prospective Investigation into Cancer and Nutrition-Norfolk in relation to phytoestrogen intake derived from an improved database. *Am J Clin Nutr*. 2010;91(2):440-448.

85. Zaineddin AK, Vrieling A, Buck K, et al. Serum enterolactone and postmenopausal breast cancer risk by estrogen, progesterone and herceptin 2 receptor status. *Int J Cancer*. 2012;130(6):1401-1410.

86. McCann SE, Wactawski-Wende J, Kufel K, et al. Changes in 2-hydroxyestrone and 16alpha-hydroxyestrone metabolism with flaxseed consumption: modification by COMT and CYP1B1 genotype. *Cancer Epidemiol Biomarkers Prev*. 2007;16(2):256-262.

87. Sturgeon SR, Volpe SL, Puleo E, et al. Effect of flaxseed consumption on urinary levels of estrogen metabolites in postmenopausal women. *Nutr Cancer*. 2010;62(2):175-180.

88. Chen J, Power KA, Mann J, Cheng A, Thompson LU. Dietary flaxseed interaction with tamoxifen induced tumor regression in athymic mice with MCF-7 xenografts by downregulating the expression of estrogen related gene products and signal transduction pathways. *Nutr Cancer*. 2007;58(2):162-170.

89. Chen J, Saggar JK, Corey P, Thompson LU. Flaxseed cotyledon fraction reduces tumour growth and sensitises tamoxifen treatment of human breast cancer xenograft (MCF-7) in athymic mice. *Br J Nutr*. 2011;105(3):339-347.

90. Saggar JK, Chen J, Corey P, Thompson LU. Dietary flaxseed lignan or oil combined with tamoxifen treatment affects MCF-7 tumor growth through estrogen receptor- and growth factor-signaling pathways. *Mol Nutr Food Res*. 2010;54(3):415-425.

91. Saggar JK, Chen J, Corey P, Thompson LU. The effect of secoisolariciresinol diglucoside and flaxseed oil, alone and in combination, on MCF-7 tumor growth and signaling pathways. *Nutr Cancer*. 2010;62(4):533-542.

92. Chen LH, Fang J, Sun Z, et al. Enterolactone inhibits insulin-like growth factor-1 receptor signaling in human prostatic carcinoma PC-3 cells. *J Nutr.* 2009;139(4):653-659.

93. Lin X, Gingrich JR, Bao W, Li J, Haroon ZA, Demark-Wahnefried W. Effect of flaxseed supplementation on prostatic carcinoma in transgenic mice. *Urology*, 2002;60(5):919-924.

94. Demark-Wahnefried W, Polascik TJ, George SL, et al. Flaxseed supplementation (not dietary fat restriction) reduces prostate cancer proliferation rates in men presurgery. *Cancer Epidemiol Biomarkers Prev.* 2008;17(12):3577-3587.

95. Yang CS, Wang X. Green tea and cancer prevention. *Nutr Cancer.* 2010; 62(7):931-937.

96. Yang CS, Wang X, Lu G, Picinich SC. Cancer prevention by tea: animal studies, molecular mechanisms and human relevance. *Nat Rev Cancer.* 2009;9(6):429-439.

97. Ellinger S, Müller N, Stehle P, Ulrich-Merzenich G. Consumption of green tea or green tea products: is there any evidence for antioxidant effects from controlled interventional studies? *Phytomedicine.* 2011;18(11): 903-915.

98. Zheng J, Yang B, Huang T, Yu Y, Yang J, Li D. Green tea and black tea consumption and prostate cancer risk: an exploratory meta-analysis of observational studies. *Nutr Cancer.* 2011;63(5):663-672.

99. Butler LM, Wu AH. Green and black tea in relation to gynecologic cancers. *Mol Nutr Food Res.* 2011;55(6):931-940.

100. Boehm K, Borrelli F, Ernst E, et al. Green tea (Camellia sinensis) for the prevention of cancer. *Cochrane Database Syst Rev.* 2009 Jul 8;(3):CD005004. doi: 10.1002/14651858.CD005004.pub2.

101. Johnson JJ, Bailey HH, Mukhtar H. Green tea polyphenols for prostate cancer chemoprevention: a translational perspective. *Phytomedicine.* 2010;17(1):3-13.

102. Bettuzzi S, Brausi M, Rizzi F, Castagnetti G, Peracchia G, Corti A. Chemoprevention of human prostate cancer by oral administration of green tea catechins in volunteers with high-grade prostate intraepithelial neoplasia: a preliminary report from a one-year proof-of-principle study. *Cancer Res.* 2006;66(2):1234-1240.

Nutrition Risk Screening and Assessment of the Oncology Patient

Rhone Levin, MEd, RD, CSO, LD

Importance of Nutrition Screening and Assessment in the Oncology Patient

Oncology treatment can create a physiologic burden that can overwhelm even a healthy person's nutritional reserve. Good nutrition during oncology treatment is fundamental to meet the increased nutritional demands required to support the healing process. The benefits of good nutrition during cancer treatment include fewer complications, better quality of life and most importantly the ability to tolerate full treatment as prescribed.

The purpose of nutrition screening and assessment is to identify patients who are at risk for malnutrition, which then leads to nutrition assessment and early intervention provided by a Registered Dietitian (RD) with oncology nutrition specialization. Access to nutrition care and early intervention that provides an individualized nutrition management plan is most effective in preserving the health and well being of the oncology patient (1).

The Effects of Malnutrition On the Oncology Patient

As many as 40% of patients experience anorexia and weight loss prior to diagnosis, and 40% to 80% are expected to experience malnutrition at some point in their treatment (2). At the time of diagnosis, up to 80% of upper gastrointestinal cancer patients and 60% of lung cancer patients have already experienced significant weight loss (3). Weight loss correlates with decreased performance status in a majority of tumor categories, and a weight loss of as little as 6% predicts a reduced response to oncology treatment, reduced survival and a reduced quality of life (4).

Patients diagnosed with gastrointestinal and head and neck cancers are at highest risk of weight loss and malnutrition, but all cancer types benefit from screening and nutrition surveillance. Several studies evaluating chemotherapy tolerance in breast, metastatic breast, renal cell, gastrointestinal and colorectal cancer demonstrate that patients losing weight and lean body mass experience increased toxicity and ultimately receive less treatment than patients who are not losing weight. In the case of renal cell carcinoma, dose reductions were observed in 13% of patients and treatment termination occurred in 21% of patients (5). Treatment dosage reduction, the holding of treatment and treatment termination have a negative impact on outcomes (6-9). Body weight and lean body mass also are considered independent risk factors for chemotherapy tolerance and survival in gastric cancer (10). Toxicity from radiation treatment can lead to unplanned treatment breaks that result in lower loco-regional control and survival rates in patients with head and neck cancer. In these patients, tumor control rate is reduced 1% for every day that the radiation therapy plan is interrupted (11).

It is vital to maintain weight and performance status as performance status scores may determine decisions about treatment modality, amount of treatment, and timing of treatment. Malnutrition is frequently underreported and its presence is often ignored, yet providing nutrition intervention that prevents and/or limits malnutrition can significantly influence treatment schedules, therapeutic efficacy and treatment outcomes.

The management of overweight and obesity during cancer treatment is an emerging area of importance, in particular in early stage breast and prostate cancers, which are usually not associated with involuntary weight loss. *Nutrition and Physical Activity Guidelines for Cancer Survivors*, published in 2012 by the American Cancer Society (12), introduced a new component of nutrition assessment and intervention for cancer survivors. These guidelines state: "for cancer survivors who are overweight or obese and who choose to pursue weight loss, there appears to be no contraindication to modest weight loss (i.e., a maximum of 2 pounds per week) during treatment, as long as the treating oncolgoists approve, weight loss is monitored closely, and it does not interfere with treatment" (12). This last criteria may disqualify many patients, as a weight loss of as little as 6% has been associated with reduced response to oncology treatment, reduced survival and reduced quality of life (4). However, evidence clearly suggests that overweight and obesity are detrimental to long term prognosis of breast cancer. Oncology RDs, when routinely reassessing nutrition risk throughout treatment, should consider this concern and at some point, perhaps in recovery, transition patients to weight management nutrition intervention. Increasing numbers of cancer programs are adding weight management programs, in particular but not limited to breast cancer survivors. The oncology RD should be involved when decisions are made for the patient to begin weight control interventions and should supervise the adequacy of the nutrition regimen that is implemented.

Nutrition Screening

Nutrition screening for malnutrition leads to early identification of patients who are experiencing malnutrition or are at risk for malnutrition. Implementation of a screening process is imperative to ensure proactive nutrition care. Early intervention is essential, as attempts to reverse severe nutrition depletion or severe malnutrition in the oncology patient are more challenging and likely to fail. The later oncology nutrition care is implemented, the more difficult it is to modify a patient's nutritional status (13).

Oncology treatment occurs over a lengthy period of time, even in early staged, curative therapy. Treatment is cumulative, with total doses achieved over weeks and months. Due to the length of cancer treatments, all oncology patients should be screened and rescreened during treatment for nutrition impact symptoms and characteristics of malnutrition. Even those identified as being at low risk for malnutrition by diagnosis may experience unpredictable barriers to nutrition, may lack basic nutrition knowledge, or may practice nutrition behaviors inappropriate or non-conducive to the healing process required during oncology therapy.

Malnutrition screening should be conducted upon admission to oncology services, and then applied routinely throughout the treatment regimen. Many facilities choose shorter nutrition screening tools that can be accomplished rapidly and accurately by properly trained para-professionals. Commonly, ambulatory cancer centers will apply a malnutrition screening tool prior to physician visits: weekly in radiation therapy, every two to three weeks during chemotherapy and at each follow up visit.

Nutrition Screening Tools

Several associations including the Academy of Nutrition and Dietetics (the Academy), the Association for Enteral and Parenteral Nutrition (A.S.P.E.N.), The Oncology Nursing Society (ONS), and the Association of Community Cancer Centers (ACCC) have recommended tools and processes for nutrition screening of ambulatory cancer patients.

According to the Oncology Nutrition Evidence Analysis Work Group, "The screening tool should be a valid identifier of malnutrition risk in adult oncology patients who would benefit from nutrition assessment and intervention by a Registered Dietitian/Nutritionist. This tool should be able to detect a measurable adverse effect on body composition, function or clinical outcome" (14).

Tools used to screen oncology patients should be a valid identifier of those who are experiencing nutrition impact symptoms and the characteristics of malnutrition. The tool itself should be: easy to use, standardized, rapid, non-invasive, valid for the intended population, reliable, sensitive and cost effective (15).

When choosing a malnutrition screening tool, several criteria should be considered:
1) who will perform the screening of the patient and how they will document the screening in the patient chart;
2) how much staff time will be required to perform a screening; and
3) how referrals generated from the screening process will be triaged.

There are many nutrition screening tools, several of which have not been validated for use in oncology patients. Most consider: height and weight or BMI, weight change, presence of appetite, disease severity and presence of co-morbidities. The Academy's Evidence Analysis Library (EAL) has compared parameters measured in the most common nutrition screening tools, collected information regarding sensitivity, specificity, and reliability, and has graded the tools. The complete chart is available at www.adaevidencelibrary.org. Four tools were found to be appropriate for use with oncology patients (14) and are summarized in Table 1.

Evidence Based Nutrition Assessment

Patients identified as being at risk of malnutrition are referred to an RD for nutrition assessment. The purpose of the oncology nutrition assessment is to perform an in-depth evaluation of factors that impact nutrition and then plan appropriate interventions. It is the first step in the Nutrition Care Process crafted by the Academy for each of the five domains/categories: Food and Nutrition Related History; Anthropometric Measurements; Biochemical Data, Medical Tests and Procedures; Nutrition–Focused Physical Findings; and Client History. The use of comparative standards provides normative values to evaluate the patient data.

Currently, definitions for nutrition assessment incorporate processes grounded in evidence for gathering clinical and biochemical data, which are then used to create a plan for intervention.

Table 1: Screening Tools Validated for Use with Oncology Patients (14)

Screening Tool	Data Points Evaluated	Comments
Patient Generated – Subjective Global Assessment (PG-SGA)	17 data points	Includes both screening and assessment criteria. Inpatient and outpatient setting.
Malnutrition Screening Tool (MST)	2 data points	Pure screening tool. Inpatient and outpatient setting.
Malnutrition Screening Tool for Cancer Patients (MSTC)	4 data points	Includes ECOG* performance status. Inpatient setting only.
Malnutrition Universal Screening Tool (MUST)	4 data points	Contains both screening and assessment criteria. Inpatient setting only.

*ECOG Eastern Cooperative Oncology Group performance status rates performance from 0-5, with 0 being able fully active and 5 being deceased.

Definitions of Nutrition Assessment:

- The Academy's 2008 definition for nutrition assessment is: "A systematic method for obtaining, verifying, and interpreting data needed to identify nutrition related problems, their causes and significance. It is an ongoing, non-linear, dynamic process that involves initial data collection, but also continual reassessment and analysis of the patient's status compared to specific criteria" (16).
- In 2008, A.S.P.E.N. defined a nutrition assessment for adults, writing that it: "characterizes a combination of clinical and biochemical parameters to create a written assessment of this data, nutrition risk stratification and specific recommendations" (17).

Assessment interpretations were analyzed by the EAL Oncology Work Group in their development of a definition of nutrition assessment specific to adult oncology patients. Their definition is:

> **Academy of Nutrition and Dietetics Evidence Analysis Library:**
>
> **"An adult oncology nutrition assessment should characterize and document the presence of (or expected potential for) altered nutrition status and nutrition impact symptoms that may result in a measurable adverse effect on body composition, function, QOL or clinical outcome, and may also include indicators of malnutrition." (18)**

Interpretation specific to the oncology experience may be useful to guide oncology nutrition practice and oncology nutrition interventions within the five domains of the Nutrition Care Process. The practice points provided below may assist in distinguishing relevant oncology data:

Food and Nutrition Related History

- **Diet History:** food allergies; food records in the setting of the treatment cycle (how does it change across the cycle); current portion size compared to usual intake; patterns of meals and snacks; use of functional foods (e.g., shakes, smoothies, bars); use of alcohol; use of a restricted diet which may be liberalized in the context of overall decreased intake (e.g., medical nutrition therapy for hypercholesterolemia, obesity, irritable bowel, diabetes), cancer prevention strategies potentially not appropriate in treatment (e.g., Gonzalez Regimen and Raw Food Diet, each of which may result in unintentional reduction in energy intake); food intolerances; food aversions; foods that are currently tolerated.

- **Medication History**: amount and frequency of prescribed medications and over-the-counter medications; narcotics; antiemetics; steroids; stool softeners and laxatives; digestive enzymes; vitamin, herbal, alternative or natural botanical products; use of probiotics; fiber supplementation; use of medical marijuana or appetite stimulants.

- **Patient Efforts**: assessment of current strategies used by the patient to overcome difficulty with nourishment; "what is working" and willingness to modify behaviors.

Anthropometric Measurements

- **Measure, categorize and assess**: height; current weight, usual weight and weight change over time; BMI; adjusted weight if obese; grip strength values; triceps skin fold and mid upper arm circumference measured over time.

Note: Any weight loss that is unintended in adult oncology patients has potential significance.

Biochemical Data, Medical Tests and Procedures

- Biochemical Assessment in the setting of chemotherapy, radiation and biotherapy: Hydration status, electrolytes, white blood cell count, red blood cell count, absolute neutrophil count, anemias (i.e., folate and B12), calcium, liver function, glucose ranges, and renal function. In the past C-reactive protein (CRP) has been used to assess inflammatory status (CRP >/= 10 can be used to indicate if inflammation is present, which determines the severity of each malnutrition characteristic) (19). It is important to monitor trends across time. Be aware that biochemical values may be altered due to oncology treatment (e.g., glucose may be elevated due to steroid use, white blood cell count may be elevated / reduced due to treatment and medications and liver function tests (LFTs) may be elevated due to chemotherapy).
  - Bioimpedence results (20), and potential future use of CT scans that document changes in fat and muscle volume over time.
  - GI function tests (e.g., gastric emptying, swallowing evaluations, stool elastase test).
  - Note regarding evaluation of hepatic proteins (e.g., albumin) to indicate overall protein status: Over the past decade nutrition research has produced evidence that inflammatory state significantly impacts traditionally utilized lab values and renders them inaccurate for nutrition decision making. Cancer and its treatments can encourage inflammatory states, thus requiring alternate nutrition assessment strategies. Currently, neither the Academy nor A.S.P.E.N. propose any specific protein or hepatic protein markers for diagnostic purposes.

Nutrition Focused Physical Findings

  - Nutrition Impact Symptoms (NIS) that impede intake, digestion, absorption or utilization include but are not limited to: anorexia, cachexia, muscle wasting, dysphasia, xerostomia, taste and smell changes, mucositis and stomatitis, nausea and vomiting, esophagitis, diarrhea, early satiety, gastroparesis, malabsorption, constipation, shortness of breath, pain, dehydration (21).
  - Assessment of vital signs: oxygenation, pulse, blood pressure, temperature.
  - Grip strength, changes in grip strength over time in the individual patient.
  - Inspection for nutrient deficiencies: pallor, stomatitis, glossitis, anemia, quality of hair (if present), appearance of nails (may be altered by chemotherapy).

- Appearance: cachexia, muscle loss, sunken eyes, presence of edema.
- Abdomen: assess for pain; bowel function and presence or absence of bowel sounds; frequency, quantity and characteristic of stool, steatorrhea; presence and health of a feeding tube site; frequency and quantity of urination; symptoms of dehydration; digestion (e.g., of fat, fiber, lactose, and other food components); digestion of pills or medication; gastrointestinal symptoms stimulated by food intake and timing at which they occur; bloating; gassiness; gastroparesis; reflux; presence of ascites.
- Dermatologic: assess for stomatitis, angular cheilitis, erythemia from chemotherapy, presence and healing status of surgical wounds and radiation burns, skin turgor, other wounds.
- Head and neck: assess for pain, movement of head, neck and face, swallowing adequacy, presence of dysphagia for solids, dry foods, pills, and liquids of varying consistency, "lump" sensation after swallowing, obstruction or compression of esophagus.
- Intra-oral cavity: assess for pain, presence of surgical or radiation sites, motor strength for jaw, movement and chewing, trismus, oral manipulation of a food bolus, tongue range of motion, oral ulcers, mucositis, infection or thrush, stomatitis, dental repair, recent edentulous status, fit of dentures, saliva quality and quantity, perceived tolerance of temperature, acidity, and texture.
- Assessment of taste: quality of taste that is present, absent or altered, perceived tolerances.

Client History / Medical / Health / Social
- Cancer diagnosis and treatment regimen, anticipated side effects, timing of the treatment cycle and timing of the side effects.
- Age > 65, other medical history, comorbidities.
- Social history, family setting, caregiver support system, food security, ability to obtain and prepare food, religious and cultural factors, financial concerns, level of literacy.

Comparative Standards
- Functional and Quality of Life assessments: Karnofsky Performance Status and Eastern Cooperative Oncology Group (ECOG), Functional Assessment of Cancer Therapy (FACT). Oncology nutrition guidelines: A.S.P.E.N., Clinical Oncology Society of Australia (COSA).

Defining Malnutrition
In oncology patients, malnutrition usually refers to undernutrition and changes in body composition, which occur due to the cancer itself or from the impact of the oncology treatment. The effects of malnutrition can impact immune response, muscle strength, level of fatigue, wound healing, psycho-social function, quality of life, tolerance of treatment regimen and ultimately treatment outcome (22). In addition, the presence of malnutrition may increase treatment and disease complications and increase frequency of hospitalizations, hospital length of stay, utilization of support services and resources, all of which contributes to increasing the cost of providing healthcare (23). Several key experts in oncology have offered definitions of adult malnutrition.

Definitions of Adult Malnutrition

"decline in lean body mass with the potential for functional impairment", and as "any nutritional imbalance" (24)

"Adult undernutrition typically occurs along a continuum of inadequate intake and/or increased requirements, impaired absorption, altered transport, and altered nutrient utilization" (25)

"a state of nutrition in which a deficiency or excess (or imbalance) of energy, protein, and other nutrients causes measurable adverse effects on tissue/body form (body shape, size and composition) and function and clinical outcome" (26)

A key feature of malnutrition in the oncology patient is that it may or may not be associated with cancer cachexia syndrome. Up to 80% of patients with advanced cancer may be diagnosed with cancer cachexia (27).

Cancer cachexia is a multifactorial syndrome characterized by an ongoing loss of skeletal muscle mass (with or without loss of fat mass) that cannot be fully reversed by conventional nutritional support and leads to progressive functional impairment (28).

Cancer cachexia is indicated as a factor in the cause of death of 30%-50% of all cancer patients (29). The pathophysiology of cachexia is characterized by a negative protein and energy balance driven by reduced food intake and/or abnormal metabolism. There are several stages of cancer cachexia: pre-cachexia, cachexia, and refractory cachexia (which occurs in the last 3 months of life) (28). Regardless of the presence of cachexia, it is important to address the direct and indirect causes of decreased intake, and intervene regarding the factors and behaviors that can be manipulated (30). Key features to be assessed include: anorexia; reduced food intake; catabolic drivers; muscle mass and strength; and changes over time.

Malnutrition Characterization
Nutrition assessment includes evaluation of the characteristics that define malnutrition. The goal is to prevent or modify the factors that influence malnutrition. Malnutrition is associated with worse outcomes in patients treated for cancer, as nutritional deficiencies can decrease response to therapy, functional capacity and even survival (31). A landmark consensus document released simultaneously in May 2012 issues of both the Journal of the Academy of Nutrition and Dietetics and the Journal of Parenteral and Enteral Nutrition proffers the newest clinical characteristics upon which to base nutrition assessment and diagnose malnutrition in adults: *Consensus Statement of the Academy of Nutrition and Dietetics/American Society for Parenteral and Enteral Nutrition: Characteristics Recommended for the Identification and Documentation of Adult Malnutrition (Undernutrition), Table 1* (32).

Table 1: Clinical Characteristics of Malnutrition

Table. Academy of Nutrition and Dietetics (Academy)/American Society for Parenteral and Enteral Nutrition (A.S.P.E.N.) clinical characteristics that the clinician can obtain and document to support a diagnosis of malnutrition [a] [b]

Clinical characteristic	Malnutrition in the Context of Acute Illness or Injury		Malnutrition in the Context of Chronic Illness		Malnutrition in the Context of Social or Environmental Circumstances	
	Non-severe (moderate) malnutrition	Severe malnutrition	Non-severe (moderate) malnutrition	Severe malnutrition	Non-severe (moderate) malnutrition	Severe malnutrition
(1) Energy intake (reference 30) Malnutrition is the result of inadequate food and nutrient intake or assimilation; thus, recent intake compared to estimated requirements is a primary criterion defining malnutrition. The clinician may obtain or review the food and nutrition history, estimate optimum energy needs, compare them with estimates of energy consumed and report inadequate intake as a percentage of estimated energy requirements over time.	< 75% of estimated energy requirement for > 7 days	50% of estimated energy requirement for ≥ 5 days	< 75% of estimated energy requirement for ≥ 1 month	< 75% of estimated energy requirement for ≥ 1 month	< 75% of estimated energy requirement for ≥ 3 months	50% of estimated energy requirement for ≥ 1 month
(2) Interpretation of weight loss (references 33, 34, 35, 36) The clinician may evaluate weight in light of other clinical findings including the presence of under- or over- hydration. The clinician may assess weight change over time reported as a percentage of weight lost from baseline.	% / Time 1-2 / 1 wk 5 / 1 mo 7.5 / 3 mos	% / Time >2 / 1 wk >5 / 1 mo >7.5 / 3 mos	% / Time 5 / 1 mo 7.5 / 3 mo 10 / 6 mo 20 / 1y	% / Time >5 / 1 mo >7.5 / 3 mo >10 / 6 mo >20 / 1y	% / Time 5 / 1 mo 7.5 / 3 mo 10 / 6 mo 20 / 1y	% / Time >5 / 1 mo >7.5 / 3 mo >10 / 6 mo >20 / 1 y
Physical findings (references 36, 37) Malnutrition typically results in changes to the physical exam. The clinician may perform a physical exam and document any one of the physical exam findings below as an indicator of malnutrition.						
(3) Body fat Loss of subcutaneous fat (eg, orbital, triceps, fat overlying the ribs).	Mild	Moderate	Mild	Severe	Mild	Severe
(4) Muscle mass Muscle loss (eg, wasting of the temples [temporalis muscle]; clavicles [pectoralis and deltoids]; shoulders [deltoids]; interosseous muscles; scapula [latissimus dorsi, trapezious, deltoids]; thigh [quadriceps] and calf [gastrocnemius]).	Mild	Moderate	Mild	Severe	Mild	Severe
(5) Fluid accumulation The clinician may evaluate generalized or localized fluid accumulation evident on exam (extremities; vulvar/scrotal edema or ascites). Weight loss is often masked by generalized fluid retention (edema) and weight gain may be observed.	Mild	Moderate to severe	Mild	Severe	Mild	Severe

(Continued)

Table 1: Clinical Characteristics of Malnutrition *(continued)*

Table. Academy of Nutrition and Dietetics (Academy)/American Society for Parenteral and Enteral Nutrition (A.S.P.E.N.) clinical characteristics that the clinician can obtain and document to support a diagnosis of malnutrition a b						
	Malnutrition in the Context of Acute Illness or Injury		Malnutrition in the Context of Chronic Illness		Malnutrition in the Context of Social or Environmental Circumstances	
Clinical characteristic	**Non-severe (moderate) malnutrition**	**Severe malnutrition**	**Non-severe (moderate) malnutrition**	**Severe malnutrition**	**Non-severe (moderate) malnutrition**	**Severe malnutrition**
(6) **Reduced grip strength** (reference 42)	N/A c	Measurably reduced	N/A	Measurably reduced	N/A	Measurably Reduced
Consult normative standards supplied by the manufacturer of the measurement device.						

a A minimum of two of the six characteristics above is recommended for diagnosis of either severe or non-severe malnutrition. Height and weight should be measured rather than estimated to determine body mass index. Usual weight should be obtained in order to determine the percentage and to interpret the significance of weight loss. Basic indicators of nutritional status such as body weight, weight change, and appetite may substantively improve with refeeding in the absence of inflammation. Refeeding and/or nutrition support may stabilize but not significantly improve nutrition parameters in the presence of inflammation. The National Center for Health Statistics defines "chronic" as a disease/condition lasting 3 months or longer (reference 12). Serum proteins such as albumin and prealbumin are not included as defining characteristics of malnutrition because recent evidence analysis shows that serum levels of these proteins do not change in response to changes in nutrient intake (references (22, 23, 52, 53).

b This table was developed by Annalynn Skipper PhD, RD, FADA. The content was developed by an Academy workgroup composed of Jane White PhD, RD, FADA, LDN, Chair; Maree Ferguson MBA, PhD, RD; Sherri Jones MS, MBA, RD, LDN; Ainsley Malone, MS, RD, LD, CNSD; Louise Merriman, MS, RD, CDN; Terese Scollard MBA, RD; Annalynn Skipper PhD, RD, FADA; and Academy staff member Pam Michael, MBA, RD. Content was approved by an A.S.P.E.N. committee consisting of Gordon L. Jensen, MD, PhD, Co-Chair; Ainsley Malone, MS, RD, CNSD, Co-Chair; Rose Ann Dimaria, PhD, RN, CNSN; Christine M. Framson, RD, PhD, CSND; Nilesh Mehta, MD, DCH; Steve Plogsted PharmD, RPh, BCNSP; Annalynn Skipper, PhD, RD, FADA; Jennifer Wooley, MS, RD, CNSD; Jay Mirtallo, RPh, BCNSP Board Liaison; and A.S.P.E.N. staff member Peggi Guenter, PhD, CNSN. Subsequently, it was approved by the A.S.P.E.N. Board of Directors. The information in the table is current as of February 1, 2012. Changes are anticipated as new research becomes available. Adapted from: Skipper A. Malnutrition coding. In Skipper A (ed). *Nutrition Care Manual.* Chicago, IL: Academy of Nutrition and Dietetics; 2012 Edition.

c N/A=not applicable.

Reprinted from *J Acad Nutr Diet*, 2012, 112(5), White J, Guenter P, Jensen G, Malone A, Schofield M. Consensus Statement: Characteristics Recommended for the Identification and Documentation of Adult Malnutrition (Undernutrition), 275-283, 2012, with permission from Elsevier

A standardized set of diagnostic characteristics are used to identify and document adult malnutrition. This document applies to all adult patients including oncology patients. The etiologically based diagnostic nomenclature incorporates the current understanding of the inflammatory response on the incidence, progression, and resolution of disease. The chief complaint and past medical history is evaluated by the RD to identify presence or absence of inflammation. The goal of the document is to facilitate more valid estimates of the prevalence of malnutrition, and ultimately guide interventions. For each characteristic, the consensus statement provides guidelines to address acute illness or injury versus chronic versus context of social or environmental circumstances. It also distinguishes between severe (inflammation present) and non-severe malnutrition (absence of inflammation) when describing the six characteristics.

Regarding the guidelines' description of *acute illness or injury* versus *chronic*; it is important to note that oncology patients may experience "acute illness" during rigorous treatment weeks, following oncologic surgery, following biotherapy treatment, during the last weeks of head and neck or gastrointestinal radiation therapy and for weeks after radiation is completed. "Chronic illness" (a disease or condition that lasts 3 months or longer) may describe many oncology patients in long term maintenance therapy.

The consensus document states that two or more of the six characteristics (below) must be present for a diagnosis of malnutrition, and documentation regarding all six characteristics represents a complete nutrition assessment. Upon review by the ON EAL Work Group, the characteristics listed in the consensus report were accepted as appropriate for use in oncology patients, and may form the outline of a nutrition assessment (32).

Additional considerations that may assist the RD when examining the six characteristics identified in the consensus document are provided below:

Insufficient energy intake:
– Consider the percentage of food eaten during each phase of the treatment cycle.

Unintended Weight Loss:
– Any weight loss has potential significance as oncology patients often experience weight loss prior to diagnosis, which is associated with poor outcomes. It is important to account for weight loss that occurred prior to diagnosis as well as weight loss experienced once admitted to an oncology service. Evaluate rate of weight loss over specified timeframes (33).
– Baseline weight is defined as usual body weight taken from medical records; if not available then usual weight recorded when admitted to oncology service; or if not available use self report of recent healthy weight.
– Assess for presence of under- or over hydration.

- Weight loss in elderly patients may have additional significance as there is an association between increased mortality and BMI <20 and / or weight loss of 5% in 30 days or any further weight loss after meeting this criteria (34).
- Analysis of body composition is helpful in determining the significance of weight change. Bioimpedence analysis and the use of CT images used to diagnose and monitor disease progression may be useful in monitoring changes in the individual regarding lean body mass and fat mass.

Loss of muscle mass:
- Reduced muscle mass is an independent predictor of loss of independence, immobility, and mortality.
- Reduced muscle mass is associated with greater toxicity during chemotherapy, which may lead to treatment delays, dose reductions and worse outcomes (5-7).
- Weight loss in obese patients can lead to sarcopenic obesity (i.e., a combination of increased fat mass and decreased muscle mass) and a negative prognosis (35-36).

Loss of subcutaneous fat:
- Weight loss in obese patients can lead to sarcopenic obesity (i.e., a combination of increased fat mass and decreased muscle mass) and a negative prognosis.
- The shortest survival times are found among obese patients with sarcopenia (37).
- Sarcopenia is found in 50% of patients with advanced cancer (35).
- Fat loss may occur with or without the presence of cachexia (37).
- If cachexia is present, lipolysis may occur even in the setting of adequate calories (37).

Localized or generalized fluid accumulation
(which may mask weight loss):
- May use girth measurements to monitor changes in abdominal ascites.
- Track changes in presence and severity of edema over time.
- Monitor frequency of interventions used to reduce fluid accumulation (i.e. tapping of fluid, drains, medications such as diuretics).
- Monitor IV fluid provision: volume and frequency may alter weight status.
- Monitor for medications that promote fluid retention (i.e., steroids).

Diminished functional status,
as measured by hand grip strength:
- Compare grip strength measured to manufacturer norms.
- Monitor changes over time as an individual performance measure.
- Use this information to aid interpretation of functional scores (i.e., Karnofsky – see Appendix 2).

Conclusion: The Oncology Dietitian Perspective

The heterogeneity of oncology illness, combined with the variety of cancer treatments, is best described and recorded by the medical tumor registration system and within nationally recognized treatment guidelines such as National Cancer Institute, National

Comprehensive Cancer Network, and the American Society of Clinical Oncology. At the time of diagnosis, a treatment regimen is determined by the oncologist to provide the best chance of cancer control or cure. Thorough knowledge of oncologic treatment and expected effects are required to guide appropriate nutrition intervention that will keep a patient healing, nourished and able to complete his/her prescribed treatment regimen. This role is best filled by the oncology specialist RD or Certified Specialist in Oncology Nutrition (CSO). Delineation of this specialty level of practice is discussed at length in the Standards of Practice, Standards of Professional Performance for Oncology Nutrition (38), published by the Academy.

Nutrition plays a significant role in helping patients meet the increased demands of healing, and becomes crucial in minimizing effects of cancer and its treatment that limit or reduce nutritional intake. Nutritional status can deteriorate during the course of treatment and weight loss is a common experience. The perspective of the RD considers the unique experience of each patient, which is influenced by a multitude of variables. The oncology RD evaluates the immediate NIS and also incorporates the following oncology specific variables into a nutrition assessment: health at time of diagnosis; effects of the cancer itself upon digestion, absorption, and utilization of nutrients; treatment strategies (surgical, chemotherapy, radiation, and biological); timing of the treatments; tolerance to each aspect of the treatment regimen; and the resilience of the patient and family to adapt the nutrition plan as each barrier to nutrition occurs. Lastly, the oncology RD evaluates the next steps of the treatment plan, and anticipates the potential nutrition challenges a patient may experience. Nutrition assessment provides a means for the oncology RD to evaluate a patient's ability to achieve adequate nutrition during treatment. When assessment is followed by evidence-based nutrition interventions, the oncology patient has a better chance of tolerating the prescribed treatment and receiving full treatment.

References

1. Strasser F, Bruera ED. Update on anorexia and cachexia. *Hematol Oncol Clin North Am.* 2002;16(3):589-617.
2. Ollenschlager G, Viell B, Thomas W, Konkol K, Burger B. Tumor anorexia: causes, assessment, treatment. *Recent Results Cancer Res.* 1991;121: 249–259.
3. Bruera E. (1997). ABC of palliative care. Anorexia, cachexia, and nutrition. *BMJ.* 1997;315(7117):1219–1222.
4. Dewys WD, Begg C, Lavin PT, et. al. Prognostic effect of weight loss prior to chemotherapy in cancer patients. Eastern Cooperative Oncology Group. *Am J Med.* 1980;69(4):491-497.
5. Antoun S, Baracos VE, Birdsell L, Escudier B, Sawyer MB. Low body mass index and sarcopenia associated with dose-limitng toxicity of sorafenib in patients with renal cell carcinoma. *Annals of Oncology.* 2010; 21(8): 1594-1598.
6. Prado CM, Baracos VE, McCargar LJ, et al. Body composition as an independent determinant of 5-fluorouracil-based chemotherapy toxicity. *Clin Cancer Res.* 2007;13(11):3264–3268.
7. Prado CM, Baracos VE, McCargar LJ, et al. Sarcopenia as a determinant of chemotherapy toxicity and time to tumor progression in metastatic breast cancer patients receiving capecitabine treatment. *Clin Cancer Res.* 2009;15(8):2920–2926.

8. Parsons HA, Baracos VE, Dhillon N, Hong DS, Kurzrock R. Body composition, symptoms, and survival in advanced cancer patients referred to a phase I service. PLoS One. 2012;7(1):e29330.

9. Andreyev HJ, Norman AR, Oates J, Cunningham D. Why do patients with weight loss have a worse outcome when undergoing chemotherapy for gastrointestinal malignancies? Eur J Cancer. 1998;34(4):503-509.

10. Aoyama T, Yoshikawa T, Shiraj J. Body weight loss after surgery is an independent risk factor for continuation for S-1 adjuvant chemotherapy for gastric cancer. Gastrointestinal Oncology. 2012;20(6):2000-2006.

11. Russo G, Haddad R, Posner M, Machtav M. Radiation treatment breaks and ulcerative mucositis in head and neck cancer. Oncologist. 2008; 13(8):886-898.

12. Rock CL. Nutrition and physical activity guidelines for cancer survivors. CA Cancer J Clin. 2012;62(4):242-274.

13. Isenring EA, Bauer JD, Capra S. Nutrition support using the American Dietetic Association medical nutrition therapy protocol for radiation oncology patients improves dietary intake compared with standard practice. J Am Diet Assoc. 2007;107(3):404-412.

14. Academy of Nutrition and Dietetics. Evidence Analysis Library: Oncology Nutrition Screening project. Found at http://andevidencelibrary.com/. Accessed 5/20/13.

15. Skipper A, Ferguson M, Thompson K, Castellanos VH, Porcari J. Nutrition screening tools: an analysis of the evidence. J Parenter Enteral Nutr. 2012;36(3):292-298.

16. Academy of Nutrition and Dietetics. Nutrition Care Process. http://www.eatright.org/HealthProfessionals/content.aspx?id=7077. Accessed 5/20/13.

17. Association for Enteral and Parenteral Nutrition: Definition of Nutrition Assessment. https://www.nutritioncare.org/lcontent.aspx?id=546. Accessed 5/20/13.

18. Evidence Analysis Library: Oncology Nutrition Assessment. Found at http://andevidencelibrary.com (currently in press). Accessed 5/20/13.

19. Ferron K, Voss A, Hustead D. Definition of cancer cachexia: effect of weight loss, reduced food intake, and systematic inflammation on functional status and prognosis. Am J Clin Nutr. 2006;83(6);1345-1350.

20. Thibault R, Pichard C. The evaluation of body composition: A useful tool for clinical practice. Ann Nutr Metab. 2013;60 :6-16. DOI:10.1159/000334879.

21. Kubrak C, Olson K, Jha N, et al. Nutrition impact symptoms: key determinants of reduced dietary intake, weight loss, and reduced functional capacity of patients with head and neck cancer before treatment. Head Neck. 2010;32(3):290-300.

22. Capuano G, Gentile PC, Bianciardi F, Tosti M, Palladino A, Di Palma M: Prevalence and influence of malnutrition on quality of life and performance status in patients with locally advanced head and neck cancer before treatment. Support Care Cancer 2010;18(4):433-437.

23. Kruizenga HM, Tulder MWV, Seidell JC, Thijs A, Ader HJ, van Bokhurst-de van der Schueren MAE. Effectiveness and cost-effectiveness of early screening and treatment of malnourished patients. Am J Clin Nutr. 2005;82(5):1082-1089.

24. Jensen G, Bistrian B, Roubenoff R, Heimburger D. Malnutrition syndromes: a conundrum vs. continuum. J Parenteral Enteral Nutrition. 2009;33(6):710-716.

25. White J, Guenter P, Jensen G, Malone A, Schofield M. Consensus Statement: Academy of Nutrition and Dietetics and American Society for Parenteral and Enteral Nutrition: Characteristics Recommended for the Identification and Documentation of Adult Malnutrition (Undernutrition). J Parenter Enteral Nutr. 2012 36(3):275-283.

26. Stratton RJ, Green CJ, Elia M. Disease Related Malnutrition: an Evidence Based Approach to Treatment. Cambridge, MA: CABI; 2003: 3.

27. Fox K, Brooks J, Gandra S, Markus R, Chiou C. Estimation of cachexia among cancer patients based on four definitions. J Oncology. 2009; Article ID 693458, 7 pages.

28. Palomares MR, Sayre JW, Shekar KC, Lillington LM, Chlebowski R. Gender influence of weight-loss pattern and survival of non-small cell lung carcinoma patients. Cancer. 1996;78(10):2119-2126.

29. Fearon K, Strasser F, Anker SD, et al. Definition and classification of cancer cachexia: an international consensus. Lancet Oncol. 2011;12(5):489-495.

30. Isenring E, Capra S, Bauer J. Nutrition intervention is beneficial in oncology outpatients receiving radiotherapy to the gastrointestinal, head or neck area. Br J Cancer. 2004;91(3):447-452.

31. Shike M. Nutrition therapy for the cancer patient. Hematol Oncol Clin N Am. 1996;10(1):221-324.

32. White J, Guenter P, Jensen G, Malone A, Schofield M. Consensus Statement: Academy of Nutrition and Dietetics and American Society for Enteral and Parenteral Nutrition: Characteristics Recommended for the Identification and Documentation of Adult Malnutrition (Undernutrition). J Acad Nutr Diet. 2012;112(5):730-738.

33. Jensen GL, Hsiao PY, Wheeler D. Adult nutrition assessment tutorial, J Parenter Enter Nutr. 2012;36(3);267-274.

34. Grabowski DC, Ellis JE. High body mass index does not predict mortality in older people: analysis of the Longitudinal Study of Aging. J Am Geriatr Soc. 2001;49(7):968-979.

35. Prado CM, Lieffers JR, McCargar LJ, et al. Prevalence and clinical implications of sarcopenic obesity in patients with solid tumours of the respiratory and gastrointestinal tracts: a population-based study. Lancet Oncol. 2008;9(7):629-635.

36. Tan BH, Birdsell LA, Martin L, Baracos VE, Fearon KC. Sarcopenia in an overweight or obese patient is an adverse prognostic factor in pancreatic cancer. Clin Cancer Res. 2009;15(22):6973-6979.

37. Fearon KC. The 2011 ESPEN Arvid Wretlind lecture: cancer cachexia: the potential impact of translational research on patient-focused outcomes. Clin Nutr. 2012;31(5):577-582.

38. Robien K, Levin R, Pritchett E, Otto M. American Dietetic Association: standards of practice and standards of professional performance for registered dietitians (generalist, specialty, and advanced) in oncology nutrition care. J Am Diet Assoc. 2006;106(6):946-951.

Nutritional Needs of the Adult Oncology Patient

Kathryn K Hamilton, MA, RD, CSO, CDN

Introduction

Nutritional status influences disease prognosis, treatment tolerance and the quality of life of individuals diagnosed with cancer (1-3). Nutrition intervention provided by a Registered Dietitian/Registered Dietitian Nutritionist (RD/RDN) utilizes a variety of strategies to manage side effects of cancer treatments and improve functional status, including provision of the most appropriate diet for meeting the patient's needs. These interventions are grounded in science that has identified nutritional needs of healthy and physically stressed adults. This chapter reviews current knowledge and research on the nutritional needs of adult oncology patients.

Metabolic Changes Associated with Cancer

Research has identified types and amounts of nutrients and bioactive compounds in food that will promote good health. Inflammatory processes such as cancer alter those requirements. These alterations are largely cytokine mediated and will persist as long as the inflammation is present (4). As often happens in individuals with cancer, when the severity or persistence of inflammation results in a decrease in lean body mass, causing functional impairment, it is considered "disease-related malnutrition". The inflammatory process may limit the effectiveness of targeted nutrition interventions and the resulting malnutrition may further compromise the clinical response to medical therapy (5). For this reason, in chronic disease-related malnutrition, successful nutrition intervention must address the underlying health condition and its nutritional needs (6-7).

Individuals with cancer often have increased requirements for macro- and micronutrients due to periods of under-nutrition before or after diagnosis (8) as well as metabolic effects from the cancer and its treatments (9). In a study looking at the resting energy expenditure (REE) of select diagnostic groups of newly diagnosed individuals with cancer, 46.7% were hypermetabolic, 43.5% were normometabolic and 9.8% were hypometabolic. People diagnosed with esophageal, gastric, pancreatic and non-small cell lung cancers had higher energy expenditures, while individuals with colorectal cancer showed no significant difference in energy expenditure from controls (9). Estimation of each cancer survivor's nutritional needs is based on clinical data as well as physical assessment and observation, and the clinician should assess needs and then reassess needs at regular intervals, based on achievement of pre-determined goals.

Over- and underfeeding can have detrimental effects. The longer-term consequences of under-feeding can lead to loss of lean body mass, immunosuppression, poor wound healing and risk of hospital acquired infections (10). Conversely, the longer-term consequences of over-feeding can lead to respiratory failure due to increased CO_2 production, hyperglycemia, azotemia, hypertryglyceridemia, electrolyte imbalances, immunosuppression, alterations in hydration status and hepatic steatosis (10).

Dietary Reference Intakes

Dietary Reference Intakes (DRI) estimate amounts of energy and nutrients needed for various life stages and gender groups (11). DRIs identify intakes that meet the needs of the majority of Americans and intakes that pose a risk of adverse effects. They include Recommended Dietary Allowances (RDA) and Adequate Intakes (AI), which estimate intakes needed for good health and Upper Intake Levels (UL), which identify intakes that pose a risk of adverse effects. Estimates of nutrient needs for various health conditions are based upon this data. DRIs were developed and are periodically revised by the Food and Nutrition Board of the Institute of Medicine, National Academy of Sciences (11).

Macronutrient Needs

Protein (see Table 1)

Protein is essential for a range of life-sustaining functions such as building and repairing cells and maintaining muscle mass. The DRI for protein for healthy individuals is 0.8g/kg/day (12). Protein needs for catabolic individuals are generally higher and in the range of 1.2 to 2.0 g/kg per day (13). According to the *ADA Pocket Guide to Nutrition Assessment, 2nd edition,* 1.5 g/kg per day protein is recommended for metabolically stressed individuals (14) while less protein is needed in cases of documented organ failure (14).

Carbohydrate and Fat

Carbohydrates and fats are the primary energy sources. Adequate calories from carbohydrates and fats are needed each day to spare protein for its essential functions and to preserve lean muscle. The RDA for carbohydrate is 130g/day for healthy adults (12,14). No estimated average requirement (EAR), AI or RDA was determined for fat, though there is a need for essential fatty acids that can usually be met when linoleic acid provides approximately 2% to 4% of total energy intake and alpha linolenic acid provides 0.25% to 0.5% of total energy intake (15). For those receiving nutrition support,

Table 1: Protein Requirements in Health and Disease (12-13)

Condition	Protein Requirement g/kg/day (actual weight unless specified)
DRI reference	0.8
Healthy adult	0.8-1.0
Older adult	1.0

Renal disease: predialysis
                     hemodialysis
                     peritoneal dialysis
	0.6-0.8
	1.2-1.3, up to 1.5-1.8
	1.5-2.5

Cirrhosis/Hepatic failure	1.0-1.2
Cancer	1.0-1.5
Cancer cachexia	1.5-2.5
Bone marrow transplant	1.5
Inflammatory bowel disease	1.0-1.5
Short bowel syndrome	1.5-2.0
BMI > 27 with normal renal and hepatic function	1.5-2.0 (of ideal body weight* with hypocaloric feeding)
Obesity class I (BMI≥30 but <35) or class II (BMI≥35 but <40), trauma (ICU)	1.9 (of ideal body weight* with hypocaloric feeding)
Obesity class III (BMI≥40), trauma (ICU)	2.5 (of ideal body weight* with hypocaloric feeding)
Pulmonary disease	1.2-1.5
Critical illness (trauma, sepsis)	1.5-2.0

*The Hamwi method has traditionally been used to estimate ideal body weight (i.e., men: 106 pounds for first 5 feet plus 6 pounds per inch for every additional inch, and women: 100 pounds for first 5 feet plus 5 pounds per inch for every additional inch).

A.S.P.E.N. Guidelines suggest limiting carbohydrate to <7 g/kg per day and fat to ≤2.5 g/kg per day, though it is still important to provide adequate calories for individual needs (16).

Fluid Requirements

Adequate hydration is important to sustain life. Thirst is the main determinant but is not always a reliable gauge for fluid needs. Under-hydration is often a problem for individuals with cancer due to decreased intake (e.g., difficulty obtaining and consuming fluids) and excessive losses (e.g., volume depletion due to vomiting and diarrhea). Adequate hydration is especially a problem in the elderly population due to impaired thirst mechanisms and access issues from decreased mobility (17). In the palliative care setting, an average of 1000mL of fluid per day is considered acceptable for adequate urine output and hydration (13,18).

Intravenous hydration (IV) may be recommended for individuals with cancer struggling to achieve adequate hydration, but need must be determined on an individual basis, taking fluid intake and output into consideration. Over-hydration can occur with excessive IV hydration and can complicate underlying conditions of congestive heart failure and pulmonary and/or renal disease.

Several methods are used to calculate fluid requirements (13):
- According to the *A.S.P.E.N. Core Curriculum*, typical fluid requirements for adults are 20-40mL/kg/day or 1 to 1.5mL/kcal of energy expended.
- *RDA Method*: 1mL per 1kcal consumed
- Body Surface Area (BSA) Method: 1500 mL/m^2 or BSA x 1500mL

The DRIs (Table 2) suggest a distribution range for macronutrients and other dietary components, which is provided in Table 3.

Table 2: Dietary Reference Intakes (DRIs): Recommended Dietary Allowances and Adequate Intakes (12,19)

Life Stage Group	Total Water L/day	Carbohydrate g/day	Total Fiber g/day	Total Fat g/day	Protein g/day
Males					
19-50y	3.7*	**130**	38*	ND	**56**
51->70y	3.7*	**130**	30*	ND	**56**
Females					
19-50y	2.7*	**130**	25*	ND	**46**
51->70y	2.7*	**130**	21*	ND	**46**

Recommended Daily Allowances (RDAs) in bold; Adequate Intakes (AI)*; Not Determined (ND)
Total Water includes all water contained in food, beverages and drinking water

Table 3: Acceptable Macronutrient Distribution Ranges for adults (12)

Macronutrient	Recommendations
Fat	20-35% total calories
Carbohydrate	45-65% total calories
Protein	10-35% total calories
Dietary cholesterol	As low as possible while consuming a nutritionally adequate diet
Trans fatty acids	As low as possible while consuming a nutritionally adequate diet
Saturated fatty acids	As low as possible while consuming a nutritionally adequate diet

Micronutrient Needs with Cancer

Micronutrients are required in small amounts, but are essential for triggering the range of biochemical reactions essential for life. Micronutrient deficiencies such as zinc, iron, selenium and vitamins A, B, and C are common in individuals who are ill (20). Deficiencies may result from suboptimal intake and extraordinary losses. In some cases decreased micronutrient levels may not indicate an actual deficiency but instead a redistribution of the micronutrients. The decrease may be an adaptive response in the body as increased levels of some vitamins function as pro-oxidants (20). Micronutrient deficiencies in an already ill person can affect various biochemical processes and enzyme functions that can lead to organ dysfunction, muscle weakness, poor wound healing and altered immunity (16). Unfortunately, supplementation in excess of the DRIs may not result in elevated serum levels and may, in fact, be detrimental (20). Unless otherwise indicated by results of a nutrition assessment, cancer patients should aim for an intake of 100% of the RDAs/AIs for micronutrients. The complete set of DRIs for vitamins and minerals can be downloaded from the United States Department of Agriculture, National Agricultural Library (21) http://fnic.nal.usda.gov/dietary-guidance/dietary-reference-intakes/dri-tables.

Effect of Inflammatory Response on Micronutrient Status

Serum levels of some micronutrients decrease with inflammation but the significance of these fluctuations is unclear. Surgical patients may experience a decrease in levels of vitamins A, C and E and septic patients may excrete higher than normal levels of vitamin A in urine (20). Thiamin, riboflavin, vitamin B12, and folate levels are usually not affected by inflammation; consequently low levels may be related to actual deficiencies.

During the inflammatory process, selenium, copper, iron and zinc levels decrease due to sequestration, possibly in the liver and reticuloendothelial system, though increased urinary losses and protein catabolism also contribute to losses (20). The decrease in serum levels of trace minerals may occasionally be beneficial as lower levels of iron help protect against bacterial infections (20). Table 4 summarizes medical conditions that influence micronutrient levels.

Estimating Energy Needs

Energy drives every biological reaction in the body and essential processes including respiration and circulation. Consequences of under- and overfeeding can be obvious, as evidenced by classic external signs of cachexia and obesity. However, body composition can mask underlying changes in lean body mass (e.g., sarcopenia) that also may influence organ function and outcomes of cancer treatment. There are several methods for predicting energy requirements:

- **Direct calorimetry**, used infrequently, and mostly employed as a research method, which measures heat from macronutrient consumption released from the subject (13).
- **Indirect calorimetry**, known as "the gold standard", uses oxygen consumption and carbon dioxide production but the equipment is not always available (7,14).
- **Predictive equations**, some validated, some not, developed for select patient populations and used to assess energy needs. The appropriate method or equation depends on an individual's clinical status and the results of available clinical data (7,22).

Indirect Calorimetry (IC)

Measuring resting metabolic rate (RMR) (7,14,22-23) with IC is thought to be a more accurate way to estimate energy requirements as compared with common prediction equations. It has been shown to closely mirror actual expenditures and account for changes in metabolic state (14).

Table 4: General Medical Conditions affecting Vitamin and Mineral Levels (20)

Medical Condition	Possible Resulting Change in Micronutrient levels
Alcoholic liver	Decrease in folate, thiamine, pyridoxine and vitamin A
Renal failure	Decrease in pyridoxine, folic acid, and vitamin C
GI fistulas and diarrhea	Decrease in all vitamins and multiple trace minerals, especially zinc and selenium
Loss of bile	Decrease in fat soluble vitamins
Pancreatitis	Decrease absorption of B12
Chylous leaks and fistulas (with large protein-rich fluid losses)	Decrease in micronutrients
Gastrectomy or terminal ileum resection	Decrease in iron and B12
Bariatric surgery (Roux-en-Y gastric bypass and gastric banding procedures)	Decrease in fat-soluble vitamins, water soluble vitamins, and minerals, such as iron and zinc
Critical illness	Decrease in vitamin C despite supplementation

Terminology (7,14,23)

BEE (Basal Energy Expenditure): minimum amount of energy expended to be compatible with life

BMR (Basal Metabolic Rate): measurement of baseline energy expended; measured early in the morning before activity and 10-12 hours after ingestion of food, beverage or nicotine; is measured in a temperate environment

RMR (Resting Metabolic Rate): energy expended at rest; measured after fasting for at least five hours, generally 10-20% higher than BMR

REE (Resting Energy Expenditure): energy needed to maintain normal body functions measured after 30 minutes of recombinant rest

EEE (Estimated Energy Expenditure): energy needed per day to maintain normal body functions

EER (Estimated Energy Requirement): average predicted nutrition intake for maintenance of energy balance and good health based on age, gender, weight, height and activity level

PAL (Physical Activity Levels): four activity levels, *sedentary, low active, active, very active,* as defined by the Institute of Medicine (IOM)

RQ (Respiratory Quotient): calculation derived from IC using carbon dioxide expended and oxygen consumed

BMI (Body Mass Index): calculation of the degree of adiposity

IC is often conducted in a clinical setting using a metabolic cart. Respiratory Therapists (RTs) and RDs are trained to conduct the test. If not already in the hospital, participants are often admitted and required to fast overnight, refraining from nicotine, alcohol and exercise the day before the test. They are to stay in bed for the 12 hours prior to the test except to use the bedside commode. The test is conducted in the morning, and requires the participant to remain under a canopy for a minimum of 30 minutes so as to collect at least one, 5-minute interval of steady state (i.e., < 10% change in VO2 and VCO2 in a five-minute interval) (22). The test measures carbon dioxide production and oxygen consumption, and provides an RQ. The RQ, a measure of CO2 produced over O2 consumed, can then be inserted into a modified *Weir formula* to determine REE in kcals/day.

Weir Formula: REE=(3.9VO$_2$+1.1VCO$_2$) x 1.44. (VO$_2$ is oxygen consumption (mL/min) and VCO$_2$ is carbon dioxide expended (mL/min)

RQ=VCO$_2$/VO$_2$

RQ readings below 0.7 and above 1.0 warrant a repeat test as according to the EAL a RQ below 0.7 suggests hypoventilation or prolonged fasting and a RQ above 1.0, in the absence of overfeeding, represents hyperventilation or inaccurate gas collection (7).

New, portable, and cost-effective indirect calorimeters are being tested for use in the hospital as well as in the ambulatory setting. One such device, a portable armband, measures sleeping energy expenditure (SEE) and in a recent study, registered a slightly higher reading than a REE measured with IC but with less deviation than using a predictive equation (24). Because of concerns regarding accuracy, energy needs of patients receiving mechanical ventilation should be measured by metabolic carts rather than new portable indirect calorimeters. Table 5 summarizes conditions that influence the accuracy of IC measurement.

Predictive Equations

When assessment with IC is not possible, predictive equations can be used to determine energy needs. Energy equations have been developed for specific medical conditions and groups, and it is important to apply the most appropriate calculations to the individual or population being assessed. In most cases, researchers compared predictive equations to IC to assess the accuracy of their equations. Formulas have been developed for use in healthy, acutely ill, critically ill and obese populations. Predictions for the latter three groups are most relevant for patients undergoing cancer treatment and in active recovery.

Table 5: Conditions That Influence Indirect Calorimetry

Conditions Required for a Valid Assessment (14)	Conditions That Influence Accuracy (7,11)	Ineligibility Criteria (7)
Hemodynamic stability	Beards	Required nasal oxygen supplementation
Cooperative or sedated patient	Thin faces and jaws on frail individuals	Complaint of upper respiratory infection symptoms
Period of rest prior to the measurement	Leaky chest tubes or other conditions preventing collection of expired gas	
Fraction of inspired oxygen (FIO2) <60%	Hemodialysis, peritoneal dialysis or continuous renal replacement therapy	
Absence of chest tubes or other sources of air leaks		
Absence of supplemental oxygen		
Absence of hyperventilation		

HEALTHY POPULATIONS

The Mifflin-St Jeor equation, the Harris Benedict equation and the DRIs for energy were initially developed to assess energy needs of healthy people. In addition, the Mifflin-St Jeor equation is a component of several equations used to assess energy needs in critically ill patients.

Mifflin-St Jeor Equation was developed, then published by Mark Mifflin, Sachiko St Jeor and colleagues from the University of Nevada School of Medicine in 1990. It was created by studying healthy men and women, then comparing the predictive equation conclusions to IC readings. According to the Academy of Nutrition and Dietetics Evidence Analysis Library (EAL), the Mifflin-St. Jeor equation, using actual weight, was best at predicting RMR in non-obese and obese populations, ages 20-82 years (7,14,25).
- **Men: RMR = (9.99 x weight in kilograms) + (6.25 x height in centimeters) – (4.92 x age in years) + 5**
- **Women: RMR = (9.99 x weight in kilograms) + (6.25 x height in centimeters) – (4.92 x age in years) – 161**

Harris-Benedict Equation was proposed in 1919 by J. Arthur Harris and Francis G. Benedict to estimate energy needs for healthy adults, taking into consideration both activity and stress levels (26). It is still used today, but should not be used to assess energy needs in the acutely or critically ill.
- **Men: BMR = 66.47 + 13.75 (weight in kilograms) + 5(height in centimeters) - 6.78(age in years)**
- **Women: BMR = 655.1 + 9.65(weight in kilograms) + 1.85(height in centimeters) - 4.68(age in years)**

DRIs for Estimated Energy Requirements (EER) are for health maintenance in healthy adults and utilize age, weight, height and gender, in addition to physical activity levels, to determine needs (12-13). *PA* represents the physical activity coefficient.

Men 19 years and older
- **EER=662 - 9.53(age in years) + PA (15.91 x weight in kilograms) + 539.6(height in meters)**

Women 19 years and older
- **EER=354 - 6.91(age in years) + PA(9.36 x weight in kilograms) +726(height in meters)**

Physical Activity (PA)

Men:	Women:
PA = 1.00 for sedentary	PA = 1.00 for sedentary
PA = 1.11 for low-activity	PA = 1.12 for low-activity
PA = 1.25 moderate activity	PA = 1.27 moderate activity
PA = 1.49 high-activity	PA = 1.45 high-activity

ACUTELY ILL

The Mifflin-St Jeor Equation (provided in the previous section) and the 1997 Ireton-Jones Equation for spontaneously breathing individuals are appropriate for use in the acutely ill population (27).

Ireton-Jones Equation

The Carol Ireton-Jones assessment equation for spontaneously breathing individuals is acceptable for the acutely ill individual (7,28).
- **Spontaneously breathing patients (1992 and 1997)**
- **EEE = 629 - 11(age in years) + 25(weight in kilograms) - 609(O) (O = obesity factor; 1 if present and 0 if absent)**

CRITICALLY ILL

According to the Academy EAL, the Penn State equation, the Swinamer equation and the Ireton-Jones 1992 ventilator-dependent equation are good predictors of energy needs in the critically ill patient population. Patients who are septic, suffering traumatic injury, have burns and who have undergone major surgery are among those considered critically ill (7,10,14).

Penn State Equation

The Penn State Equation was developed by David Frankenfield and colleagues at Pennsylvania State University. Clinical measurements taken in the early 1990's were reviewed retrospectively to compare energy expenditure under a number of clinical conditions including trauma, surgery, medical and intensive care (29). According to a conversation with D Frankenfield (2/6/2013), it was determined that the most significant factor was not the medical condition but whether the patient was febrile before the energy expenditure measurement was taken.

The Penn State Equation (2003a) has been invalidated and should not be used.
The Penn State Equation (2003b) was validated in 2009 and is called the Penn State Equation.
- **RMR=Mifflin (0.96) + (minute ventilation in L/min)(31) + (maximum daily body temp in C)(167)-6212 (requires use of Mifflin-St Joer equation)**

A third Penn State Equation was validated in 2010 and is also referred to as the Modified Penn State Equation.
- **RMR=Mifflin (0.71) + (minute ventilation in L/min)(64) + (maximum daily body temp in C)(85)-3085 (requires use of Mifflin-St Joer equation)**

Swinamer Equation

Developed, then published by DL Swinamer and colleagues from the University of Alberta in Edmonton Canada in 1990, the Swinamer Equation was developed to accurately assess the needs of the mechanically ventilated critically ill patient (30).
- **BMR (kcals/day) = (Body Surface Area in m²)(945) - age in years(6.4) + (body temp in C)(108) + (respiratory rate)(24.2) + (tidal volume in L/min)(81.7) - 4349**

Ireton-Jones Equation for ventilator-dependent patients

The 1997 Ireton-Jones Equation for spontaneously breathing individuals **is not** suggested for use in the critically ill population.

The 1992 Ireton-Jones equation for estimated energy expenditure can be used for ventilator-dependent critically ill patients and is:

Ventilator-dependent patients (1992)
- **(1992) EEE = 1925 - 10(age in years) + 5(weight in kilograms) +281(G) + 292(T) + 851(B)**

EEE in kilocalories per day
O= presence of obesity >27kg/m² (use *0* if absent, use *1* if present)
T=diagnosis of trauma (use *0* if absent, use *1* if present)
B=diagnosis of burn (use *0* if absent, use *1* if present)
G=gender (*use 1 for males, use 0 for females*)

OBESE POPULATION

Hypocaloric Regimen (BMI ≥30)
Formulas and arguments put forward by Choban et al, Dickerson et al, A.S.P.E.N. and The Society of Critical Care Medicine suggest safe and effective strategies to permissively underfeed this patient population. In addition to obesity, additional indications for use of these equations include: Chronic Obstructive Pulmonary Disease (COPD), acute respiratory distress syndrome, systemic inflammatory response syndrome, sepsis with hemodynamic instability, multiple organ dysfunction syndrome, hypercapnia, hyperglycemia and hypertriglyceridemia (31-33).

The best way to assess energy needs for an obese patient is to use IC, but if it is not available, predictive equations such as Ireton-Jones 1992 or hypocaloric formulas are suggested. Use of hypocaloric formulas in the critically ill overweight/obese population have been shown to positively affect protein anabolism and minimize complications from overfeeding such as hyperglycemia (14,28).

- **11-14 kcalories/kilogram of actual body weight (in hypometabolic disease states without renal or hepatic dysfunction)**
- **14-18 kcalories/kilogram of actual body weight (without renal or hepatic dysfunction)**
- **22 kcalories/kilogram of ideal body weight (without renal or hepatic dysfunction)***
  * tested in both acutely ill and critically ill

A.S.P.E.N. Energy Expenditure formulas (kcals/kg)
A.S.P.E.N. suggests providing a range of between 25 and 35 kcal/kg/day for adults. The initial assessment generally starts at 25 kcal/kg and is followed by adjustments based on the patient's clinical response (16). This formula lacks evidence-based validation and is not an accurate method to assess energy needs of the critically ill (10,16), though it is frequently used as a baseline estimate and then adjusted after comparison to outcome goals (see table 7).

Table 7: Estimated Energy Needs based on Body Weight (10,16)

Medical Condition	Estimated Energy Needs in kcals/kg
Cancer, repletion, weight gain	30-35
Cancer, inactive, non-stressed	25-30
Cancer, hypermetabolic, stressed	35
Sepsis	25-30
Hematopoietic cell transplant	30-35

Actual, Ideal or Adjusted Body Weight

Some predictive equations use actual weight, some ideal weight, and some adjusted weight. Unless specified, it is suggested to use actual weight as several of the predictive equations already adjust for obesity. Overfeeding is problematic in any patient population, but most assuredly in the critically ill patient population, and calculations for estimated needs are of particular importance in the overweight and obese patient. Determination of needs using adjusted weight becomes increasingly less accurate as BMI increases. Furthermore, predictive equations, such as the Harris Benedict equation, that are based on normal, healthy individuals can underestimate the energy expenditure of obese individuals if ideal body weight is used and overestimate energy expenditure if actual body weight is used (27).

Refeeding Syndrome

Significant, potentially life-threatening, metabolic changes can occur when aggressively refeeding an individual with starvation-related malnutrition or substantial weight loss. During starvation, insulin secretion decreases due to limited carbohydrate intake and the energy source converts from glucose to ketones and fatty acids (34). Phosphorus, magnesium, and potassium levels are depleted from cells but serum levels remain normal due to regulation by the kidneys. The restart of feeding introduces carbohydrates into the system and the compensatory release of insulin, which drives phosphorus, magnesium and potassium back into the cells. Hypophosphatemia, one sign of refeeding syndrome, usually occurs within three days of starting nutrition intervention (34) and can derail recovery, increase length of stay in the hospital and complicate the weaning process from the vent.

Conditions such as anorexia, alcoholism, prolonged starvation, morbid obesity with substantial weight loss, and chronic diseases that impact nutritional status like cancer and cirrhosis are risk factors for refeeding syndrome (34).

For individuals at risk for refeeding syndrome, calorie repletion should start at low levels, estimated at 20 kcal/kg or no more than 1000 kcal per day and advance as tolerated while monitoring electrolyte levels (35). Another recommendation is to start with 25% of estimated needs and advance to goal slowly over 3-5 days while monitoring electrolyte levels and for signs of refeeding (36).

References

1. Huhmann MB, Cunningham RS: Importance of nutritional screening in treatment of cancer-related weight loss. *Lancet Oncology*. 2005;6(5): 334-343.

2. Ottery FD. Definition of standardized nutritional assessment and interventional pathways in oncology. *Nutrition*.1996;12(1):S15-S19.

3. Davies M. Nutritional screening and assessment in cancer-associated malnutrition. *Eur J Oncol Nurs*. 2005;9(Suppl 2):S64-S73.

4. Jensen GL, Mirtallo J, Compher C et al. Adult Starvation and Disease-related Malnutrition: A Proposal for Etiology-based Diagnosis in the Clinical Practice Setting from the International Consensus Guideline Committee. *J Parenter Enteral Nutr*. 2010;34(2):156-159.

5. Mueller C, Compher C, Druyan ME and the ASPEN Board of Directors. A.S.P.E.N Clinical Guidelines: Nutrition Screening, Assessment, and Intervention in Adults. *J Parenter Enteral Nutr*. 2011; 35(1):16-24.

6. White JV, Guenter P, Jensen G, et al. Consensus State: Academy of Nutrition and Dietetics and American Society for Parenteral and Enteral Nutrition: Characteristics Recommended for the Identification and Documentation of Adult Malnutrition (Under-nutrition). *J Parenter Enteral Nutr*. 2012;36(3):275-283.

7. Academy of Nutrition and Dietetics Evidence Analysis Library. Available at http:www.eatright.org (subscription or membership required).

8. Van Bokhorst-de van der Schueren MAE. Nutritional support strategies for malnourished cancer patients. *Eur J Oncol Nurs*. 2005;9(Suppl 2): S74-S83.

9. Cao D, Wu G, Zhang B, et al. Resting Energy Expenditure and Body Composition in Patients with Newly Detected Cancer. *Clin Nutr*. 2010; 29(1):72-77.

10. Loh NH, Griffiths RD. The curse of overfeeding and the blight of underfeeding. In: *Intensive Care Medicine*. New York; Springer New York; 2009;675-682.

11. Background Information: Dietary Reference Intakes Tables and Application. Institute of Medicine of the National Academies. http://www.iom.edu/Activities/Nutrition/SummaryDRIs/DRI-Tables.aspx. Last updated 9/12/2011. Accessed 7/10/2013.

12. Dietary Reference Intakes for Energy, Carbohydrate, Fiber, Fat, Fatty acids, Cholesterol, Protein and Amino acids. Institute of Medicine of the National Academies, The National Academies Press, Washington DC 2002/2005. Available at www.nap.edu Accessed July 2013.

13. Forchielli ML, Miller SJ. Nutritional goals and requirements. In Merritt R (ed). *A.S.P.E.N. Nutrition Support Practice Manuel*. 2nd ed. Silver Spring, MD: ASPEN Publishing; 2005;50-51.

14. Russell M, Malone AM. Nutrient Requirements. In: Charney P, Malone AM, ed. *ADA Pocket Guide to Nutrition Assessment*, Second Edition. Chicago IL: American Dietetic Association Publications; 2009:167-191.

15. Task Force for the Revision of Safe Practice for Parenteral Nutriiton: Mirtallo J, Canada T, Johnson D, et al. Safe practices for parenteral nutrition. *J Parenter Enteral Nutr*. 2004;28(6):S39-S70.

16. ASPEN Board of Directors and Clinical Guidelines Task Force. A.S.P.E.N Guidelines for the Use of Parenteral and Enteral Nutrition in Adult and Pediatric Patients. *J Parenter Enteral Nutr*. 2001;26(1)Supplement:22SA.

17. Popkin BM, D'Anci KE, Rosenberg IH. Water, hydration and health. *Nutr Rev*. 2010;68(8):439-458.

18. Steiner N, Bruera E. Methods of hydration in palliative care patients. *J Palliat Care*. 1998;14(2):6-13.

19. Dietary Reference Intakes for Water Potassium, Sodium, Chloride and Sulfate. Institute of Medicine of the National Academies, The National Academies Press, Washington DC 2005. Available at www.nap.edu. Accessed July 2013.

20. Sriram K, Lonchyna VA. Micronutrient Supplementation in Adult Nutrition Therapy Practical Considerations. *J Parenter Enteral Nutr*. 2009; 33(5):548-562.

21. United States Department of Agriculture. National Agricultural Library. DRI Tables. http://fnic.nal.usda.gov/dietary-guidance/dietary-reference-intakes/dri-tables Last modified Sept 17, 2013. Accessed 9/17/2013.

22. Haugen HA, Chan LN, Li F. Indirect Calorimetry: a Practical Guide for Clinicians. *Nutrition in Clinical Practice*. 2007;22(4):377-388.

23. Ireton-Jones CS Intake: Energy in Mahan K, Escott-Stump S, and Raymond JL (ed) *Krause's Food and the Nutrition Care Process, 13th edition*. United Stated: Elsevier Publishing; 2012: 19-31.

24. Elbelt U, Schuetz T, Lochs H. Estimating Resting Energy Expenditure With a Portable Armband Devise in an Ambulatory Setting. *Nutr Clin Pract*. 2012; 27(6):825-831.

25. Mifflin MD, St Jeor ST, Hill LA, Scott BJ, Daugherty SA, Koh YO. A new predictive equation for resting energy expenditure in healthy individuals. *Am J Clin Nutr*. 1990;51(2):241-247.

26. Harris JA, Benedict FG. Monograph: A Biometric Study of Human Basal Metabolism in Man. Carnegie Institute of Washington. Publication No 279. Philadelphia, PA: Lippincott Publishing; 1919:

27. Russell M, Malone AM. Nutrient Requirements. In Charney P, Malone A. *ADA Pocket Guide to Nutrition Assessment, second edition*. Chicago, Ill. American Dietetic Association; 2009:167-191.

28. Ireton-Jones C, Jones JD. Improved equations for predicting energy expenditure in patients: the Ireton-Jones Equations. *Nutr Clin Pract*. 2002;17(1):29-31.

29. Frankenfield D. Validation of an equation for resting metabolic rate in older obese critically ill patients. *J Parenter Enteral Nutr*. 2011;35(2): 264-269.

30. Swinamer DL, Grace MG, Hamilton SM, Jones RL, Roberts P, King EG. Predictive equation for assessing energy expenditure in mechanically ventilated critically ill patients. *Crit Care Med*. 1990;18(6):657-661.

31. Choban PA, Dickerson RN. Morbid obesity and nutrition support: is bigger different? *Nutr Clin Pract* 2005;20(4):480-487.

32. Dickerson RN. Hypocaloric feeding of obese patients in the intensive care unit. *Curr Opin Clin Nutr Metabol Care*. 2005;8(2):189-196.

33. Magnuson B, Peppard A, Flomenhoft DA. Hypocaloric considerations in patients with potentially hypometabolic disease states. *Nutr Clin Pract*. 2011;26(3):253-260.

34. Walker RN, Heuberger RA. Predictive Equations for Energy Needs for the Critically Ill. *Respir Care*. 2009; 54(4): 509-521

35. Crook MA, Hally V, Panteli JV. The importance of the refeeding syndrome. *Nutrition*. 2001;17(7-8):632-637.

36. Kraft MD, Btaiche IF, Sacks GS. Review of the refeeding syndrome. *Nutr Clin Pract*. 2005;20(6):625-633.

Energetics, Exercise and Cancer

Mary Marian, MS, RD, CSO

Introduction

Energy balance is important for health and quality of life, and integral to avoiding the many chronic diseases associated with excess body weight. Energy intake is a primary factor, in addition to physical activity, in the regulation of body weight. While there may be some limitations to using BMI as an indicator of "healthy" body weight for all adults, the healthcare community has accepted the BMI range of 18.5 kg/m^2 – 24.9 kg/m^2 as a healthy body weight range.

Prior to the advent of early cancer screening and detection, cancer patients were usually diagnosed at advanced stages, a time when malnutrition, cachexia and inadequate intake from nutrition-impact symptoms such as anorexia, nausea and early satiety were common (1). Exacerbation of pre-existing nutrition-related impact symptoms as well as new challenges associated with treatment (e.g., xerostomia, mucositis, diarrhea, etc.) further contributed to inadequate oral intake and the risk of malnutrition (1). Today, cancer is more often diagnosed at early stages when cancer is most treatable and curable. Moreover, cancer survivors today, and in particular those who are diagnosed by screening tests, are more likely to be overweight or obese at the time of diagnosis (2). Additionally, weight gain during treatment of these cancers is becoming more common (2).

Evidence is growing that being overweight or obese at the time of diagnosis of some cancers is associated with adverse outcomes including increased risk of disease recurrence and reduced survival (3). It is therefore recommended that cancer survivors be encouraged to prevent involuntary weight loss and also to avoid weight gain during cancer treatment (2). Conversely, intentional weight loss post-treatment for overweight or obese survivors may reduce cancer recurrence and also risk of other health-related conditions such as cardiovascular disease, diabetes and hypertension (2,4).

Obesity and Cancer Risk

A growing body of evidence shows that obesity, sedentary lifestyle, energy imbalance and diet are modifiable risk factors associated with the development of many different types of cancer as well as risk of recurrence and survival from some cancers (5). Convincing evidence reveals that obesity, particularly abdominal obesity, increases the risk for breast (postmenopausal), cervical, colon and rectal, endometrial, esophageal, pancreatic, and renal cancers (6). Evidence also suggests that obesity increases risk for aggressive forms of prostate cancer and non-Hodgkins lymphoma and cancers of the gallbladder, liver, ovary and thyroid (7). Obesity is associated with an increased risk for recurrence of colorectal and breast cancers (in postmenopausal women); it also promotes the development of chronic diseases and reduces survival and quality of life.

If current trends in obesity continue, approximately 500,000 new cancer cases due to obesity may be diagnosed by 2030 (8). The American Cancer Society (ACS) estimates that one third of cancer-related deaths annually are associated with body weight, diet and physical activity habits (see Table 1) (2).

Table 1: Cancers Associated with Lifestyle Habits (2)

Lifestyle Habit	Increased Cancer Risk Associated with Lifestyle Habit
Excess Body Weight	Breast Cervical Colon & Rectal Endometrial Esophageal (Adenocarcinoma) Gallbladder Pancreatic Renal Thyroid
Physical Inactivity	Breast Colon Endometrial
Lifestyle Habit	**Decreased Cancer Risk Associated with Lifestyle Habit**
Less Weight Gain, Energy Balance, and Physical Activity	Breast Prostate (advanced disease)

Physiological Impact of Body Weight

Excess body weight generally reflects an imbalance between energy intake and calories expended, and calorie consumption in excess of energy expenditure is usually the underlying culprit. The precise mechanisms related to how adiposity increases the risk for cancer or its recurrence are unknown and experts in the field acknowledge that the interactions are complex and involve a number of factors. Moreover, different cancers are likely to develop from different underlying pathways. Estrogens promote breast and endometrial cancers whereas alterations in insulin pathways have been implicated in colon and prostate cancer development; inflammation may be the underlying culprit for other malignancies (9). Numerous interactions involving the role of insulin, insulin-like growth factor-1, vascular endothelial growth factor (VEGF) (in addition to other growth factors), mammalian target of rapamycin (mTOR), phosphatidylinositol 3-kinase and AMP-activated kinase are driven by energy intake and physical activity (10).

Adipokines are cytokines, growth factors, proteins and other bioactive substances secreted by adipocytes. Two adipokines, leptin and adiponectin, are hormones influenced by adiposity that may modulate carcinogenesis. Adiponectin promotes an anti-inflammatory environment; levels are inversely associated with insulin and inflammation (9). However, an inverse relationship also is seen between increasing body weight and adiponectin levels. Leptin is a key regulator of energy balance and appetite control. In obese individuals, leptin levels increase, potentially resulting in "leptin resistance" (10). Leptin has been implicated in tumorgenesis through its promotion of angiogenesis via increased VEGF synthesis and expression of other growth factors. It may alter insulin signaling that interferes with insulin pathways thereby leading to cell proliferation and migration. Additionally, leptin has been found to influence the production of inflammatory mediators including cytokines (e.g., interleukins 6 and 1, and tumor necrosis factor-α), which in turn activate the transcription factor nuclear factor-kappa beta (NFκB) (11). Downstream cell signaling is then modulated through NFκB activation via the mammalian target of rapamycin (mTOR) (11). The sex hormones testosterone and estradiol modulate this cascade through alterations in steroid hormone balance. Adiposity enhances aromatase enzymatic activity, leading to higher estrogen levels (11). Alterations in the insulin and IGF-1 balance associated with obesity also reduce sex protein-binding globulin levels, resulting in greater bioavailability of free estrogen. This has been linked with an increased risk for breast, ovarian, and endometrial cancers (12). In addition to excess body weight, a sedentary lifestyle also leads to elevated circulating levels of insulin, thereby increasing the risk for breast cancers and also colorectal, pancreatic, and endometrial cancers (13).

Guidelines for cancer prevention published by a variety of organizations typically emphasize the importance of consuming a healthy diet, maintaining a healthy weight and engaging in regular physical activity as these lifestyle habits are associated with risk reduction for not only cancer but also other chronic diseases such as heart disease, hypertension, metabolic syndrome and diabetes. In fact, McCullough et al. reported that following the 2006 American Cancer Society recommendations for weight control, physical activity and alcohol intake reduced the risk of dying from cancer or heart disease (14). Despite the plethora of nutrition guidelines that reinforce these guidelines, obesity continues to be a significant problem worldwide.

Weight and Cancer Outcomes

The impact of obesity (and overweight) on disease-related survival has been investigated in only a few trials; data are primarily from studies investigating breast or colorectal cancer survivors, some of which suggest a poorer quality of life for obese cancer survivors in general (15-17). Rock et al. report that being overweight or obese at the time of diagnosis adversely affects prognosis (2). A meta-analysis found a statistically significant and clinically relevant increase in breast cancer-specific as well as all cause mortality for obese women compared with non-obese women, not altered by menopausal status (15). For breast cancer survivors, maintaining a healthy body weight profoundly improves clinical outcomes and survival. Additionally, intentional weight loss has been linked with a reduced risk for postmenopausal breast cancer (18) and may also reduce the risk for other types of cancers (19).

Evidence in the colorectal population is mixed and the strongest data reflects that excess body weight may increase the risk of recurrence in survivors with class II or III obesity (BMI > 35 kg) (2,20). Overall, studies reflect that obesity pre-cancer diagnosis is more likely to influence recurrence and survival compared with a post-cancer diagnosis (4).

The relationship between body weight and prostate cancer is less clear. Many prospective studies have demonstrated an increased mortality rate from prostate cancer in men with higher BMIs (21-22). Obesity also appears to be associated with more biologically aggressive forms of prostate cancer. Gong et al. noted that men with a BMI over 30 kg/m^2 had a 2.6 increased risk for dying from prostate cancer after controlling for confounding factors including age, race, Gleason grade, stage, primary treatment and smoking status (23). Additionally, Ma and colleagues found a 1.4 and 2.6 fold (respective) increased risk for prostate cancer mortality among men with a prediagnostic BMI >25-29 kg/m^2 and >30 kg/m^2 (24). Conversely, three large prospective cohort studies did not report associations between BMI and prostate cancer outcomes (25-27).

Prostate cancer treatment may profoundly impact body composition. Men undergoing androgen deprivation therapy (ADT) commonly experience an increase in fat mass and reduced lean body mass (28). These body composition changes, when combined with ADT-related weight gain and subsequent hyperinsulinemia, potentially may enhance aggressive androgen-independent disease progression. Because a number of factors can influence cancer progression, well-designed prospective trials are needed to assess the impact of body weight in prostate cancer.

Studies suggest that obesity pre-cancer diagnosis may have an unfavorable impact on surgical and cytotoxic outcomes (29) and may increase ovarian cancer-related mortality (30-31). Obesity also has been associated with a poorer prognosis of survivors undergoing hematopoietic stem cell transplantation for hematological malignancies (32).

The issue of whether it is safe for overweight and obese cancer survivors to lose weight during treatment is controversial. Several studies reflect poor outcomes related to treatment-related weight loss for individuals with ovarian, head-and-neck cancers (HNC), and gastrointestinal cancers (33-35). Most studies failed to distinguish between the impact of intentional versus involuntary weight loss, however weight loss that occurs during chemotherapy treatment is rarely intentional.

Weight During Treatment and Post-Treatment

Many cancer patients are overweight or obese at the time of diagnosis. In a representative sample of cancer survivors in the Behavior Risk Factor Surveillance System, 27.5% of respondents were obese and 31.5% reported no physical activity in the last 30 days (36). The issue and management of weight loss in overweight and obese patients during treatment is changing. Historically, weight loss was not recommended during treatment primarily because weight loss was associated with cachexia and poor survival. However, guidelines from the ACS state that for individuals who wish to pursue intentional weight loss during treatment, there may be no contraindication in doing so (2). The ACS guidelines state that up to 2 lbs/week may be safely lost through close monitoring via consumption of a healthy diet together with regular physical activity, as long as the oncologist concurs and weight loss does not interfere with treatment (2).

While being overweight or obese has been associated with adverse outcomes (2-3,6), data also indicate that weight loss during cancer treatment is associated with increased toxicity from chemotherapy, incomplete cancer treatment, and decreased survival rates (37). A weight loss of as little as six percent predicts a reduced response to oncology treatment and reduced survival and quality of life (1,38). It is important to evaluate the etiology of weight loss that occurs during treatment. When weight loss is the result of nutrition impact symptoms associated with treatment toxicity, appropriate nutrition intervention to control or limit symptoms is essential. Clearly, whether weight loss during treatment is advisable needs to be individualized based on the patient's health status, patient goals, and agreed upon between the treating physician(s), the RD, and the patient.

Given that a weight loss of 5% to 10% is associated with a number of health benefits, some degree of weight loss may be appropriate in overweight and obese survivors who have recovered from treatment (39-40). Certainly energy restricted diets can be effective in promoting weight loss, and a plethora of diets are available to choose from. However, the success rate with long-term adherence to a calorie-controlled diet is poor in general and the critical challenge is how to maintain weight loss without weight "cycling".

Calorie Restriction and Cancer Prevention

Energy modulation through calorie restriction (CR), a 20-40% reduction in calorie intake and also known as deprivation (41), has been explored as a mechanism to prevent carcinogenesis. CR may be effective through the modulation of a host of hormones such as insulin, insulin-like growth factor 1, proinflammatory cytokines,

adiponectin and leptin while also increasing antioxidant defenses and DNA-repairing mechanisms (42). In addition, preclinical studies suggest that fasting for 2-3 days protected healthy cells and mice from cytotoxic drugs while the cancer cells were left unprotected – referred to as differential stress resistance (41). In a very small study including older cancer patients, voluntarily fasting before and during chemotherapy resulted in less reports of fatigue, weakness, and gastrointestinal issues (43). It is difficult to ferret out the true impact of CR as an anti-cancer intervention given that avoidance of excess body weight and regular physical activity also have anti-carcinogenic benefits by favorably impacting inflammatory pathways through the reduction of proinflammatory cytokine, fasting insulin, and leptin levels (42).

Because of the challenge of restricting calories, attention has turned to using pharmacological agents such as mTOR inhibitors, including rapamycin and metformin, as adjunct therapies to diet in order to obtain similar advantages seen in CR alone (4).

Exercise and Cancer Survivors

The numerous benefits of regular physical activity have been widely reported by health organizations throughout the world. Physical activity reduces the risk for cardiovascular disease, type 2 diabetes, and hypertension, and evidence is accruing regarding benefits related to cancer. Data from prospective observational studies suggests that exercise helps reduce the risk of breast, colon, prostate and ovarian cancers (12,18,44). Although the precise mechanisms involved have not been clearly elucidated, the benefits are thought to be associated with reduced levels of circulating insulin and proinflammatory mediators as well as alterations in inflammatory pathways (15,21,42).

Guidelines for cancer survivors published by the American College of Sports Medicine provide recommendations for safe and effective physical activity modalities (see Table 2) (45). Additionally, data suggest that clinically relevant outcomes such as improved quality of life are associated with regular physical activity (46-47). While considered safe for most survivors, a preclinical assessment is recommended prior to beginning any exercise program (45).

Table 2: Summary of the American College of Sports Medicine Recommendations for Physical Activity for Cancer Survivors (45)

Type of Activity*	Goals

Aerobic Physical Activity
  Moderate intensity
  Vigorous intensity
  Or Combination of above
	
	150 minutes/week
	75 minutes/week

Weight resistance training utilizing all muscle groups	Twice weekly

* Guidelines are for adults aged 18 to 64 years and recommend patients be evaluated for presence of peripheral neuropathies, musculoskeletal and/or fracture risk based on disease and treatment history. Morbidly obese individuals could require an additional medical assessment.

Exercise During Cancer Treatment

Evidence reflects that exercising during and post treatment is safe and may be associated with improvements in physical functioning, fatigue, exercise tolerance, body composition, cardiopulmonary fitness, muscular strength, depression, anxiety, and quality of life (2,22,44-46,48). Despite these benefits, many cancer survivors are sedentary. Cancer survivors with established physical activity patterns prior to diagnosis are more likely to continue exercising through treatment (2). While beginning an exercise program during treatment may be difficult for some, any exercise should be encouraged to obtain the reported benefits.

The type of treatment, stage of disease, and current health status are possible factors that impact whether an exercise program will be followed although studies reflect that patients can safely exercise through treatment (2,46-48). Recommendations should be individualized based on the patient's current clinical and functional status.

The strongest evidence that regular physical activity may play a positive role in oncological care comes from studies enrolling cancer survivors with breast and colorectal cancers. In the breast cancer population, physical activity during treatment, particularly weight resistance training, has been shown to help preserve lean body mass while decreasing the risk for gaining adipose tissue (47,49). Data from cohort studies enrolling colon cancer survivors noted that physical activity after diagnosis may reduce the risk of recurrence, colon cancer-related mortality as well as overall mortality up to 50% (2). Studies show that cancer patients are willing to exercise through treatment, including those who are very old. In a study by Sprod et al., older patients (mean = age 73; range 65-92) who exercised during treatment (46% of 408 study participants) reported less shortness of breath and fatigue and improved self-related health (50).

Effects of Post-Treatment Exercise on Cancer Outcomes

Current available data regarding exercise and post-treatment outcomes is derived from studies of breast cancer survivors. Much of the evidence reflects an inverse association between self-reported regular physical activity and cancer-specific mortality as well as all-cause mortality. Risk reduction ranged from 15% to 67% and 18% to 67% for cancer-specific and all-cause mortality, respectively. About 180 minutes per week of exercise of moderate intensity to ≥500 minutes/week of moderate intensity activity may be required to obtain those benefits (51). The type of activity should be individualized based on treatment history, current disease status, and ability to exercise. For example, aerobic activity in addition to weight resistance activity is recommended as an effective strategy to combat and reduce lymphedema in breast cancer survivors (52-53).

Evidence reflects a positive association between improvements in muscular strength and lean body mass, functional status and quality of life in prostate cancer survivors (21. Resistance training may be

beneficial; 24 weeks of aerobic or resistance training resulted in long-term improvements in fatigue in one study (54). Prostate cancer survivors who participated in vigorous physical activity ≥ 3 hours/week experienced reductions of 61% for prostate specific mortality and 49% for all-cause mortality (55).

ACS guidelines on nutrition and physical activity recommend that cancer survivors in all phases of the cancer-care spectrum (e.g., treatment, recovery and life after recovery) be as physically active as possible (2). The ACS expert panel reiterated the recommendations provided previously by the American College of Sports Medicine (see Table 2). (2,45). The ACS review also noted that observational studies reflect a favorable association between post-diagnosis physical activity level and the risk for recurrence, cancer-related deaths and overall mortality for individuals diagnosed with breast, colorectal, ovarian and prostate cancers, with higher activity levels being associated with lower risk for recurrence and mortality (2). Additional benefits that may be derived from regular physical activity include lower risk for chronic diseases including heart disease, diabetes, and hypertension, which also affect cancer survivors.

In summary, data regarding physical activity for improved survival is promising however these observations should be confirmed with randomized trials. Indeed, a number of clinical trials are now underway to further investigate these findings and address our current gaps in knowledge.

Promoting Physical Activity

While a number of barriers may preclude regular activity (see Table 3), a variety of methods can be used to encourage cancer survivors to become more physically active. Cancer survivors have found written materials on using exercise to manage treatment-related fatigue to be helpful (56). In the RENEW (Reach Out to Enhance Wellness) trial, Demark-Wahnefried et al. found that a home-based diet-exercise intervention delivered by tailored mailed-print materials, quarterly newsletters and telephone counseling sessions resulted in significant weight loss, improvements in quality of life and physical functioning for long-term cancer survivors (>5 years after cancer diagnosis) (57). Other studies have found both individual as well as group counseling to be effective approaches to promoting weight loss (58-59). Nevertheless, studies suggest that adherence to dietary and physical activity recommendations decreased as the time from study completion increased. Because

Table 3: Benefits and Barriers to Exercise (2,17,56)

Benefits	Barriers
Reduced fatigue	Chemotherapy
Improved physical functioning	Fatigue
Improved mood and less depression	Tender wounds
Increased coping skills	Age
Improved quality of life	Economic status
Lean body mass	
Long-term health benefits	

sustaining weight loss is challenging, successful programs must include elements that not only address energy intake and physical activity but also behavioral strategies, cognitive restructuring and social support to promote long-term adherence to changes.

Further research is clearly needed to elucidate how physical activity impacts tumor growth and progression. Moreover, much of the evidence to date comes from epidemiological studies where exercise behaviors are self-reported. Self-reported data is subject to several limitations including subjectivity, poor reliability and validity and lack of sensitivity. Prospective randomized controlled trials with diverse populations are needed to explore the benefits of physical activity as it relates to prevention and to recurrence and survival for all cancers.

Conclusion

The majority of Americans are either overweight or obese with a low activity level, including cancer survivors. Excess energy intake and sedentary lifestyle lead to excess body weight, which are important modifiable risk factors for cancer prevention and risk reduction for recurrence. The consensus report, "From Cancer Patient to Cancer Survivor: Lost in Translation", published by The Institute of Medicine recommends that all cancer survivors have an individualized cancer survivorship plan developed including a detailed history of their oncology history and also recommendations for having a healthy lifestyle and how to prevent a recurrence (60). Given the data available supporting the positive impact of weight loss and physical activity for risk reduction, energy balance is a critical area in clinical practice.

References

1. DeWys WD, Begg C, Lavin PT, et al. Prognostic effect of weight loss prior to chemotherapy in cancer patients: Eastern Cooperative Oncology Group. *Am J Med.* 1980;69(4):491-497.
2. Rock CL, Boule C, Demark-Wahnerfried W, et al. Nutrition and physical activity guidelines for cancer survivors. *CA Cancer J Clin.* 2012;62(4): 243-274.
3. Institute of Medicine. The Role of Obesity in Cancer Survival and Recurrence: Workshop Summary. Washington, DC: The National Academies Press; 2012.
4. Demark-Wahnefried W, Platz EA, Ligibel JA, et al. The role of obesity in cancer survival and recurrence. *Cancer Epidemiol Biomarkers Prev.* 2012; Aug;21(8):1244-1259.
5. Haslam D. Obesity a medical history. *Obes Rev.* 2008;8(Suppl1):31-36.
6. World Cancer Research Fund/American Institute for Cancer Research. Food, Nutrition, Physical Activity, and the Prevention of Cancer: A Global Perspective. Washington, DC: World Cancer Research Fund/American Institute for Cancer Research; 2007.
7. Kushi LH, Coyle C, McCullough M, et al. American Cancer Society Guidelines on Nutrition and physical Activity for cancer prevention: reducing the risk of cancer with healthy food choices and physical activity. *CA Cancer J Clin.* 2012;62(1):30-67.
8. Obesity and Cancer Risk. National Cancer Institute. Available at: http://www.cancer.gov/cancertopics/factsheet/Risk/obesity. Reviewed 1/03/12. Accessed June 28, 2012.
9. Wolin KY, Caron K, Colditz GA. Obesity and cancer. *The Oncologist.* 2010;15(6):556-565.
10. Pittas AG, Joseph NA, Greenberg AS. Adipocytokines and insulin resistance. *J Clin Endocrinol Metab.* 2004;89(2):447-452.
11. Parekh N, Chandran U, Bandera EV. Obesity in cancer survival. *Ann Rev Nutr.* 2012;32:311-342.
12. Beral V, Banks E, Reeves G, Appleby P. Use of HRT and the subsequent risk of cancer. *J Epidemiol Biostat.* 1999;4(3):191-210.
13. Eheman C, Henley SJ, Ballard-Barbash R, et al. Annual report to the nation on the status of cancer, 1975-2008, featuring cancers associated with excess weight and lack of sufficient physical activity. *Cancer.* 2012; 118(9):2338-2366.
14. McCullough ML, Patel AV, Kushi LH, *et al.* Following cancer prevention guidelines reduces risk of cancer, cardiovascular disease, and all-cause mortality. *Cancer Epidemiol Biomarkers Prev.* 2011;20(6):1089-1097.
15. Ibrahim EM, Al-Homaidh A. Physical activity and survival after breast cancer diagnosis: meta-analysis of published studies. *Med Oncol.* 2011: 28(3):753-765.
16. Meyerhardt JA, Giovannucci EL, Ogino S, et al. Physical activity and male colorectal cancer survival. *Arch Intern Med.* 2009;169(22):2102-2108.
17. Protani M, Coory M, Martin JH. Effect of obesity on survival or women with breast cancer: systematic review and meta-analysis. *Breast Cancer Res Treat.* 2010;123(3):627-635.
18. Harvie M, Howell A, Vierkant RA, et al. Association of gain and loss of weight before and after menopause with risk of postmenopausal breast cancer in the Iowa women's health study. *Cancer Epidemiol Biomarkers Prev.* 2005;14(3):656-661.
19. Parker ED, Folsom AR. Intentional weight loss and incidence of obesity-related cancers: the Iowa Women's Health Study. *Int J Obes Relat Metab Disord.* 2003;27(12):1447-1452.
20. Campbell PT, Newton CC, Dehal AN, Jacobs EJ, Patel AV, Gapstur SM. Impact of body mass index on survival after colorectal cancer diagnosis: the Cancer Prevention Study-II Nutrition Cohort. *J Clin Oncol.* 2012; 30(1):42-52.
21. Meyerhardt JA, Ma J, Courneya. Energetics in colorectal and prostate cancer. *J Clin Oncol.* 2010;28(26):4066-4073.
22. Fowke JH, Motley SS, Concepcion RS, Penson DF, Barocas DA. Obesity, body composition, and prostate cancer. *BMC Cancer.* 2012 Jan 18;12:23. doi: 10.1186/1471-2407-12-23.
23. Gong Z, Agalliu I, Lin DW, et al. Obesity is associated with increased risks of prostate cancer metastasis and death after initial cancer diagnosis in middle-aged men. *Cancer.* 2007;109(6):1192-1202.
24. Ma J, Li H, Giovannucci E, et al. Prediagnostic body-mass index, plasma C-peptide concentration, and prostate cancer-specific mortality in men with prostate cancer: A long-term survival analysis. *Lancet Oncol.* 2008; 9(11):1039-1047.
25. Siddiqui SA, Inman BA, Sengupta S, et al. Obesity and survival after radical prostatectomy: A 10-year prospective cohort study. *Cancer.* 2006;107(3):521-529.
26. Davies BJ, Smaldone MC, Sadetsky N, et al. The impact of obesity on overall and cancer specific survival in men with prostate cancer. *J Urol.* 2009;182(1):111-117.
27. Giovannucci E, Liu Y, Platz EA, et al. Risk factors for prostate cancer incidence and progression in the health professionals follow-up study. *Int J Cancer.* 2007;121(7):1571-1578.
28. Van Londen GJ, Levy ME, Perera S, Nelson JB, Greenspan SL. Body composition changes during androgen deprivation therapy for prostate cancer;a 2-year prospective study. *Crit Rev Oncol Hematol.* 2008;68(2): 172-177.
29. Modesitt SC, van Nagell JR Jr. The impact of obesity on the incidence and treatment of gynecologic cancers: A review. *Obstet Gynecol Surv.* 2005;60(10):683-692.
30. Calle EE, Rodriguez C, Walker-Thurmond KW, Thun MJ. Overweight, obesity and mortality from cancer in a prospectively studied cohort of U.S. adults. *N Engl J Med.* 2003;348(17):1625-1638.
31. Reeves GK, Pirie K, Beral V, et al. Million women study collaboration. Cancer incidence and mortality in relation to body mass index in the Million Women Study: cohort study. *BMJ.* 2007;Dec 1;335(7630):1134. Epub 2007 Nov 6.
32. Meloni G, Proia A, Capria S, et al. Obesity and autologous stem cell transplantation in acute myeloid leukemia. *Bone Marrow Transplant.* 2001;28(4):365-367.

33. Hess LM, Barakat R, Tian C, Ozols RF, Alberts DS. Weight change during chemotherapy as a potential prognostic factor for stage III epithelial ovarian carcinoma: a Gynecologic Oncology Group study. *Gynecol Oncol.* 2007;107(2):260-265.

34. Datema FR, Ferrier MB, Baatenburg de Jong RJ. Impact of severe malnutrition on short-term mortality and overall survival in head and neck cancer. *Oral Oncol.* 2011;47(9):910-914.

35. Hill A, Kiss N, Hodgson B, Crowe TC, Walsh AD. Associations between nutritional status, weight loss, radiotherapy treatment toxicity and treatment outcomes in gastrointestinal cancer patients. *Clin Nutr.* 2011; 30(1):92-98.

36. UnderwoodJM, Townsend JS, Stewart SL, et al. Division of Cancer Prevention and Control, National Center for Chronic Disease Prevention and Health Promotion, Centers for Disease Control and Prevention (CDC). Surveillance of demographic characteristics and health behaviors among adult cancer survivors – Behavioral Risk Factor Surveillance System. United States, 2009. MMWR Surveill Summ. 2012;20;61(1):1-23.

37. Suzuki H, Cancer cachexia-pathophysiology and management. *J Gastroenterol.* 2013;48(5):574-594.

38. Shike M. (1996). Nutrition therapy for the cancer patient. *Hematol Oncol Clin N Am.* 10:221-234

39. Look AHEAD Research Group, Wing RR. Long-term effects of a lifestyle intervention on weight and cardiovascular risk factors in individuals with type 2 diabetes mellitus: four-year results of the Look AHEAD trial. *Arch Intern Med.* 2010;170(17):1566-1575.

40. Centers for Disease Control and Prevention. Healthy Weight-it's not a diet, it's a lifestyle! Atlanta, GA: Centers for Disease Control and Prevention: 2011. http://www.cdc.gov/healthyweight/losing_weight/index.html. Access June 14,2012.

41. Lee C, Raffaghello L, Brandhorst S, et al. Fasting cycles retard growth of tumors and sensitize a range of cancer cell types to chemotherapy. *Sci Transl Med.* 2012;4(124):124ra27.

42. Harvey AE, Lashinger LM, Hursting SD. The growing challenge of obesity and cancer: an inflammatory issue. *Ann NY Acad Sci.* 2011:1229:45-52. doi: 10.1111/j.1749-6632.2011.06096.x.

43. Lee C, Lee C, Longo VD. Fasting vs. dietary restriction in cellular protection and cancer treatment: from model organisms to patients. *Oncogene.* 2011;30(30):3305-3316.

44. Moorman PG, Jones LW, Akushevich L, Schildkraut JM. Recreational physical activity and ovarian cancer risk and survival. *Ann Epidemiol.* 2011;21(3):178-187.

45. Schmitz KH, Courneya KS, Matthews C, et al. American College of Sports Medicine roundtable on exercise guidelines for cancer survivors. *Med Sci Sports Exerc.* 2010;42(7):1409-1426.

46. Granger CL, McDonald CF, Berney S, Chao C, Denehy L. Exercise intervention to improve exercise capacity and health related quality of life for patients with non-small cell lung cancer: a systematic review. *Lung Cancer.* 2011;72(2):139-153.

47. Herman DR, Ganz PA, Petersen L, Greendale GA. Obesity and cardiovascular risk factors in younger breast cancer survivors: The Cancer and Menopause Study (CAMS). *Breast Cancer Res Treat.* 2005;93:13-23.

48. Brown JC, Huedo-Medina TB, Pescatello LS, Pescatello SM, Ferrer RA, Johnson BT. Efficacy of exercise interventions in modulating cancer-related fatigue among adult cancer survivors: a meta-analysis. *Cancer Epidemiol Biomarkers Prev.* 2011;20(1):123-133.

49. Schmitz KH, Ahmed RL, Hannan PJ, Yee D. Safety and efficacy of weight training in recent breast cancer survivors to alter body composition, insulin, and insulin-like growth factor axis proteins. *Cancer Epidemiol Biomarkers Prev.* 2005;14(7):1672-1680.

50. Sprod LK, Mohile SG, Demark-Wahnefried W, et al. Exercise and cancer treatment symptoms in 408 newly diagnosed older cancer patients. *J Geriatr Oncol.* 2012;3(2):90-97.

51. Betof AS, Dewhirst MW, Jones LW. Effects and potential mechanisms of exercise training on cancer progression: A translational perspective. *Brain Behav Immun.* 2013 Mar;30 Suppl:S75-87. doi: 10.1016/j.bbi.2012.05.001.

52. Schmitz KH, Ahmed RL, Troxel AB, et al. Weight lifting for women at risk for breast cancer-related lymphedema: a randomized trial. *JAMA.* 2010;304(24):2699-2705.

53. Schmitz KH, Ahmed RL, Troxel A, et al. Weight lifting in women with breast-cancer-related lymphedema. *N Engl J Med.* 2009;361(7):664-673.

54. Wolin KY, Yan Y, Colditz GA, et al. Physical activity and colon cancer prevention: A meta-analysis. *Br J Cancer.* 2009;100(4):611-616.

55. Haydon AM, Macinnis RJ, English DR, et al: Effect of physical activity and body size on survival after diagnosis with colorectal cancer. *Gut.* 2006;55:689-694.

56. Haydon AM, Macinnis RJ, English DR, et al: Physical activity, insulin-like growth factor 1, insulin-like growth factor binding protein 3, and survival from colorectal cancer. *Gut.* 2006;55(5):689-694.

57. Segal RJ, Reid RD, Courneya KS, et al: Randomized controlled trial of resistance or aerobic exercise in men receiving radiation therapy for prostate cancer. *J Clin Oncol.* 2009;27(3):344-351.

58. Kenfield SA, Chang ST, Chan JM: Diet and lifestyle interventions in active surveillance patients with favorable-risk prostate cancer. *Curr Treat Options Oncol.* 2007;8(3):173-196.

59. Windsor PM, Potter J, McAdam K, McCowan C. Evaluation of a fatigue initiative: information on exercise for patients receiving cancer treatment. *Clin Oncol* (R Coll Radiol). 2009;21(6):473-482.

60. Demark-Wahnefried, Morey MC, Sloane R, et al. Reach out to enhance wellness home-based diet-exercise intervention promotes reproducible and sustainable long-term improvements in health behaviors, body weight, and physical functioning in older, overweight/obese cancer survivors. *J Clin Oncol.* 2012;30(19);2354-2361.

61. Djuric Z, Ellsworth JS, Weldon AL, et al. A diet and exercise intervention during chemotherapy for breast cancer. *Open Obes J.* 2011;3:87-97.

62. Greenlee HA, Crew KD, Mata JM, et al. A pilot randomized controlled trial of a commercial diet and exercise weight loss program in minority breast cancer survivors. *Obesity.* 2013 Jan;21(1):65-76. doi: 10.1002/oby.20245.

63. Institute of Medicine. From cancer patient to cancer survivor: lost in translation. http://iom.edu/Reports/2005/From-Cancer-Patient-to-Cancer-Survivor-Lost-in-Transition.aspx Accessed July 7, 2012.

Defining and Developing an Oncology Nutrition Program in a Cancer Center

Shari Oakland Schulze, RD, CSO

Introduction

Cancer care has moved from the inpatient setting to the outpatient setting, with an estimated 90% of patients receiving treatment in outpatient cancer centers and clinics. In 2012, the American College of Surgeons Commission on Cancer (ACOS CoC) added a standard to address nutrition as a component of cancer care. The standard, which states, "A policy or procedure is in place to access nutrition services either on-site or by referral", recognizes that *"nutrition services are essential components of comprehensive cancer care and patient rehabilitation. These services provide safe and effective nutrition care across the cancer continuum (prevention, treatment, and survivorship) and are essential to promoting quality of life"* (1). The Joint Commission (TJC) ambulatory standards for nutrition and functional screening state that nutrition screening needs to be performed when warranted by a patient's needs or condition while inpatient screenings must be completed within 24 hours after inpatient admission (2). And the Center for Medicare and Medicaid Services (CMS) include nutrition care in their patient care standards, recognizing the importance of nutrition and the role of the registered dietitian (RD) in addressing the nutritional needs of cancer patients. In addition, the National Cancer Institute (NCI) and the Association of Community Cancer Centers (ACCC) report nutrition to be a highly desired service as part of a cancer center program (3).

Malnutrition is reported in approximately 15-20% of cancer patients at the time of diagnosis, and up to 80% over the course of care (4). It impairs the ability to complete treatment, reduces cancer survival and quality of life, and increases the risk of cancer recurrence (5-8). Patients receiving multi-modality treatments experience multiple side effects, from both the cancer and its treatment, which may result in inadequate intake and weight loss. In contrast, undesirable weight gain is increasingly seen after some cancer treatments, specifically in breast cancer.

Medical nutrition therapy is aimed at managing symptoms, preventing weight loss, and maintaining optimal nutrition status during cancer treatment. Studies demonstrate the value of nutrition interventions on functional outcomes including improved tolerance to treatment, reduced treatment breaks, decreased weight loss, decreased muscle loss, and increased quality of life (5-8). RDs are uniquely qualified to screen for nutritional risk; assess nutritional needs; implement appropriate and effective nutrition care plans; and educate patients about using nutrition as a treatment ally and how nutrition can impact the outcome of cancer care (9).

Defining an Oncology Nutrition Program

A comprehensive cancer center is defined by the NCI as an institution that provides state-of-the-art cancer care and service that includes a strong research base along with a variety of prevention, care, and educational activities that serve the community (10). Services include medical oncology, surgical oncology and radiation oncology, along with support services such as psychology, social work, and nutrition. Likewise, comprehensive oncology nutrition programs are those that include multiple intervention strategies targeting nutrition and nutrition related outcomes. This comprehensive view addresses all of the needs of the patients and their families throughout the cancer continuum.

In the past, oncology patients treated in cancer centers or clinics were referred to RDs for nutrition care only after experiencing malnutrition and/or cancer cachexia. When nutrition problems are addressed reactively, a patient's nutrition status may already be severely compromised. The optimal nutrition program is proactive. Early nutrition intervention and aggressive management of symptoms provides the best opportunity to interrupt the deterioration in nutrition status, resulting in positive outcomes and increased quality of life. Proactive nutrition care is only achieved by having a dedicated oncology RD available who can provide these essential services.

Essential Components of a Nutrition Program

A comprehensive oncology nutrition program should be modeled after the Nutrition Care Process and include nutrition screening, nutrition assessment, intervention, education, and nutrition monitoring. All components of nutrition care should be provided throughout the cancer continuum: prevention, treatment, survivorship, palliative care, and hospice.

Nutrition programs need to establish a routine method of screening for nutrition risk during an initial patient visit and at subsequent defined intervals. Nutrition screening tools traditionally are either completed by a nurse or are patient self-generated, and identify parameters indicative of nutrition risk. Unintentional weight changes, anorexia or difficulty eating, and nausea or vomiting are common parameters used. The Patient Generated Subjective Global Assessment (PG-SGA) is a validated nutrition screening tool for use in the oncology setting (11), but diagnoses associated with a high risk of nutrition problems; co-morbidities with known clinical nutrition needs; and treatments that may result in eating difficulties also can serve as indicators for nutrition risk. For more information on nutrition screening see chapter 3 of this book.

Once patients at nutrition risk have been identified, a standardized process should trigger a referral to the RD. Referrals can easily be generated via an electronic medical record (EMR), resulting in timely nutrition assessment and implementation of a nutrition plan. When an EMR is not in place there must be a defined referral process to ensure the RD is promptly notified of patients at nutrition risk. By repeating the screening process during subsequent treatment visits, changes in the patient's nutrition status can be identified and addressed before a nutrition crisis occurs.

Nutrition assessment and subsequent interventions should be appropriate, individualized, and specific to best meet the patient's needs. The Academy of Nutrition and Dietetics (The Academy) Evidence Based Analysis Library and the Oncology Nutrition-Dietetic Practice Group (ON-DPG) Oncology Tool Kit are two resources that can be utilized to guide interventions appropriate to the nutrition care plan and desired outcomes (12).

Education is an essential component of nutrition intervention. Education can occur at chair-side during a clinic visit, in the nutrition counseling office, over the phone, or in a classroom. Because multiple support services vie to deliver care during the patient's treatment, the RD must consider multiple options to quickly identify and address nutrition issues.

The Association of Community Cancer Centers (ACCC), in collaboration with oncology dietitians and practitioners, developed guidelines for nutrition care in a cancer center. These guidelines offer a general framework for what an oncology program should entail and can be used when developing a proposal for a comprehensive nutrition program (13).

Guideline I A nutrition professional is available to work with patients and their families, especially patients identified at nutrition risk for having nutritional problems or special needs.

Guideline II The nutrition professional with the patient, family, and the oncology team manages issues involving the patient's nutrition and hydration status through appropriate nutrition screening, assessment, and intervention across the care continuum.

Guideline III The nutrition professional serves as a resource and provides nutrition and diet information about reducing cancer risk and cancer recurrence risk through educational program materials and services to the community.

Guideline IV The nutrition professional manages nutrition and diet-related needs specific to each patient's individualized survivorship plan.

Process for Developing a Nutrition Program

To successfully implement a nutrition program within a cancer center, it is essential to obtain support from key decision-makers within the organization. RDs need to identify administrators and clinicians who recognize the medical benefits and financial impact of evidence-based nutrition interventions provided by a qualified (i.e., RD) professional. Identifying and including impacted departments from budgeting to process flow is essential. It is also important to ensure Nutrition is represented on institutional committees and in planning institution-related events.

To obtain support for an oncology nutrition program, it is important to increase institutional awareness of the value of nutrition in a cancer center and to inform administrators and key decision-makers of accreditation agency nutrition standards. All members of the care team, from registration clerks to treatment providers, should be encouraged to identify nutrition issues and to refer at-risk patients to the RD. Nutrition services can be marketed to patients and providers with brochures and flyers. Care providers can be educated about the importance of informing the RD of nutrition problems. And nutrition programs can be included in grand rounds, practice group meetings, and other organizational events. As part of an organization's quality control program, the RD should present outcome data on compliance with the nutrition screening process, effectiveness of nutrition care, and overall impact of the nutrition program.

Staffing

The type of cancer treatment center (e.g., teaching hospital, private practice, independent radiation facility) influences staffing structure and needs. There are currently no standards on RD staffing across the spectrum of care, however having a dedicated RD is optimal. The scope of practice, standards of care, and desired points of nutrition intervention can be used to develop staffing models. It is also important to consider baseline data regarding patient acuity and number of new analytical cases (i.e., patients who were diagnosed and/or received their first course of therapy at the facility) per year. The Clinical Nutrition Service should lobby the administration to meet standards developed by accreditation agencies (e.g., CoC and TJC), which are considered a measure of quality to which the department should aspire to meet. It may also be helpful to examine benchmarking of specialized (e.g., renal or diabetes) nutrition care.

Organizational Structure

When considering the organizational structure of the cancer center, the RD can fit into several different areas, as outlined in Table 1.

Regardless of where the RD/nutrition team is placed within the organizational structure, the RD needs to be recognized as the dedicated nutrition professional and representative for nutrition issues. Due to the specialization of the RD working in a cancer center as part of a multi-disciplinary team, the position needs to have a well-defined set of job skills.

Table 1: Potential Organizational Structures for Clinical Nutrition Services

Organization	Supervision	Competency Assessment	Benefits
Nutrition Service or Department	Director	Immediate Supervisor	Professional networking with hospital system
Pharmacy Department	Pharmacy Director	Clinical RD Manager if available	Strong clinical focus
Other: Department of Psychosocial Oncology, Patient Navigation, or Support Services	Department Director	Clinical RD Manager if available	Improved collaboration and research opportunities
Cancer Center	Cancer Center Administrator or Nursing Administrator	Clinical RD Manager if available	Direct relationship to cancer center leadership

Job Description

In 2010, the Academy and the ON-DPG revised the Standards of Practice (SOP) and Standards of Professional Performance (SOPP) for the Oncology RD (14). These standards provide RDs in oncology nutrition with a tool to evaluate their practice, identify areas for professional development, and demonstrate competency in their specialty. The SOP and SOPP standardize the quality of oncology nutrition services and can be used as a basis for job descriptions and professional competencies. They also establish an expectation of continual learning and specialization for providing high quality nutrition care to cancer patients.

Standards of Practice in Oncology Nutrition Care (14):

1. Nutrition Assessment: RDs use accurate and relevant data and information to identify nutrition-related problems.
2. Nutrition Diagnosis: RDs identify and label specific nutrition problem(s) that the RD is responsible for treating.
3. Nutrition Intervention: RDs identify and implement appropriate, purposefully planned actions designed with the intent of changing a nutrition-related behavior, risk factor, environmental condition, or aspect of health status for an individual, target group, or the community at large.
4. Nutrition Monitoring and Evaluation: RDs monitor and evaluate indicators and outcomes data directly related to the nutrition diagnosis, goals, and intervention strategies to determine the progress made in achieving desired outcomes of nutrition care and whether planned interventions should be continued or revised.

Standards of Professional Performance (14):

1. Provision of Services: RDs provide quality service based on customer expectations and needs.
2. Application of Research: RDs apply, participate in, or generate research to enhance practice.
3. Communication and Application of Knowledge: RDs effectively apply knowledge and communicate with others.

4. Utilization and Management of Resources: RDs use resources effectively and efficiently.
5. Quality in Practice: RDs systematically evaluate the quality of services and improve practice based on evaluation results.
6. Competence and Accountability: RDs engage in lifelong learning.

The job description should include essential functions of the position, standards of professional practice (above), and required knowledge, skills, abilities, and education and certification requirements (below).

- A minimum of a Bachelor's degree in Nutrition and Dietetics and is an RD with preference for an RD experience or familiar with oncology nutrition.
- Knowledge of clinical nutrition with emphasis on nutrition needs of the cancer patient. Can specify requirement for Certified Specialist in Oncology Nutrition (CSO) certification or CSO certification within 2 years (see box below).
- Excellent counseling skills, cultural competency, and ability to communicate within varied learning levels.
- Ability and interest in developing and implementing programs and educational tools.
- Strong interpersonal skills.
- Basic computer skills.
- Effective written and verbal communication skills.
- Knowledge of nutrition care process.
- Knowledge of charting formats.
- Organizational skills and ability to accomplish work without direct daily supervision.

The Certified Specialist in Oncology (CSO) certification from the Commission of Dietetic Registration (CDR) is a value-added credential for nutrition professionals working in oncology care. The credential identifies the RD as an expert in oncology with specialized knowledge and enhanced understanding of cancer care and nutrition. The CSO certification is recognized in the ACOS COC standards in 2012 and in the ACCC guidelines revised in 2012.

Cost of Services: Billing and Reimbursement

Before detailing the workflow of the clinical process, the program must decide whether to charge for nutrition services. Clinical nutrition services improve patient care, engagement, and satisfaction, which may, in turn, help improve medical treatment outcomes. Many cancer centers recognize this and consider nutrition intervention a value added service or benefit and an integral part of the patient's cancer treatment. Other cancer centers believe that charging a fee for nutrition services emphasizes the importance of nutrition intervention by the RD, therefore potentially improving compliance. Understandably, the question of who is going to pay for these services can influence RD staffing.

Systems can be put in place to bill for medical nutrition therapy. Historically, the reimbursement process of public and private payers has been tedious and requires planning to ensure compliance with federal standards. To answer the "who pays" question, it is critical to partner with reimbursement and compliance specialists in the institution to fully understand the billing and coding process and to assure adherence with standards and acceptable billing practices. Successful reimbursement comes from proving outcomes and demonstrating the cost-benefit of oncology nutrition services. Other options to financially support the role of an RD in a cancer center include grant and charity funding. Patient targeted programming has the potential to produce revenue through grant funding, foundation funding, and/or participant fees. While these resources may not always be reliable, they might help sustain a nutrition program when funding is limited.

Systems of Operation

Most organizations function within a framework of systems that standardize ways of completing tasks within set guidelines. Developing the nutrition program within this model can facilitate a well-functioning service. Systems may include standards and guidelines, policies and procedures, standards of care, nutrition protocols and nutrition algorithms. The Joint Commission and CMS have established standards that guide health care facilities and practitioners in providing safe care. The Academy's Quality Management department also provides resources that will help determine efficient, effective, and safe processes.

Once the workflow, program systems and best processes are determined, they must be translated into written policies and procedures that are approved by the institution. Cancer center specific nutrition policies and procedures would include nutrition screening and assessment, nutrition education, diet orders, and provision of supplements. Policies and procedures should be reasonable and realistic. Regulatory agencies do give some freedom to define parameters but policies must be achievable with current staffing and practice models.

A clinical protocol is a pre-determined course of action or treatment ordered by a physician for a particular patient. Protocols may only be implemented by an authorized licensed healthcare professional after receipt of a patient-specific order. The protocol must be consistent with hospital policy, medical staff rules and regulations, and scope of practice. Oncology nutrition protocols may address recommendations for individual nutrient supplements, provision of sample products, indications for diet supplements, and adjustment of feeding schedules. The scope of RD care can be expanded in the protocol to include ordering supplemental nutrition products or changing an enteral nutrition order.

An algorithm is used to manage an operation such as assessing use of enteral or parenteral nutrition or determining an appropriate enteral formula. Implementation of nutrition algorithms can standardize many clinical nutrition care decisions.

Developing the Specifics of Nutrition Programming

The first consideration in designing oncology nutrition programming is to assess the needs of the population served including age, ethnic, cultural and socioeconomic backgrounds. To improve efficacy, nutrition classes and programs should be designed to meet the needs of patients and their families. Educational materials and community resources can be tailored to match literacy levels or translated into different languages. Within a comprehensive cancer center, the goal is to integrate nutrition programs and services throughout the cancer continuum.

Nutrition Classes are a way to reach a large number of individuals including patients, families, and community members. Cancer prevention, healthy eating on a budget, cancer nutrition myths, and many other topics can be presented at monthly classes and special events. Cooking classes are increasingly popular and provide a way for patients and caregivers to participate in learning while experiencing healthy eating recommendations. And weight loss programs for breast cancer survivors can be a valuable resource that promotes survival.

Prevention and survivorship programs are essential to include in a nutrition program. Anyone with a cancer diagnosis is considered a survivor, but most survivorship programs begin after treatment has ended. When patients enter periods of remission, RDs should promote nutritional strategies that decrease the risk of recurrence and help survivors manage co-morbidities such as cardiovascular disease or diabetes. Survivorship care plans are a newly required component of cancer care per ACOS CoC guidelines. Nutrition can be integrated into care plans with referrals to the RD for weight management strategies, behavioral modification to promote healthy behavior change, management of late effects of treatment, and guidance on complementary and alternative nutrition modalities. Survivor celebrations, seminars, newsletters, and websites are methods that help meet the needs of this patient group. Nutrition programs and services within the center can be introduced in new patient orientation and treatment classes.

Educational Materials and Community Resources: From the inception of the nutrition program, it is important to obtain or develop uniform and professional educational materials. Materials can be developed to meet the needs of certain patient groups such as chemotherapy and radiation-specific nutrition needs. Nutrition handouts should utilize a template that includes the cancer center logo and contact information. The "Management of Nutrition Impact Symptoms in Cancer and Educational Handouts", which is available from the Academy, is a helpful resource to get started with evidence-based education materials.

Demonstration Kitchen: Many cancer centers are able to include a resource or demonstration kitchen for classes and education. Stock the kitchen with nutrition information, including handouts, as well as examples of food packaging to teach patients what to look for on a label when purchasing cancer fighting foods. Supplemental nutrition products can be safely stored and sampled. If a kitchen is not available, consider a cooking demonstration cart, which can be used for spotlight cooking demonstrations.

Online Presence: The Internet has become a research tool that allows patients to find information to guide them in their care decisions. Most cancer centers have a web page to highlight their program and the services offered. Make sure that nutrition has a strong presence on the website. Work with the website development team to make the nutrition section accessible and "user friendly." Provide resources, class schedules, and links to approved sites for additional nutrition information. The Internet is also a great venue to post podcasts and webinars on popular nutrition topics. Consider video clips of cooking demonstrations or "how to" demonstrations. Continually check with your marketing and IT team for other opportunities to highlight the nutrition program.

Integrative Medicine: Integrative medicine combines conventional with safe, effective complementary and alternative medical care. Many cancer centers are developing programs that incorporate integrative medicine practices such as meditation, yoga, and massage. The RD can play a role in integrative medicine by addressing the safety and possible effectiveness of dietary supplements and the use of functional foods to treat disease. Access to databases such as the Natural Medicine Comprehensive Database (http://naturaldatabase.therapeuticresearch.com) or other reputable sites can help provide patients with evidenced based information to help make informed decisions about their care.

Community Relations: Newsletters and articles in newspapers and journals provide information to the local community that can help market the benefits of good nutrition. Participating in community and business health fairs advertises the services of the RD and promotes the role of nutrition in cancer care. Radio and television stations often feature segments on cancer care, and nutrition is a popular topic for viewers. RDs always need to be ready to comment on current research on nutrition and cancer.

Creative and Innovative Programming: When it comes to nutrition, creativity abounds. Herb gardens, cancer victory gardens, partnerships with local healthy food stores, grocery store tours, and retreats can showcase the versatility of using food in health promotion. Food service departments can work with the oncology RD team to feature cancer preventive nutrition in their service area. Innovations with technology can expand the ability to reach more patients through computer teleconferencing, DVD education series, or through journals or blogs.

Measuring Outcomes of Nutrition Care and Programs

With any program, it is critical to demonstrate efficacy and to help refine the focus of oncology nutrition care to best meet the needs of the population served. The challenge of identifying desired outcomes can be simplified by identifying goals in the following categories:

- Clinical: Clinical outcome measures focus on the end result of a medical intervention.
- Practice: Practice based outcome measures look at best practice and meeting established guidelines.

- Program: Program focused outcomes measure the success of a program and can be determined through patient satisfaction surveys. Press Ganey, Gallup, or a program specific survey can generate data that is used to better meet the needs and requests of patients served.

Results of outcome measures can be used as evidence to support the nutrition program within the cancer center, increase staffing, and improve services and overall nutrition care.

Over the past several decades significant evidence has identified the risks of ignoring malnutrition. As now acknowledged by accreditation agencies of cancer programs, it is essential to provide clinical nutrition services provided by a qualified health professional. The RD holds the only credential backed by education and accreditation that meets the standard for the term "qualified."

References

1. Commission on Cancer: Cancer Program Standards 2012: Ensuring Patient-Centered Care, Chicago, IL: American College of Surgeons. Page 38. http://www.facs.org/cancer/coc/programstandards2012.pdf. Published 2012. Accessed August 17, 2012.
2. The Joint Commission Standards for Nutrition, Functional, and Pain Assessments and Screens. Revised November 24, 2008. http://www.jointcommission.org/standards_information/jcfaqdetails.aspx?StandardsFAQId=208&StandardsFAQChapterId=12. Accessed August 17, 2012.
3. Association of Community Cancer Centers. Cancer Nutrition Services: A Practice Guide for Cancer Programs. Available at: http://www.accc-cancer.org/education/NutritionPrograms-Overview.asp. Published March 2012. Accessed November 20, 2012.
4. Haehling S, Anker SD. Cachexia as a major underestimated and unmet medical need: facts and numbers. *J Cachexia Sarcopenia Muscle.* 2010;1-5.
5. Ravasco, P, Monteiro-grillo, I, Marques Vidal, P, ErmelindaCamilo, M. Dietary Counseling Improves Patient Outcomes: A Prospective, Randomized, Controlled Trial in Colorectal Cancer Patients Undergoing Radiotherapy. *J Clin Oncology.* 2005;23(7):1431-1438.
6. Isenring EA, Capra S, Bauer JD. Nutrition intervention is beneficial in oncology outpatients receiving radiotherapy to the gastrointestinal or head and neck area. *Br J Cancer.* 2004;91(3):447-452.
7. Rock C. Dietary counseling is beneficial for the patient with cancer. *J Clin Oncology.* 2005;23(7):1348-1349.
8. Halfdanarson TR, Thordardottir E, West CP, Jatoi A. Does dietary counseling improve quality of life in cancer patients? A systematic review and meta-analysis. *J Support Oncol.* 2008;6(5):234-237.
9. Robien, K, Snyder D, Elliot, L, Frankmann, C. Dietary Counseling and Quality of Life. *J Support Oncol.* 2008;6(8):353-354.
10. National Cancer Institute. NCI Guidelines for Comprehensive Designation. Available at: http://cancercenters.cancer.gov/documents/CCSG_Guidelines.pdf. Published January 2013. Accessed September 16, 2013.
11. Huhmann MB and Cunningham RS. Importance of nutritional screening in treatment of cancer-related weight loss. *Lancet Oncol.* 2005;6(5):334-343.
12. Academy of Nutrition and Dietetics. Evidence Analysis Library/Oncology Toolkit: Evidence-Based Nutrition Practice Guideline. Chicago, IL: American Dietetic Association. www.eatright.org/shop/product.aspx?id=6442472065. Published 2012. Accessed August 17, 2012.
13. Association of Community Cancer Centers. Cancer Program Guidelines. http://accc-cancer.org/publications/CancerProgramGuidelines-4.asp#section 8. Published 2012. Accessed August 17, 2012.
14. Robien K, Bechard L, Elliott L, Fox N, Levin R, Washburn S. American Dietetic Association: Revised Standards of Practice and Standards of Professional Performance for Registered Dietitians (Generalist, Specialty, and Advanced) in Oncology Nutrition Care. *J Am Diet Assoc.* 2010;110(2):310-317.

Integrative Oncology: The Role of Nutrition

Donald I. Abrams, MD

Overview

Integrative medicine provides relationship-centered care with an emphasis on addressing the needs of the whole person — body, mind, spirit and community. The Consortium of Academic Health Centers for Integrative Medicine defines it as "the practice of medicine that reaffirms the importance of the relationship between practitioner and patient, focuses on the whole person, is informed by evidence, and makes use of all appropriate therapeutic approaches, health care professionals and disciplines to achieve optimal health and healing (1)". In integrative medicine, the patient and the practitioner are partners in the healing process with the relationship being a centerpiece of the paradigm. Open and honest bidirectional communication that establishes a mutually respectful trusting relationship is a key component of the integrative medicine consultation (2). In the words of an integrative therapist — "Research suggests that our presence as medical or mental health clinicians, the way we bring ourselves fully into connection with those for whom we care, is one of the most crucial factors supporting how people heal — how they respond to our therapeutic efforts (3).

Patients with cancer and cancer survivors are increasingly seeking integrative medicine practitioners to complement their conventional cancer care. Integrative oncology is an emerging subspecialty (4-5). Integrative oncologists strive to combine the best of conventional interventions with evidence-informed complementary therapies into a personalized treatment regimen. Integrative oncology should not be equated with the popular acronym CAM, short for complementary and alternative medicine. CAM as a term is a self-contradiction as alternative therapies are used *instead of* and complementary therapies are used *in addition* to conventional therapies. The role of the integrative oncologist is to assist the patient in creating a treatment regimen that safely incorporates complementary therapies with their conventional treatment, using evidence-informed data where it exists. One could ask whether a new subspecialty in oncology is necessary — could not the conventional oncologist serve this function? In these days of the exploding knowledge base in cancer therapeutics, it is difficult enough to keep up with all of the treatment algorithms and interventions for breast cancer. To expect the conventional oncologist to stay up-to-date with the rapidly expanding field of integrative oncology would be asking too much.

A diagnosis of cancer removes the locus of control from the patient. Often we find previously highly functional individuals, stunned to hear the very word, at the mercy of the surgeon, the radiation oncologist, the medical oncologist and the chemotherapy nurse. Consultation with an integrative oncologist often serves to return to the patient a sense that they may, in fact, have some control. The integrative oncologist may equate cancer to a weed and the patient to a garden. The role of the integrative oncology consultation is to make the garden soil as inhospitable to growth and spread of the weed. This may be accomplished by advising the patient on ways to decrease inflammation, enhance their own immunity and decrease stress. All of these together provide the patient with increased control and return a sense of hope, which, in and of itself, may have therapeutic value.

Essential Components of an Integrative Oncology Program

The opportunity to receive both conventional and integrative oncology care from a single practitioner is rare as few conventional oncologists have yet received adequate training in integrative medicine. Most patients see both a conventional oncologist and a second practitioner — an oncologist, general internist or family medicine physician with an integrative medicine background — who recommends additional complementary therapies to consider. The National Institute of Health's National Center for Complementary and Alternative Medicine (NCCAM) recognizes four main categories of complementary therapies (6). Mind and body medicine approaches include meditation, deep-breathing exercises, hypnotherapy, guided imagery, yoga, tai chi, qi gong and other spiritual practices. Manipulative and body-based practices include massage and spinal manipulation as performed by chiropractors, osteopathic physicians, naturopathic physicians, massage therapists and physical therapists. The energy-based therapies are Reiki, healing touch and qi gong. Natural products therapies include dietary interventions and dietary supplements such as antioxidants, probiotics and botanicals. These four modalities are utilized by the "whole systems" practices recognized by NCCAM — traditional Chinese medicine, Ayurveda, naturopathy and homeopathy. The integrative oncologist, who may often have expertise in one of the complementary modalities, assists the patient in devising a personalized treatment regimen that combines appropriate integrative interventions safely with their conventional cancer care.

Although a small percentage of patients may come to an integrative oncologist seeking truly alternative therapy for their malignant diagnosis, eschewing surgery, radiation, chemotherapy, hormones and targeted therapies, the data supporting the utility of any such interventions is lacking. Patients are counseled that conventional cancer therapy has made significant progress in being able to prolong survival, if not cure, and that the pursuit of exclusively seeking alternative therapies is a waste of valuable time and resources. Most cancer patients choose to integrate complementary therapies into their regimen with a goal of ameliorating the symptoms associated with the cancer or its treatment. Many hope that by decreasing inflammation and enhancing their innate immunity in the fight against cancer that they may improve their chances for obtaining and maintaining a disease-free status.

Complementary interventions may also have a role in reducing the risk of cancer. Hypnosis and acupuncture may assist in helping tobacco smokers break their habit. Lifestyle interventions such as nutrition and physical activity can also play a role in decreasing the risk of developing a number of malignant diagnoses. Unfortunately, although most of the general public recognizes the hazard of tobacco consumption as a cause of cancer, far fewer appreciate that what we eat and what we don't eat contributes to an equivalent number of avoidable malignant diagnoses.

Anti-Cancer Nutrition

Few physicians obtain any nutrition training during medical school or in their post-graduate years. When asking their oncologist what they should eat during treatment, patients are often told that "it doesn't matter" or they may be asked to avoid antioxidant rich foods for fear that they may interfere with their radiation or chemotherapy. Many integrative oncologists focus a significant portion of their patient consultation on reviewing available information on nutrition and cancer. Fortunately, the American Institute for Cancer Research (AICR) and the American Cancer Society are at the forefront of the issue, publishing updated guidelines pertaining to cancer risk reduction, but also relevant to the person diagnosed with cancer and survivors as well (7-8). In fact, the tenth and last of the AICR guidelines states that "After treatment, cancer survivors should follow the recommendations for cancer prevention."

The American Cancer Society's nutrition and physical activity guidelines are summarized as four main recommendations: 1) achieve and maintain a healthy weight throughout life; 2) adopt a physically active lifestyle; 3) choose a healthy diet with an emphasis on plant foods; and 4) if you drink alcoholic beverages, limit consumption. The AICR estimates that obesity-related excesses of seven cancers — postmenopausal breast, esophagus, pancreas, gallbladder, colorectal, endometrial and kidney — account for 105,000 preventable deaths in the United States each year (9). Numerous mechanisms have been suggested for how obesity increases the risk of cancer (9-11). Fat secretes cytokines that promote inflammation. An excess in body fat may impair immunity. Obesity leads to insulin resistance, elevating levels of insulin, insulin-like growth factor-1 and other growth factors that foster malignant transformation and proliferation (12). Finally, fat produces estrogen which is especially relevant in the increased risk of post-menopausal estrogen-receptor positive breast cancer and endometrial carcinoma. Obesity is also associated with a poorer prognosis in a number of malignancies with evidence accumulating that intentional weight loss after a cancer diagnosis may improve survival (11,13-15).

Physical activity is a key component of the integrative approach. An active lifestyle has been shown to reduce the risk of breast, colon and prostate cancers (16). Increasing evidence suggests that even in patients with a cancer diagnosis, three to six hours of vigorous exercise each week may prolong survival (17). Exercise also helps to reduce fatigue and depression by way of endorphin release and may also improve sleep. Some physical activities — yoga, tai chi and qi gong — have a significant mind-body component that also serves to help reduce stress above and beyond the effect of the exercise itself. These practices are increasingly being associated with improvement in quality of life measures in cancer patients and survivors (18-19).

The third AICR recommendation, the first to mention food, advises to avoid sugary drinks and limit consumption of energy-dense foods. This links to the body weight guideline as sugary drinks contribute many empty calories to the standard American diet. In addition, the contribution of insulin and insulin-like growth factor type 1 to the development of malignant disease is being increasingly appreciated in a number of cancers (12,20). Many integrative oncologists caution their patients to avoid refined sugars. Additional strategies to improve glycemic control include a high fiber diet with healthy fats, exercise, and adequate sleep.

Although one can measure fasting glucose and levels of insulin and insulin-like growth factor-1, a more relevant and practical bioassay might be measurement of hemoglobin A1C. This provides a picture of the patient's glycemic control over the past 3 months. Patients with an elevated level of hemoglobin A1C could be appropriate for nutrition counseling and the use of adjuvant metformin, the oral hypoglycemic agent that has been associated with decreased risk of various malignancies and with in vitro activity against a number of cancer cell lines (21-22). Finally, measurement of high sensitivity C-reactive protein (hs-CRP) provides information on the patient's ongoing level of systemic inflammation (23). Results from this assay might focus the integrative oncologist towards recommending a more anti-inflammatory diet and, possibly, supplements with anti-inflammatory effects.

AICR suggests eating more of a variety of fruits, vegetables, whole grains and legumes such as beans. Data from the U.S. Centers for Disease Control demonstrates that the American public falls far short of the conservative recommendation to consume at least 5 servings of fruits and vegetables daily with only 14% of adults meeting the guideline. The importance of consuming plant products is being increasingly appreciated as the developed world combats the obesity epidemic. Plants provide an alternate source of calories to animal fat, protein and processed foods. Plants are also rich sources of fiber, antioxidants and phytonutrients, many of which are felt to be useful in cancer risk reduction. For example, a recent pooled analysis of 8 prospective studies demonstrated that women with high levels of plant-derived carotenoids had significant reductions in the risk of breast cancer, with some associations appearing stronger for estrogen receptor negative tumors (24). The authors suggest that their observations highlight carotenoids as one of the first modifiable risk factors for this poor prognosis tumor type.

A British meta-analysis reported no statistically different concentration of macronutrients between organic and conventional produce. The organic foodstuffs, however, were higher in phytochemical content, such as phenolic compounds and flavonoids, the very potent health-promoting phytonutrients that one seeks from the consumption of organic produce (25). AICR recommendations include limiting consumption of red meats (beef, pork and lamb) and avoiding processed meats. Epidemiologic studies suggest that consumption of red meats is directly proportional to the risk of developing colon cancer (26). Conversely, consumption of higher levels of omega-3 or marine fatty acids has been shown to be inversely correlated with the development of a number of malignancies (27). Patients with cancer are best advised to obtain their animal fats and proteins from wild, deep cold-water fish and organic poultry products while avoiding red and processed meats and dairy products.

The AICR alcohol guideline recommends that, if consumed at all, alcoholic drinks be limited to two for men and one for women per day. Although moderate alcohol consumption may be associated with cardiovascular benefits, alcohol use has been associated with an increased risk of a number of malignancies.

In summary, these nutrition guidelines suggest Americans eat at least 2.5 cups of fruits and vegetables each day, choose whole grains instead of refined grain products, avoid sugary drinks and limit consumption of red meats while avoiding processed meats. These recommendations are attuned to the ultimate goal of achieving and maintaining a healthy weight that will serve to decrease the risk of cancer as well as diabetes, heart disease and other degenerative diseases that plague our overweight society. Epidemiologic studies in patients participating in cancer clinical trials have shown that cancer patients who adhere to these more prudent dietary recommendations as opposed to consuming the standard American diet benefit with regards to more prolonged disease-free and overall survival (13-15).

A recent study also suggests that patients with a genetic predisposition to develop colon cancer can modify their risk significantly by what they eat. Among 486 people with Lynch syndrome followed for a median of 20 months, a statistically significant increased risk of adenomas was observed in individuals eating in the highest tertile of what was called the "Snack" pattern (heavy on chips, fried snacks, fast food, diet soda, etc.) compared to the lowest tertile (28). A modest non-statistically significant inverse association with colorectal adenomas was seen in those adhering to the "Prudent" pattern which included heavy consumption of fruits and vegetables, whole grains, poultry, fish and green tea. These exciting findings support healthy nutrition as a lifestyle factor that may modify risk of cancer development even among people with a genetic predisposition.

Dietary Supplements

Most conventional medical and radiation oncologists recommend that cancer patients avoid all supplements, especially during active radiation or chemotherapy. Much of this recommendation is based on the concern that evidence to support the use of any of these agents is lacking and, as a specialty, oncologists rely heavily on evidence before recommending any of the very potent therapies used against malignant disease. In the absence of convincing data supporting benefit, the conventional oncologist takes the path of least resistance and advises patients to avoid all supplements. Three other valid concerns about supplement use include the potential for supplement:drug interactions via a pharmacokinetic or pharmacodynamics pathway, the oxidant:antioxidant issue and the impact of the supplement on clotting, a particular problem for patients with hematologic malignancies, those receiving cytotoxic chemotherapy and those on anticoagulants.

Concurrent use of a supplement — particularly a botanical — with chemotherapy could lead to a clinically important interaction which might translate into an increase or decrease in the effects of either component. As 35% of currently prescribed oncology drugs are metabolized by the CYP3A4 isoform of the hepatic cytochrome p450 enzyme system, use of supplements that either induce or inhibit the pathway can be problematic (29). For example, the botanical supplement St. John's wort used for the treatment of mild depression is a strong inducer of many CYP isoforms. In a classic pharmacokinetic interaction study, ten healthy volunteers were administered a single 400 mg oral dose of imatinib (30). The investigators found that the pharmacokinetics of imatinib were significantly altered by St. John's wort, with significant reductions in the median area under the concentration-time curve, in the maximum observed concentration, and the half-life. The conclusion was that co-administration of St. John's wort could compromise the clinical efficacy of imatinib. Because of the potential for the same effect when taken with a number of anti-cancer drugs metabolized by this system, it is recommended that cancer patients receiving any chemotherapeutic intervention avoid taking St. John's wort.

Radiation therapy, and many chemotherapeutic interventions, damage tumor cell DNA via production of reactive oxygen species. The alkylating agents (cyclophosphamide, ifosfamide and melphalan) and the antitumor antibiotics (daunorubicin, doxorubicin and bleomycin) are strongly oxidative chemotherapeutic agents. Many patients are interested in taking antioxidants to protect themselves from the toxic effects of cytotoxic chemotherapy on non-malignant cells. Radiation oncologists and medical oncologists are reluctant to go along with this desire for fear that the antioxidant will negate the anti-tumor effect of their radiation or chemotherapy. A study looking at alpha-tocopherol as a radioprotectant in patients being treated for head and neck cancer demonstrated a reduction in overall adverse events in the supplemented arm during acute therapy (31). However, with prolonged follow-up, the group receiving the alpha-tocopherol supplementation was found to have a non-significant increased risk of local recurrence but a significant increase in all-cause mortality at 6.5 years of follow-up (32). Despite this being the only evidence available on the topic, oncologists feel comfortable using this data to advise patients to avoid all antioxidants during acute cancer therapy. Perhaps a more rational approach might be to consider that patients who are being treated with a goal of cure or in an adjuvant setting should abstain from use of antioxidants until completion of their acute therapy while those being treated with palliative intent could consider concomitant use. In any event, consumption of an antioxidant rich diet should never be contraindicated.

Patients with malignancies are often at increased risk for bleeding problems, either from their underlying disease or treatment with cytotoxic agents that also lead to myelosuppression. There has been a long-standing tendency to attribute thrombocytopenias of unclear etiology in cancer patients to botanical supplements that they are taking, particularly traditional Chinese medicine herbs. Warfarin is a frequently prescribed anticoagulant, itself derived from a botanical, which can be impacted in a number of ways by diet and dietary supplements. Inappropriate control of anticoagulation due to fluctuation in warfarin effect exposes the patient to increased bleeding or thromboembolic complications. The anticoagulant effect of warfarin can be antagonized by vitamin K intake. Patients placed on warfarin are often advised to limit green leafy and cruciferous vegetables or not to consume green tea as they are all rich in vitamin K and might interfere with the anticoagulant effect. A more integrative approach is to recommend that the patient consume a healthful diet and adjust the warfarin dose accordingly to maintain the desired International Normalization Ratio (INR).

Useful Nutraceuticals

Omega 3 Fatty Acids
In view of the epidemiologic data suggesting an inverse relationship between the intake of marine omega-3 fatty acids and the development of a number of malignancies and the good risk:benefit profile, integrative oncologists may recommend that cancer patients might consider a daily omega-3 supplement. Fish oil supplements contain oils from cod, krill, salmon, sardines and other species that are high in long-chain polyunsaturated fatty acids. The omega-3 fatty acids eicosapentaenoic acid (EPA) and docosahexaenoic acid (DHA) are most abundant. Fish oil reduces inflammation through changes in membrane fluidity, cell signaling and production of anti-inflammatory eicosanoids (33). These effects may retard cancer progression. Fish oil may increase apoptosis by suppressing NF-kappa B (34). A phase II clinical trial investigating the potential benefits of omega-3 supplementation involved 48 men scheduled for radical prostatectomy (35). Preclinical studies had suggested that decreased dietary fat and a decreased ratio of omega-6 to omega-3 fatty acids might lower risk and slow progression of prostate cancer. Participants in the study were randomized to a low fat (15%) diet and 5 grams of fish oil (yielding an omega-6:omega-3 ratio of 2:1) or a control Western diet (40% fat, omega-6:omega-3 ratio of 15:1) for 4 to 6 weeks pre-operatively. All the food prepared was prepared by UCLA chefs and delivered to the patients. At the end of the trial, men in the lower fat, omega-3 supplemented group had lower omega-6:omega-3 ratios in both blood and prostate, a decreased volume of prostate tissue (both benign and malignant) and reduced cancer cell proliferation as measured by the Ki-67 index. In addition, blood from the experimental group added to prostate cancer cells in culture reduced proliferation more than the blood from the control group. In a non-randomized trial of fish oil supplementation in lung cancer patients receiving chemotherapy, higher rates of response and clinical benefit with a tendency toward longer survival were observed with no increase in dose-limiting toxicities (36). Omega-3 supplements are felt to be safe; there is concern of increased bleeding tendencies at doses above 4000 milligrams daily.

Vitamin D3
Vitamin D has hormone-like action that controls calcium, phosphorus and bone metabolism. It is the only vitamin that the body manufactures from sunlight. An increasing proportion of the global population is deficient in vitamin D because of indoor living, distance from the equator, clothing styles, avoidance of sunlight for fear of cutaneous malignancies and widespread use of sunscreen (37). An early suggestion that vitamin D was related to cancer risk came from an observation that colon cancer mortality rates were lower in the southwestern United States compared to the northeast (38). Subsequent studies have supported the finding that lower serum 25-hydroxyvitamin D levels are associated with increased risks of breast and prostate as well as colorectal and possibly other cancers, although the data is considered inconclusive (39-40). An increasing body of evidence suggests that lower serum levels are also related to poorer prognoses in patients diagnosed with various malignancies (41). Administration of vitamin D analogues produce antiproliferative effects, can activate apoptotic pathways and inhibit angiogenesis. Additional benefits of vitamin D may be by way of enhancing the anti-cancer effects of cytotoxic agents. Vitamin D supplementation is generally safe with few side effects, most commonly gastrointestinal. Excess vitamin D supplementation can lead to hypercalcemia.

Measurement of serum 25-hydroxyvitamin D level should guide dosing (42). The Institute of Medicine guideline that a level greater than 20 ng/mL is adequate for maintaining bone health may not be appropriate in the care of patients with malignant diagnoses although conclusive evidence of the optimal 25-hydroxyvitamin D level in these patients is lacking (43). A safe recommendation would be to achieve a 25-hydroxyvitamin D level in the range of 40-80 ng/mL. Although some food products (eggs, fortified dairy, mushrooms and fish) may provide small amounts of vitamin D2 (ergocalciferol), ultraviolet light from the sun is the best source of vitamin D3 (cholecalciferol). However, production is impaired with age, obesity and pigmentation, and oral supplementation is advised. In severe deficiency, each 1000 IU dose increment should increase 25-hydroxyvitamin D levels by 10 ng/mL; effects of supplementation decrease as optimal levels are achieved (44).

Curcumin

Curcumin, the major component of the Indian spice turmeric (*Curcuma longa*) and widely used in Indian cuisine as a coloring and flavoring additive, has anti-inflammatory properties. Epidemiological evidence suggests that the incidence of certain cancers is less in people who consume curcumin than in those who do not. *In vitro* and *in vivo* data indicate that curcumin is a potent anti-inflammatory and antioxidant with broad antibiotic activity as well (45). It can inhibit tumor initiation, promotion, invasion, angiogenesis and metastasis and also acts as a chemosensitizer and radiosensitizer for some tumors (46). The chemopreventive effects of turmeric appear most promising for colorectal and pancreatic cancers.

Although there is no clear dosage recommendation for curcumin, doses up to 12 grams have been employed in clinical trials with no major adverse effects. Curcumin has poor bioavailability, so it stays in the gastrointestinal tract and has local action on the mucosa since it is poorly absorbed systemically in transit. This action may suggest why curcumin may have potential benefit in reducing the risk of colon cancers. In order to increase the systemic availability, curcumin is frequently combined with black pepper or its active component, piperine (47). Consuming curcumin with fatty foods — olive oil, avocado, fish oil, milk and seeds — will also increase the absorption. Trials have shown curcumin supplementation to be safe with gemcitabine and perhaps synergistic with taxanes by sensitizing tumor cells. There is a suggestion that turmeric could reduce the toxicities of a number of chemotherapeutic agents, but it remains unclear as to whether the effectiveness of the chemotherapy may also be compromised as well (48).

Green tea (Camellia sinensis)

Tea is the second most widely consumed beverage in the world after water. Green tea is brewed from the unfermented tea leaves of *Camellia sinensis* which contains polyphenols with chemopreventive properties. Epigallocatechin gallate (EGCG) is the major catechin in green tea. Green tea has multiple mechanisms of action against cancer including pro-apoptotic effects, inhibition of NF-kappaB and other signaling molecules, antimetastatic, and antioxidant effects. In animal studies, green tea has a protective effect against tumors of the colon, prostate, esophagus, liver, stomach, lung, breast, pancreas and skin. In the Iowa Women's Health Study, catechin intake from tea was associated with a lower incidence of digestive tract cancers. The epidemiology suggests that Chinese tea drinking men have half the risk of developing stomach or esophageal cancer, and a significantly lower risk of prostate cancer. A recent meta-analysis evaluated 13 studies providing data on green tea and black tea consumption and the risk of prostate cancer (49). The findings supported that green tea but not black tea may have a protective effect against prostate cancer, especially in Asian populations where a 40% reduction in risk was appreciated. Another meta-analysis concluded that observational data support a protective role of green tea, but not black tea, on the development of ovarian (32% reduction in risk) and endometrial (23% reduction in risk) cancers (50).

Decaffeinated green tea may not have the same effectiveness as caffeinated forms as some of the chemopreventive chemicals may be extracted along with the caffeine. Although generally regarded as safe, gastrointestinal distress and mild elevation of liver function tests have been noted in clinical trials. A canine study suggested that taking green tea supplements on an empty stomach increased toxicity (51). Green tea may antagonize warfarin due to vitamin K content. *In vitro* and *in vivo* studies suggest that EGCG could inhibit the activity of bortezomib in multiple myeloma (52). However, the concentration of polyphenols necessary to reproduce the in vitro and animal model results is not readily achievable from drinking green tea alone. Consumption of no more than 5 large cups of green tea daily is likely adequate for desired benefits with low risk of adverse effects.

Medicinal Mushrooms

Medicinal mushrooms have a long history of use especially in Asia where hot water fractions (decoctions and essences) are used for treating a number of conditions. Most *Basidiomycetes* mushrooms contain biologically active polysaccharides in their fruit bodies, culture mycelia or culture broth. Mushroom polysaccharides exert their antitumor action by activation of the host immune response. The mushroom β-glucans, resembling bacterial cell walls, complex with complement on macrophages and activate an immune response leading to release of various cytokines that are active in tumor inhibition (53). An intact T-cell immune system is essential for the antitumor activity of medicinal mushrooms. Interest in the West in the investigation of medicinal mushrooms as potential anti-cancer agents was piqued by epidemiology studies from Japan and Brazil suggesting that long-term exposure to local medicinal mushroom species was associated with lower cancer mortality rates (54-55).

Some of the mushroom species with immune enhancing and possible anti-cancer activity are edible, such as *Grifola frondosa* (maitake), *Lentinus edodoes* (shiitake) and *Flammulina velutipes* (enokitake). Dried varieties may have higher concentrations of the beneficial nutrients than the fresh mushrooms. Although available as edibles, pharmaceuticalized extracts of these mushrooms are also available as supplements and used by many cancer patients. Other varieties that may have potential immune modulating and anticancer activity – *Ganoderma lucidum* (reishi) and *Trametes* or *Coriolus versicolor* (turkey tail) can be consumed as an infusion, but more commonly are taken in capsules or as extracts. The common *Agaricus bisporus* (white button) may contain significant amounts of a hydrazine derivative, agaritine, that is carcinogenic in animal models (56). As heating inactivates the agaritine and allows for better utilization of mushroom nutrients, all edible mushrooms should be cooked. A Chinese case control study demonstrates the concept that individual components of the diet are less critical than the whole diet overall, with synergy seen between nutritional components. A thousand women with breast cancer were matched with controls. Women who consumed fresh (white button) and dried (shiitake) mushrooms daily had a decreased risk of developing breast cancer compared to those who did not (57). However, when the diet included green tea as well, the risk reduction was even more dramatic.

Additional Integrative Oncology Interventions

Stress Management

The integrative oncologist appreciates that patients with cancer are often very stressed, leading to sympathetic nervous system excess with overproduction of epinephrine and cortisol, both of which are immunosuppressant. Consultation with an integrative oncologist who can outline steps that the patient can take themselves — nutrition, exercise, supplements — allows patients to regain some of the sense of control that they feel they have lost once they have been diagnosed with cancer. This patient empowerment serves to reduce stress and increase a sense of hope. However, some patients actually become upset attempting to incorporate recommended dietary changes into their lifestyle, relating that eating healthfully and adhering to dietary guidelines becomes a stressful event. Some become fearful that they will precipitate a recurrence if they veer from recommendations. These patients should be reminded that they should embrace the nutrients they ingest and not fear them. Occasional divergence from a healthful anti-cancer diet is to be expected and tolerated without generating additional angst.

A controlled study in mice with breast cancer confined for three hours a day to reproduce stress showed that after three weeks, the stressed cohort had increased size and number of metastatic lesions while the primary lesions were similar to the unstressed control group (58). Evidence now suggests that women with higher stress levels and less social support have ovarian tumors that are more aggressive due to higher expression of vascular endothelial growth factor (VEGF) compared to women with better social support (59). A similar finding has been described in head and neck cancer patients where the stressed cohort also experienced shorter survival (60).

The broad field of mind-body interventions includes mindfulness-based stress reduction (MBSR), biofeedback, hypnosis, guided imagery, art therapy, music therapy, yoga, tai chi and other relaxation techniques (19,61-62). These mind-body interventions work by increasing parasympathetic tone, and lowering epinephrine and cortisol levels. Mindfulness meditation is being increasingly utilized in the treatment of eating disorders and may ultimately become a useful tool in managing obesity in patients with malignant diagnoses where weight loss may be desirable in improving prognosis (62).

Acupuncture and Traditional Chinese Medicine

An NIH consensus panel in 1997 recognized the benefit of acupuncture for the treatment of chemotherapy-induced nausea and vomiting (63). Since that time, a number of controlled clinical trials have shown additional benefits in the treatment of cancer or treatment-related symptoms such as xerostomia following radiation therapy for head and neck tumors; musculoskeletal complaints related to aromatase inhibitor therapy; hot flashes in both men and women with hormone ablation therapies and chemotherapy-induced peripheral neuropathy. Perhaps most relevant to the discussion of the importance of nutrition in integrative oncology is the potential for patients undergoing radiation for head and neck cancers to maintain better salivary flow with the use of acupuncture (64-65).

Traditional Chinese medicine (TCM) practitioners are valuable members of the integrative oncology team. These practitioners also employ herbs, attention to diet, moxibustion (the application of heat resulting from the burning of a small bundle of tightly bound herbs, or moxa, to targeted acupoints) and qi gong in their armamentarium of therapies. They use a diagnostic system based on examination of the tongue and palpation of 12 pulses to devise a unique treatment plan for each patient. Cancer patients seeking consultation with TCM practitioners are often advised to avoid foods suggested by the integrative oncologist or oncology nutrition professional. Rather than focusing on macronutrient and phytonutrient contents, TCM practitioners recommend food on the basis of the patient's TCM diagnosis. The patient with "excess heat", for example, would be instructed to favor foods with cooling properties. Similarly, patients who see an Ayurvedic practitioner will have their dietary recommendations based on their type, or dosha. Conflicting nutritional advice from their Eastern and Western-focused integrative practitioners can become a source of confusion and stress for the patient attempting to optimize their anticancer diet.

Summary and Conclusion

Body weight, physical activity and nutrition are the cornerstones of many integrative oncologists' practices and recommendations. The American Society of Clinical Oncology has now also recognized the importance of lifestyle discussion and counseling with cancer patients and survivors to improve outcomes (66). They, like the American Cancer Society, are promoting the consumption of a healthy diet as a more appropriate way to ensure ingestion of nutrients as opposed to turning to supplements to do the job when, in fact, they usually fall short or, worse, can be detrimental (7,67). Perhaps with more widespread attention to the importance of lifestyle modification, especially the adoption of a healthy organic, plant-based, antioxidant rich, anti-inflammatory whole foods diet, the health of the nation be can improved and sustained for future generations with a marked decline in the epidemic of chronic illness and the flourishing of health and well-being, even in patients living with and beyond cancer.

References

1. Kligler B, Maizes V, Schachter S, et al. Core competencies in integrative medicine for medical school curricula: a proposal. *Acad Med.* 2004;79(6):521-531.
2. Abrams DI. Communication issues in integrative oncology. In: Surbone A, Zwitter M, Rajer M, Stiefel R, eds. *New Challenges in Communication with Cancer Patients.* New York: Springer; 2012 pp 81-90.
3. Siegel D. *The Mindful Therapist*, New York: WW Norton & Co; 2010.
4. Abrams DI. An overview of integrative oncology. *Clin Adv Hematol Oncol.* 2007;5(1):45-47.
5. Deng GE, Frenkel M, Cohen L, et al. Evidence-based clinical practice guidelines for integrative oncology: complementary therapies and botanicals. *J Soc Integr Oncol.* 2009;7(3):85-120.
6. CAM Basics: What is complementary and alternative medicine? National Center for Complementary and Alternative Medicine. http://nccam.nih.gov/health/whatiscam Published October 2008. Updated May 2012. Accessed January 20, 2013.
7. Kushi LH, Doyle C, McCullough M, et al. American Cancer Society guidelines on nutrition and physical activity for cancer prevention. *CA Cancer J Clin.* 2012;62(1):30-67.

8. Food, nutrition, physical activity, and the prevention of cancer: a global perspective. Washington DC: World Cancer Research Fund/American Institute for Cancer Research; 2007.

9. Calle EE, Kaaks R. Overweight, obesity and cancer: epidemiologic evidence and proposed mechanisms. *Nature Reviews Cancer.* 2004;4:579-591. doi:10.1038/nrcl1408

10. Wolin KY, Carson K, Colditz GA. Obesity and cancer. *The Oncologist.* 2010;15(6):556-565.

11. Ligibel J. Obesity and breast cancer. *Oncology.* 2011;25(11):994-1000.

12. Wolpin BM, Meyerhardt J, Chan AT, et al. Insulin, insulin-like growth factor axis, and mortality in patients with nonmetastatic colorectal cancer. *J Clin Oncol.* 2008;27(2):176-185.

13. Li CI, Daling JR, Porter PL, et al. Relationship between potentially modifiable lifestyle factors and risk of second primary contralateral breast cancer among women diagnosed with estrogen receptor-positive invasive breast cancer. *J Clin Oncol.* 2009;27(32):5312-5318. doi: 10.1200/JCO.2009.23.1597.

14. Meyerhardt JA, Niedzwiecki D, Hollis D, et al. Association of dietary patterns with cancer recurrence and survival in patients with stage III colon cancer. *JAMA.* 2007;298(7):754-764.

15. Dolecek TA, McCarty BJ, Joslin CE, et al. Prediagnosis food patterns are associated with length of survival from epithelial ovarian cancer. *J Am Diet Assoc.* 2010;110(3):369-382.

16. Stevinson C, Courneya K. Physical activity and cancer. In: Abrams DI, Weil A, eds. *Integrative Oncology.* New York: Oxford University Press; 2009: 215-231.

17. Meyerhardt JA, Heseltine D, Niedzwiecki, et al. Impact of physical activity on cancer recurrence and survival in patients with stage III colon cancer: findings from CALGB 89803. *J Clin Oncol.* 2006;24(22):3535-3541.

18. Chandwani KD, Thronton B, Perkins GH, et al. Yoga improves quality of life and benefit finding in women undergoing radiotherapy for breast cancer. *J Soc Integr Oncol.* 2010;8(2)43-55.

19. Stan DL, Collins NM, Olsen MM, Croghan I, Pruthi S. The evolution of mindfulness-based physical interventions in breast cancer survivors. *Evid Based Complement Alternat Med.* 2012;2012:758641. doi: 10.1155/2012/758641.

20. Gallagher EJ, LeRoith D. Minireview: IGF, insulin and cancer. *Endocrinology.* 2011;152(7):2546-2551.

21. Soranna D, Scotti L, Zambon A, Bosetti C, Grassi G, Catapano A, et al. Cancer risk associated with use of metformin and sulfonylurea in type-2 diabetes: a meta-analysis. *The Oncologist.* 2012;17(6):813-822.

22. Dowling RJO, Niraula S, Stambolic V, Goodwin PJ. Metformin in cancer: translational challenges. *J Mol Endocrinol.* 2012;48(3):R31-R43.

23. Windgassen EB, Funtowicz L, Lunsford TN, Harris LA, Mulvagh SL. C-reactive protein and high-sensitivity C-reactive protein: an update for clinicians. *Postgrad Med.* 2011;123(1):114-119.

24. Eliassen AH, Hendrickson SJ, Brinton LA, Buring JE, Camos H, Dai Q, et al. Circulating carotenoids and risk of breast cancer: Pooled analysis of eight prospective studies. *J Natl Cancer Inst.* 2012;104(24):1905-1916.

25. Dangour A, Dodhia S, Hayter A, et al. Comparison of composition (nutrients and other substances) of organically and conventionally produced foodstuffs: a systematic review of the available literature. Report for the Food Standards Agency. *London School of Hygiene and Tropical Medicine.* (http://www.food.gov.uk/multimedia/pdfs/organicreviewappendices.pdf Published July 2009. Accessed 9/2011.

26. Meyerhardt JA. Beyond standard adjuvant therapy for colon cancer: role of nonstandard interventions. *Semin Oncol.* 2011;38(4):533-541.

27. Bartsch H, Nair J, Owen RW. Dietary polyunsaturated fatty acids and cancers of the breast and colorectum: emerging evidence for their role as risk modifiers. *Carcinogenesis.* 1999;20(12):2209-2218.

28. Botma A, Vasen HFA, van Duijnhoven FJB, Kleibeuker JH, Nagengast FM, Kampman E. Dietary patterns and colorectal adenomas in Lynch syndrome: The GEOLynch Cohort Study. *Cancer.* 2013;119(3):512-521.

29. Sparreboom A, Baker SD. CAM:chemo interactions- what is known. In: Abrams DI, Weil A, eds. *Integrative Oncology.* New York: Oxford University Press; 2009: 171-194.

30. Smith P, Bullock JM, Booker BM, et al. The influence of St. John's wort on the pharmacokinetics and protein binding of imatinib mesylate. *Pharmacotherapy.* 2004;24(11):1508-1514.

31. Bairati I, Meyer F, Gelinas M, et al. Randomized trial of antioxidant vitamins to prevent acute adverse effects of radiation therapy in head and neck cancer patients. *J Clin Oncol.* 2005;23(24):5805-5813.

32. Bairati I, Meyer F, Jobin E, et al. Antioxidant vitamins supplementation and mortality: a randomized trial in head and neck cancer patients. *Int J Cancer.* 2006;119(9):2221-2224.

33. Calder PC. Fatty acids and inflammation: the cutting edge between food and pharma. *Eur J Pharmacol.* 2011;668 Suppl1:S50-S58.

34. Shaikh IA, Brown I, Wahle KW, Heys SD. Enhancing cytotoxic therapies for breast and prostate cancers with polyunsaturated fatty acids. *Nutr Cancer.* 2010;62(3):284-296.

35. Aronson WJ, Kobayashi N, Barnard RJ. Phase II prospective randomized trial of a low-fat diet with fish oil supplementation in men undergoing radical prostatectomy. *Cancer Prev Res.* 2011;4(12):2062-2071.

36. Murphy RA, Mourtzakis M, Chu QS, Baracos VE, Reiman T, Mazurak VC. Supplementation with fish oil increases first-line chemotherapy efficacy in patients with advanced non-small cell lung cancer. *Cancer.* 2011;117(16):3774-3780.

37. Kennel KA, Drake MT, Hurley DL. Vitamin D deficiency in adults: when to test and how to treat. *Mayo Clin Proc.* 2010;85(8):752-758.

38. Deeb KK, Trump DL, Johnson CS. Vitamin D signaling pathways in cancer: potential for anticancer therapeutics. *Nature Reviews/Cancer.* 2007;7(9):684-700.

39. Davis CD, Hartmuller V, Freedman M, Hartge P, Picciano MF, Swanson CA, Milner JA. Vitamin D and cancer: current dilemmas and future needs. *Nutrition Reviews.* 2007;65(s2):S71-S74.

40. Jenab M, Bueno-de-Mesquita HB, Ferrari P, et al. Association between pre-diagnostic circulating vitamin D concentration and risk of colorectal cancer in European populations: a nested case-control study. *BMJ.* 2010;340:b5500.

41. Rheem DS, Baylink DJ, Olafsson S, Jackson CS, Walter MH. Prevention of colorectal cancer with vitamin D. *Scand J Gastroenterol.* 2010;45(7-8):775-784.

42. Holick MF, Binkley NC, Bischoff-Ferrari HA, Gordon CM, Hanley DA, Heaney RP, et al. Evaluation, treatment, and prevention of vitamin D deficiency: an Endocrine Society Clinical Practice Guideline. *J Clin Endocrinol Metab.* 2011; 96(7):1911-1930.

43. Institute of Medicine. Food and Nutrition Board. *Dietary Reference Intakes for calcium and vitamin D.* Washington, DC: National Academy Press. 2010.

44. Garland CF, French CB, Baggerly LL, Heaney RP. Vitamin D supplement doses and serum 25-hydroxyvitamin D in the range associated with cancer prevention. *Anticancer Research.* 2011;31(2):617-622.

45. Schaffer M, Schaffer PM, Zidan J, Bar Sela G. Curcuma as a functional food in the control of cancer and inflammation. *Curr Opin Clin Nutr Metab Care.* 2011;14(6):558-597.

46. Goel A, Aggarwal BB. Curcumin, the golden spice from Indian saffron, is a chemosensitizer and radiosensitizer for tumors and chemoprotector and radioprotector for normal organs. *Nutr Cancer.* 2010;62(7):919-930.

47. Shoba G, Joy D, Joseph T, Majeed M, Rajendran R, Srinivas PS. Influence of piperine on the pharmacokinetics of curcumin in animals and human volunteers. *Planta Med.* 1998;64(4):353–356.

48. Stargrove MB, Treasure J, McKee DL. *Herb, Nutrient, and Drug Interactions.* St. Louis, MO, Mosby; 2008:160,165-166.

49. Zheng J, Yang B, Huang T, Yu Y, Yanq J, Li D. Green tea and black tea consumption and prostate cancer risk: An exploratory meta-analysis of observational studies. *Nutrition and Cancer.* 2011;63(5):663-672.

50. Butler LM, Wu AH. Green and black tea in relation to gynecologic cancers. *Mol Nutr Food Res.* 2011;55(6):931-940.

51. Schönthal AH. Adverse effects of concentrated green tea extracts. *Mol Nutr Food Res.* 2011; 55(6):874-885.

52. Golden EB, Lam PY, Kardosh A, et al. Green tea polyphenols block the anticancer effects of bortezomib and other boronic acid-based proteasome inhibitors. *Blood.* 2009;113(23):5927-5937.

53. Stamets P. Potentiation of cell-mediated host defense using fruitbodies and mycelia of medicinal mushrooms. *Int J Med Mushrooms.* 2003;5:179-191.

54. Wasser SP. Medicinal mushrooms as a source of antitumor and immunomodulating polysaccharides. *Appl Microbiol Biotechnol.* 2002;60(3):258-274.

55. Sullivan R, Smith JE, Rowan NJ. Medicinal mushrooms and cancer therapy: translating a traditional practice into Western medicine. *Perspect Biol Med.* 2006;49(2):159-170.

56. Grube B, Eng ET, Kao Y-C, Kwon A, Chen S. White button mushroom phytochemicals inhibit aromatase activity and breast cancer cell proliferation. *J Nutr.* 2001;131(12):3288-3293.

57. Zhang M, Huang J, Xie X, Holman CD. Dietary intakes of mushrooms and green tea combine to reduce the risk of breast cancer in Chinese women. *Int J Cancer.* 2009;124(6):1404-1408.

58. Sloan EK, Priceman SJ, Cox BF, et al. The sympathetic nervous system induces a metastatic switch in primary breast cancer. *Cancer Res.* 2010;70(18):7042-7052.

59. Lutgendorf SK, Johnsen EL, Cooper B, et al. Vascular endothelial growth factor and social support in patients with ovarian carcinoma. *Cancer.* 2002;95(4):808-815.

60. Fang CY, Ridge JA, Lango MN, et al. Biobehavioral pathways in head and neck cancer [abstract # 2051]. Society of Behavioral Medicine 32nd Annual Meeting and Scientific Sessions. April 28, 2011.

61. Hoffman CJ, Ersser SJ, Hopkinson JM, et al. Effectiveness of mindfulness-based stress reduction in mood, breast- and endocrine-related quality of life, and well-being in stage 0 to III breast cancer: A randomized, controlled trial. *J Clin Oncol.* 2012;30(12):1335-1342.

62. Sojcher R, Gould Foerite S, Perlman A. Evidence and potential mechanism for mindfulness practices and energy psychology for obesity and binge-eating disorder. *Explore.* 2012;8(5):271-276.

63. NIH Consensus Conference. Acupuncture. *JAMA.*1998;280(17):1518-1524.

64. O'Sullivan EM, Higginson IJ. Clinical effectiveness and safety of acupuncture in the treatment of irradiation-induced xerostomia in patients with head and neck cancer: A systematic review. *Acupunct Med.* 2010; 28(4):191-199.

65. Wong RK, James JL, Sagar S, et al. Phase 2 results from Radiation Therapy Oncology Group Study 0537: a phase 2/3 study comparing acupuncture-like transcutaneous electrical nerve stimulation versus pilocarpine in treating early radiation-induced xerostomia. *Cancer.* 2012;118(17):4244-4252.

66. Anderson V. Improving outcomes: discussing healthy lifestyle choices with your patients. *ASCO Connection.* 2013;4:12-16. Published online December 12, 2012 at https://connection.asco.org/Magazine/Article/id/3402/Improving-Outcomes-Discussing-Healthy-Lifestyle-Choices-with-Your-Patients.aspx.

67. Byers T. Anticancer vitamins de jour: the ABCED's so far. *Am J Epidemiol.* 2010;172(1):1-3.

Diets, Functional Foods and Dietary Supplements for Cancer Prevention and Survival

Sarah O'Brien, MS, RD, CSO
Maureen Leser, MS, RDN, CSO, LD
Natalie Ledesma, MS, RDN, CSO

Introduction

The nutritional core of cancer prevention is a plant-based diet dominated by whole foods. A body of research has identified cancer-preventive benefits in whole grains, fruits, vegetables and beans/legumes; these foods are fundamental components of a varied, healthful diet. Evidence also suggests that consuming excess amounts of solid fats and added sugars as well as processed meats and excess calories may increase cancer risk. This research is reflected in evidence-based guidelines (1) including the 2010 Dietary Guidelines for Americans (DGA) (2) as well as nutrition recommendations published by the American Cancer Society (ACS) (3) and the World Cancer Research Fund/American Institute for Cancer Research (WCRF/AICR) (4).

For cancer prevention and survival, there is no known substitute for the wide array of nutrients, fibers, phytonutrients, prebiotics, antioxidants and anti-inflammatory compounds that act independently and synergistically to deter carcinogenesis. Functional foods, which are conventional foods that have been enhanced to benefit health beyond the effects of basic nutrition, can provide versatile options for meeting nutrition and health needs. Their benefits may be particularly valuable when matched to the unique needs of each cancer survivor and when someone is unable to consume certain conventional foods. Dietary supplements, in particular vitamin and/or mineral supplementation, may fill gaps in nutrient intake and be essential for replenishing deficient states, but have not proved to be valuable for cancer prevention and in some cases may increase cancer risk (5). Emerging research suggests that some bioactive compounds available in supplement form may help manage side effects of cancer treatments or improve treatment efficacy. However, effective and safe doses of these supplements are still unknown. Using dietary supplements during cancer treatment may have potential benefits but also presents risks, and may be most appropriate in research settings or when closely monitored by the medical team.

With approximately one-third of cancers being attributed to a poor diet, efforts to modify cancer risk by appropriate dietary changes,

Figure 1: Role of Functional Foods in the Health Care Continuum

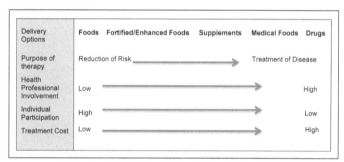

Reprinted courtesy of the Institute of Food Technologists, www.ift.org

facilitated by the use of functional foods, and followed by appropriate dietary supplementation to achieve specific health goals may prove to be an effective and efficient model that enhances health care of the cancer survivor. Figure 1 describes the therapeutic roles of foods, functional foods, dietary supplements and drugs in the health care continuum and the relative role of health professionals and individuals in this model.

This chapter critiques alternative diets marketed for cancer treatment and prevention; examines the significance of the emerging functional food market to oncology nutrition; and reviews the popularity, safety and efficacy of dietary supplements commonly used by cancer survivors. To navigate the intersections among these categories, nutrition intervention should be directed by results of a nutrition assessment. Intervention should begin with dietary improvements and modifications, incorporate functional foods as indicated, and utilize dietary supplements when dietary and functional foods interventions are inadequate for meeting nutrition needs. The registered dietitian (RD) should discuss findings regarding use of herbal and botanical supplements with the multidisciplinary team, who will discuss research and safety issues before jointly making a recommendation for each patient.

References

1. King JC. An evidence-based approach for establishing dietary guidelines. *J Nutr.* 2007;137(2):480-483.
2. U.S. Department of Agriculture and U.S. Department of Health and Human Services. Dietary Guidelines for Americans, 2010. 7th Edition, Washington, DC: U.S. Government Printing Office, December 2010.
3. Kushi LH, Doyle C, McCullough M. American Cancer Society Guidelines on nutrition and physical activity for cancer prevention: reducing the risk of cancer with healthy food choices and physical activity. *CA Cancer J Clin.* 2012;62(1):30-67.
4. World Cancer Research Fund/American Institute for Cancer Research. Food, Nutrition, Physical Activity, and the Prevention of Cancer: a Global Perspective. Washington DC: AICR 2007.
5. Marra MV, Boyar AP. Position of the American Dietetic Association: Nutrient Supplementation. *J Am Diet Assoc.* 2009;109(12):2073-2085.

Integrative Use of Diets in Cancer Treatment and Survival

Overview

All cancers involve the malfunction of genes that control cell growth and division. While some inherited gene mutations can increase cancer risk, a variety of biological and environmental events also may alter genes and gene expression. Researchers increasingly recognize that nutrients and by-products of nutrient metabolism may turn genes on and off, a role that, depending upon one's diet, may decrease or increase cancer risk.

Increased recognition of the role of diet in preventing and treating cancer has raised the profile of nutrition screening, assessment and intervention among those undergoing cancer treatment. Nutrition assessment provided by an RD includes assessing dietary intake and addressing whether and which dietary patterns may be appropriate and beneficial for cancer treatment and long-term cancer survival. This review critiques alternative diets marketed for cancer treatment.

Alternative Diets for Cancer Prevention and Survival

Approximately three-fourths of all cancers are diagnosed in persons 55 years and older; therefore, it is clear that increasing age is an important risk factor for cancer. Nevertheless, lifestyle habits are also important; approximately one-third of cancers are related to overweight/obesity, physical inactivity and poor nutrition (1). Cancer survivors are aware of this association, and are very interested in using diet to improve short and long-term cancer outcomes. Several evidence-based diet and nutrition recommendations fit this purpose, including the 2010 Dietary Guidelines for Americans (DGA) (2) and MyPlate (3), the latter of which provides visual and practical tools that help consumers implement the DGA. Diets including a range of whole foods provide bioactive compounds that have complementary biological effects on health promotion and disease prevention. Studies suggest that adhering to nutrition recommendations proposed by ACS and WCRF/AICR can reduce cancer risk (5-6).

Even though evidence-based nutrition recommendations are available and effective, a cancer diagnosis increases vulnerability to claims that an alternative dietary pattern may provide a cure. Most alternative dietary patterns marketed as cancer cures do not originate from science but from an individual's efforts to cure or treat his/her own medical ailments or a philosophical ideology. Max Gerson, M.D. originally developed the Gerson Therapy to self-treat migraine headaches (7). The Macrobiotic Diet is based on a philosophical ideology that applies a conception of the universe to diet and biology (8). Alternative anti-cancer diets are commonly purported to work via cleansing the body of toxins or boosting the immune system.

A number of anti-cancer diets have gained a following, though only one has undergone rigorous scientific investigation. For seven years, pancreatic cancer patients adhering to the Gonzalez regimen (without conventional treatment) were followed along with a group who received conventional chemotherapy treatment for pancreatic cancer. Survivors treated with standard chemotherapy reported a better quality of life and survived 10 months longer than those treated with the Gonzalez regimen alone (9-10).

Often developed decades ago, very few alternative anti-cancer diets have evolved their recommendations as research has revealed new discoveries. The macrobiotic diet has eased restrictions since it was first developed and when carefully planned can be nutritionally adequate. Recognizing that the original diet plan posed a high risk of nutrient deficiencies, The Gerson Therapy now advises nutrient supplementation, which was shunned by the original program. However, many alternative diet plans ignore new research findings, and do a disservice to cancer survivors who are open to integrative nutrition recommendations but also expect them to be respectful of science.

Although scientific evidence supporting most alternative anti-cancer diet plans is lacking, it is important to recognize that cancer survivors may achieve a sense of hope and control from these plans. Armed with a scientific understanding of anti-cancer nutrition and alternative diets for cancer treatment, RDs should offer suggestions and support to guide patients in making positive health and quality of life decisions. Examining the adequacy of usual dietary intake and use of alternative dietary practices is an important component of a nutrition assessment. When committed to an alternative dietary plan, survivors can still be encouraged to continue health-promoting components of the plan while avoiding harmful practices. Table 1, posted on the next few pages, summarizes several commonly promoted anti-cancer diets and critiques their nutritional adequacy.

References

1. U.S. Department of Agriculture and U.S. Department of Health and Human Services. Dietary Guidelines for Americans, 2010. 7th Edition, Washington, DC: U.S. Government Printing Office, December 2010.
2. U.S. Department of Agriculture. MyPlate. Washington, DC: http://www.choosemyplate.gov/ Accessed 7-20-13.

3. Kushi LH, Coyle C, McCullough M, et al. American Cancer Society guidelines on nutrition and physical activity for cancer prevention. *CA: A Cancer Journal for Clinicians.* 2012;62(1):30-67.
4. World Cancer Research Fund/American Institute for Cancer Research. Food, Nutrition, Physical Activity, and the Prevention of Cancer: a Global Perspective. Washington DC: AICR 2007.
5. McCullough ML, Patel AV, Kushi LH, et al. Following cancer prevention guidelines reduces risk of cancer, cardiovascular disease, and all-cause mortality. *Cancer Epidemiol Biomarkers Prev.* 2011;20(6):1089-1097.
6. Cerhan JR, Potter JD, Gilmore JM, et al. Adherence to the AICR cancer prevention recommendations and subsequent morbidity and mortality in the Iowa Women's Health Study cohort. *Cancer Epidemiol Biomarkers Prev.* 2004;13(7):1114-1120.
7. American Cancer Society. Gerson Therapy. http://www.cancer.org/treatment/treatmentsandsideeffects/complementaryandalternativemedicine/dietandnutrition/gerson-therapy Accessed 7-20-13.
8. American Cancer Society. Macrobiotic Diet. http://www.cancer.org/treatment/treatmentsandsideeffects/complementaryandalternativemedicine/dietandnutrition/macrobiotic-diet Accessed 7-20-13.
9. Chabot JA, Tsai WY, Fine RL, et al.: Pancreatic proteolytic enzyme therapy compared with gemcitabine-based chemotherapy for the treatment of pancreatic cancer. *J Clin Oncol.* 2010;28(12):2058-2063.
10. National Cancer Institute. Gonzalez Regimen. http://www.cancer.gov/cancertopics/pdq/cam/gonzalez/patient/page2/AllPags. Last modified 5/24/12. Accessed 7/22/13.

Table 1: Comparison of Alternative Diets Proposed For Cancer Treatment

Diet	Alkaline Diet (1-4)	Budwig Diet (5-6)	Essiac and Flor-Essence (7-8)
General Description	Claims that an acidic environment is toxic to the body and increases cancer risk. The version promoted by the Acid-Alkaline Association (AAA) is intended to balance pH by consuming 80% alkaline foods (e.g., vegetables, fruits, legumes) and 20% acid-forming foods (e.g., beef and poultry, dairy foods, eggs, coffee, sugar and alcohol). AAA describes ten levels of the alkaline diet with additional restrictions as the diet approaches the tenth level (i.e., a 100% raw food vegan diet). AAA states that some food combinations should be avoided (e.g., bananas and oranges). Unusual dietary habits may be recommended, such as eating at specified times. Drinking 2+ quarts of water daily is also recommended.	Emphasizes natural, unrefined foods. Sweeteners allowed include raw non-pasteurized honey, dates, figs, berry, fruit juices and stevia. Whole grains are allowed. A flaxseed oil and cottage cheese (FOCC) or quark recipe is consumed twice a day. It blends flaxseed oil, low-fat quark or cottage cheese, whole flax seeds and honey with optional ingredients. Because some become nauseous after consuming this, advocates are asked to eat papaya immediately afterwards. Avoids refined foods, hydrogenated oils, trans fats, animal fats, pork (some reports say all meats), seafood, dairy products (other than cottage cheese used to make Budwig Muesli), soy, and corn. For cancer treatment, the diet is combined with specific breathing exercises and enemas if tolerated.	Proponents claim it strengthens the immune system, improves quality of life, shrinks tumors and lengthens life. Essiac is an herbal mixture developed in Canada in the 1920s. The herbs are brewed into a tea. Burdock root, inner bark of slippery elm and sheep sorrel are included in essiac; Flor essence also includes Indian rhubarb root, watercress, blessed thistle, red clover and kelp. The tea may be prepared with spring or non-fluoridated water and is kept refrigerated. One-ounce is consumed one to three times daily. Proponents drink Essiac tea on an empty stomach, 2 hours before or after meals, for one to two years; consuming up to 12 ounces daily may be recommended.
Major Food Groups Avoided	Red meat, sugar, white rice, refined flours, coffee and alcohol. Some versions of the alkaline diet also omit dairy foods. The diet may over-restrict protein, calcium, and vitamin D and it may be difficult to consume adequate calories. The diet becomes more deficient in nutrients as it progresses to level 10.	Dairy (except for cottage cheese) and complete protein sources are avoided, so the diet may be limited in protein and calcium. It also may be limited in calories.	No dietary restrictions
Recommends Supplements?	No	No	No
Clinical trials?	There is no scientific evidence available that supports the effectiveness or safety of this diet in humans.	No	No published clinical trials. Animal studies showed no anti-tumor effects. Individually, Indian rhubarb and burdock may have anti-tumor effects.
Other	Calcium and/or vitamin D supplements are likely needed. Other supplements (or a multivitamin-mineral supplement) also may be needed. When kidney function is normal the body will maintain pH balance regardless of diet. The pH of urine (used to assess this diet's efficacy) changes as the body regulates pH.	The diet encourages use of essiac tea and allows one glass of red wine and some champagne.	Essiac tea has a laxative effect but also may cause nausea, vomiting, diarrhea, constipation, and headaches. An investigation by the Cancer Commission found there was limited evidence this product is effective.

(Continued)

Table 1: Comparison of Alternative Diets Proposed For Cancer Treatment *(continued)*

Diet	Fasting (9-11)	Gerson Therapy (12)	Gonzalez Regimen (13-14)
General Description	Proponents claim that fasting allows the body to focus energy on cleansing and healing itself. Additional claims: fasting supports the immune system, starves tumors and stimulates cellular repair. Adherents avoid all food and drink only water for several days at a time. Dry fasts avoid all liquids and juice fasts may allow only water and juice for several days, though broths and teas are sometimes allowed.	Described as a natural treatment that activates the body's ability to heal itself. It includes a vegetarian diet, raw juices, coffee enemas (for detoxification) and natural supplements. Three vegetable meals and fruits and vegetables for snacking are also recommended. Advises intake of 15 to 20 pounds of organically grown fruits and vegetables each day, most of which are juiced. One cup of juice is consumed each hour, 13 times per day. Raw carrot/apple and green-leaf juices are often recommended. This therapy also incorporates natural supplements and up to five coffee enemas daily. This diet also limits salt and fat	Describes itself as a metabolic therapy and includes dietary modifications, dietary supplements including pancreatic supplements for cancer patients and detoxification routines such as coffee enemas. Dietary patterns are individualized and may range from vegan diets to plans including red meat several times per day. Organic foods are preferred and processed foods such as white flour and white sugar are avoided. It includes animal organ extracts and digestive enzymes. From 130 to 175 capsules per day are taken.
Major Food Groups Avoided	No food or just juice, so diet is deficient in all or most food groups and nutrients	Avoids fat and many complete protein sources.	Varies according to individual recommendations
Recommends Supplements?	No	Yes; program includes supplements of vitamin B12 and potassium as well as pancreatic enzymes and thyroid hormone.	Yes; recommends large doses of vitamin and mineral supplements, animal glandular products (primarily for pancreatic enzymes) and food concentrates.
Clinical trials?	Animal studies suggest that fasting may make cancer cells more susceptible to treatment while protecting non-cancerous cells. A study of fasting in 10 elderly cancer patients found fewer treatment-related side effects.	No randomized clinical trials (RCTs) have been conducted with this diet. A retrospective review conducted in 1995 by the Gerson Research Organization reported positive results. Non-randomized efforts to examine this diet were poorly designed and suffered from high drop-out rates. The ACS urges cancer patients to avoid this and other metabolic therapies.	In a non-randomized, clinical trial, quality of life was better and survival time was greater in patients on conventional chemotherapy rather than the Gonzalez regimen.
Other	Total fasting limits all nutrient intake and results in malnutrition if used for an extensive time. Dry fasting can lead to dehydration and death if continued for long periods. Fasting may temporarily result in headaches, dizziness, fatigue and low blood pressure. Food intake may improve bioavailability of some cancer drugs, raising a question about effective dosing during fasting.	Poses a risk for malnutrition (from severe dietary restrictions), dehydration, and colitis (from frequent enemas). The Gerson Institute is a non-profit located in San Diego, CA.	The U.S. FDA has not approved the Gonzalez regimen for cancer treatment. *(Continued)*

References

1. Schwalfenberg GK. The alkaline diet: Is there evidence that an alkaline pH diet benefits health? *J Environmental Public Health.* 2012; 2012: 727630. Published online 2011 October 12. doi: 10.1155/2012/727630.
2. The Acid Alkaline Association. Acid alkaline balance diet. http://www.acidalkalinediet.net/acid-alkaline-diet.php Accessed 7/20/13.
3. Acid Alkaline Association. http://www.acidalkalinediet.net/acid-alkaline-diet.php Accessed June 20, 2013.
4. Collins S. Alkaline diet: what to know before trying it. *Web*MD. http://www.webmd.com/diet/features/alkaline-diets-what-to-know?page=2Now 7 Kaegi E. Unconventional therapies for cancer: 1.
5. Dana Farber Cancer Institute. The Budwig Diet. http://www.dana-farber.org/Health-Library/Budwig-Diet-During-Chemotherapy.aspx Accessed 7/20/13
6. The Budwig Diet. http://www.budwigcenter.com/anti-cancer-diet.php Accessed 7/20/13
7. Kaegi E. Unconventional therapies for cancer: 1. *Essiac. CMAJ.* 1998;158:897-902.
8. American Cancer Society. Essiac Tea. Last Revised 10/14/2011. http://www.cancer.org/treatment/treatmentsandsideeffects/complementaryandalternativemedicine/herbsvitaminsandminerals/essiac-tea Accessed 7/20/13.
9. Fasting: American Cancer Society. Fasting. http://www.cancer.org/treatment/treatmentsandsideeffects/complementaryandalternativemedicine/dietandnutrition/fasting Last revised 2/27/12. Accessed June 20, 2013
10. Babbage (science and technology). Starving the beast. *The Economist.* February 9th, 2012. Accessed June 20, 2013.

Table 1: Comparison of Alternative Diets Proposed For Cancer Treatment *(continued)*

Diet	Livingston-Wheeler (15)	Macrobiotic Diet (16-17)	Raw Food Plan (18-19)
General Description	Livingston Wheeler is considered a metabolic treatment. The program combines a vegetarian diet supplemented with vitamins, minerals and digestive enzymes with antibiotic treatment. The patients also received an individualized vaccine usually derived from the patient's own blood or urine.	A philosophy and diet based on avoidance of toxins. Emphasizes organic and primarily vegetarian foods with a typical daily distribution of: 50%-60% organic whole grains, 20%-25% organic, locally grown fruits and organic vegetables, and 5%-10% soup prepared with beans, miso, and vegetables. Fruit not locally grown is excluded, as are some vegetables (e.g., potatoes, tomatoes, eggplant, asparagus, and others). Seeds and nuts are allowed. Refined sugars are excluded and naturally sweetened desserts are limited. Specific cooking methods and utensils are recommended.	The "Living Foods Diet" allows only raw foods or foods heated to 105 degrees F (40.5 degrees C). About 75% of foods consumed are fruits and vegetables but proponents also eat seaweed, sprouts, seeds, beans, whole grains and nuts. Sprouting and dehydration are common. Supporters claim that less processed foods and fewer added ingredients preserve enzymes in food and provide health benefits
Major Food Groups Avoided	This diet excludes poultry, meat, eggs, and milk. A vegetarian diet can provide all required nutrients.	Avoids all meat, dairy, eggs and processed sweeteners. The earliest version of this diet advised eating only whole grains and was linked to multiple nutritional deficiencies and death.	Avoids all meat, dairy foods and eggs.
Recommends Supplements?	Yes	No	Yes; the diet recommends vitamin B12, vitamin D, and calcium supplements.
Efficacy studied in clinical trials	There is no scientific evidence available that supports the effectiveness or safety of this diet.	No RCTs; limited research shows no evidence of improved survival. The National Center for Complementary and Alternative Medicine (NCCAM) at the NIH has funded a study to examine cancer-preventive benefits of the macrobiotic diet.	Studies on health and nutrition aspects of raw foods or living food diets are limited.
Other	The diet may be deficient in protein, calcium, iron, vitamins D and B12 and protein. In 1990 the California Department of Health Services ordered the clinic to stop giving the vaccine. When open, ACS strongly advised cancer patients to avoid this treatment. The clinic that offered this therapy is no longer in operation but some proponents still follow the diet.	The current version of the macrobiotic diet is plant based and when planned carefully can meet nutrition needs. Proponents do not use microwaves or electricity to cook food. Food is chewed until fluid. The diet may be deficient in vitamin B12 and potentially deficient in protein, zinc, calcium, vitamin D and iron. Cancer patients experiencing involuntary weight loss from inadequate intake are at risk of additional nutrient insufficiencies and deficiencies.	The diet may be deficient in calories, protein, iron, calcium, vitamin B12 and zinc.

11. National Cancer Institute (NCI). NCI Cancer Bulletin. To eat or not to eat: with cancer therapies, that is the questions. http://www.cancer.gov/ncicancerbulletin/071012/page5 Accessed June 20, 2013.

12. American Cancer Society. Gerson Therapy. http://www.cancer.org/treatment/treatmentsandsideeffects/complementaryandalternativemedicine/dietandnutrition/gerson-therapy Accessed June 20, 2013.

13. Gonzalez treatment. National Cancer Institute. http://www.cancer.gov/cancertopics/pdq/cam/gonzalez/patient/page1 Last modified May 24, 2012. Accessed June 20, 2013.

14. Dr-Gonzalez.com: individualized nutritional protocols. http://www.dr-gonzalez.com/index.htm Accessed June 20, 2013.

15. The American Cancer Society. Livingston-Wheeler Therapy. http://www.cancer.org/treatment/treatmentsandsideeffects/complementaryandalternativemedicine/pharmacologicalandbiologicaltreatment/livingstone-wheeler-therapy Accessed 7/20/13.

16. American Cancer Society. Macrobiotic Diet. http://www.cancer.org/treatment/treatmentsandsideeffects/complementaryandalternativemedicine/dietandnutrition/macrobiotic-diet Accessed June 20, 2013.

17. Russell NC. The University of Texas MD Anderson Center. Nutrition and Special Diets: Macrobiotics. http://www.mdanderson.org/education-and-research/resources-for-professionals/clinical-tools-and-resources/cimer/therapies/nutrition-and-special-diets/macrobiotics.html Accessed June 20, 2013.

18. Raw Food diet. WebMD. http://www.webmd.com/food-recipes/guide/raw-food-diet. Acessed June 20, 2013.

19. Raw food reference from the Academy of Nutrition and Dietetics. Accessed June 20, 2013.

Integrative Use of Functional Foods in Cancer Treatment and Survival

History and Definition

Whole foods are prized for their natural array of nutrients, phytonutrients and other health-promoting bioactive compounds; however, for nearly one hundred years food and health agencies have recognized the need to enrich, fortify, and/or enhance food to improve public health. Since the early 20th century food manufacturers have fortified or enriched food, sometimes to replace what had been removed during processing (e.g., enriching grains with niacin and iron to prevent pellagra and iron deficiency, respectively) and at other times to achieve a public health goal (e.g., fortifying milk with vitamin D to prevent rickets and improve bone health and fortifying grains with folic acid to prevent neural tube defects) (1). Today, food manufacturers replace nutrients lost in food processing (i.e., food enrichment); add nutrients not normally found in some foods (i.e., food fortification) and enhance foods with a variety of physiologically active compounds that provide consumers with a means to self-treat a condition or disease (2).

The Academy of Nutrition and Dietetics (the Academy) defines functional foods as "whole foods along with fortified, enriched, or enhanced foods that have a potentially beneficial effect on health when consumed as part of a varied diet on a regular basis at effective levels based on significant standards of evidence" (2). Definitions vary among organizations, but most emphasize that benefits of functional foods go beyond those provided by basic nutrition (3-4).

While whole foods should be considered the ideal functional foods, the term is used more often to describe foods enhanced with ingredients chosen for specific health purposes. The Academy states

Table 1: Categories of Functional Foods (2)

Category	Examples
Conventional Foods	Vegetables, fruits, grains, dairy and fish provide a variety of non-nutritive bioactive compounds (e.g., antioxidant vitamins, isoflavones and prebiotics) that influence health
Modified Foods	Ready-to-eat cereals fortified and enriched with vitamins, minerals and phytonutrients including lycopene and lutein
	Margarines and spreads fortified or enhanced with bioactive substances such as n-3 fatty acids
Food Ingredients	Indigestible carbohydrates such as resistant starch that provide prebiotic benefits

that functional foods fall into three general categories, as indicated in Table 1 (2).

Regulations

FDA regulations for functional foods fall under those for conventional foods. Health claims must meet requirements of the Nutritional Labeling and Education Act of 1990, which characterize relationships between bioactive substances and disease risk reduction based on a "standard of significant scientific agreement" (5). Qualified health claims also describe diet-disease relationships but are used when research results do not reach the highest level of evidence. Claims are allowed between food (including functional foods) and six disease categories, cancer being one (5).

Health Benefits

A food developed for a specific condition or disease (e.g., a food product developed for phenylketonuria) is considered a medical food rather than a functional food. On the other hand, foods providing general health benefits, including medical nutrition beverages supplemented with protein, vitamins, minerals and sometimes other compounds such as glutamine fall under the functional food umbrella. Yogurts with added fibers and probiotics, juices fortified with added calcium and snack bars fortified with isoflavones also are functional foods. Ready-to-eat cereals are a vehicle for many bioactive compounds including B vitamins, iron, calcium, vitamin D, lutein, lycopene and zeaxanthin. Snack bars are a common source of soy isoflavones as well as indigestible carbohydrates that promote a variety of gastrointestinal effects; resistant starch is digested slowly and may help maintain the right balance of microbes in the digestive system. Functional food ingredients are selected for their versatility in food processing in addition to their health effects, as manufacturers are interested in marketing functional foods that are likely to be popular (e.g., snack bars and ready-to-eat cereals).

Dietary improvement, dietary fortification/enrichment and dietary supplementation can prevent nutrient insufficiencies and deficiencies. While dietary improvement is the first goal, functional foods are a valid and versatile source of nutrients and other bioactive compounds when conventional food sources are not appropriate or effective and when nutrient needs may be greater than usual (e.g., malabsorption, vegan lifestyle, cultural preferences, presence of nutrition impact symptoms).

The sheer number of health-promoting substances in whole foods poses a daunting task for researchers, making it difficult to identify the optimal dose of each compound for a specific purpose. Consumers are unlikely to anticipate adverse effects that may arise when consuming identical or similar compounds in foods, functional foods and dietary supplements. While soyfoods consumed in moderate amounts are generally considered safe for breast cancer survivors, consuming genistein in conventional foods, functional foods, and dietary supplements can potentially provide far more of this compound than would be consumed by several servings of conventional soyfoods per day. Table 2 lists the bioactive

Table 2: Functional Food Sources of Select Cancer-Fighting Compounds (6-20)

Compound	Potential Anti-Cancer Function	Conventional Food Sources	Functional Food Sources
Beta-Carotene*	Antioxidant activity	Carrots and other bright orange, red and yellow foods	Beta-carotene rich juice
β-glucans	Natural polysaccharide and soluble fiber that may boost the immune system	Barley, oats, fruits, vegetables and seaweed	β-glucan-enriched breakfast cereals, breads, snack bars, bran products and milk beverages
Genistein	May block estrogen receptors; early exposure to genistein may decrease breast cancer risk	Soyfood, including edamame, tofu and soymilk	Genistein added to a variety of foods including snack bars
Inulin and fructo-oligosaccharides (FOS), a by-product of inulin	Exhibits prebiotic activity, which can enhance intestinal health	Onions, shallots, Jerusalem artichokes	Inulin can be incorporated into food as a fat replacement FOS and inulin added to beverages and jellies
Lignans	Phytoestrogen; associated with reduced risk of breast cancer	Flaxseed is the richest source; grind flaxseed to improve digestion (whole seeds sometimes pass through the digestive system intact); sesame seeds, chickpeas, oats and barley	Flaxseed added to snack bars and muffins
Lutein	Lutein is a xanthophyll, has antimutagenic and anticarcinogenic properties	Dark green leafy vegetables including spinach and kale, broccoli, squash, green peas, lettuce, onions, corn, pumpkin and egg yolk	Lutein added to some ready-to-eat cereals
Lycopene	Antioxidant; blocks activity of free radicals	Tomatoes and tomato products (i.e., tomato sauce, tomato paste, tomato juice) as well as other red, yellow and orange fruits and vegetables	Lycopene added to some ready-to-eat cereals; tomato lycopene complexes developed for functional foods
Omega-3 fats	Anti-inflammatory activity	Fatty fish	Eggs fortified with omega-3 fats
Soluble fibers (e.g., guar gum, pectin, acacia gum and psyllium)	Promote intestinal health	Oats, lentils, apples, oranges, bananas, pears, strawberries, nuts, flaxseeds, beans, dried peas, blueberries	Soluble fiber available in banana flakes; soluble fibers added to some ready-to-eat cereals and other functional foods

* Regular intake of spreads containing plant sterols may decrease carotenoid levels by 10-20%; consuming an extra serving per day of carotenoid-rich food can prevent this effect (21)

compounds naturally found in food and available in functional foods; in many cases they are also sold in dietary supplements. Dietary intake assessment should determine use of functional foods and dietary supplements in order to assess total intake of all nutritive and bioactive compounds.

Summary

Many consumers and cancer survivors are interested in merging health benefits of food with traditional medical approaches to combat disease (3); functional foods may be viewed as an additional means to reduce disease risk and promote good health. RDs educate and counsel cancer survivors on cancer-preventive nutrition, sometimes using meal plans, recipes and food lists to demonstrate how functional and conventional foods can be integrated within a diet to provide overall health and cancer-preventive value. At times, this education may eliminate the need for (and cost of) dietary supplements. When a nutrition assessment reveals that diet alone, even with evidence-based dietary modifications, cannot meet nutrition needs, the availability of functional foods provides an additional route of intervention. It is important to stay current with

functional foods entering the marketplace and their potential benefits for cancer survivors.

References

1. Backstrand JR. The history and future of food fortification in the United States: a public health perspective. *Nutr Rev.* 2002;60(1):15-26.
2. The Academy of Nutrition and Dietetics. Position of the Academy of Nutrition and Dietetics: Functional Foods. *J Acad Nutr Diet.* 2013; 113:1096-1103.
3. Institute of Food Technologists. Functional foods: Opportunities and challenges. March 2005. http://www.ift.org/Knowledge-Center/Read-IFT-Publications/Science-Reports/Scientific-Status-Summaries/~/media/Knowledge%20Center/Science%20Reports/Expert%20Reports/Functional%20Foods/Functionalfoods_expertreport_full.pdf Accessed 8-11-13.
4. Health Canada. Policy paper—Nutraceuticals/functional foods and health claims on foods. http://www.hc-sc.gc.ca/fn-an/label-etiquet/claims-reclam/nutra-funct_foods-nutra-fonct_aliment-eng.php#2. (now archived) .Published November 1998. Accessed October 24, 2012.
5. Food and Drug Administration. Guidance for industry: A food labeling guide. http://www.fda.gov/Food/GuidanceCompliance Regulatory Information/GuidanceDocuments/ FoodLabelingNutrition/Food LabelingGuide/ http://www.fda.gov/downloads/Food/Guidance Regulation/UCM265446.pdf Revised October 2009. Accessed October 24, 2012.

6. Michaud DS, Feskanich D, Rimm EB, et al. Intake of specific carotenoids and risk of lung cancer in 2 prospective US cohorts. *Am J Clin Nutr*. 2000; 72(4):990-997.

7. Omenn GS, Goodman GE, Thornquist MD, et al. Effects of a combination of beta-carotene and vitamin A on lung cancer and cardiovascular disease. *New Engl J Med*. 1996;334(18):1150-1155.

8. Holick CN, Michaud DS, Stolzenberg-Solomon R, et al. Dietary carotenoids, serum beta-carotene, and retinol and risk of lung cancer in the alpha-tocopherol, beta-carotene cohort study. *Am J Epidemiol*. 2002;156(6): 536-547.

9. Noakes M, Clifton P, Ntanios F, Shrapnel W, Record I, McInerney J. An increase in dietary carotenoids when consuming plant sterols or stanols is effective in maintaining plasma carotenoid concentrations. *Am J Clin Nutr*. 2002;75(1):79-86.

10. B-glycan reference: Chan GCF, Chan WK, Man-Yuen D. The effects of B-glucan on human immune and cancer cells. *J Hematol Oncol*. 2009; 2: 25. Published online 2009 June 10. doi: 10.1186/1756-8722-2-25

11. Warri A, Saarinen NM, Makela S, Hilakivi-Clarke L. The role of early life genistein exposures in modifying breast cancer risk. *Br J Cancer*. 2008; 98(9):1485-1493.

12. Borromei C, Careri M, Cavazza A, et al. Evaluation of fructooligosaccharides and inulins as potentially health benefiting food ingredients by HPAEC-PED and MALDI-TOF MS. *Int J Analytical Chem*. 2009. Article ID 530639, 9 pages http://dx.doi.org/10.1155/2009/530639.

13. Patterson RE. Flaxseed and breast cancer: What should we tell our patients? *J Clin Oncol*. 2011;29(28):3723-3724.

14. McCann SE, Hootman KC, Weaver AM. Dietary intakes of total and specific lignans are associated with clinical breast tumor characteristics. *J Nutr*. 2012;142(1):91-98.

15. Ribaya-Mercado JD, Blumberg JB. Lutein and zeaxanthin and their potential roles in disease prevention. *J Am College Nutr*. 2004;23(6): 567S-587S.

16. Memorial Sloan-Kettering Cancer Center. Integrative Medicine. Lutein. http://www.mskcc.org/cancer-care/herb/lutein Last updated 4-23-13. Accessed 8-15-13.

17. American Cancer Society. Lycopene. http://www.cancer.org/treatment/ treatmentsandsideeffects/complementaryandalternativemedicine/ dietandnutrition/lycopene. Last revised 5-10-13. Accessed 8-15-13.

18. Murphy RA, Mourtzakis M, Mazurak VC. N-3 polyunsaturated fatty acids: the potential role for supplementation in cancer. *Curr Opin Clin Nutr Metab Care*. 2012;15(2):246-251.

19. Shaikh IA, Brown I, Wahle KW, Heys SD. Enhancing cytotoxic therapies for breast and prostate cancers with polyunsaturated fatty acids. *Nutr Cancer*. 2010;62(3):284-296.

20. Negri E, Franceschi S, Parpinel M, LaVecchia C. Fiber intake and risk of colorectal cancer. *Cancer Epidemiol Biomarkers Prev*. 2991;7(8):667-671.

21. Ntanios FY, Duchateau GS. A healthy diet rich in carotenoids is effective in maintaining normal blood carotenoid levels during the daily use of plant sterol-enriched spreads. *Int J Vitam Nutr Res*. 2002;72(1):32-39.

Dietary Supplements for Cancer Survivors

Introduction

Interest in herbal/botanical, vitamin and mineral supplements surged in the latter half of the 20th century with many Americans considering these products natural, and therefore safer than prescription medicines. By the 1980s, with sales skyrocketing, it was clear that new legislation was needed to define dietary supplements. When debating legislation, the U.S. Senate Committee on Labor and Human Resources summarized a widely held consumer view of herbal products, stating "Unlike many drugs, the role of herbal

dietary supplements is to enhance the diet by adding safe and natural plants and their constituents to support and protect bodily functions and processes" (1).

In 1994, the U.S. Congress, when passing the Dietary Supplement Health and Education Act (DSHEA), defined and established a regulatory framework for dietary supplements (2). Dietary supplements were defined as products taken by mouth that provide ingredients intended to supplement the diet; they may include vitamin and minerals, herbal and botanical products, amino acids and other nutritive and dietary substances (2). The regulatory framework assigned responsibility for ensuring that products are safe before being marketed to the manufacturer. The burden of taking action against any unsafe dietary supplement was assigned to the FDA (2). Today, healthy Americans and those with chronic and acute conditions can purchase dietary supplements over the Internet and in supermarkets, drug stores and other retail outlets across the U.S. Although there is significant concern in the healthcare community that cancer survivors are vulnerable to unsubstantiated anti-cancer claims made for some dietary supplements, use of these products is widespread and growing.

The objective of *Dietary Supplements for Cancer Survivors* is to arm RDs with knowledge and resources to help them become proficient in this field.

Prevalence

The percentage of Americans using at least one dietary supplement increased from 42% in 1988–1994 to 54% in 2003–2006 (3). These numbers jump to 64% and 81% among cancer patients and long-term cancer survivors, respectively (4). While vitamin and mineral products are the most popular supplements used in the U.S., approximately 20% of Americans and 23% of cancer patients take herbal/botanical supplements (5-6). Cancer survivors are interested in exploring all options for managing their disease and treatment-related side effects, including use of dietary supplements to "help themselves" and to "boost their immunity" (7).

Dietary supplements fuel a multi-billion dollar industry; the 2007 National Health Interview Survey (NHIS) reported that Americans spent $15 billion dollars annually on non-vitamin non-mineral natural products alone (8). In 2011, U.S. sales of all dietary supplements totaled approximately $30 billion, an amount that included $12.4 billion for all vitamin- and mineral-containing supplements, of which $5.2 billion was for multi-vitamins and minerals (9).

Plants and Pharmaceuticals

Approximately 40% of pharmaceutical products are derived from plants (10). Thirty plant-derived compounds are currently being investigated for use in cancer therapy (10) and many other active but perhaps untested plant compounds are widely available in dietary supplements.

Plants and dietary supplements made from their parts (e.g., leaves and stems) possess a variety of active compounds that influence carcinogenesis. Some help regulate cell cycles; others modulate inflammation, promote DNA repair and reduce oxidative stress. They may influence drug metabolism, and by increasing or decreasing a drug's blood level can influence its therapeutic effect. Interactions can result from alterations in absorption, bioavailability and/ or drug clearance (11). Because dietary supplements are not required to undergo premarket evaluation, adverse side effects may not be recognized until reported by consumers.

Safety Profile of Dietary Supplements

By law, dietary supplement packaging must provide contact information for reporting adverse events, and in turn manufacturers and distributors of dietary supplements are required to forward reports of serious adverse effects to the FDA (12). Consumers can report adverse effects associated with dietary supplements to the MedWatch program (14). In 2011, the FDA reported receipt of 1,777 adverse event reports from the dietary supplement industry (15), though U.S. Poison Control Centers reported receiving 29,000 calls regarding adverse effects experienced after taking a dietary supplement (16). Chaparral, ephedra and comfrey are inherently unsafe and have been banned in the U.S. Pennyroyal is also unsafe but is still available in the marketplace. These products have been linked with serious liver toxicity and should never be consumed. The National Library of Medicine, under the auspices of the National Institute of Diabetes and Digestive and Kidney Diseases (NIDDK) of the National Institutes of Health (NIH) has established a resource to identify herbal and dietary supplements as well as conventional medications linked with liver toxicity (17). This website also includes a Case Submission Registry that allows users to submit case reports.

Select Interactions Between Cancer Treatments and Dietary Supplements

Researchers are examining effects of various plant-derived and nutrient supplements on the biological activity of cancer treatments and their side effects. Curcumin, which is found in the spice turmeric, can inhibit cyclooxygenase-2 (COX-2), an enzyme that stimulates synthesis of types of prostaglandins that increase inflammation (18).

Quercetin is a flavonoid found in a variety of foods including citrus fruits, apples, onions, parsley and tea. It is also sold as a dietary supplement. While flavonoids are now well known for their anti-inflammatory properties, quercetin (in doses sometimes found in dietary supplements) also can bind with iron and thereby decrease iron bioavailability, potentially increasing the risk of iron deficiency in vulnerable individuals undergoing cancer treatment (19).

The cytochrome P450 enzyme system is important to drug metabolism. Genetics, prescription drugs, food and dietary supplements may influence the activity of these enzymes, potentially decreasing drug efficacy or resulting in adverse effects. St. John's wort may influence the P450 system and can potentially reduce concentrations of some drugs including imatinib and irinotecan, which are commonly used in cancer treatments (20);

garlic, ginseng and gingko also may interact with cytochrome P450 substrates (20).

Aloe vera has a strong laxative effect; a case report revealed that an RD, during a nutrition reassessment, correctly identified an aloe vera beverage as the cause of diarrhea experienced by a hospitalized cancer patient, saving the post-stem cell transplant survivor from undergoing a lengthy work-up for the symptom (21-22). Coenzyme-Q10 (Co-Q10) has shown potential for limiting cardiac and renal toxicity of the chemotherapy agent Doxorubicin (Adriamycin®). A small, randomized study with 20 children supports this potential (23).

Researchers are examining whether selenium-based compounds may synergistically improve treatment efficacy of Taxol in triple-negative breast cancer, one of the most aggressive forms of this disease (24). A number of studies suggest that glutamine, which is essential for gastrointestinal health and wound healing (25), may lessen the degree of mucositis, stomatitis, esophagitis and diarrhea resulting from some cancer therapies (26-27), though not all studies support this benefit (28).

Research is just beginning to uncover the myriad of interactions among dietary supplements and cancer treatments, some of which promote while others may blunt desired outcomes. Until more is known about the most effective and safe formulation and dose of each supplement, it is unsafe to make recommendations for using these products during cancer treatment. However, cancer survivors undergoing treatment are using dietary supplements and perhaps unknowingly influencing the effectiveness of cancer treatment in one way or another.

Addressing dietary supplement use as part of a nutrition assessment should be the first step in comprehensive dietary supplement care management and should be followed by documenting types and doses of supplements taken. The RD should then share findings with the multidisciplinary team and participate in discussions to determine patient recommendations. Table 1 summarizes potential interactions between select dietary supplements and cancer treatments, and suggests appropriate RD actions and messages.

Vitamin-Mineral Supplements

Research examining the role of vitamin and mineral supplementation in cancer prevention has failed to consistently demonstrate a benefit. However, cancer survivors having difficulty eating because of nutrition impact symptoms may be at risk of malnutrition and/or nutrient deficiency and thus may benefit from a multivitamin/mineral supplement. An intake analysis of 19 micronutrients from natural foods, fortified and enriched food and nutrient-based dietary supplements found that vitamin and mineral supplements made important contributions to total micronutrient intake, thus demonstrating their benefit (42). Multi-vitamin/mineral supplements providing 100% of the Daily Value for each nutrient can be considered safe and likely adequate for healthy individuals, but it is important to evaluate individual needs per each cancer

Table 1: Select Drug: Supplement Interactions of Interest to Cancer Survivors

Dietary Supplement	Side Effects, Interactions, and RD Messages
Aloe Vera (21)	• Has a laxative effect • May exacerbate diarrhea in those at risk and may intensify action of laxatives • Inform medical team of noted associations; cross-check concurrent use of laxatives; develop a unified message
Coenzyme-Q10 (22, 29-30)	• May reduce renal and cardio-toxicity of Doxorubicin (Adriamycin®), but research is insufficient for recommending a specific dose • Initiate multi-disciplinary discussion on this research; help develop a unified message for patients taking coenzyme-Q10 supplements
Curcumin (31-32)	• In doses available in dietary supplements, may sensitize Cisplatin-resistant tumor cells to Cisplatin, thus improving its efficacy • May reduce Cisplatin-induced neurotoxicity • Incorporating turmeric within a varied diet is reasonable and safe • Initiate a multi-disciplinary discussion on available research and participate in developing a unified message
Melatonin (33-34)	• When simultaneously administered with tamoxifen, melatonin may improve anti-cancer response of women with metastatic breast cancer who did not respond to tamoxifen alone • Melatonin is also being investigated as a potential treatment for limiting oxidative damage to normal tissue during radiotherapy • Initiate a multi-disciplinary discussion on potential anti-cancer effects of melatonin and assist with the development of a unified message
Oleic acid (35-36)	• Oleic acid is a natural component of olive oil and avocado; it may provide cytotoxic synergism with Herceptin • Other bioactive components of olive oil also may improve sensitivity of Herceptin • At this time oleic acid is not sold as a dietary supplement • Advise the cancer survivor that olive oil and avocado are healthy foods that may have cancer-preventive benefits and are acceptable within tenets of a varied diet
Omega-3 fats (37-40)	• May reduce toxicity of Irinotecan and Paclitaxel • May enhance clinical benefit of Doxorubicin (Adriamycin®), Cisplatin and Vincristine • May enhance clinical benefit of pro-oxidant chemotherapies • Inclusion of food sources of omega-3 fats in the diet is appropriate as recommended in the 2010 Dietary Guidelines for Americans. Help develop and deliver a unified message on use of omega-3 fat supplements (i.e., usually fish oil)
Quercetin (19)	• Offers anti-inflammatory effects • May decrease bioavailability of iron • Initiate a multi-disciplinary discussion on available research and assist with the development of a unified message

survivor's diagnosis, symptoms and treatments. When a diet includes many fortified, enriched and functional foods, it may already be providing recommended nutrient needs.

Antioxidant Supplements and Cancer

There are two main controversies regarding the use of antioxidants: whether they are safe and provide any health benefit (or risk) when used during conventional cancer treatment, and whether long-term use of antioxidant supplements provides any protection against the development or recurrence of cancer and its mortality.

Taking Antioxidant Supplements While Receiving Conventional Treatment:
One school of thought proposes that taking antioxidant supplements during cancer treatments may reduce the effectiveness of therapy. Another school believes that antioxidant supplements may protect healthy cells and decrease side effects of treatment while also augmenting therapy. The literature has yielded mixed results. A review of 52 clinical trials examining effects of combining antioxidant supplementation (e.g., glutathione compounds, vitamin E, selenium, Co-Q10 and zinc) with conventional treatment found that a number of antioxidants studied conferred a benefit (e.g., reduced side effects) but no conclusion could be reached because of the wide variability in type of compound tested, dosage, and method of administration (e.g., at least five different types of vitamin

E have been tested, in doses ranging from 100 mg to 3200 IU) (43). Well-designed studies that consider the "complexity and diversity" (44) of antioxidants are needed before clinicians can confidently provide cancer survivors undergoing active treatment with much needed evidence-based advice on this controversy.

Antioxidants For Cancer Prevention:
The "5 a day" campaign resulted from research suggesting an inverse relationship between vegetable and fruit intake and risk of disease, including cancer (45). Vitamins, minerals, and phytonutrients in these foods likely act independently and synergistically to impart a wide range of cancer-preventive effects (46). While an early study suggested some cancer-preventive benefit from selenium (47), other trials found no benefit (48-49). RCTs examining effects of antioxidant supplements on cancer risk are summarized in Table 2.

Vitamin D, Calcium and Cancer

Observations revealing lower rates of certain cancers, including breast cancer, in regions with greater yearly sun exposure (54) led to research exploring biologic associations between vitamin D and cancer. Discoveries that the vitamin D receptor (VDR) is found in most cells including many cancer cells and that vitamin D helps regulate genes that modulate cell proliferation, differentiation and apoptosis support a biologic role in carcinogenesis (55).

Table 2: RCTs on Antioxidant Supplementation and Cancer Risk

Study	Antioxidant Supplement	Results
AATBC, 1994 (48)	Vitamin E 50 mg B-carotene 20 mg	Decreased risk of prostate cancer* Increased risk of lung cancer*
CARET (49)	B-carotene 30 mg Retinol (retinyl palmitate) 2500 IU	Increased risk of lung cancer in active treatment group*
Physicians Health Study II (50)	Vitamin C 500 mg Vitamin E 400 IU every other day	No effect on prostate cancer risk No effect on total cancer risk
SELECT (51)	Vitamin E 400 IU Selenium 200 mcg	Increased risk of prostate cancer (vitamin E alone)
SU.VI MAX (52)	Vitamin C 120 mg Vitamin E 30 mg B-carotene 6 mg Selenium 100 mcg Zinc 20 mg	No effect on cancer incidence or mortality between treatment and placebo groups. When stratified by sex, men in the treatment group had a lower risk of cancer and all-cause mortality than men receiving a placebo**
WACS (53)	Vitamin C 500 mg daily Vitamin E 60 IU every other day B-carotene 50 mg every other day	No effect on total cancer incidence or mortality (from single supplements or combinations)

ATBC: alpha-Tocopherol, Beta Carotene Cancer Prevention Study, CARET: The Carotene and Retinol Prevention Trial, WACS: Women's Antioxidant Cardiovascular Study, SU.VI.MAX: Supplementation en Vitamines et Mineraux Antioxydants Trial
*Results are statistically significant ($P < 0.05$)
** Results are statistically significant ($P = 0.004$)
Source: Adapted with permission from *Oncology Nutrition Connection* (2009;17(3):3-9) the newsletter of the Oncology Nutrition Dietetic Practice Group of the Academy of Nutrition and Dietetics

Associations between vitamin D intake and/or 25(OH)D levels and risk of breast, colorectal and prostate cancer are of particular interest to researchers. A number of observational studies have supported an inverse association between these vitamin D parameters and breast cancer (56-57) while others have not (58-59). The body of evidence examining 25(OH)D intake and blood levels and colorectal cancer risk weighs in favor of an inverse association (60-62) and a number of researchers have recommended specific 25(OH)D levels for reducing colorectal cancer risk (63-64). Most observational studies examining relationships between vitamin D (intake or circulating levels) and prostate cancer have reported null results (65-66). As additional studies examining the chemo-preventive role of vitamin D are published, RDs need to monitor results to keep abreast of this active research area.

Calcium exerts a variety of biologic effects that may be protective against certain cancers such as colorectal cancer but also may increase risk of other cancers such as prostate cancer. Observational studies examining associations between calcium intakes and prostate cancer risk have yielded mixed results (67-70). Only one randomized, controlled, double blind trial has investigated the effect of calcium supplementation on prostate cancer risk. After 10 years, risk of prostate cancer did not differ between research subjects randomized to 1,200 mg calcium per day or those randomized to placebo (71).

Few RCTs have examined the role of vitamin D and/or calcium on risk of breast, colon, and prostate cancer; Table 3 summarizes those that have been conducted (71-73).

Table 3: RCTs on Vitamin D/Calcium Supplements and Colon, Breast, and Prostate Cancer

Study	No.	Subject Characteristics	Vitamin D/ Calcium (daily)	Dose	Results
Nebraska Trial (72)	1,179	Postmenopausal women 55 years	Elemental calcium Elemental calcium plus Vitamin D3	1.4 g/1.5g 1.4 g/1.5g 1100 IU	There were fewer total cancer cases in the Ca/D group than the placebo group (p<0.05) but the small number (13) of breast cancer cases prevents interpretation
Women's Health Initiative (73)	36,282	Postmenopausal women 50-79 years	Calcium Vitamin D	1 g 400 IU	Intervention with calcium and vitamin D did not alter risk of colorectal, breast, or overall cancer incidence
Randomized Clinical Trial of Calcium Supplementation (71)	672	Men	Calcium	1200 mg	Null findings; calcium supplements did not reduce incidence of prostate cancer

Vitamin D Adequacy

With few natural food sources of vitamin D and cultural emphasis on safe sun exposure, fortified foods and dietary supplements have become increasingly important for maintaining vitamin D sufficiency and/or correcting a deficiency. Because of its longer half-life [15 days versus 15 hours for 1,25(OH)D], 25(OH)D is used to assess vitamin D status (55). The Institute of Medicine (IOM) concluded that for every 100 IU vitamin D consumed, 25(OH)D levels increase by 1.0 to 2.0 mmol/L, with smaller increments seen when 25(OH)D level is greater than 40 nmol/L. Complicating the determination of ideal 25(OH)D levels is the observation that vitamin D is sequestered in fat and therefore may not be as readily available in overweight and obese persons as in persons of healthy weight (55). Key research findings are shown below:

- The IOM found that 25(OH)D levels greater than 20 ng/mL are generally required for bone health (55).
- The IOM found that almost all people (i.e., 97% of the population) have sufficient vitamin D stores when 25(OH)D level is > 20ng/mL (>50 nmol/L) (55).

Table 3: Resources on Dietary Supplements

Resources
Herbs, botanicals, and other products Memorial Sloan-Kettering Cancer Center http://www.mskcc.org/mskcc/html//11570.cfm
Dietary supplement fact sheets Office of Dietary Supplements, National Institutes of Health http://ods.od.nih.gov/healh_information/information_about_individual_dietary_supplements.aspx
Dietary supplements during cancer care Caring 4 Cancer http://www.caring4cancer.com/go/cancer/nutrition/dietary-supplements
Nutrient Supplementation (position paper) Academy of Nutrition and Dietetics http://www.eatright.org/
Natural ingredients monographs including interactions that could be problematic for individuals receiving cancer treatment Natural Comprehensive Database http://naturaldatabase.com
Micronutrient Information Center Linus Pauling Institute, Oregon State University http://Lpi.orst.edu/infocenter
Food and Drug Administration Dietary supplement alerts and safety information and adverse event reporting www.fda.gov/Food/DietarySupplements/default.htm
Position paper on dietary supplements American Society of Health-System Pharmacists (ASHP) http://www.ashp.org/DocLibrary/BestPractices/SpecificStDietSuppl.aspx
Livertox: Clinical and Research Information on Drug-Induced Liver Injury United States National Library of Medicine http://livertox.nlm.nih.gov/index.html

- Research has suggested that optimal calcium absorption occurs at approximately 32 ng/mL (80 nmol/L) in postmenopausal women (75).
- It has been suggested that vitamin D levels in the range of 60-80 ng/ml are needed to reduce cancer risk (76). This recommendation is in contrast to results of the third NHANES survey (1988-1994), which showed a significant inverse relationship between vitamin D level and colorectal but not other cancers (77).

Vitamin D_2 (ergocalciferol) from plant sources and Vitamin D_3 (cholecalciferol) from animal sources (and synthesized in the skin) are available in over-the-counter supplements. Each form can raise respective 25(OH)D_2 and 25(OH)D_3 levels by 10 ng/mL per 1000 IU taken (75). The IOM states that D_2 and D_3 appear to be equally effective at low doses. At high doses D_2 is likely less effective than D_3 but animal research also suggests that at high doses D_2 is likely less toxic than D_3 (55).

Disagreement over optimal and safe 25(OH)D levels for overall health and cancer prevention remains widespread. The IOM used research on vitamin D and bone health to set 2010 Dietary Reference Intakes (DRIs) for vitamin D (74).

Omega-3 Fatty Acids

The long-chain polyunsaturated omega-3 fatty acids (n-3 fats) eicosapentaenoic acid (EPA) and docosahexaenoic acid (DHA) influence a wide range of chronic diseases through their ability to direct eicosanoid metabolism towards anti-inflammatory pathways. They also may limit neuro-toxic symptoms of the chemotherapy agent Paclitaxel. A randomized, double-blind placebo controlled trial found that seventy percent of those enrolled in the n-3 fatty acid arm (640 mg with 54% DHA and 10% EPA three times a day) but only 40.7% of those enrolled in the placebo arm did not experience peripheral neuropathy. The study was small but suggested a benefit without adverse effects and supports the need for additional studies with larger numbers (32).

A meta-analysis of prospective cohort studies did not show an association between n-3 fatty acid intake and colorectal cancer risk (78) and efforts to associate n-3 fatty acid intake with prostate cancer risk are mixed (79-80). Data from the WHEL study suggested that consuming more than 73 g/day of EPA and DHA from food reduced breast cancer events and all-cause mortality (81). Fish intake recommendations in the Dietary Guidelines for Americans (82) provide amounts of n-3 fatty acids found to be beneficial. Fish oil supplements, though not found beneficial in the WHEL study, are a source of n-3 fatty acids and are considered safe (from adverse affects) by the FDA at intakes up to 3 grams daily (83), and up to 4 grams daily when under care of a physician who can monitor the potential for abnormal bleeding function (84).

Summary

Most cancer survivors use dietary supplements, some of which may be safe and others unsafe and may interfere with cancer treatments.

RDs should integrate questions regarding supplement use into the nutrition assessment process. Findings should then be discussed with the multidisciplinary team, who can jointly develop a management plan. RDs also can recommend conventional and functional foods that may meet the survivor's desired health goals.

RDs already educate and counsel cancer survivors on diets that meet their unique needs. It is equally important for RDs to become leaders in advising the medical team on potential effects of dietary supplements on cancer treatment and on educating cancer survivors on evidence-based and appropriate use of dietary supplements. Table 3 provides resources on dietary supplements. Table 4 follows the list of references and summarizes evidence on select supplements commonly used by the cancer population.

References

1. Committee on Labor and Human Resources, S. Rep. No 410, 103d Cong., 2d Sess, at 16 (1994). Dietary Supplement Health and Education Act of 1994, Pub. L. No. 103–417, 103rd Congress (Oct. 25, 1994).
2. Gauche J, Bailey R, Burt V, et al. Dietary supplement use among U.S. adults has increased since NHANES III (1988–1994). NCHS data brief, no 61. Hyattsville, MD: National Center for Health Statistics. 2011.
3. Velicer C, Ulrich C. Vitamin and mineral supplement use among US adults after cancer diagnosis: a systematic review. *J Clin Oncol.* 2008;26(4):665-73.
4. Bardia A, Greeno E, Bauer BA. Dietary supplement usage by patients with cancer undergoing chemotherapy: does prognosis or cancer symptoms predict usage? *J Support Oncol.* 2007;5(4):195-198.
5. Bailey RL, Gahche JJ, Lentino CV, et al. Dietary supplement use in the United States, 2003-2006. *J Nutr.* 2011;141(2):261-266.
6. Ferrucci LM, McCorkle R, Smith T, Stein KD, Cartmel B. Factors related to the use of dietary supplements by cancer survivors. *J Alt Complement Med.* 2009;15(6):673-680.
7. Barnes PM, Bloom B, Nahin RL. Complementary and Alternative Medicine Use Among Adults and Children: United States, 2007 [360KB PDF]. *National health statistics reports; no 12.* Hyattsville, MD: National Center for Health Statistics. 2008
8. *Nutrition Business Journal.* NBJ's Supplement Business Report 2012. Penton Media, Inc., 2012.
9. Cassileth BR, Heitzer M, Wesa K. The public health impact of herbs and nutritional supplements. *Pharm Biol.* 2009;47(8):761-767.
10. Nirmala MJ Samundeeswari A, Sankar PD. Natural plant resources in anti-cancer therapy - a review. *Research in Plant Biology.* 2011;1(3):1-14.
11. Boullata JI, Hudson LM. Drug-nutrient interactions: a broad view with implications for practice. *J Acad Nutr Dietetics.* 2012;112(4):506-517.
12. U.S. Food and Drug Administration. For Industry: Dietary supplements. Reporting an Adverse Event, At A Glance. Available at http://www.fda.gov/downloads/Food/DietarySupplements/UCM267417.pdf Accessed 6-5-13.
13. U.S. Food and Drug Administration. Dietary Supplements – Adverse Event Reporting. Last Updated 5/21/13. http://www.fda.gov/Food/DietarySupplements/ReportAdverseEvent/default.htm Accessed 7-18-13.
14. U.S. Food and Drug Administration. Medwatch online voluntary reporting form. https://www.accessdata.fda.gov/scripts/medwatch/ Accessed 09-1-13.
15. Federal Register volume 77, number 57 (Friday, March 23, 2012). From the Federal Register Online via the Government Printing Office (www.gpo.gov).
16. Bronstein AC, Spyker DA, Cantilena LR Jr, et al. 2009 Annual Report of the American Association of Poison Control Centers' National Poison Data System (NPDS): 27th Annual Report. *Clinical Toxicology.* 2010;48(10):979–1178.
17. United States National Library of Medicine. LiverTox: Clinical and Research Information on Drug-Induced Liver Injury. http://livertox.nlm.nih.gov/index.html Last updated 06/03/2013. Accessed 08/27/2013.
18. Aggarwal BB, Harikumar K. Potential therapeutic effects of curcumin, the anti-inflammatory agent, against neurodegenerative, cardiovascular, pulmonary, metabolic, autoimmune and neoplastic diseases. *Int J Biochem Cell Biol.* 2009;41(1):40-59.
19. Guo M, Perez C, Wei Y, et al. Iron-binding properties of plant phenolics and cranberry's bio-effects. *Dalton Trans.* 2007;43:4951-4961.
20. Mathijssen RHJ, Verweij J, de Bruijn P, Loos WJ. Effects of St. John's wort on irinotecan metabolism. *J Natl Cancer Inst.* 2002;94(16):1247-1249.
21. National Center for Complementary and Alternative Medicine (NCCAM). Herbs at a glance: aloe vera. http://nccam.nih.gov/health/aloevera. Updated April 2012. Accessed July 7, 2013.
22. Fox N. Using nutrition intervention to resolve nutrition impact symptoms and save healthcare dollars. *Oncology Nutrition Connection.* 2013;21(1):15-17.
23. Iarussi E, Auricchio U, Agretto A, et al. Protective effect of coenzyme Q10 on anthracyclines cardiotoxicity. *Mol Aspects Med.* 1994;15(Suppl):s207-212.
24. Qi Y, Fu X, Xiong Z. Methylseleninic acid enhances paclitaxel efficacy for the treatment of triple-negative breast cancer. PLoS One. 2012;7(2):e31539. doi: 10.1371/journal.pone.0031539. Epub 2012 Feb 14.
25. Iizuka M, Konna S. Wound healing of intestinal epithelial cells. *World J Gastroenterol.* 2011;17(17):2161-2171.
26. Anderson PM, Schroeder G, Skubitz. Oral glutamine reduces the severity and duration of stomatitis after cytotoxic cancer chemotherapy. *Cancer.* 1998;83(7);1433-1439.
27. Topkan E, Yavuz MN, Onal C, Yavuzz AA. Prevention of acute radiation-induced esophagitis with glutamine in non-small cell lung cancer patients treated with radiotherapy: evaluation of clinical and dosimetric parameters. *Lung Cancer.* 2008;63(3):393-399.
28. Pytlik R, Benes P, Patorkova M, et al. Standardized parenteral alanyl-glutamine dipeptide supplementation is not beneficial in autologous transplant patients: a randomized, double-blind, placebo-controlled study. *Bone Marrow Transplant.* 2002;30(12):953-961.
29. Conlin KA. Coenzyme Q10 for prevention of anthracycline-induced cardiotoxicity. *Integr Cancer Ther.* 2005;4(2):110-130
30. El-Sheikh AAK, Morsy MA, Mahmoud MM, Rafaai, Abdelrahman AM. Effect of coenzyme-Q10 on doxorubicin-induced nephrotoxicity in rats. *Adv Pharmacol Sci.* 2012;2012: 981461. Doi: 10.1155/2012/981461.
31. Zhou B, Huang J, Zuo Y. 1a, a novel curcumin analog, sensitizes cisplatin-resistant A549 cells to cisplatin by inhibiting thioredoxin reductase concomitant oxidative stress damage. *Eur J Pharmacol.* 2013;707(1-3):130-139.
32. Mendonca LM, da Silva Machado C, Correia Teixeira CC, Pedro de Freitas LA, Pires Bianchi Mde L, Greggi Antunes LM. Curcumin reduces cisplatin-induced neurotoxicity in NGF-differentiated PC12 cells. *Neurotoxicology.* 2013;34:205-211. doi: 10.1016/j.neuro.2012.09.011
33. Chen CQ, Fichna J, Bashashati M, Li YY, Stor M. Distribution, function and physiological role of melatonin in the lower gut. *World J Gastroenterol.* 2011;17(34):3888-3898.
34. Lissoni P, Barni S. Meregalli S. Fossati V, Cazzaniga M. Esposti D, et al. Modulation of cancer endocrine therapy by melatonin: a phase II study of tamoxifen plus melatonin in metastatic breast cancer patients progressing under tamoxifen alone. *Br J Cancer* 1995;71(4):854–856.
35. Menendez JA, Vellon L, Colomer R, Lupu R. Oleic acid, the main monounsaturated fatty acid of olive oil, suppresses Her-2/neu (erb B-2) expression and synergistically enhances the growth inhibitory effects of trastuzumab (Herceptin) in breast cancer cells with Her-2/neu oncogene amplification. *Ann Oncol.* 2005;16(3):359-371.
36. Menendez JA, Vazquez-Martin A, Colomer R. Olive oil's bitter principle reverses acquired autoresistance to trastuzumab (Herceptin™) in HER-2-overexpressing breast cancer cells. *BMC Cancer.* 2007, 7:80. doi:10.1186/1471-2407-7-80.
37. Ghoreishi Z, Esfahani A, Djazayeri A. Omega-3 fatty acids are protective against paclitaxel-induced peripheral neuropathy: A randomized double-blind placebo controlled trial. *BMC Cancer.* 2012;12:355. doi: 10.1186/1471-2407-12-355).
38. Hardman WE, Moyer MP, Cameron IL. Consumption of an omega-3 fatty acids product, INCELL AAFATM reduced side-effects of CPT-11 (irinotecan) in mice. *Br J Cancer.* 2002;86(6):983-988.

39. Pougnoux P, Hajjaji N, Ferrasson MN, Giraudeau B, Couet C, Le Floch O. Improving outcome of chemotherapy of metastatic breast cancer by docosahexaenoic acid: a phase II trial. Br J Cancer. 2009;101(12): 1978-1985.

40. Murphy RA, Mourtzakis M, Chu QSC, Baracos VE, Reiman T, Mazurak VC. Supplementation with fish oil increases first-line chemotherapy efficacy in patients with advanced nonsmall cell lung cancer. Cancer. 2011; 117(16):3774-3780

41. Hu H, Jiang C, Ip C, Rustum YM, Lu J. Methylseleninic acid potentiates apoptosis induced by chemotherapeutic drugs in androgen-independent prostate cancer cells. Clin Cancer Res. 2005;11(6):2379-2388.

42. Fulgoni VL, Keast DR, Bailey RL, Dwyer J. Foods, fortificants, and supplements: where do Americans get their nutrients? J Nutr. 2011; 141(10):1847-1854.

43. Nakayama A, Alladin K, Igbokwe O, White J. Systematic review: generating evidence-based guidelines on the concurrent use of dietary antioxidants and chemotherapy or radiotherapy. Cancer Invest. 2011;29(10):655-667.

44. Lawenda BD, Kelly KM, Ladas EJ, Sagar SM, Vickers A, Blumgerg JB. Should supplemental antioxidant administration be avoided during chemotherapy and radiation therapy? J Natl Cancer Inst. 2008;100(11): 773-783.

45. Block G, Patterson B, Subar A. Fruit, vegetables, and cancer prevention: a review of the epidemiological evidence. Nutr Cancer. 1992;18(1):1–29.

46. Bratton M, Datta M, Gewecke A, et al. Whole food, phytochemicals, and cancer. Oncology Nutrition Connection. 2010;14(2):4-12.

47. Clark L, Combs G, Turnbull BW, et al. Effects of selenium supplementation for cancer prevention for cancer prevention in patients with carcinoma of the skin: a randomized controlled trial. JAMA. 1996;276(24):1957–1963.

48. The effect of vitamin E and beta carotene on the incidence of lung cancer and other cancers in male smokers. The Alpha-Tocopherol, Beta Carotene Cancer Prevention Study Group. N Engl J Med. 1994;330(15):1029–1035.

49. Omenn GS, Goodman GE, Thornquist MD, et al. Effects of a combination of beta-carotene and vitamin A on lung cancer and cardiovascular disease. New Engl J Med. 1996;334(18):1150-1155.

50. Gaziano JM, Glynn RJ, Christen WG, et al. Vitamins E and C in the prevention of prostate and total cancer in men: the Physicians' Health Study II randomized controlled trial. JAMA. 2009;301(1):52-62.

51. Lippman SM, Klein EA, Goodman PJ, et al. Effect of Selenium and vitamin E on risk of prostate cancer and other cancers: the Selenium and Vitamin E Cancer Prevention Trial (SELECT). JAMA. 2009;301(1):39-51.

52. Hercerg S, Galan P, Preziosi P, et al. The SU.VI.MAX study-a randomized, placebo-controlled trial of the health effects of antioxidant vitamins and minerals. Arch Intern Med. 2004;164(21):2335–2342.

53. Lin J, Cook NR, Albert C, et al. Vitamins C and E and beta-carotene supplementation and cancer risk: a randomized controlled trial. J Natl Cancer Inst. 2009;191(1):14-23.

54. Garland FC, Garland CF, Gorham ED, et al. Geographic variation in breast cancer mortality in the United States: A hypothesis involving exposure to solar radiation. Prev Med. 1990;19(6):614–622.

55. Institute of Medicine, Food and Nutrition Board. Dietary Reference Intakes for Calcium and Vitamin D. Washington, DC: National Academy Press, 2010.

56. Robien K, Cutler GJ, Lazovich D. Vitamin D intake and breast cancer risk in postmenopausal women: the Iowa Women's Health Study. Cancer Causes & Control. 2007;18(7):775-782.

57. Yousef FM, Jacobs ET, Kang PT, et al., Vitamin D status and breast cancer in Saudi Arabian women: case-control study. Am J Clin Nutr. 2013; 98(1):105-110.

58. Chlebowski RT, Johnson KC, Kooperberg C. Calcium plus vitamin D supplementation and the risk of breast cancer. J Natl Cancer Inst. 2008; 100(22):1581-1591

59. Gissel T, Rejnmark L, Mosekilde L, Vestergaard P. Intake of vitamin D and risk of breast cancer—a meta-analysis. Journal of Steroid Biochemistry and Molecular Biology 2008;111(3-5):195-199.

60. Feskanich D, Ma J, Fuchs, et al. Plasma vitamin D metabolites and risk of colorectal cancer in women. Cancer Epidemiol Biomarkers Prev. 2004; 13(9):1502–1508

61. Ma Y, Zhang P, Wang F, Yang j, Liu Z, Qin H. Association between vitamin D and risk of colorectal cancer: a systematic review of prospective studies. J Clin Oncol. 2011;29(28):3775-3582.

62. Jenab M, Bueno-d-Mesquita HB, Ferrari P, et al. Association between pre-diagnostic circulating vitamin D concentration and risk of colorectal cancer in European populations: a nested case-control study BMJ. 2010; 340: b5500.

63. Gorham ED, Garland CF, Garland FC, et al. Optimal vitamin D status for colorectal cancer prevention: a quantitative meta analysis. Am J Prev Med. 2007;32(3):210–216.

64. Gilbert R, Martin RM, Beynon R. Associations of circulating and dietary vitamin D with prostate cancer risk: a systematic dose-response meta-analysis. Cancer Causes Control. 2011;22(3):319-340.

65. Tseng M, Breslow RA, Graubard BI, Ziegler RG. Dairy, calcium, and vitamin D intakes and prostate cancer risk in the National Health and Nutrition Examination Epidemiologic Follow-up Study cohort. Am J Clin Nutr. 2005;81(5):1147-1154.

66. Kristal AR, Arnold KB, Neuhouser ML. Diet, supplement use, and prostate cancer risk: results from the Prostate Cancer Prevention Trial. Am J Epidemiol. 2010;172(5):566-577.

67. Chan JM, Stampfer MJ, Ma J, Gann PH, Gaziano JM, Giovannucci EL. Dairy products, calcium, and prostate cancer risk in the Physicians' Health Study. Am J Clin Nutr. 2001;74(4):549-554.

68. Rodriguez C, McCullough ML, Mondul AM, et al. Calcium, dairy products, and risk of prostate cancer in a prospective cohort of United States men. Cancer Epidemiol Biomarkers Prev. 2003;12(7):597-603.

69. Koh KA, Sesso HD, Paffenbarger RS, Lee I-M. Dairy products, calcium and prostate cancer risk. Br J Cancer. 2006;95(11):1582-1585.

70. Berndt SI, Carter HB, Landis PK, et al. Calcium intake and prostate cancer risk in a long-term aging study: the Baltimore Longitudinal Study of Aging. Urology. 2002;60(6):1118-1123.

71. Baron JA, Beach M, Wallace K, et al. Risk of prostate cancer in a randomized clinical trial of calcium supplementation. Cancer Epidemiol Biomarkers Prev. 2005;14(3):586-589.

72. Lappe JM, Travers-Gustafson D, Davies KM, Recker RR, Heaney RP. Vitamin D and calcium supplementation reduces cancer risk: results of a randomized trial. Am J Clin Nutr. 2007;85(6):1586-1591.

73. Wactawski-Wende J, Kotchen JM, Anderson GL. Calcium plus vitamin D supplementation and the risk of colorectal cancer. New Engl J Med. 2006;354(7):684-696.

74. Ross AC, Manson JE, Abrams SA, et al. The 2011 report on dietary reference intakes for calcium and vitamin D from the Institute of Medicine: What clinicians need to know. J Clin Endocrinol Metab. 2011;96(1):53–58.

75. Holick MF, Chen TC. Vitamin D deficiency: A worldwide problem with health consequences. Am J Clin Nutr. 2008;87(4):1080S–1086S.

76. Garland CF, French CB, Baggerly LL, Heaney RP. Vitamin D supplement doses and serum 25-hydroxyvitamin D in the range associated with cancer prevention. Anticancer Research. 2011;31(2):617-622.

77. Freedman DM, Looker AC, Abnet CC, Linet MS, Graubard BI. Serum 25-hydroxyvitamin D and cancer mortality in the NHANES III study. Cancer Res. 70(21):8587-8597.

78. Shen XJ, Zhou JD, Ding WQ, Wu JC. Dietary intake of n-3 fatty acids and colorectal cancer risk: a meta-analysis of data from 489,000 individuals. Br J Nutr. 2012;108(9):1550-1556.

79. Crowe FL, Allen NE, Appleby PN, et al. Fatty acid composition of plasma phospholipids and risk of prostate cancer in a case-control analysis nested within the European Prospective Investigation into Cancer and Nutrition. Am J Clin Nutr. 2008;88(5):1353-1363.

80. BraskyTM, Darke AK, Song X, et al. Plasma phospholipid fatty acids and prostate cancer risk in the SELECT trial. J Natl Cancer Inst. 2013. doi: 10.1093/jnci/djt174

81. Patterson RE, Flatt SW, Newman VA, et al. Marine fatty acid intake is associated with breast cancer prognosis. J Nutr. 2011;141(2):201-206.

82. U.S. Department of Agriculture and U.S. Department of Health and Human Services. Dietary Guidelines for Americans. 2010. 7th Edition, Washington, DC: U.S. Government Printing Office, December 2010.

83. Department of Health and Human Services, US Food and Drug Administration. Substances affirmed as generally recognized as safe: menhaden oil. Federal Register. June 5, 1997. Vol. 62, No. 108: pp 30751-30757. 21 CFR Part 184 (Docket No. 86G-0289).

84. Kris-Etherton PM, Harris WS, Appel LJ. American Heart Association. Nutrition Committee. Fish consumption, fish oil, omega-3 fatty acids, and cardiovascular disease. Circulation. 2002;106(21):2747-2457.

Table 4: Select Supplements used by Cancer Survivors: Evidence and Messages

Dietary Supplement	Reported Anti-cancer Benefits and Concerns	Evidence	Messages
Black Cohosh (Cimmicifua Racemosa): Rhizome and roots are used in herbal treatments; Remifemin®, a commercial preparation of black cohosh, provides 10 mg root/rhizome per tablet	**Reported Benefits:** Suppresses symptoms (e.g., hot flashes) associated with menopause; used as a cancer treatment **Potential Concerns:** May be toxic to the liver (1)	• Meta-analysis concluded that black cohosh is not effective for treating menopausal symptoms (2) • Black cohosh was more effective than fluoxetine for treating hot flashes associated with menopause (3) • German Commission E has found black cohosh to be effective at treating tension secondary to menopause (4) • May interfere with Tamoxifen (5); increases toxicity of Doxorubicin and Docetaxel (6)	• Black Cohosh may reduce menopausal symptoms but evidence is equivocal (2) • No evidence supports the use of black cohosh in cancer treatment • Black cohosh may interfere with some conventional cancer treatments and the activity of Atorvastatin, Azathioprine and Cyclosporine (5-6)
Coenzyme 10 (Co-Q10): A bioactive substance found in every cell in the body; body levels decline with aging	**Reported Benefits:** • Involved in cellular energy production • May reduce renal and cardio-toxicity of Doxorubicin (Adriamycin®) (7-8) **Potential Concerns:** • Structurally similar to vitamin K-2; has procoagulant effects (9) • Mild nausea, vomiting and diarrhea (10)	• Animal study suggested that low and high doses of Co-Q10 reduced nephrotoxicity from Doxorubicin (7) • Preclinical studies suggest that Co-Q10 may help prevent cardiotoxic effects of Doxorubicin (8)	• May reduce toxicity of some chemotherapy agents, however evidence is insufficient for recommending C0-Q10 for this purpose (7-8) • Is contraindicated in those who take warfarin (9) • As with other antioxidants, there is concern that it could interfere with chemotherapy treatments (10)
Curcumin (cucurma longa): The rhizome (i.e., root) of turmeric contains curcumin; the common dose used in clinical trials is 4 grams of curcumin daily for 30 days	**Reported Cancer Benefits:** • May inhibit growth of cancer cells (11) • Has anti-inflammatory and antioxidant properties (12) **Potential Concerns:** • May prolong activated partial thromboplastin time (aPTT) and prothrombin time (PTT) (13)	• Inhibited growth of esophageal cancer cells in vitro (11) • In a phase I trial for advanced/metastatic breast cancer, 8,000 mg/day was the maximal tolerated dose (14) • Not well absorbed but piperine, a spice in black pepper, improves its absorption and bioavailability without adverse effects (15) • Piperine may slow clearance of Phenytoin, Propranolol, and Theophylline (16)	• The bioavailability of curcumin is low, thus increasing the pill burden. Piperine improves curcumin absorption but slows clearance of several drugs (15-16) • Evidence shows promise but is currently insufficient for recommending curcurmin for cancer treatment
EPA/DHA: (Omega-3 fatty acids) Found in fatty fish and in dietary supplements (i.e., fish oil pills)	**Reported Cancer Benefits:** • May reduce inflammation (17) • May reduce toxicity of Irinotecan and Pacetaxel (18) • May enhance clinical benefit of Doxorubicin, Cisplatin and Vincristine (19) **Potential Concerns:** • EPA/DHA may increase bleeding risk if taken in high doses (>4 grams daily)	• Omega-3 fats influence genes that modulate inflammation (17) • Preclinical studies suggest that omega-3 supplements may increase apoptosis (20) • Randomized double-blind placebo controlled trial demonstrated that DHA/EPA supplement reduced incidence of peripheral neuropathy from Paclitaxel (18)	• Fish intake recommendations from the 2010 Dietary Guidelines for Americans provide amounts of EPA/DHA found to be beneficial in clinical trials (21-22) • Fish oil supplements up to 3 grams daily are considered safe (23) • Fish oil doses up to 4 grams daily are safe if monitored by a physician for bleeding risk (24)
Flaxseed: Ground flaxseed may be better absorbed than whole flaxseeds, which may pass through the gastrointestinal tract undigested	**Reported Benefits (25-27)** • Provides lignans, fiber and alpha-linolenic acid, which may protect against cancer • Has weak estrogenic activity and may enhance efficacy of Tamoxifen **Potential Concerns:** • May cause nausea, gas and diarrhea • Contraindicated in inflammatory bowel disease • May influence absorption of some drugs	• Flaxseed may inhibit growth of breast and prostate cancers (25) • Consuming 25 grams flaxseed daily may reduce tumor growth in breast cancers (28)	• Flaxseed oil does not contain lignans • Take medications one or two hours before or after consuming flaxseed (to reduce effects of flaxseed on drug absorption) • Lignans, fiber and alpha-linolenic acid in flaxseed have cancer-preventive properties (25-27) • Ground flaxseed can be added to cereals, muffins, yogurt, and salads • One to two tablespoons of flaxseed daily are considered acceptable and safe (27)

(Continued)

Table 4: Select Supplements used by Cancer Survivors: Evidence and Messages (continued)

Dietary Supplement	Reported Anti-cancer Benefits and Concerns	Evidence	Messages
Garlic: This perennial bulb is used in cooking and as an herbal treatment	**Reported Cancer Benefits:** • May stimulate apoptosis and help regulate cell cycles (29) **Potential Concerns:** • May interfere with function of some prescription drugs, including Saquinavir and may increase risk of bleeding (30)	• Study suggested that 200 mg synthetic allitridum and 100 mcg selenium reduced risk for all tumors by 33% and for stomach cancer by 52% vs. placebo (31) • Ajoene, a compound found in crushed garlic, stimulated apoptosis in promyeloleukemic cells (32) • Allyl sulfides, which comprise 94% of compounds in garlic, may promote apoptosis and cell cycle arrest (33)	• Compounds in garlic demonstrate anti-cancer activity but current evidence is insufficient for recommending garlic supplements for cancer treatment • Garlic may interfere with the activity of some medications, in particular anticoagulant drugs
Ginger: The rhizome is used as an herbal treatment	**Reported Cancer Benefits:** • Manage nausea associated with chemotherapy **Potential Concerns:** • May interfere with the activity of anticoagulant drugs, but evidence is equivocal (34)	• Study suggested that 0.5-1.0 g ginger/day reduced severity of acute chemotherapy-induced nausea and vomiting (CINV) in adult cancer patients (35) • Study suggested that 1.0-2.0 g ginger taken daily for 3 days, given with antiemetic medicine, did not reduce the prevalence or severity of acute or delayed nausea (36)	• Evidence examining effects of ginger on CINV is mixed; current evidence is insufficient for confidently recommending ginger supplements for anti-emetic treatment
Gingko Biloba: Seeds and leaves of the gingko tree	**Reported Cancer Benefits:** • May inhibit proliferation of cancer cells **Potential Concerns:** • Side effects uncommon but may increase bleeding risk (37)	• Study found that those who received gingko (vs. placebo) did not have lower cancer risk - when followed for six years (38) • Treatment of pancreatic cell lines with 70uM kaempferol (an active component of gingko) for 4 days significantly inhibited cell proliferation (39)	• Cell studies are promising but at this time evidence is insufficient for recommending gingko for cancer treatment • May interfere with activity of anticoagulant drugs (37) and anti-seizure medications (40)
Glutamine: The most prevalent amino acid in the body	**Reported Cancer Benefits:** • May reduce degree of mucositis, stomatitis, esophagitis and diarrhea associated with cancer treatment (41) **Potential Concerns:** • May decrease efficacy of lactulose (42)	• May reduce severity of stomatitis secondary to cytotoxic chemotherapy (41) • May reduce severity of radiation-induced esophagitis (43) • Not beneficial in autologous transplant patients (44) • May interact with seizure medication (45)	• Evidence suggests it may reduce stomatitis, mucositis and esophagitis secondary to chemotherapy; use should be evaluated by the medical team • Is contraindicated in those taking anti-seizure medication (46) and lactulose (42)
Silymarin: Silymarin is an extract of milk thistle	**Reported Cancer Benefits:** • Antioxidant (47) • May reduce side effects of Cisplatin (rat study) (48) **Potential Concerns:** • Allergic reactions (> 1500 mg/d) (49)	• May regulate cell cycles, induce apoptosis, and reduce angiogenesis (50) • May reduce inflammation and oxidative stress and may protect DNA (51)	• May promote anti-cancer activity, but research is inadequate to support recommending it for patients undergoing cancer treatment
St. John's Wort (Hypericum perforatum): Yellow flowers are used as herbal remedies	**Reported Cancer Benefits:** • May make cancer cells more sensitive to photodynamic (light) therapies (52) **Potential Concerns:** • May interact with many medications including warfarin (53)	• VITAL study: use of St. John's Wort was inversely associated with risk of colorectal cancer (54) • Cell and animal studies suggest that St. John's wort may make cancer cells more sensitive to photodynamic (light) therapies; may have potential to improve anti-cancer effects of these modalities (52)	• At this time evidence is insufficient for recommending St. John's wort for cancer treatment • Induces CYP3A4, resulting in lower plasma levels of drugs that are CYP3A4 substrates, including Cyclosporine, Simvastatin, Warfarin, and Amitriptyline (53)
Theanine: An amino acid; common dosage is 200 to 400 mg QD/BID; maximum dose 1200 mg (55)	**Reported Cancer Benefits** • Antioxidant • Enhances benefits/reduces toxicity of Doxorubicin and Idarubicin (56-57) **Potential Concerns:** • May reduce blood pressure (55)	• Cell studies suggest that theanine suppresses growth of non-small cell lung cancer cells (56) • At a concentration of 0-125 µM, theanine suppresses migration of tumor cells (58)	• Theanine is a natural component of tea. • May enhance some chemotherapies but there is no evidence that supplements are superior to tea • May reduce blood pressure and thus interact with anti-hypertensive medications

References

1. Mahady GB, Dog TL, Barrett ML, Chaavez ML, Gardiner P, Ko R. United States Pharmacopeia review of the black cohosh case reports of hepatotoxicity *Menopause*. 2008;15(4 Pt 1):628-638.

2. Leach MJ, Moore V. Black cohosh (Cimicifuga spp.) for menopausal symptoms. *Cochrane Database Syst Rev*. 2012 Sep 12;9:CD007244.

3. Oktem M, Eroglu D, Karahan HB, Taskintuna N, Kuscu E, Zeyneloglu y HB. Black cohosh and fluoxetine in the treatment of postmenopausal symptoms: a prospective, randomized trial. *Adv Ther*. 2007;24(2):448-461.

4. *Bundesanzeiger* (Cologne, Germany): January 5, 1989

5. Li J, Gödecke T, Chen SN, Imai A, Lankin DC, Farnsworth NR, et al. In vitro metabolic interactions between black cohosh (Cimifuga racemosa) and tamoxifen via inhibition of cytochromes P450 2D6 and 3A4. *Xenobiotica*.2011;41(12):1021-1030.

6. Rockwell S, Liu Y, Higgins SA. Alteration of the effects of cancer therapy agents on breast cancer cells by the herbal medicine black cohosh. *Breast Cancer Res Treat* 2005;90(3):233-239.

7. Colas S, Mahéo K, Denis F, et al. Sensitization by dietary docosahexaenoic acid of rat mammary carcinoma to anthracycline: a role for tumor vascularization. *Clin Cancer Res*. 2006;12(19):5879–5886.

8. Conlin KA. Coenzyme Q10 for prevention of anthracycline-induced cardiotoxicity. *Integr Cancer Ther*. 2005;4(2):110-130

9. Heck AM, Dewitt BA, Lukes AL. Potential Interations between alternative therapies and warfarin. AM J Health Syst Pharm. 2000;57(13). http://www.medscape.com/viewarticle/406896_3. Accessed 8-11-13

10. Medline Plus. Coenzyme Q10. http://www.nlm.nih.gov/medlineplus/druginfo/natural/938.html. Last reviewed 10-21-11. Accessed 8-11-13.

11. Subramaniam D, Ponnurangam S, Ramamoorthy P, Standing D, Battafarano RJ, Anant S, et al. Curcumin induces cell death in esophageal cancer cells through modulating notch signaling. PLoS One. 2012; 7(2): e30590. Published online 2012 February 17. doi: 10.1371/journal.pone.0030590.

12. American Cancer Society. Tumeric. http://www.cancer.org/treatment/treatmentsandsideeffects/complementaryandalternativemedicine/herbsvitaminsandminerals/turmeric. Accessed 8-11-13.

13. Kim DC, Ku SK, Bae JS. Anticoagulant activities of curcumin and its derivative. *BMB Reports* Online (*Korean Society for Biochemistry and Molecular Biology*). 2012;45(4):221-226.

14. Bayet-Robert M, Kwiatkowski F, Leheurteru M, Gachon F, Planchat E, Abrial C, et al. Phase I dose escalation trial of docetaxel plus curcumin in patients with advanced and metastatic breast cancer. *Cancer Biology & Therapy*. 2010;9(1):8-14.

15. Bano G, Raina RK, Zutshi U, Bedi KL, Johri RK, Sharma SC. Effect of piperine on bioavailability and pharmacokinetics of propranolol and theophylline in healthy volunteers. *Eur J Clin Pharmacol*. 1991;41(6): 615-617.

16. Velpandian T, Jasuja R, Bhardwaj RK, Jaiswal J, Gupta SK. Piperine in food: interference in the pharmacokinetics of phenytoin. *Eur J Drug Metab Pharmacokinet*. 2001;26(4):241-247.

17. Vedin I, Cederholm T, Freund-Levi Y, et al. Effects of DHA- rich n-3 fatty acid supplementation on gene expression in blood mononuclear leukocytes: the OmegAD study. PLoS One. 2012; 7(4): e35425. Published online 2012 April 24. doi: 10.1371/journal.pone.0035425

18. Ghoreishi Z, Esfahani A, Djazayeri A. Omega-3 fatty acids are protective against paclitaxel-induced peripheral neuropathy. A randomized double-blind placebo controlled trial. *BMC Cancer*. 2012;12:355. doi: 10.1186/1471-2407-12-355).

19. Pardini R. Nutritional intervention with omega-3 fatty acids enhances tumor response to anti-neoplastic agents. *Chemico-Biological Interactions*. 2006;162(2):89-105.

20. Shaikh IA, Brown I, Wahle KW, Heys SD. Enhancing cytotoxic therapies for breast and prostate cancers with polyunsaturated fatty acids. *Nutr Cancer*. 2010;62(3):284-296.

21. Patterson RE, Flatt SW, Newman VA, et al. Marine fatty aid intake is associated with breast cancer prognosis. *J Nutr*. 2011;141(2):201-206.

22. U.S. Department of Agriculture and U.S. Department of Health and Human Services. Dietary Guidelines for Americans. 2010. 7th Edition, Washington, DC: U.S. Government Printing Office, December 2010.

23. Department of Health and Human Services, US Food and Drug Administration. Substances affirmed as generally recognized as safe: menhaden oil. Federal Register. June 5, 1997. Vol. 62, No. 108: pp 30751-30757. 21 CFR Part 184 (Docket No. 86G-0289).

24. Kris-Etherton PM, Harris WS, Appel LJ. American Heart Association. Nutrition Committee. Fish consumption, fish oil, omega-3 fatty acids, and cardiovascular disease. *Circulation*. 2002;106(21):2747-2457.

25. Memorial Soan-Kettering. Flaxseed. http://www.mskcc.org/cancer-care/herb/flaxseed

26. American Cancer Society. Flaxseed. http://www.cancer.org/treatment/treatmentsandsideeffects/complementaryandalternativemedicine/herbsvitaminsandminerals/flaxseed

27. WebMD. The Benefits of Flaxseed. http://www.webmd.com/diet/features/benefits-of-flaxseed

28. Thompson LU, Chen JM, Li T,Strasser-Weippi K, Goss PE. Dietary flaxseed alters tumor biological markers in postmenopausal breast cancer. *Clin Cancer Res*. 2005. 11:3828. doi: 10.1158/1078-0432.CCR-04-2326.

29. Pinto JT, Rivlin RS. Antiproliferative effects of allium derivaties from garlic. *J Nutr*. 2001;131(3):10585-10605.

30. Medline Plus. Garlic. http://www.nlm.nih.gov/medlineplus/druginfo/natural/300.html. Last reviewed 12-24-11. Accessed 8-11-13.

31. National Center for Complementary and Alternative Medicine (NCCAM). Herbs at a glance: Garlic. http://nccam.nih.gov/health/garlic/ataglance.htm Updated April 12, 2012, Accessed 8-11-13.

32. Li H, Li HQ, Wang Y, et al. An intervention study to prevent gastric cancer by micro-selenium and large dose of allitridum. *Chinese Medical Journal (English)*. 2004;117(8):1155-1160.

33. Wang H-C, Pao J, Lin S-Y, Sheen L-Y. Molecular mechanisms of garlic-derived allyl sulfides in the inhibition of skin cancer progression. *Ann NY Acad Sci*. 2012;1271(1):44-52.

34. Janssen PL, Meyboom S, van Staveren WA et al. Consumption of ginger (Zingiber officinale Roscoe) does not affect ex vivo platelet thromboxane production in humans. *Eur J Clin Nutr*. 1996;50:772-774.

35. Ryan JL, Heckler CE, Roscoe JA, Dakhil SR, Kirshner J, Flynn PJ. Ginger (zingiber officinale) reduces acute chemotherapy-induced nausea: A URCC CCOP study of 576 patients. *Support Care Cancer*. 2012;20(7): 1479-1489.

36. Zick SM, Ruffin MT, Lee J, Normolle DP, Siden R, Alrawi S, et al. Phase II trial of encapsulated ginger as a treatment for chemotherapy-induced nausea and vomiting. *Support Care Cancer*. 2009;17(5):563-572.

37. Roland PD, Nergard CS. Ginkgo biloba-effect, adverse events and drug interactions. *Tidsskr Nor Laegeforen*. 2012.143(8):956-959.

38. Biggs ML, Sorkin BC, Nahin RL, Kuller LH, Fitzpatrick AL. Ginkgo biloba and risk of cancer: secondary analysis of the ginkgo evaluation of memory (GEM) study. *Pharmacoepidemiol Drug Saf*. 2010;19(7):694-698.

39. Zhang Y, Chen AY, Chen C, Yao Q. Ginkgo biloba extract kaempferol inhibits cell proliferation and induces apoptosis in pancreatic cancer cells. *J Surg Res*. 2008;148(1):17-23.

40. U.S. Food and Drug Administraiton. Avoiding Drug Interactions. http://www.fda.gov/ForConsumers/ConsumerUpdates/ucm096386.htm Developed 11-8-08. Accessed 8-11-13.

41. Sipahi S, Gungor O, Gunduz M, Cilci M, Demirci MC, Tamer A. The effect of oral supplementation with a combination of beta-hydroxy-beta-methylbutyrate, arginine and glutamine on wound healing: a retrospective analysis of diabetic haemodialysis patients. *BMC Nephrol*. 2013; 14: 8. Published online 2013 January 12. doi: 10.1186/1471-2369-14-8

42. *WebMD*. Glutamine. http://www.webmd.com/vitamins-supplements/ingredientmono-878-GLUTAMINE.aspx?activeIngredientId=878&activeIngredientName=GLUTAMINE. Accessed 8-11-13.

43. Anderson PM, Schroeder G, Skubitz. Oral glutamine reduces the severity and duration of stomatitis after cytotoxic cancer chemotherapy. *Cancer*. 1998;83(7);1433-1439.

44. Topkan E, Yavuz MN, Onal C, Yavuzz AA. Prevention of acute radiation-induced esophagitis with glutamine in non-small cell lung cancer patients treated with radiotherapy: evaluation of clinical and dosimetric parameters. *Lung Cancer* 2008;63(3):393-399.

45. Pytlik R, Benes P, Patorkova M, et al. Standardized parenteral alanyl-glutamine dipeptide supplementation is not beneficial in autologous transplant patients: a randomized, double-blind, placebo-controlled study. *Bone Marrow Transplant*. 2002;30(12):953-961.

46. Chapman AG. Glutamate and epilepsy. *J Nutr*. 2000;130(4S Suppl): 1043S-1045S.

47. National Cancer Institute. Milk Thistlte. http://www.cancer.gov/cancertopics/pdq/cam/milkthistle/Patient/page3

48. Abdelmeguide NE. Silymarin ameliorates cisplatin-induced hepatotoxicity in rats: histopathological and ultrastructural studies. *Pak J Biol Sci*. 2010'13(10):463-479.

49. *Web*MD. Milk Thistle: Benefits and Side Effects. http://www.webmd.com/heart-disease/milk-thistle-benefits-and-side-effects. 2012. Accessed 8-11-13.

50. Ramasamy K, Agarwal R. Multitargeted therapy of cancer by silymarin. Cancer Letter. 2008;269(2):352-362.

51. Feher J, Lengyel G. Silymarin in the prevention and treatment of liver diseases and primary liver cancer. Current Pharmaceutical Biotechnology, 2012;13(1):210-217.

52. Wessels JT, Busse AC, Rave-Fränk M, Zänker S, Hermann R, Grabbe E, et al. Photosensitizing and radiosensitizing effects of hypericin on human renal carcinoma cells in vitro. *Photochem Photobiol*. 2008;84(1):228-35.

53. Roby CA, Anderson GD, Kantor E, Dryer DA, Burstein AH. St John's Wort: effect on CYP3A4 activity. *Clin Pharmacol Ther*. 200;67(5):451-457.

54. Satia JA, Littman A, Slatore CG, Galanko JA, White E. Associations of herbal and specialty supplements with lung and colorectal cancer risk in the VITamins And Lifestyle(VITAL) study. *Cancer Epidemiol Biomarkers Prev*. 2009;18(5):1419-1428.

55. Clevelanad Clinic Wellness. L-Theanine Supplement Review. http://www.clevelandclinicwellness.com/Features/Pages/l-theanine-pro-con.aspx

56. Sugiyama T, Sadzuka Y. Combination of L-theanine with doxorubicin inhibits hepatic metastasis of M5076 ovarian sarcoma. *Clin Cancer Res*. 1999;5(2):413-6.

57. Sadzuka Y, Sugiyama T, Sonobe T. Improvement of idarubicin induced antitumor activity and bone marrow suppression by L-theanine, a component of tea. *Cancer Lett*. 2000;158(2):119-24.

58. Liu Q, Duan H, Luan J, Yagasaki K, Zhang G. Effect of theanine on growth of human lung cancer and leukemia cells as well as migration and invasion of human lung cancer cells. *Cytotechnology*. 2009;59(3): 211-217.

Nutrigenomics and Cancer

Colleen K. Spees PhD, MEd, RD
Elizabeth M. Grainger, PhD, RD

Drs. Spees and Grainger would like to acknowledge the contributions of Steven K. Clinton, MD, PhD to this manuscript.

Nutritional Genomics

Nutritional genomics is the scientific investigation of the composite interactions between nutrients, **bioactive food components**, and the genome as they impact host health and risk of disease (definitions of bolded terms are found in Table 1) (1–6). Recent advances are improving our understanding of biological responses to nutrients and bioactive food components, and genetic variation and population heterogeneity in regards to nutrient requirements. The broad field of nutritional genomics is complex in regards to cancer because critical questions involve the inherited genetics of the host and the multiple and often heterogeneous acquired genetic defects of the developing and ever-evolving cancer. One goal of nutritional genomics is that based on an individual's unique genotypic profile, the healthcare team will eventually tailor diet and nutritional recommendations to prevent, delay, halt, or possibly reverse carcinogenesis. As the evidence continues to expand, registered dietitians (RDs) will be better equipped to provide personalized recommendations for cancer prevention and survivorship.

Carcinogenesis

Carcinogenesis is a complex evolutionary process in which accumulating genetic and epigenetic alterations drive the transformation of normal cells to malignant cancer cells with increasingly dysfunctional behavior. Hanahan and Weinberg (7-8) reviewed the history of carcinogenesis research and conceptually defined critical hallmarks, which are characteristic of possibly all cancerous cells. These hallmarks include the following: growth signal autonomy; evading apoptosis; insensitivity to anti-growth signals; tissue invasion and metastasis; unlimited proliferation potential (immortality); and sustained angiogenesis. After a decade of new discoveries, four additional molecular characteristics of cancer cells were recently recognized: avoidance of immune destruction; tumor-promoting inflammation; genome instability; and deregulating cellular energetics (8).

The progression of a cancer is enhanced by genetic instability of cancer cells, often due to defective DNA repair processes. These defective DNA repair processes increase the frequency of mutational events and allow for aggressive clones to evolve in spite of initially effective therapy. Damage to the genome, particularly in solid tumors, is complex and can be extensive; this damage may manifest as chromosomal **deletions, duplications**, and **large translocations**.

Cancers typically contain multiple **point mutations** in genes and their regulatory elements, both of which directly contribute to carcinogenesis. Mutations in these critical genes are termed **oncogenes** (gain-of-function genes) and **tumor suppressor genes** (loss-of-function genes) (9). In addition to the chromosomal defects and specific mutations, cancers acquire additional defects in gene regulation that impact carcinogenesis. **Epigenetic** changes, such as **methylation** and **acetylation**, are heritable and potentially reversible modifications in DNA that affect gene expression and function without altering the nucleotide sequence (10-11).

Defective gene regulation is the foundation of cancer biology. Importantly, the potential for nutrients and bioactive food components to modify the accumulation of genetic defects—or the downstream biological impact of such defects—is a critical thrust of nutrigenomics research. Nutrients and bioactive food components may interact with the evolving genetic damage of cancer in a number of ways. Examples include: (1) influence susceptibility to chemical carcinogens such as those found in tobacco smoke by altering their metabolism; (2) impact sensitivity to UV-light and other forms of irradiation; (3) modulate DNA repair processes; (4) impact metabolism and the production of genotoxic reactive oxygen species such as superoxide anion and hydroxyl radicals; (5) alter the severity and character of inflammation; (6) change the hormonal environment or a cell's sensitivity to hormones thereby impacting expression of oncogenes and tumor suppressor genes; (7) influence the pathogenesis of carcinogenic infections such as hepatitis B or human papilloma virus; and (8) alter the interaction of the emerging cancer with the host to thwart anti-cancer immune surveillance.

A classic example of nutrigenomics in human carcinogenesis is illustrated by the role of all-trans retinoic acid (ATRA) in acute promyelocytic leukemia (APL). This disease typically has a chromosomal translocation (t(15;17)(q24;q21)) involving the retinoic acid receptor-alpha gene on chromosome 17 with a reciprocal translocation with the promyelocytic leukemia gene on chromosome 15. This defect creates a hybrid protein with altered function and prevents the differentiation of normal blood leukocytes. Remarkably, APL is unique among leukemias due to its sensitivity to the administration of ATRA, a derivative of vitamin A. The ATRA binds the mutant protein and prevents its aberrant procarcinogenic action, causing the terminal differentiation and

Table 1: Glossary of Terms

Term	Definition
Acetylation	Modification of histones by attachment of acetyl groups.
Acquired (or somatic) mutation	A change in the genetic structure that is neither inherited nor passed to offspring; occurs after conception.
Bioactive food components	Substances in foods which are not essential nutrients, but may have biologic effects. These include phytochemicals (plants), zoochemicals (animal), fungochemicals (mushrooms) and bacterochemicals (gut bacteria).
Chromatin remodeling	Changes in chromatin structure that occur during regulatory processes and alter the nuclease sensitivity of a region of chromatin.
Deletion	A type of mutation in which genetic information has been lost.
Duplication	A type of mutation that involves the production of one or more copies of a gene or region of a chromosome.
Epigenetics	Modifications in DNA that affect gene expression and function without altering the nucleotide sequence. Examples of epigenetics include altering the proteins that control gene expression through methylation or acetylation, or regulation of microRNA's which can then regulate gene expression.
Epigenomics	The study of epigenetic changes in a cell or entire organism.
Genomewide association study (GWAS)	An approach that looks for associations between many specific genetic variations and particular diseases.
Haplotype	A group of gene variants that occur together.
Histone	A protein around which DNA is wrapped.
Histone modificaton	A variety of modifications (i.e., acetylation, methylation, phosphorylation, ADP-ribosylation) that occur on histones and may augment gene transcription and translation.
Inherited mutation	A change in the genetic structure that is inherited or passed to offspring.
Methylation	The addition of methyl (-CH$_3$) groups to DNA. DNA methylation patterns can be inherited and impact patterns of gene expression.
MicroRNAs	Small fragments of cytosolic RNA, usually about 22 nucleotides in size, which bind to mRNA and function as post transcriptional regulators. Also called miRNA.
Noncoding RNAs	RNA that does not encode a protein but appears to play a role in both oncogenic and tumor suppressive pathways.
Nutritional genomics	The scientific investigation of the composite interactions between nutrients, bioactive food components and the genome as they impact host health and disease.
Oncogenes	A gene whose product is involved either in transforming cells in culture or inducing cancer in animals. Most are mutant forms of normal genes involved in control of cell growth or division.
Phenotype	The physical and observable properties, or traits, of an organism.
Point mutations	Change of a single nucleotide in DNA, especially in a region coding for protein.
Polymorphisms	The minor variations, among individuals, in the sequence of DNA bases in specific genes.
Translocation	Movement of a segment of a chromosome from its normal site to another chromosome.
Tumor suppressor gene	Genes that normally restrain cell growth but, when missing or inactivated by mutation, allow cells to grow uncontrolled.
Xenobiotics	Chemicals found in an organism but not produced by it, such as drugs or pollutants.

spontaneous apoptosis of leukemia cells (12), often leading to dramatic remission for the affected individual. Another example (13-14) is the potential impact of diets rich in omega-3 fatty acids in slowing the progression of a specific type of breast cancer. Her2neu is a gene encoding a protein within the epidermal growth factor receptor family. Amplification or over-expression of this gene plays a role in aggressive subtypes of human breast cancer. Laboratory models with over expressed Her2neu develop breast cancer, a process that is significantly inhibited by diets rich in omega-3 containing lipid sources (14). These clinical and pre-clinical examples represent the beginning of our understanding of how nutrients and bioactive food components may have specific benefits for emerging and progressing cancers with unique genetic signatures.

Nutrigenomics in Non-Cancer Conditions: Lessons Learned

Successful dietary interventions for other types of heritable diseases exist and can serve as poignant examples of applied nutritional genomics. For example, phenylketonuria (PKU) is an inborn error of metabolism which results from a mutation in the gene encoding the enzyme phenylalanine hydroxylase. Newborns who test positive for PKU can successfully avoid the serious consequences of this disease by maintaining a diet very low in phenylalanine (15). Other inherited diseases, such as galactosemia, maple syrup urine disease, and lactose intolerance, also can be successfully treated with dietary modifications alone (16). Clinicians also provide specific diet interventions in conjunction with pharmacologic interventions for patients with genetically defined hyperlipidemias that predispose affected individuals to atherosclerosis. Persons with familial hypercholesterolemia (FH) have a mutation in the low density lipoprotein receptor gene which results in premature cardiovascular disease (17). Although the primary treatment for individuals with FH is statins and weight control, a diet low in total fat, saturated fat, and dietary cholesterol; high in fiber and a diet that incorporates soy foods are also key pillars of treatment (18). These examples illustrate the potential and the promise of nutrition therapy for those with genetic diseases relevant to cancer.

Genetic Variation and Cancer Risk

Each individual begins life with an inherited genome of over 20,000 protein-coding genes (19), some of which will define how a person responds to insults contributing to carcinogenesis. Most of our genes contain **polymorphisms**, which are typically minor variations in nucleotide sequence that may impact the function of corresponding proteins to varying degrees and thereby modify cancer risk. Single nucleotide polymorphisms (SNPs) are variations in a single nucleotide in the DNA sequence. There are an estimated ten million SNPs in the human genome (20-21), most of which result in what appears to be a normal or slightly variable **phenotype**. SNPs account for approximately 90% of all gene polymorphisms and occur, in humans, at a frequency of every 100 to 300 bases throughout our three billion nucleotide sequence (22). Because SNPs are common and typically not problematic, many researchers focus on **haplotypes**, or statistically related groups of SNPs present along a segment of a chromosome. Additional information can be attained with **genome-wide association studies** (GWAS), which map disease risk loci. Future studies focusing upon dietary patterns and genetic status based upon haplotype studies and GWAS will be valuable for defining nutrient-gene interactions.

The literature on smoking and lung cancer provides examples of gene polymorphisms interacting with diet to determine risk of cancer. The GST gene encodes glutathione S-transferase, a key enzyme in the Phase II detoxification pathway for carcinogens (23). In provocative studies (24-25), diet and genotype had no significant impact on lung cancer risk in non-smokers. However, in smokers, the null GST polymorphism increased lung cancer risk. Interestingly, in this genetic subgroup exposed to tobacco carcinogens, the consumption of isothiocyanate rich cruciferous vegetables reduced lung cancer risk. These studies illustrate a three-way interaction among carcinogen exposure, genotype, and diet with regards to risk of cancer (24-25).

Perhaps the most informative evidence of a dietary impact on cancer is found with colorectal cancer (CRC) (1). CRC is the second most common cancer in Americans and is thought to have many modifiable risk factors, such as intake of red meat, processed meat, body fatness, exercise, and alcohol among others (1,26). Alcohol intake has been found to be a risk factor for CRC in many epidemiological studies (1,26). Several polymorphisms impacting the metabolism of dietary components are proposed to modify CRC risk. A meta-analysis of 29 studies found a common polymorphism

in the methylenetetrahydrofolate reductase (MTHFR) gene, which encodes an enzyme that is critical in folate metabolism. This particular mutation has been associated with a 17% lower risk of CRC in non-Hispanic whites and Asians, but not Latinos or African Americans. Interestingly, this relationship was significant only when the analysis was limited to persons with the gene variant who were regular alcohol consumers, whom are often deficient in folate (27).

Epidemiological studies have implicated mutagens formed during high temperature cooking and excessive meat browning to be risk factors for colon cancer. In the Health Professionals Follow Up Study (HPFS), intake of meat mutagens was associated with adenoma of the distal colon independent of total meat intake (28). A large cohort of men and women enrolled in the NIH-AARP Diet and Health study reported similar findings (29). It is possible that persons with polymorphisms in genes for phase I or phase II **xenobiotic** metabolizing enzymes are particularly susceptible to meat mutagens. A recent case-control study within the Prostate, Lung, Colorectal and Ovarian Cancer Screening Trial evaluated the dietary intake of meat mutagens and reported an interaction between SNPs and dietary intake. Investigators found that the highest dietary intake of one particular type of heterocyclic amine was significantly associated with advanced colon adenoma among persons with a N-acetyltransferase 1 (NAT1) polymorphism. This is one of the genes that encodes for xenobiotic enzymes and therefore impacts carcinogen metabolism and detoxification (30).

Inherited Cancer Syndromes

Less common, but of critical importance, are gene mutations associated with defined inherited cancer syndromes. Familial cancer predisposition syndromes are passed from one generation to another and are also known as germline, hereditary, or inherited cancer syndromes. Typically, the original genetic predisposition is inherited in one allele and additional mutations or 'hits' in the second allele are often required to induce the carcinogenic process (31). Many inherited cancer syndromes are observed at a younger age, because affected individuals already possess one of the two allelic mutations necessary to activate the cancer process. Thus, genotype determines susceptibility to disease, and a second mutational event determines the initiation of the cancer phenotype.

Inherited defects in TP53 are associated with Li-Fraumeni Syndrome (LFS) (32), predisposing individuals to multiple primary cancers at an early age. The TP53 gene serves as the "guardian of the genome" (33) and is critical for normal cell senescence and programmed cell death, particularly when genetic damage and genotoxic stress has occurred (34). Although no human studies have addressed dietary intake and the patterns, frequency, or age of onset of specific malignancies in those with LFS, murine models have revealed that tumor development is inhibited in energy restricted TP53 null mice (35-36). Radiation-induced malignancies have also been observed among LFS individuals and validation of cancer secondary to radiation sensitivity has been confirmed in TP53 deficient mice (37). These animal study results suggest that in the LFS genotype, modifiable environmental exposures appear to impact the observed phenotype.

Familial adenomatous polyposis (FAP) is an autosomal dominant inherited cancer predisposition syndrome in which the colon of affected persons predictably develops adenomatous polyps and eventually CRC at an earlier age than observed in the general population (38). The gene associated with FAP is adenomatous polyposis coli (APC), located on chromosome 5. This tumor suppressor gene encodes a protein involved in cell adhesion and migration, signal transduction, cytoskeletal structure, and cell cycle regulation (39). Many FAP murine studies have shown that dietary variables can suppress carcinogenesis (40-42). For example, an increased caloric intake was correlated with a greater risk of CRC after six months of consuming a Western-type diet in preclinical murine models (40). These findings warrant future investigation in human trials. Pilot feasibility studies in humans with FAP have investigated eicosapentaenoic acid (EPA) (43), curcumin (44), quercitin (45) vitamin C (46), fiber (46) and calcium (47). EPA, curcumin alone and curcumin plus quercitin is associated with a significantly reduced number and size of rectal polyps (EPA and curcumin plus quercitin) or stabilized disease (curcumin alone) compared with controls; however, these studies are limited in both sample size and study duration (43). Larger randomized trials are critically needed to define effective and safe interventions that will reduce cancer risk and enhance quality of life for those with inherited cancer syndromes (47).

Epigenetics and Cancer

We now appreciate the existence of heritable changes in gene expression independent of alterations in the nucleotide sequence of DNA (49). There are two ways in which diet impacts epigenetics: (1) host somatic cell mitosis and (2) germ cell transgenerational inheritance (50-51). The known epigenetic mediators that are implicated in carcinogenesis include DNA methylation, **histone modification**, **chromatin remodeling**, and **noncoding RNAs** (ncRNAs) (52-53). Elucidation of the role that non-coding DNA plays in the regulation of gene expression, particularly **microRNAs**, has led to new concepts regarding how nutrients and bioactive food components may impact cell biology and carcinogenesis (54).

Dysregulation of epigenetic control of gene expression can influence cancer risk and, in turn, phenotype (55-56). The classic agouti mice studies provided the first evidence that maternal bioactive food components interact with fetal epigenetic gene expression to alter phenotype and disease risk in offspring (57). The wild type agouti mouse model (A^{vy}) is phenotypically characterized by a yellow agouti coat color and obesity. Supplementation of the pregnant females' diet with genistein, a soy phytochemical, resulted in hypermethylation and an altered offspring phenotype. Descendants of supplemented agouti mice were born with a pseudoagouti (brown) coat color and a healthy body weight. Interestingly, the genistein-induced epigenetic methylation patterns persevered into adulthood for all offspring (57). This landmark study illustrates a dietary impact on phenotype that is mediated by a heritable alteration in gene expression, ultimately reducing the risk of obesity-related chronic disease.

Epigenetic imprints (signatures) can persist transgenerationally even in the absence of the original environmental exposure (51). The first reported evidence of transgenerational epigenetics related to human nutrition was published in the 1980s (58). Using meticulous historical agriculture, environmental, and death records of Swedish citizens over several generations, investigators determined that abundant food intake during periods of 'feast' were correlated with higher mortality rates up to two generations later (58). This landmark observation suggested that certain environmental exposures, including nutrition, led to immediate germline epigenetic alterations that are passed, and may persist, for subsequent generations (59).

Diet and Nutrition Recommendations for Cancer Prevention and Survivorship

For many individuals, it can be challenging to navigate through the overwhelming amount of available nutrition information and to discriminate between reliable and unreliable information. This is particularly challenging due to the plethora of information-and misinformation-found on the Internet and in the popular press. Physicians and genetic counselors frequently lack adequate training in nutrition and are unaware of public health guidelines or specific recommendations for those with a family history of cancer, known genetic predisposition syndromes, or established premalignant conditions. Individuals who have been diagnosed with cancer may be more motivated to make behavior changes regarding tobacco, diet, and exercise to reduce the risk of cancer recurrence or the development of a second malignancy (60-61). However, many studies investigating behavior change after a cancer diagnosis suggest that cancer survivors have a difficult time achieving healthy dietary patterns and only a minority meet the public health guidelines for diet, physical activity and cancer prevention (3,62-63). Cancer survivors are a vulnerable population and are often more likely than non-cancer survivors to fall prey to purveyors of unproven or untested interventions or supplements, all of which can become a financial burden (64-65). Therefore, RDs serve as a critical resource to complement the care provided by physicians and genetic counselors in these high-risk populations.

In the absence of data from diet and nutritional studies undertaken in those with known genetic conditions, counseling for cancer prevention and survivorship should focus on the evidence-based guidelines established by numerous reputable organizations for chronic disease prevention (**Appendix 1** (10-11,66-69). These frequently updated guidelines from various organizations are often very similar and can be briefly summarized as the following major concepts: (1) maintain a healthy body weight; (2) consume a largely plant-based diet; (3) reduce consumption of processed meats; (4) reduce the amount of added sugars, refined carbohydrates, and calorically dense foods; and (5) limit alcohol intake. As the complex field of nutritional genomics continues to expand and the number of preclinical and clinical studies of diet and gene mutations increases, nutritional scientists will be able to develop specific diet recommendations for high-risk populations.

Current Limitations and Future Research Priorities

Research challenges continue to exist in studies of diet, exercise, and other modifiable lifestyle habits. For example, new strategies to reduce high attrition rates and poor compliance with long-term behavior changes are needed (70-71). Poor compliance also has been reported in persons with known high-risk genotypes (72). DeCosse et al. conducted a randomized, double-blinded study of 58 men and women with FAP who were randomized to either a high fiber supplement or a low fiber placebo for four years (46). Although all the subjects were aware of their high risk for colon cancer, adherence to the dietary intervention was approximately 40% for the placebo group and 70% for the high-fiber group (46,72). RDs can play a key role in the clinical trial team and help patients make diet and lifestyle changes that are both meaningful and achievable. Furthermore, research regarding novel strategies to enhance compliance among people who begin diet or behavior modification programs are needed.

One possible approach to improving compliance to certain dietary interventions is the development of novel functional foods that, like pharmaceuticals, are easy to deliver and readily incorporated into daily life. Examples of such interventions that have been developed are soy-tomato juice (73) and soy pretzels (74) that deliver doses of isoflavones comparable to other soy foods. The soy pretzel has a lower glycemic index than traditional pretzels and sensory testing found it to be highly acceptable, thereby illustrating the potential for use by diabetics (74). Functional foods may be able to target genetic defects with specific phytochemicals and deliver them in a formula that can be easily incorporated into a busy life. However, more research is needed in this relatively new area.

Research priorities should also include using the current infrastructure of large ongoing cohort and cross-sectional studies where dietary data is routinely collected. Use of existing cohorts, such as the Nurses' Health Study, HPFS, and the National Health and Nutrition Examination Survey to identify gene polymorphisms and correlate these with the diet and lifestyle information already collected would be a reasonable way to discover links between nutrients, diet, and genes.

There also is an opportunity to collect diet, nutrition, and lifestyle data in emerging cohorts at risk for various genetically predisposed cancers. For example, the Li-Fraumeni Exploration Research Consortium (LiFE) was created to generate evidence for the most effective cancer prevention and risk-reducing strategies for future LFS family members (75). The future inclusion of dietary and lifestyle questionnaires, as well as biological samples, to the routine collection of cancer incidence profiles and clinical data could serve as the foundation for understanding critical factors that impact cancer development. Banked biospecimens for the evaluation of specific nutrients and biomarkers of relevant modifiable variables will ultimately provide algorithms that integrate genetic and environmental data and impact survival and quality of life for those with genetic syndromes. In parallel, the development of animal models that reflect human genetic disease and facilitate the screening of effective dietary and nutritional interventions is paramount to progress.

The field of nutrition and cancer is rapidly moving forward. Human nutritional genomic and cancer research is needed in order to elucidate the role of nutrition and dietary patterns as factors which can interact with host genetics and cancer genomics to impact biology and cancer risk. Personalized dietary and lifestyle interventions, as an adjunct to therapy, may lessen cancer risk. Diet also has potential to enhance survivorship, though more research is warranted. RDs can position themselves as experts in the field of nutritional genomics and be comfortable in discussing genetic concepts with their clients and incorporate this information into individualized clinical recommendations when strong evidence exists.

References

1. World Cancer Research Fund / American Institute for Cancer Research. *Food, Nutrition, Physical Activity and the Prevention of Cancer: a Global Perspective*. Washington DC: AICR; 2007.
2. Joint WHO/FAO Expert Consultation on Diet, Nutrition and the Prevention of Chronic Diseases. *Diet, nutrition and the prevention of chronic diseases: report of a joint WHO/FAO expert consultation*. Geneva, Switzerland; 2002. Available at: http://whqlibdoc.who.int/trs/who_trs_916.pdf.
3. Rock CL, Doyle C, Demark-Wahnefried W, et al. Nutrition and physical activity guidelines for cancer survivors. *CA Cancer J Clin*. 2012. Available at: http://www.ncbi.nlm.nih.gov/pubmed/22539238 [Accessed July 11, 2012].
4. American Cancer Society. Nutrition for the Person With Cancer During Treatment. *American Cancer Society: Find Support and Treatment*. 2012. Available at: http://www.cancer.org/Treatment/SurvivorshipDuringandAfterTreatment/NutritionforPeoplewithCancer/NutritionforthePersonwithCancer/nutrition-during-treatment-plan-for-treatment [Accessed September 11, 2012].
5. National Comprehensive Cancer Network. Nutrition for Cancer Survivors. *National Comprehensive Cancer Network*. 2012. Available at: http://www.nccn.com/index.php?option=com_content&view=article&id=129:nutrition-for-cancer-survivors&catid=66 [Accessed September 11, 2012].
6. National Comprehensive Cancer Network. Exercise for Life. 2012. Available at: http://www.nccn.com/index.php?option=com_content&view=article&id=127:exercise-for-life&catid=66 [Accessed September 11, 2012].
7. Hanahan D, Weinberg RA. The hallmarks of cancer. *Cell*. 2000;100(1):57–70.
8. Hanahan D, Weinberg RA. Hallmarks of cancer: the next generation. *Cell*. 2011;144(5):646–674.
9. Croce CM. Oncogenes and Cancer. New Engl J Med. 2008;358(5):502–511.
10. Barnes S. Nutritional genomics, polyphenols, diets, and their impact on dietetics. *J Am Diet Assoc*. 2008;108(11):1888–1895.
11. Fenech M, El-Sohemy A, Cahill L, et al. Nutrigenetics and nutrigenomics: viewpoints on the current status and applications in nutrition research and practice. *J Nutrigenet Nutrigenomics*. 2011;4(2):69–89.
12. Siddikuzzaman, Guruvayoorappan C, Berlin Grace VM. All trans retinoic acid and cancer. *Immunopharmacol Immunotoxicol*. 2011;33(2):241–249.
13. Yee LD, Lester JL, Cole RM, et al. Omega-3 fatty acid supplements in women at high risk of breast cancer have dose-dependent effects on breast adipose tissue fatty acid composition. *Am J Clin Nutr*. 2010;91(5):1185–1194.
14. Yee LD, Young DC, Rosol TJ, Vanbuskirk AM, Clinton SK. Dietary (n-3) polyunsaturated fatty acids inhibit HER-2/neu-induced breast cancer in mice independently of the PPARgamma ligand rosiglitazone. *J Nutr*. 2005;135(5):983–988.
15. Filiano JJ. Neurometabolic diseases in the newborn. *Clin Perinatol*. 2006;33(2):411–479.

16. Trahms C, Verona M. Nutrition Management of Inborn Errors of Metabolism. In: Nevin-Folino N, ed. *Pediatric Manual of Clinical Dietetics.* Second ed. Pediatric Nutrition Practice Group, American Dietetic Association; 2008:341–359.

17. Rader DJ, Cohen J, Hobbs HH. Monogenic hypercholesterolemia: new insights in pathogenesis and treatment. *J Clin Invest.* 2003;111(12):1795–1803.

18. Sjouke B, Kusters DM, Kastelein JJP, Hovingh GK. Familial hypercholesterolemia: present and future management. *Curr Cardiol* Rep. 2011;13(6):527–536.

19. Gibb EA, Brown CJ, Lam WL. The functional role of long non-coding RNA in human carcinomas. *Mol Cancer.* 2011;10:38.

20. National Center for Biotechnology Information. dbSNP. 2012. Available at: http://www.ncbi.nlm.nih.gov/snp [Accessed August 24, 2012].

21. Altshuler DM, Gibbs RA, Peltonen L, et al. Integrating common and rare genetic variation in diverse human populations. *Nature.* 2010;467(7311):52–58.

22. Human Genome Project Information. SNP Fact Sheet. 2008. Available at: http://www.ornl.gov/sci/techresources/Human_Genome/faq/snps.shtml [Accessed July 11, 2012].

23. Hecht SS, Kassie F, Hatsukami DK. Chemoprevention of lung carcinogenesis in addicted smokers and ex-smokers. *Nat Rev Cancer.* 2009;9(7):476--488.

24. Herr I, Büchler MW. Dietary constituents of broccoli and other cruciferous vegetables: implications for prevention and therapy of cancer. *Cancer Treat Rev.* 2010;36(5):377--383.

25. Spitz MR, Duphorne CM, Detry MA, et al. Dietary intake of isothiocyanates: evidence of a joint effect with glutathione S-transferase polymorphisms in lung cancer risk. *Cancer Epidemiol Biomarkers Prev.* 2000;9(10):1017–1020.

26. Chan AT, Giovannucci EL. Primary prevention of colorectal cancer. *Gastroenterology.* 2010;138(6):2029–2043.e10.

27. Taioli E, Garza MA, Ahn YO, et al. Meta- and pooled analyses of the methylenetetrahydrofolate reductase (MTHFR) C677T polymorphism and colorectal cancer: a HuGE-GSEC review. *Am J Epidemiol.* 2009;170(10):1207–1221.

28. Zhang X, Giovannucci EL, Smith-Warner SA, et al. A prospective study of intakes of zinc and heme iron and colorectal cancer risk in men and women. *Cancer Causes Control.* 2011;22(12):1627–1637.

29. Cross AJ, Ferrucci LM, Risch A, et al. A large prospective study of meat consumption and colorectal cancer risk: an investigation of potential mechanisms underlying this association. *Cancer Res.* 2010;70(6):2406–2414.

30. Gilsing A, Berndt S, Ruder E, et al. Meat-related mutagen exposure, xenobiotic metabolizing gene polymorphisms and the risk of advanced colorectal adenoma and cancer. *Carcinogenesis.* 2012. Available at: http://www.ncbi.nlm.nih.gov/pubmed/22552404 [Accessed July 12, 2012].

31. Knudson AG. Two genetic hits (more or less) to cancer. *Nat Rev Cancer.* 2001;1(2):157–162.

32. Ognjanovic S, Olivier M, Bergemann TL, Hainaut P. Sarcomas in TP53 germline mutation carriers: a review of the IARC TP53 database. *Cancer.* 2012;118(5):1387–1396.

33. Lane DP. Cancer. p53, guardian of the genome. *Nature.* 1992;358(6381):15–16.

34. Whibley C, Pharoah PDP, Hollstein M. p53 polymorphisms: cancer implications. *Nat Rev Cancer.* 2009;9(2):95–107.

35. Hursting SD, Lavigne JA, Berrigan D, et al. Diet-gene interactions in p53-deficient mice: insulin-like growth factor-1 as a mechanistic target. *J Nutr.* 2004;134(9):2482S–2486S.

36. Hursting SD, Smith SM, Lashinger LM, Harvey AE, Perkins SN. Calories and carcinogenesis: lessons learned from 30 years of calorie restriction research. *Carcinogenesis.* 2010;31(1):83–89.

37. Kleinerman RA. Radiation-sensitive genetically susceptible pediatric sub-populations. *Pediatr Radiol.* 2009;39 Suppl 1:S27–31.

38. Ribeiro RC, Pinto EM, Zambetti GP. Familial predisposition to adrenocortical tumors: clinical and biological features and management strategies. *Best Pract Res Clin Endocrinol Metab.* 2010;24(3):477–490.

39. Heinen CD. Genotype to phenotype: analyzing the effects of inherited mutations in colorectal cancer families. *Mutat Res.* 2010;693(1-2):32–45.

40. Itano O, Fan K, Yang K, et al. Effect of caloric intake on Western-style diet-induced intestinal tumors in a mouse model for hereditary colon cancer. *Nutr Cancer.* 2012;64(3):401–408.

41. Bommareddy A, Zhang X, Schrader D, et al. Effects of dietary flaxseed on intestinal tumorigenesis in Apc(Min) mouse. *Nutr Cancer.* 2009;61(2):276–283.

42. Murphy EA, Davis JM, McClellan JL, Gordon BT, Carmichael MD. Curcumin's effect on intestinal inflammation and tumorigenesis in the ApcMin/+ mouse. *J Interferon Cytokine Res.* 2011;31(2):219–226.

43. West NJ, Clark SK, Phillips RKS, et al. Eicosapentaenoic acid reduces rectal polyp number and size in familial adenomatous polyposis. *Gut.* 2010;59(7):918–925.

44. Sharma RA, McLelland HR, Hill KA, et al. Pharmacodynamic and pharmacokinetic study of oral Curcuma extract in patients with colorectal cancer. *Clin Cancer Res.* 2001;7(7):1894–1900.

45. Cruz-Correa M, Shoskes DA, Sanchez P, et al. Combination treatment with curcumin and quercetin of adenomas in familial adenomatous polyposis. *Clin Gastroenterol Hepatol.* 2006;4(8):1035–1038.

46. DeCosse JJ, Miller HH, Lesser ML. Effect of wheat fiber and vitamins C and E on rectal polyps in patients with familial adenomatous polyposis. *J Natl Cancer Inst.* 1989;81(17):1290–1297.

47. Kim B, Giardiello FM. Chemoprevention in familial adenomatous polyposis. *Best Pract Res Clin Gastroenterol.* 2011;25(4-5):607–622.

48. Thomas MG, Thomson JP, Williamson RC. Oral calcium inhibits rectal epithelial proliferation in familial adenomatous polyposis. *Br J Surg.* 1993;80(4):499–501.

49. Berger SL, Kouzarides T, Shiekhattar R, Shilatifard A. An operational definition of epigenetics. *Genes Dev.* 2009;23(7):781–783.

50. Daxinger L, Whitelaw E. Understanding transgenerational epigenetic inheritance via the gametes in mammals. *Nat Rev Genet.* 2012;13(3):153–162.

51. Skinner MK. Environmental epigenetic transgenerational inheritance and somatic epigenetic mitotic stability. *Epigenetics.* 2011;6(7):838–842.

52. Sharma A, Heuck CJ, Fazzari MJ, et al. DNA methylation alterations in multiple myeloma as a model for epigenetic changes in cancer. *Wiley Interdiscip Rev Syst Biol Med.* 2010;2(6):654–669.

53. Dawson MA, Kouzarides T. Cancer epigenetics: from mechanism to therapy. *Cell.* 2012;150(1):12–27.

54. Iorio MV, Croce CM. microRNA involvement in human cancer. *Carcinogenesis.* 2012;33(6):1126–1133.

55. Ross SA, Milner JA. Epigenetic modulation and cancer: effect of metabolic syndrome? *Am J Clin Nutr.* 2007;86(3):s872–877.

56. Walker CL, Ho S-M. Developmental reprogramming of cancer susceptibility. *Nat Rev Cancer.* 2012;12(7):479–486.

57. Dolinoy DC. The agouti mouse model: an epigenetic biosensor for nutritional and environmental alterations on the fetal epigenome. *Nutr Rev.* 2008;66 Suppl 1:S7–11.

58. Bygren LO, Kaati G, Edvinsson S. Longevity determined by paternal ancestors' nutrition during their slow growth period. *Acta Biotheor.* 2001;49(1):53–59.

59. Faulk C, Dolinoy DC. Timing is everything: the when and how of environmentally induced changes in the epigenome of animals. *Epigenetics.* 2011;6(7):791–797.

60. Hawkins NA, Smith T, Zhao L, Rodriguez J, Berkowitz Z, Stein KD. Health-related behavior change after cancer: results of the American Cancer Society's studies of cancer survivors (SCS). *J Cancer Surviv.* 2010;4(1):20–32.

61. Park ER, Japuntich SJ, Rigotti NA, et al. A snapshot of smokers after lung and colorectal cancer diagnosis. *Cancer.* 2012;118(12):3153–3164.

62. Ollberding NJ, Maskarinec G, Wilkens LR, Henderson BE, Kolonel LN. Comparison of modifiable health behaviours between persons with and without cancer: the Multiethnic Cohort. *Public Health Nutr.* 2011;14(10):1796–1804.

63. Blanchard CM, Courneya KS, Stein K. Cancer survivors' adherence to lifestyle behavior recommendations and associations with health-related quality of life: results from the American Cancer Society's SCS-II. *J Clin Oncol.* 2008;26(13):2198–2204.

64. Miller PE, Vasey JJ, Short PF, Hartman TJ. Dietary supplement use in adult cancer survivors. *Oncol Nurs Forum.* 2009;36(1):61–68.

65. Miller MF, Bellizzi KM, Sufian M, Ambs AH, Goldstein MS, Ballard-Barbash R. Dietary supplement use in individuals living with cancer and other chronic conditions: a population-based study. *J Am Diet Assoc.* 2008;108(3):483–494.

66. Nelms M, Sucher KP, Lacey K, Roth SL. *Nutrition Therapy and Pathophysiology.* 2nd ed. Brooks Cole; 2010.

67. DeBusk RM, Ph D. *Genetics: The Nutrition Connection.* 1st ed. Amer Dietetic Assn; 2003.

68. Feero WG, Guttmacher AE, Collins FS. Genomic medicine-an updated primer. *N Engl J Med.* 2010;362(21):2001–2011.

69. Lodish H, Berk A, Kaiser CA, et al. *Molecular Cell Biology.* 7th ed. W. H. Freeman; 2012.

70. Foster GD, Wyatt HR, Hill JO, et al. Weight and metabolic outcomes after 2 years on a low-carbohydrate versus low-fat diet: a randomized trial. *Ann Intern Med.* 2010;153(3):147–157.

71. Shiffman S, Brockwell SE, Pillitteri JL, Gitchell JG. Use of smoking-cessation treatments in the United States. *Am J Prev Med.* 2008;34(2): 102–111.

72. Greenwald P, Witkin KM. Familial adenomatous polyposis: a nutritional intervention trial. *J Natl Cancer Inst.* 1989;81(17):1272–1273.

73. Bohn T, Blackwood M, Francis D, Tian Q, Schwartz SJ, Clinton SK. Bioavailability of phytochemical constituents from a novel soy fortified lycopene rich tomato juice developed for targeted cancer prevention trials. *Nutr Cancer.* 2011. Available at: http://www.ncbi.nlm.nih.gov/pubmed/22098224 [Accessed September 26, 2012].

74. Simmons AL, Miller CK, Clinton SK, Vodovotz Y. A comparison of satiety, glycemic index, and insulinemic index of wheat-derived soft pretzels with or without soy. *Food Funct.* 2011;2(11):678–683.

75. Mai PL, Malkin D, Garber JE, et al. Li-Fraumeni syndrome: report of a clinical research workshop and creation of a research consortium. *Cancer Genet.* 2012. Available at: http://www.ncbi.nlm.nih.gov/pubmed/22939227 [Accessed September 26, 2012].

Nutrition and Cancer Survivorship

Cynthia A. Thomson, PhD, RD, CSO
Ashley J. Vargas, PhD, RD, CSG

The Cancer Survivor

Cancer survivorship is an expanding area of clinical dietetics practice. Approximately 13.6 million Americans are living with a history of a cancer diagnosis (1) primarily because survival rates have improved steadily for many cancers over the past few decades. Close to 70% of patients diagnosed with cancer survive beyond the five-year monitoring period, which is a benchmark for studies of survivorship (1). Cancer survivorship encompasses individuals in active treatment and recovery as well as those with advanced disease commonly receiving palliative care; however, for the purpose of this chapter the focus is on those living after cancer therapy, primarily those who are disease-free or who have stable disease. The *National Action Plan for Cancer Survivorship* led by the Centers for Disease Control and Prevention calls for an even broader definition that encompasses caregivers, family and friends who support individuals diagnosed with cancer (2).

While cancer survivors have been diagnosed with a wide variety of neoplasms, breast, prostate and colon cancer survivors represent the vast majority of survivors. These cancers are more commonly diagnosed through early detection screening plans, and survival rates are high. For example over 98% of women diagnosed with early stage breast cancer will be living 10 years post diagnosis; they comprise approximately 40% of female cancer survivors (3).

Importantly, cancer survivors represent a highly motivated segment of the clinical care population that actively seek counseling and information to improve their overall health, quality of life and survival (4). More importantly, survivors report personal attempts to improve dietary selections at the time of or shortly after diagnosis, which indicates that survivors are highly motivated candidates for dietary change (5). The usual dietary behavior of patients at the time of cancer diagnosis is increasingly identified as an indicator of survival after cancer. This suggests that those at risk for cancer, including family members of cancer patients, would benefit from adopting healthy eating habits in an effort to reduce risk and improve outcomes if diagnosed with cancer (6-8).

Early Survival Period

The weeks and months post-therapy leave many oncology patients at nutritional risk. A significant number of patients lose lean mass due to surgery and/or chemotherapy, suffer fatigue related to radiation therapy, or become depressed as a result of having a life-threatening illness (9). These treatment-associated problems can compromise a person's nutritional status but these concerns are, fortunately, responsive to dietary counseling (10-12). As body weight is regained during this period, many patients increase their fat mass without concomitantly increasing their lean mass, placing them at risk for sarcopenic obesity (13). It is, therefore, important for the dietetic professional to perform a thorough nutritional assessment when therapy ends to identify any compromise in nutritional status. Assessments should include anthropometric evaluation to identify changes in central adiposity by measuring waist circumference, and assessing lean and fat mass status by using bioelectrical impedance or dual-xray absorptiometry. Serial assessments are important to assure that lean mass is maintained and to implement a nutrition and activity plan if lean mass is depleted. Many patients who have undergone extensive surgery or long-term therapies will require ample protein intake and regular physical activity in order to increase lean mass (14). Partnering registered dietitians (RDs) with exercise physiologists will promote optimal body composition in these patients.

Additionally, early in the survivorship period many dietetic professionals recommend patients complete a comprehensive symptom report to identify issues that alter eating such as changes in taste, nausea, irregular bowel or gastrointestinal function, and dysgeusia and/or dysphagia. Long term survivors of head and neck cancer (15) and bone marrow transplantation may be at higher risk for sustained problems with eating and food tolerance and will require more comprehensive and frequent nutritional evaluations (16).

The early survival period post-therapy is generally up to 12 months; during that time eating may be difficult due to persistent issues such as nausea, xerostomia, loss of dentition and/or radiation enteritis. During this period efforts to reduce persistent therapy-related side effects should be a primary focus of nutritional care. Table 1 lists many of the more common symptoms and health issues of survivors during this period, as well as several appropriate nutritional approaches that can be used to effectively intervene. Further, numerous reliable resources for information on coping with other symptoms and side effects that result from cancer therapy are available. Several of these resources are described in Table 2. Chapter 12 also addresses management strategies for nutrition impact symptoms.

Table 1: Long-term nutrition-related complications of common cancers by cancer site

Common Cancer Site	Common Nutrition Complications	Nutrition Diagnoses	Common Nutritional Approaches (modify approaches per results of nutrition assessment)
Breast	Impaired bone health (1)	NB-2.3 NI-55.1	• Ensure adequate intake of calcium and vitamin D • Promote weight bearing exercises, if appropriate
	Weight gain/metabolic syndrome (2)	NI-1.3 NI-5.5	• Adjust calorie, carbohydrate, fat and whole grain intake to promote healthy weight, blood glucose, and circulating insulin and lipid levels. • Promote physical activity to meet current guidelines for survivors
	Cardiovascular complications (1)	NI-5.5	• Recommend a heart healthy diet • Promote weight control
Prostate	Impaired bone health (1)	NI-55.1 NB-2.3	• Ensure adequate intake of calcium and vitamin D • Promote weight bearing exercises, if appropriate
	Enteritis/chronic diarrhea (1)	NI-3.1 NC-1.4	• Increase fluid intake and balance electrolytes • Decrease fat intake, alter fiber intake and limit dairy intake as needed
Lung & bronchus	Esophageal pain/dysphagia (1)	NC-1.1 NC-1.2	• Alter food/beverage consistency and use medical nutrition beverages as needed • Alter food temperature and avoid alcohol, spicy foods and other irritant-containing foods (e.g., acidic foods)
	Respiratory failure (1)	NI-5.5 NI-5.8	• Monitor and correct fluid balance • Decrease carbohydrate intake, if needed
Colon & rectum	Malabsorption (3)	NC-2.1 NC-3.2	• Increase intake or modify sources of nutrients that are malabsorbed • Monitor nutrition status and weight
	Altered liver function/cirrhosis (3)	NC-2.1	• Increase intake of nutrients that are malabsorbed • Monitor liver enzymes • If cirrhotic, follow evidence-based medical nutrition therapy for liver cirrhosis
	Weight change (4)	NC-3.2 NC-3.4 NI-1.1 NI-1.3	• Monitor weight • Ensure balanced nutrient intake for maintaining and/or achieving a healthy weight • Balance calorie intake with physical activity
	Irregular bowel movements (1)	NC-1.4	• Alter fiber intake as needed • Consume adequate fluids; monitor fluid intake • Use probiotics/prebiotics, if appropriate
	Enteritis/chronic diarrhea (1)	NI-3.1 NC-1.4	• Increase fluid intake and balance electrolytes • Decrease fat intake, alter fiber intake and limit dairy intake as needed
	Bowel strictures/obstructions (3)	NC-1.4	• If bowel sounds: enteral or parenteral nutrition support as appropriate • If no bowel sounds: enteral or parental nutrition support as appropriate
Urinary bladder	Irregular bowel movements (1)	NC-1.4	• Alter fiber intake as needed • Consume adequate fluids, monitor fluid status
Uterine corpus	Impaired bone health (5)	NB-2.3 NI-55.1	• Ensure adequate intake of calcium and vitamin D • Promote weight bearing exercises, if appropriate
Thyroid	Hypothyroidism (1)	NI-1.3	• Adjust calorie intake to maintain a healthy weight
Non-Hodgkin lymphoma	Metabolic syndrome (6)	NI-1.3 NI-5.5	• Adjust calorie, carbohydrate, fat and whole grain intake to promote healthy weight, blood glucose, and circulating insulin and lipid levels • Promote physical activity to meet current guidelines for survivors
	Hypothyroidism (6)	NI-1.3	• Adjust calorie intake to maintain a healthy weight • Promote physical activity to meet current guidelines for survivors
Kidney	Decreased creatinine clearance (3)	NC-2.2	• Monitor renal labs and adjust nutrient intake as needed
	Hypertension (3)	NI-5.5	• Monitor sodium intake and adjust (most commonly reduce) sodium intake as needed • Promote weight control • Promote adequate intake of potassium and calcium
	Renal failure (3)	NI-5.5	• Monitor renal labs and adjust nutrient intake as needed

(Continued)

Table 1: Long-term nutrition-related complications of common cancers by cancer site *(continued)*

Common Cancer Site	Common Nutrition Complications	Nutrition Diagnoses	Common Nutritional Approaches (modify approaches per results of nutrition assessment)
Oral cavity & pharynx	Xerostomia (7)	NI-2.1 NC-1.1 NC-1.2	• Ensure nutrient requirements are met via oral intake, if possible • Promote consumption of "wet" foods • Promote good oral care • Alter food/beverage consistency as needed, use medical nutrition beverages and supplemental calorie, protein, and nutrient products, consider nutrition support, if indicated
	Dysphagia (7)	NC-1.1	• Alter food/beverage consistency as needed and use medical nutrition beverages and supplemental calorie, protein, and nutrient products as needed • Consult with Speech-Language Pathologist
	Tooth decay/periodontal disease (7)	NC-1.2	• Alter food/beverage consistency as needed and use medical nutrition beverages and supplemental calorie, protein, and nutrient products as needed • Alter food temperature, if tooth sensitivity is an issue • Alter types of food consumed, if dysgeusia is an issue
Leukemia	Kidney stones (8)	NI-3.1	• Increase fluid intake to recommended levels
	Impaired bone health (9)	NI-55.1 NB-2.3	• Ensure adequate intake of calcium and vitamin D • Promote weight bearing exercises, if appropriate
	Metabolic syndrome (6)	NI-1.3 NI-5.5 NI-1.3	• Adjust calories, sugar and fat intake to promote healthy weight, blood glucose and insulin level and circulating lipid levels • Promote physical activity to meet current guidelines for survivors
	Hypothyroidism (6)	NI-55.1	• Adjust calorie intake to maintain a healthy weight
Ovary	Impaired bone health (10)	NB-2.3	• Ensure adequate intake of calcium and vitamin D • Promote weight bearing exercises, if appropriate
Pancreas	Anorexia (11)	NI-1.4 NC-3.2	• Increase nutrient intake using nutrient-dense foods and medical nutrition beverages as needed • Modify meal schedule as needed
	Malabsorption (11)	NC-2.1 NC-3.2	• Modify intake of nutrients that are malabsorbed, if indicated • Consider use of pancreatic enzymes • Monitor weight, nutrition and fluid status
	Irregular bowel movements (11)	NC-1.4	• Alter fiber intake • Use probiotics/prebiotics, if appropriate
All sites (1,12)	Fatigue	NB-2.3 NB-2.4 NC-3.2	• Develop an eating plan and encourage caretakers to get involved in eating plan • Use foods easy to prepare and easy to eat • Use medical nutrition beverages as needed • Monitor weight • Promote physical activity as tolerated
	Weight change	NC-3.2 NC-3.4 NI-1.1 NI-1.3	• Monitor weight • Ensure nutrient intake is balanced to maintain/achieve a healthy weight • Promote physical activity as needed
	Appetite change/nausea	NC-3.2 NC-3.4 NI-1.1 NI-1.3	• Increase/decrease nutrient intake using nutrient-dense foods and medical nutrition beverages as appropriate • If nauseous: select bland, cool, light foods and avoid foods with strong odors • Take anti-nausea medications, if prescribed and as prescribed
	Secondary cancer/recurrence (13)	NB-1.1 NB-1.7	• General interventions for cancer prevention (see Appendix 1) • Achieve/maintain healthy weight • Increase physical activity • Eat a diet that is high in fruit, vegetables and whole grains • Increase intake of foods high in omega-3 fatty acids, like fish (13) • Recommend appropriate dietary supplements when a deficiency is noted

Table 2: Resources for Cancer Survivors

Organization	Website	Synopsis
The Academy of Nutrition and Dietetics	http://www.eatright.org	Provides information on medical nutrition therapy and reference materials
American Cancer Society	http://www.cancer.org/	Provides information for cancer patients at all stages
American Cancer Society: Cancer Survivors Network	http://csn.cancer.org/	Connects survivors for support via the internet
American Institute for Cancer Research	http://www.aicr.org/reduce-your-cancer-risk/physical-activity/reduce_physical_getting_started.html	Information on increasing physical activity
American Society of Clinical Oncologist	http://www.cancer.net/patient/Survivorship	Medical association that provides information about survivorship and cancer
Cancer Care	http://www.cancercare.org/	Connects survivors with social workers, financial support and support groups
Cancer.net	http://www.cancer.net/survivorship	Introduction to life changes following cancer treatment.
Center for Disease Control: and Prevention	http://www.cdc.gov/cancer/survivorship/	Provides information on cancer survivorship-related prevalence, support for caregivers and general information
National Cancer Institute: Office of Cancer Survivorship	http://dccps.nci.nih.gov/ocs/	Provides information on cancer survivorship-related research and prevalence
National Coalition for Cancer Survivorship	http://www.canceradvocacy.org/	Cancer survivor advocacy organization with a "toolbox" and other information for survivors
Physician's Committee for Responsible Medicine Cancer Survivor's Guide	http://www.pcrm.org	Resource guide written by physician and registered dietitian that includes healthy eating tips as well as recipes.
World Cancer Research Fund/ American Institute for Cancer Research	http://www.dietandcancerreport.org/	Expert panel review of nutrition, physical activity and cancer risk research

Post-symptom Diet Therapy

After a patient's symptoms have generally improved and they are able to tolerate all food groups and textures, nutrition therapy shifts toward health promotion and cancer prevention. In this longer-term period, many cancer patients gain weight and put themselves at risk for chronic disease and cancer recurrence. Figure 1 summarizes the metabolic and physical concerns that can result in increased chronic disease risk and decreased quality of life in individuals treated for cancer.

During the 12-month post-treatment/post-symptom time period, many survivors will express interest in improving lifestyle choices to enhance health. Convincing evidence suggests that obesity is associated with a poorer prognosis and a decreased survival for patients of several cancer types (17-20), including breast and gynecological (21-22), colorectal (23), and prostate cancers (24). This association is particularly apparent in the presence of co-morbid obesity-related disease, such as diabetes (25).

Obesity in the Post-treatment Setting

Obesity is associated with several cancers including post-menopausal breast cancer, endometrial cancer, aggressive prostate cancer, colorectal cancer, cancers of the pancreas, esophagus, kidney gallbladder, liver, cervix and ovary, non-Hodgkin lymphoma and multiple myeloma (26). Central adiposity is particularly problematic.

Interesting data from the SUCCEED trial of obese endometrial cancer survivors suggests that women seek high-calorie foods as a reward (27). Other research has shown that fatigue may be a significant driver of high-calorie food seeking behavior in cancer survivors (28). In order to decrease cancer recurrence and other disease risk, survivors with excess body weight and/or body fat should be counseled to achieve a healthy body weight. Several small studies have been completed demonstrating the efficacy of weight loss interventions in cancer survivors. Overweight and obese women who lose modest amounts of body weight can experience improvements in metabolic and cardiovascular biomarkers and quality of life (29-31). For survivors who are eating to reward themselves, six-months of lifestyle coaching may lower response to high-calorie food cues (27). For survivors who are suffering fatigue, weight loss success may require fatigue intervention. The ideal weight loss approach should establish energy balance by promoting healthy food choices, portions and meal patterns and incorporating physical activity. Most cancer survivors should be encouraged to undertake a regular activity regimen that includes both aerobic and weight bearing activity. Variety in the types of physical activity pursued will promote a healthy body composition post-therapy (32). Weight lifting and weight bearing activity supports adequate bone health, which is commonly compromised after cancer therapy (14,33), and is considered safe and effective for controlling lymphedema after breast cancer (34-36). While face-to-face counseling is the most common approach, evidence from a home-based lifestyle intervention suggested mailed materials are also efficacious in promoting increased physical activity and diet in cancer survivors (37-38) and may provide a less time consuming approach to counseling.

Dietary Intervention Studies in Cancer Survivors

Several studies have been conducted in the past two decades to determine the effects of post-therapy lifestyle interventions on cancer survival. Most have been conducted in breast cancer survivors, as this is the most commonly diagnosed cancer in women, and survival rates provide a sufficient population for a large-scale study. While findings may not be generalized to all cancer survivors, the results do provide early evidence that 1) cancer survivors can make substantial changes in eating behavior and 2) healthy eating and lifestyle choices may promote overall health in survivors including such outcomes as improvements in functional health, weight control, and quality of life. Evidence relating diet and lifestyle

changes to increased progression-free survival has not generally been demonstrated. Table 3 describes the currently published and ongoing U.S. trials that enrolled or plan to enroll 100 or more cancer survivors and the key findings reported, or in the case of active trials, the *a priori* outcomes of interest.

Most of the intervention trials conducted have been developed with a strong theoretical underpinning to promote behavioral change. Behavioral strategies for improving diet and physical activity in survivors that have performed well include self-efficacy (39), motivational interviewing (40) and self-determination theory (41).

The dietary and lifestyle habits of women prior to a cancer diagnosis appear to have a significant influence on survival and recurrent disease. This relationship has been demonstrated in prospective epidemiological studies and additionally in analyses conducted using baseline lifestyle habits to predict survival in women entering lifestyle intervention trials. As an example, Dolecek *et al.* evaluated the eating habits of 341 women diagnosed with epithelial ovarian

Figure 1: Biology of Weight Change in Cancer Survivors

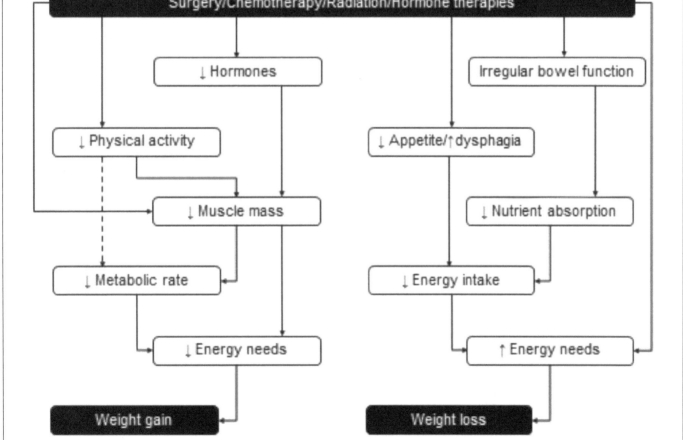

The acute and long-term consequences of cancer treatment commonly lead to weight change. For example gastrointestinal cancer survivors who have had bowel resections often experience altered bowel function and impaired nutrient absorption which causes acute weight loss. Another example is the long-term use of estrogen receptor antagonist for secondary breast cancer prevention which alters hormone metabolism and energy needs with a resulting long-term increase in body weight. A third example is the radiation damage to the esophagus that is common in lung cancer survivors and results in chronic or acute dysphagia and weight loss.

Table 3: Summary of Select Randomized Nutrition and Cancer Survivorship Clinical Trials

Study	n	Population	Intervention(s)	Primary outcome(s)	Significant finding(s)
WHEL (14)	3,088	Pre- and postmenopausal breast cancer survivors	High vegetable and fruit, low fat diet	↓ Breast cancer and related deaths	No main effect of dietary intervention
WINS (15)	2,347	Postmenopausal women with a recent history of early stage breast cancer	Reduced dietary fat intake	↑ relapse-free survival rates	Participants on the intervention diet had ↑ relapse-free survival breast cancer rates, with particular efficacy in those with hormone receptor-negative breast cancer
RENEW (16)	641	Older, overweight survivors of colorectal, breast and prostate cancer	Healthy eating counseling and physical activity	↑ levels of physical function	Participants on the intervention had ↑ levels of physical function in addition to improvements in diet, physical activity and weight loss
LEAD (17)	160	Older breast and prostate cancer survivors	Healthy eating counseling and physical activity	↑ levels of physical function	Participants on the intervention had ↑ levels of physical function in addition to improvements in diet and physical activity
FRESH START (18)	543	Early stage breast and prostate cancer survivors	High fruit and vegetables, reduced fat and increased physical activity with written material	↑ healthy lifestyle (diet and physical activity)	Participants on the intervention had ↑ in healthy lifestyle components, including increased physical activity and healthier diet compositions
SUCCEED (19)	75	Early stage overweight and obese endometrial cancer survivors	Improved nutrition and physical activity	↑ healthy lifestyle (diet and physical activity)	Participants on the intervention had ↑ in healthy lifestyle components, including increased physical activity, healthier diet compositions and weight loss
ONE (20)	51	Stage II-IV ovarian cancer survivors	Low fat/high fiber diet versus a healthy diet with soy	↓ anthropometrics and ↑ health-related quality of life	Healthy dietary choices improved in both intervention groups but no changes in anthropometrics were observed
CHOICE (21)	~370	Overweight and obese postmenopausal breast cancer survivors	Low fat versus low carbohydrates weight loss diets	Weight loss and inflammatory biomarkers	Ongoing
BONEII (22)	~279	Childhood acute lymphoblastic leukemia survivors	Nutrition counseling with vitamin D and calcium supplements	↑ bone mineral density	Ongoing
ENERGY (13)	~800	Overweight and obese breast cancer survivors	Diet and physical activity counseling	↑ healthy lifestyle (diet and physical activity)	Ongoing
LIVES	~1,080	Ovarian cancer survivors	Diet and physical activity coaching over the phone	↑ relapse-free survival rates and quality of life	Ongoing

cancer who were participating in an epidemiological cohort study. Survival was significantly increased in women who reported that their usual diets were higher in green vegetables, orange-yellow vegetables and cruciferous vegetables prior to their diagnosis. Overall mortality was significantly higher in women reporting higher red and processed meat and milk intake (6). Additionally, women previously treated for invasive breast cancer and enrolled in the control arm of the Women's Healthy Eating and Living (WHEL) study showed a significant ~50% reduction in mortality rate if they entered the study reporting dietary habits that included > 5 servings of vegetables and fruit daily combined with 30 minutes of moderate physical activity five to six days a week (42).

Dietary Guidance: A Role for Specific Foods?

In addition to weight control, dietary guidance for cancer survivors should address an overall healthy eating plan that targets increased intake of select foods and food groups while concurrently reducing or restricting other foods/food groups.

Alcohol

Alcohol consumption is generally not advised for the post-diagnosis survivor. Alcohol is a concentrated caloric source at 7 calories per gram and alcohol intake may serve as a replacement for nutrient-dense food selections that are important to health promotion. The evidence suggesting that alcohol increases risk for cancer recurrence or reduced survival is modest and has only been evaluated in women with breast cancer. Results have been mixed as the dose and type of alcohol consumed may be important determinants in the response to alcohol. In a study of ~1000 women diagnosed with early stage breast cancer, alcohol intake prior to diagnosis of any type was associated with poorer prognosis in breast cancer (43). Intakes of alcohol after breast cancer diagnosis was associated with recurrence in a study of over 1,800 women (15). However, in the WHEL study, alcohol was not associated with recurrent disease (44), possibly due to the overall low intake of alcohol and the healthier lifestyle habits of some alcohol consumers. Of note, wine was the more common alcoholic beverage consumed and red wine is known to have aromatase inhibitory effects that may play a role in reducing disease (45). Alcohol intake has been convincingly associated with primary risk for breast, head and neck, pancreatic, pharyngeal, laryngeal, esophageal, and hepatic cancers (46). Alcohol avoidance may be a prudent approach after a cancer diagnosis. Alcohol avoidance may be particularly relevant for patients diagnosed with head and neck (47) and esophageal cancers, where alcohol intake after diagnosis is predictive of poorer overall survival (48).

Vegetables/fruit
The role of vegetables and fruit in cancer survivorship is not clearly established. Intervention trials such as the WHEL study, wherein survivors consumed increased amounts of plant foods on a regular basis, showed no survival advantage versus the control condition, which included 5 servings of fruits and vegetables daily (44). However, vegetables and fruit may improve the health of cancer survivors for non-cancer outcomes and overall mortality. In a subgroup analysis, eating five servings of vegetables and fruits daily along with 30 minutes of moderate activity reduced overall mortality in breast cancer survivors by 44% (44). Vegetables and, to a slightly lesser extent, fruit are nutrient dense, low calorie options that may promote increased satiety. These foods also support increased exposure to numerous bioactive food components with chemopreventative activity such as carotenoids, allylic sulfides, isothiocyanates, and anthocyanins (49).

Fat
The role of dietary fat in cancer survivorship is also not well established. Intriguing evidence from the Women's Intervention Nutrition Study (WINS) did suggest that very low fat diets were associated with lower breast cancer recurrence in women with estrogen receptor negative disease. However, the low fat diet consumed by women enrolled in the WHEL study was not associated with reduced recurrence of breast cancer (44). Higher fat intake may contribute to increased recurrence risk for cancer because high fat diets often include more omega-6 but, not necessarily more omega-3 fatty acids. Lower omega-3 to omega-6 ratio of fat intakes generally translates to greater inflammatory status (50) and inflammation has been associated with increased cancer risk (51).

The Role of Energy Balance
As stated in the American Cancer Society (ACS) Guidelines for Nutrition and Physical Activity, maintaining a healthy body weight is integral to improved quality of life and reduced obesity-related co-morbidity. Energy balance also may influence recurrence and survival after cancer. Calorie intake should be balanced with energy expenditure to achieve a healthy body weight over time. Weight control interventions in survivors have been effective (Table 3). Several interventions have integrated physical activity to promote weight loss (19) and/or improve physical function (6,17). Most survivors will tolerate physical activity well; however, efforts to increase activity should be gradual and also consider alternative approaches beyond walking as indicated. This is particularly important in survivors who report significant fatigue, neuropathy or myalgia.

Dietary Interventions for Bone and Muscle Health
Age is the leading risk factor for cancer with over 75% of cancers diagnosed in people over 55 years of age (52). Age is also a primary risk factor for increased loss of bone mineral density, reduced physical function and in the advanced stage, sarcopenia. Obesity also increases with age although rates reduce after age 75 years (52) possibly related to survival bias (i.e., normal weight individuals survive more often over time than their obese counterparts). However, for individuals who survive beyond age 75 years there is a common and steady reduction in skeletal muscle mass, an increase in fat to lean mass ratio, and an increase in osteopenia/osteoporosis risk (53). These clinical consequences of aging are more prominent in those who have experienced a cancer diagnosis (54).

While physical activity that includes weight-bearing, resistance and balance are central to improving musculoskeletal health, dietary selections also influence musculoskeletal health. Adequate protein to reduce frailty is an important first-line nutritional therapy. In a recent study of healthy post-menopausal women, protein intake up to 1.2 grams/kilogram/day was associated with reduced frailty (55). This same level of protein intake is recommended to meet the protein requirements of cancer survivors who are over age 50 years. Further, selection of foods with higher quality protein (i.e., low fat animal protein or plant proteins paired to be "complete" sources of protein) also may promote improved musculoskeletal health (56), although this has not been sufficiently tested in cancer survivors.

Dietary Supplementation for Survivors
It has been reported that 64-81% of cancer survivors consume dietary supplements, which is a higher frequency of use than the overall population (57). However, there is limited evidence that multivitamin-mineral supplementation or individual nutrient supplements are protective against recurrence or mortality. A meta-analysis in 2006 and a cohort analysis in 2009 found no protection of antioxidant supplementation despite these nutrients being a common choice among supplementing cancer survivors (58-59). In breast cancer survivors no specific or multivitamin supplement was shown to reduce recurrence or improve survival (60-61) and similar null associations were reported in a cohort of colorectal cancer survivors (21). On the other hand, a study found that beta-carotene supplementation reduced survival in colorectal cancer patients who reported regular use of alcohol and cigarettes (62). Dietetic professionals should closely evaluate the quality of

micronutrient intake in individual survivors and make informed judgments as to how to best advise cancer survivors on the use of dietary supplementation based on the evidence. Every effort should be made to obtain nutrient needs through food selections. Chapter 8 provides additional information on dietary supplements for cancer survivors.

Resources for Supporting Dietary Lifestyle Change in Survivors

Table 2 provides a listing of select resources available to healthcare providers to support lifestyle behavior change in their patients/clients. In addition to web-based information several evidence-based books from organizations such as ACS have been published that address the role of diet and physical activity in cancer care as well as provide specific tips to survivors related to achieving optimal health through lifestyle behaviors.

References for Text

1. Eheman C, Henley SJ, Ballard-Barbash R, et al. Annual Report to the Nation on the status of cancer, 1975-2008, featuring cancers associated with excess weight and lack of sufficient physical activity. *Cancer.* 2012;118(9):2338-2366.
2. Arceci R, Ettinger A, Forman E, et al. National action plan for childhood cancer: report of the national summit meetings on childhood cancer. *CA Cancer J Clin.* 2002;52(6):377-379.
3. American Cancer Society. Breast Cancer Facts and Figures 2011-2012. 2011-2012; http://www.cancer.org/acs/groups/content/@ epidemiologysurveilance/documents/document/acspc-030975.pdf. Accessed July 16, 2012.
4. Jones LW, Demark-Wahnefried W. Diet, exercise, and complementary therapies after primary treatment for cancer. *Lancet Oncol.* 2006;7(12):1017-1026.
5. Thomson CA, Flatt SW, Rock CL, Ritenbaugh C, Newman V, Pierce JP. Increased fruit, vegetable and fiber intake and lower fat intake reported among women previously treated for invasive breast cancer. *J Am Diet Assoc.* 2002;102(6):801-808.
6. Dolecek TA, McCarthy BJ, Joslin CE, et al. Prediagnosis food patterns are associated with length of survival from epithelial ovarian cancer. *J Am Diet Assoc.* 2010;110(3):369-382.
7. Duffy SA, Ronis DL, McLean S, et al. Pretreatment health behaviors predict survival among patients with head and neck squamous cell carcinoma. *J Clin Oncol.* 2009;27(12):1969-1975.
8. Shen GP, Xu FH, He F, et al. Pretreatment lifestyle behaviors as survival predictors for patients with nasopharyngeal carcinoma. *PLoS One.* 2012;7(5):e36515.
9. Sunga AY, Eberl MM, Oeffinger KC, Hudson MM, Mahoney MC. Care of cancer survivors. *Am Fam Physician.* 2005;71(4):699-706.
10. Ravasco P, Monteiro Grillo I, Camilo M. Cancer wasting and quality of life react to early individualized nutritional counselling! *Clin Nutr.* 2007; 26(1):7-15.
11. Ravasco P, Monteiro-Grillo I, Vidal PM, Camilo ME. Dietary counseling improves patient outcomes: a prospective, randomized, controlled trial in colorectal cancer patients undergoing radiotherapy. *J Clin Oncol.* 2005;23(7):1431-1438.
12. Rock CL. Dietary counseling is beneficial for the patient with cancer. *J Clin Oncol.* 2005;23(7):1348-1349.
13. Demark-Wahnefried W, Peterson BL, Winer EP, et al. Changes in weight, body composition, and factors influencing energy balance among premenopausal breast cancer patients receiving adjuvant chemotherapy. *J Clin Oncol.* 2001;19(9):2381-2389.
14. Winters-Stone KM, Dobek J, Nail L, et al. Strength training stops bone loss and builds muscle in postmenopausal breast cancer survivors: a randomized, controlled trial. *Breast Cancer Res Treat.* 2011;127(2):447-456.
15. Kwan ML, Kushi LH, Weltzien E, et al. Alcohol consumption and breast cancer recurrence and survival among women with early-stage breast cancer: the life after cancer epidemiology study. *J Clin Oncol.* 2010; 28(29):4410-4416.
16. Lenssen P, Sherry ME, Cheney CL, et al. Prevalence of nutrition-related problems among long-term survivors of allogeneic marrow transplantation. *J Am Diet Assoc.* 1990;90(6):835-842.
17. Arem H, Irwin ML. Obesity and endometrial cancer survival: a systematic review. *Int J Obes (Lond).* Jun 19 2012 doi: 10.1038/ijo.2012.94.
18. Freedland SJ. Obesity and prostate cancer: a growing problem. *Clin Cancer Res.* 2005;11(19 Pt 1):6763-6766.
19. Patterson RE, Flatt SW, Saquib N, et al. Medical comorbidities predict mortality in women with a history of early stage breast cancer. *Breast Cancer Res Treat.* 2010;122(3):859-865.
20. Protani M, Coory M, Martin JH. Effect of obesity on survival of women with breast cancer: systematic review and meta-analysis. *Breast Cancer Res Treat.* 2010;123(3):627-635.
21. McTiernan A, Irwin M, Vongruenigen V. Weight, physical activity, diet, and prognosis in breast and gynecologic cancers. *J Clin Oncol.* 2010;28(26): 4074-4080.
22. Vance V, Mourtzakis M, McCargar L, Hanning R. Weight gain in breast cancer survivors: prevalence, pattern and health consequences. *Obes Rev.* 2011;12(4):282-294.
23. Siegel EM, Ulrich CM, Poole EM, Holmes RS, Jacobsen PB, Shibata D. The effects of obesity and obesity-related conditions on colorectal cancer prognosis. *Cancer Control.* 2010;17(1):52-57.
24. Efstathiou JA, Bae K, Shipley WU, et al. Obesity and mortality in men with locally advanced prostate cancer: analysis of RTOG 85-31. *Cancer.* 2007; 110(12):2691-2699.
25. Erickson K, Patterson RE, Flatt SW, et al. Clinically defined type 2 diabetes mellitus and prognosis in early-stage breast cancer. *J Clin Oncol.* 2011; 29(1):54-60.
26. Kushi LH, Doyle C, McCullough M, et al. American Cancer Society Guidelines on nutrition and physical activity for cancer prevention: reducing the risk of cancer with healthy food choices and physical activity. *CA Cancer J Clin.* 2012;62(1):30-67.
27. Nock NL, Dimitropoulos A, Tkach J, Frasure H, von Gruenigen V. Reduction in neural activation to high-calorie food cues in obese endometrial cancer survivors after a behavioral lifestyle intervention: a pilot study. *BMC Neurosci.* 2012 Jun 25;13:74. doi: 10.1186/1471-2202-13-74.
28. Guest DD, Evans EM, Rogers LQ. Diet components associated with perceived fatigue in breast cancer survivors. *Eur J Cancer Care (Engl).* 2013; 22(1):51-59.
29. Befort CA, Klemp JR, Austin HL, et al. Outcomes of a weight loss intervention among rural breast cancer survivors. *Breast Cancer Res Treat.* 2012;132(2):631-639.
30. Campbell KL, Van Patten CL, Neil SE, et al. Feasibility of a lifestyle intervention on body weight and serum biomarkers in breast cancer survivors with overweight and obesity. *J Acad Nutr Diet.* 2012;112(4): 559-567.
31. Thompson HJ, Sedlacek SM, Paul D, et al. Effect of dietary patterns differing in carbohydrate and fat content on blood lipid and glucose profiles based on weight-loss success of breast-cancer survivors. *Breast Cancer Res.* 2012;14(1):R1. doi: 10.1186/bcr3082.
32. Vallance JK, Courneya KS, Taylor LM, Plotnikoff RC, Mackey JR. Development and evaluation of a theory-based physical activity guidebook for breast cancer survivors. *Health Educ Behav.* 2008; 35(2):174-189.
33. Winters-Stone KM, Schwartz A, Nail LM. A review of exercise interventions to improve bone health in adult cancer survivors. *J Cancer Surviv.* 2010;4(3):187-201.
34. Schmitz KH, Ahmed RL, Troxel A, et al. Weight lifting in women with breast-cancer-related lymphedema. *N Engl J Med.* 2009;361(7):664-673.
35. Schmitz KH, Ahmed RL, Troxel AB, et al. Weight lifting for women at risk for breast cancer-related lymphedema: a randomized trial. *JAMA.* 2010;304(24):2699-2705.

36. Schmitz KH, Troxel AB, Cheville A, et al. Physical Activity and Lymphedema (the PAL trial): assessing the safety of progressive strength training in breast cancer survivors. *Contemp Clin Trials*. 2009;30(3):233-245.

37. Christy SM, Mosher CE, Sloane R, Snyder DC, Lobach DF, Demark-Wahnefried W. Long-term dietary outcomes of the FRESH START intervention for breast and prostate cancer survivors. *J Am Diet Assoc*. 2011;111(12):1844-1851.

38. Ottenbacher AJ, Day RS, Taylor WC, et al. Long-term physical activity outcomes of home-based lifestyle interventions among breast and prostate cancer survivors. *Support Care Cancer*. 2012;20(10):2483-2489.

39. Nelson RL, Turyk M, Kim J, Persky V. Bone mineral density and the subsequent risk of cancer in the NHANES I follow-up cohort. *BMC Cancer*. 2002;2(1):22. doi:10.1186/1471-2407-2-22

40. Bennett JA, Lyons KS, Winters-Stone K, Nail LM, Scherer J. Motivational interviewing to increase physical activity in long-term cancer survivors: a randomized controlled trial. *Nurs Res*. 2007;56(1):18-27.

41. Patrick H, Williams GC. Self-determination theory: its application to health behavior and complementarity with motivational interviewing. *Int J Behav Nutr Phys Act*. 2012;9:18. doi: 10.1186/1479-5868-9-18.

42. Pierce JP, Stefanick ML, Flatt SW, et al. Greater survival after breast cancer in physically active women with high vegetable-fruit intake regardless of obesity. *J Clin Oncol*. 2007;25(17):2345-2351.

43. Holm M, Olsen A, Christensen J, et al. Pre-diagnostic alcohol consumption and breast cancer recurrence and mortality: Results from a prospective cohort with a wide range of variation in alcohol intake. *Int J Cancer*. 2013;132(3):686-694

44. Pierce JP, Natarajan L, Caan BJ, et al. Influence of a diet very high in vegetables, fruit, and fiber and low in fat on prognosis following treatment for breast cancer: the Women's Healthy Eating and Living (WHEL) randomized trial. *JAMA*. 2007;298(3):289-298.

45. Eng ET, Williams D, Mandava U, Kirma N, Tekmal RR, Chen S. Suppression of aromatase (estrogen synthetase) by red wine phytochemicals. *Breast Cancer Res Treat*. 2001;67(2):133-146.

46. Food, nutrition, physical activity, and the prevention of cancer: a global perspective. Washington DC: World Cancer Research Fund/American Institute for Cancer Research; 2007. http://www.dietandcancerreport.org/. Accessed July 12, 2012.

47. Fortin A, Wang CS, Vigneault E. Influence of smoking and alcohol drinking behaviors on treatment outcomes of patients with squamous cell carcinomas of the head and neck. *Int J Radiat Oncol Biol Phys*. 2009;74(4):1062-1069.

48. Barrera S, Demark-Wahnefried W. Nutrition during and after cancer therapy. *Oncology (Williston Park)*. 2009;23(2 Suppl Nurse Ed):15-21.

49. Mates JM, Segura JA, Alonso FJ, Marquez J. Anticancer antioxidant regulatory functions of phytochemicals. *Curr Med Chem*. 2011;18(15):2315-2338.

50. Patterson E, Wall R, Fitzgerald GF, Ross RP, Stanton C. Health implications of high dietary omega-6 polyunsaturated Fatty acids. *J Nutr Metab*. 2012; doi:10.1155/2012/539426

51. Chow MT, Moller A, Smyth MJ. Inflammation and immune surveillance in cancer. *Semin Cancer Biol*. 2012;22(1):23-32.

52. Centers for Disease Control. The National Action Plan for Cancer Survivorshop. 2004; http://www.cdc.gov/cancer/survivorship/what_cdc_is_doing/action_plan.htm. Accessed April 12, 2012.

53. Bijlsma AY, Meskers CG, Westendorp RG, Maier AB. Chronology of age-related disease definitions: osteoporosis and sarcopenia. *Ageing Res Rev*. 2012;11(2):320-324.

54. Wickham R. Osteoporosis related to disease or therapy in patients with cancer. *Clin J Oncol Nurs*. 2011;15(6):E90-E104.

55. Beasley JM, LaCroix AZ, Neuhouser ML,, et al. Protein intake and incident frailty in the Women's Health Initiative Observational Study. *J AM Geriatr Soc*. 2010;58(6):1063-1071.

56. Ward K. Musculoskeletal phenotype through the life course: the role of nutrition. *Proc Nutr Soc*. 2012;71(1):27-37.

57. Velicer CM, Ulrich CM. Vitamin and mineral supplement use among US adults after cancer diagnosis: a systematic review. *J Clin Oncol*. 2008;26(4):665-673.

58. Davies AA, Davey Smith G, Harbord R, et al. Nutritional interventions and outcome in patients with cancer or preinvasive lesions: systematic review. *J Natl Cancer Inst*. 2006;98(14):961-973.

59. Pocobelli G, Peters U, Kristal AR, White E. Use of supplements of multivitamins, vitamin C, and vitamin E in relation to mortality. *Am J Epidemiol*. 2009;170(4):472-483.

60. Kwan ML, Greenlee H, Lee VS, et al. Multivitamin use and breast cancer outcomes in women with early-stage breast cancer: the Life After Cancer Epidemiology study. *Breast Cancer Res Treat*. 2011;130(1):195-205.

61. Saquib J, Rock CL, Natarajan L, et al. Dietary intake, supplement use, and survival among women diagnosed with early-stage breast cancer. *Nutr Cancer*. 2011;63(3):327-333.

62. Baron JA, Cole BF, Mott L, et al. Neoplastic and antineoplastic effects of beta-carotene on colorectal adenoma recurrence: results of a randomized trial. *J Natl Cancer Inst*. 2003;95(10):717-722.

References for Tables 1 and 3

1. Fossa SD, Vassilopoulou-Sellin R, Dahl AA. Long term physical sequelae after adult-onset cancer. *J Cancer Surviv*. 2008;2(1):3-11.

2. Ness KK, Oakes JM, Punyko JA, Baker KS, Gurney JG. Prevalence of the metabolic syndrome in relation to self-reported cancer history. *Ann Epidemiol*. 2005;15(3):202-206.

3. Ganz PA. Late effects of cancer and its treatment. *Semin Oncol Nurs*. 2001;17(4):241-248.

4. Sinicrope FA, Foster NR, Yoon HH, et al. Association of obesity with DNA mismatch repair status and clinical outcome in patients with stage II or III colon carcinoma participating in NCCTG and NSABP adjuvant chemotherapy trials. *J Clin Oncol*. 2012;30(4):406-412.

5. Nelson RL, Nelson RL, Turyk M, Kim J, Persky V. Bone mineral density and the subsequent risk of cancer in the NHANES I follow-up cohort. *BMC Cancer*. 2002;2(1):22. doi:10.1186/1471-2407-2-22

6. Steffens M, Beauloye V, Brichard B, et al. Endocrine and metabolic disorders in young adult survivors of childhood acute lymphoblastic leukaemia (ALL) or non-Hodgkin lymphoma (NHL). *Clin Endocrinol (Oxf)*. 2008;69(5):819-827.

7. Epstein JB, Huhmann MB. Dietary and nutritional needs of patients after therapy for head and neck cancer. *J Am Dent Assoc*. 2012;143(6):588-592.

8. Kaste SC, Thomas NA, Rai SN, et al. Asymptomatic kidney stones in long-term survivors of childhood acute lymphoblastic leukemia. *Leukemia*. 2009;23(1):104-108.

9. Kaste SC, Jones-Wallace D, Rose SR, et al. Bone mineral decrements in survivors of childhood acute lymphoblastic leukemia: frequency of occurrence and risk factors for their development. *Leukemia*. 2001;15(5):728-734.

10. Mahon SM, Williams MT, Spies MA. Screening for second cancers and osteoporosis in long-term survivors. *Cancer Pract*. 2000;8(6):282-290.

11. Richter E, Denecke A, Klapdor S, Klapdor R. Parenteral nutrition support for patients with pancreatic cancer - improvement of the nutritional status and the therapeutic outcome. *Anticancer Res*. 2012;32(5):2111-2118.

12. Robien K, Demark-Wahnefried W, Rock CL. Evidence-based nutrition guidelines for cancer survivors: current guidelines, knowledge gaps, and future research directions. *J Am Diet Assoc*. 2011;111(3):368-375.

13. Rock CL, Doyle C, Demark-Wahnefried W, et al. Nutrition and physical activity guidelines for cancer survivors. *CA Cancer J Clin*. 2012;62(4):242-274.

14. Pierce JP, Natarajan L, Caan BJ, et al. Influence of a diet very high in vegetables, fruit, and fiber and low in fat on prognosis following treatment for breast cancer: the Women's Healthy Eating and Living (WHEL) randomized trial. *JAMA*. 2007;298(3):289-298.

15. Chlebowski RT, Blackburn GL, Thomson CA, et al. Dietary fat reduction and breast cancer outcome: interim efficacy results from the Women's Intervention Nutrition Study. *J Natl Cancer Inst*. 2006;98(24):1767-1776.

16. Morey MC, Snyder DC, Sloane R, et al. Effects of home-based diet and exercise on functional outcomes among older, overweight long-term cancer survivors: RENEW: a randomized controlled trial. *JAMA*. 2009;301(18):1883-1891.

17. Demark-Wahnefried W, Clipp EC, Morey MC, et al. Lifestyle intervention development study to improve physical function in older adults with cancer: outcomes from Project LEAD. *J Clin Oncol.* 2006;24(21):3465-3473.

18. Demark-Wahnefried W, Clipp EC, Lipkus IM, et al. Main outcomes of the FRESH START trial: a sequentially tailored, diet and exercise mailed print intervention among breast and prostate cancer survivors. *J Clin Oncol.* 2007;25(19):2709-2718.

19. von Gruenigen V, Frasure H, Kavanagh MB, et al. Survivors of uterine cancer empowered by exercise and healthy diet (SUCCEED): a randomized controlled trial. *Gynecol Oncol.* 2012;125(3):699-704.

20. Paxton RJ, Garcia-Prieto C, Berglund M, et al. A randomized parallel-group dietary study for stages II-IV ovarian cancer survivors. *Gynecol Oncol.* 2012;124(3):410-416.

21. Sedlacek SM, Playdon MC, Wolfe P, et al. Effect of a low fat versus a low carbohydrate weight loss dietary intervention on biomarkers of long term survival in breast cancer patients ('CHOICE'): study protocol. *BMC Cancer.* 2011;11:287. doi: 10.1186/1471-2407-11-287.

22. Rai SN, Hudson MM, McCammon E, et al. Implementing an intervention to improve bone mineral density in survivors of childhood acute lymphoblastic leukemia: BONEII, a prospective placebo-controlled double-blind randomized interventional longitudinal study design. *Contemp Clin Trials.* 2008;29(5):711-719.

Nutritional Effects of Cancer Treatment: Chemotherapy, Biotherapy, Hormone Therapy and Radiation Therapy

Barbara L. Grant, MS, RDN, CSO, LD

Expert Technical Reviewers:
Juanita Bilbao, RT(R)(T), Maria Lee, RT(T) and Misti Ross, RN, OCN

OVERVIEW
Conventional methods of cancer treatment include medical oncology, radiation oncology, and surgeries used alone or in combination to prevent, cure, control or palliate cancer. Specifically, medical oncology is the diagnosis and treatment of cancer using antineoplastic therapies, which encompass several classifications of agents including chemotherapy and hormone therapy. In addition, recent advances in cancer treatment and improved understanding of the immune system, malignant transformation and metastasis have led to the emergence of biotherapy, molecularly-targeted agents and promising novel agents. Radiation oncology is the diagnosis and treatment of cancer utilizing a spectrum of ionizing radiation to a localized area. Radiation therapy modalities include teletherapy (external beam radiation therapy machines), brachytherapy (sealed sources of radiation), and radiopharmaceutical therapy (unsealed sources of radiation).

This chapter provides a comprehensive overview for all of these therapies, as well as their mechanisms of action, routes of administration, and systemic-specific and/or site-specific side effects and their impact on nutritional status for persons with cancer throughout the continuum of care. Recommendations to manage cancer treatment-related symptoms and side effects is available in *Chapter 12: Symptom Management of Cancer Therapies.*

Evidence-Based and Consensus-Driven Cancer Treatment and Care
Cancer diagnosis and treatment in the United States (U.S.) is guided by evidence-based standards known as the *National Comprehensive Cancer Network (NCCN) Clinical Practice Guidelines in Oncology.* The NCCN guidelines are based on current evidence-based and consensus-driven sequential treatment and supportive (e.g., cancer related pain, nausea and fatigue) management decisions and interventions to improve the care of persons with cancer (1). These guidelines continually undergo review and are updated to ensure that individuals receiving cancer treatment are receiving the most efficacious "standard of care" for their disease.

Seventy-one percent of all people diagnosed and treated for cancer in the U.S. receive care in the over 1,500 cancer centers accredited by the American College of Surgeons' (ACOS) Commission on Cancer (2). Eligibility standards require that all accredited programs include the provision of nutrition services. To help address the needs of the over 12 million cancer survivors in the U.S., the ACOS's accreditation standards now include patient-centered initiatives recommending every person with cancer treated in a ACOS-accredited center be provided with an individualized survivorship care plan that summarizes their treatment and cancer care, as well as a guide for monitoring and maintaining their personal health and possible continuing side effects of cancer and its treatment (2).

To guide nutrition practice, the Academy of Nutrition and Dietetics (Academy) provides dietetic professionals with evidence- and consensus-based resources and validated materials for the cancer care setting throughout the care continuum. These Academy resources include: the Evidence Analysis Library's Oncology Nutrition Evidence-Based Nutrition Practice Guidelines, the *International Dietetics & Terminology: Reference Manual, Standardized Language for the Nutrition Care Process, 4th edition,* and the *Oncology Toolkit* (3-5).

Cancer Treatment: Goals of Therapy and Factors Affecting Response
Table 11 - 1 provides an overview of the goals and types of cancer therapy used to prevent, cure, control or palliate cancer. Table 11-2 outlines factors affecting response to cancer treatment.

Antineoplastic agents can be administered in a variety of ways. Routes of administration include oral, intravenous (IV), intrathecal/intraventicular (IT), intrapleural (IP), intra-arterial (IA), subcutaneous

Table 11 - 1: Goals of Cancer Therapy (1,6-9)

Type of Therapy	Goals of Therapy
Chemoprevention	• The use of medicines, vitamins, minerals or other agents to reduce the risk of, or delay the development of cancer; • *Example:* hormone therapy (an anti-estrogen agent) prescribed to reduce risk of breast cancer for a woman determined to be at high risk for developing the disease.
Adjuvant Therapy	• The use of additional cancer treatment given after the primary therapy; • To reduce the risk of cancer recurrence and to decrease the incidence of metastatic disease; • *Example:* chemotherapy given after a lobectomy for treatment of lung cancer. • *Example:* chemotherapy, hormone therapy, and monoclonal antibody therapy given after lumpectomy for treatment of breast cancer.
Definitive Therapy	• The use of radiation therapy prescribed as the primary treatment modality, with or without chemotherapy. • *Example:* radiation therapy given for the treatment of prostate cancer.
Neoadjuvant Therapy	• The use of one or more treatment modalities given before the primary therapy; • To reduce the size of the primary tumor to improve the effectiveness of the surgery and to decrease the incidence of metastatic disease; • *Example:* chemotherapy and external beam radiation therapy given before an esophagectomy for treatment of esophageal cancer.
Palliation	• The use of cancer treatment modalities when cure and control of disease cannot be achieved; • The relief of side effects and symptoms caused by cancer and other serious illnesses to improve quality of life; • *Example:* external beam radiation therapy given to palliate painful bony lesions related to metastatic prostate cancer.
Prophylaxis Therapy	• The use of radiation therapy for the relief of symptoms such as pain, bleeding, neurological compromise, or airway obstruction to improve quality of life or to treat life-threatening problems. • *Example:* whole brain irradiation given for asymptomatic individuals diagnosed with cancers that have a high risk of occurrence of metastases (e.g., small cell lung cancer).

Table 11 - 2: Factors Affecting Response to Cancer Treatment (6-7)

Tumor Burden or Tumor Load	• Refers to the size of the tumor or the amount of cancer in the body. As the tumor mass increases in size, its growth rate can slow, thus reducing the effectiveness of the cancer treatment.
Tumor Growth Rate	• Refers to what proportion of cancer cells within the tumor are growing and dividing to form new cancer cells. Rapidly growing tumors are usually more responsive to treatment.
Drug Resistance	• Refers to the failure of cancer cells to respond to a drug used to kill or weaken them. The cancer cells may be resistant at the beginning of the treatment, or may become resistant after being exposed to the treatment.

(SC) or intramuscular (IM), and topically. Antineoplastic therapy is given in cycles. By giving agents (or a combination of agents) at specific times cancer cells can be the most susceptible and normal cells are allowed to recover from the damage. There are three important factors in the delivery of these agents:

- Frequency of cycles: daily, weekly, every 14 days, every 21 days, monthly, or continuously
- Length of cycles: injection, a bolus infusion or a continuous infusion
  o Treatments can last for minutes, hours, days or years
- Number of cycles – determined by research and clinical trials. (7)

SECTION ONE: CHEMOTHERAPY

Principles of Therapy

Chemotherapy is the use of chemical agents or drugs to systemically kill cancer cells. Chemotherapy has a cytotoxic effect on all cells (i.e., both healthy and malignant) and side effects and toxicities are often a result of damage to rapidly dividing cells. However, normal cells are able to better repair themselves, and most toxicities are reversible. Body cells with rapid turnovers that are susceptible to the effects of chemotherapy agents include bone marrow, hair follicles, gonads (e.g., testes and ovaries), and gastrointestinal mucosa.

Specifically, the actions of chemotherapy agents interfere with cell division and ultimately lead to cell death. Chemotherapy agents affect the cell during a specific phase of the cell cycle, the period of time and activities that take place between cell divisions. There are five phases of the cell cycle as outlined below.

G0 – Resting Phase: Cells are temporarily out of the cycle and have stopped dividing.

G1 – Post-Mitotic Phase: Cells begin the first phase of reproduction by synthesizing protein and RNA necessary for cell division.

S – Synthesis phase: DNA is synthesized.

G2 – Pre-Mitotic Phase: Cells prepare to divide.

M – Mitosis Phase: Cell growth and protein production stops. Cellular energy is focused on the orderly division of two daughter cells.

Classification of Agents

Chemotherapy agents are classified according to their mechanism of action and effect on cellular reproduction:

- *Cell cycle non-specific agents*: damage cells in all phases of the cell cycle; classifications include alkylating agents, antitumor antibiotics, hormone therapies, and nitrosoureas, and others (10).
- *Cell cycle-specific agents*: exert their effect within a specific phase of the cell cycle; classifications include antimetabolites and camptothecins (synthesis phase), plant alkaloids and taxanes (mitosis phase), and miscellaneous agents (10).

Side Effects and Nutritional Implications

Just as chemotherapy agents differ, short- and long-term side effects can differ depending upon the agent and its prescribed treatment regimen. Whether an individual experiences a specific side effect and how long the side effects can last depend on several factors such as personal health history, the amount of the agent given, the way it is given, how long it is given, and other agents and drugs that may have been given. Most side effects are temporary and resolve quickly. However, in some cases it can take weeks, months, and even years for treatment-related side effects to resolve. In other instances, long-term side effects occur; permanent effects may include damage to the lungs, heart, liver, kidneys, reproductive organs, nerves, and bone marrow.

Table 11 – 3 Chemotherapy: Classification, Mechanisms of Action, Possible Side Effects and Nutritional Implications provides a comprehensive overview of the chemotherapy agents and is located at end of the chapter.

SECTION TWO: BIOTHERAPY

Principles of Therapy

Biotherapy is defined as treatment to boost or restore the ability of the immune system to fight cancer, infection, and other diseases by inducing, enhancing, or suppressing an individual's own immune response (6). This type of therapy is also called immunotherapy or biological response modifier (BMR) therapy and represents monoclonal antibodies, protein-targeted therapies, angiogenesis inhibitors, cytokines, and therapeutic cancer vaccines.

Biotherapy has revolutionized cancer treatment by utilizing the body's immune system to either directly or indirectly fight the disease (11). The National Cancer Institute (NCI) outlines biotherapy's functions and uses in cancer treatment as follows:

- To stop, control, or suppress processes that allow cancer growth;
- To make malignant cells more recognizable and thus more susceptible to destruction by the immune system;
- To boost the killing ability of immune system's cells (e.g., T cells, natural killer [NK] cells, and macrophages);
- To prevent malignant cells from metastasizing to other locations in the body.
- To eliminate malignant cells that have not been killed by other modalities of cancer treatment such as chemotherapy or radiation therapy (11).

Categories of Biotherapy Agents

Biotherapy agents are classified according to their innate or adaptive effects on the immune system and whether they specifically target a tumor antigen (7). Innate or passive agents do not generate immunological memory and necessitate continued administration to impart a lasting effect. In comparison, adaptive or active biotherapy agents engage an individual's own immune system to mount a specific immune response against a tumor. The action of biotherapy agents may also be short-term (e.g., monoclonal antibodies and cytokines) or long-lasting (e.g., therapeutic cancer vaccines).

Genes influence the molecular transformation of normal to malignant cells and then to metastatic disease. By "targeting" or focusing on molecular changes that are specific to cancer, molecularly-targeted therapies show promise in being more effective than systemic (chemotherapy) or localized (radiation therapy) cancer treatments and less toxic to normal cells (12). However, this observation has not been shown to be entirely the case. Rather, as the use of targeted agents increase, their actual side effects are not less toxic to normal cells—they are just very different (13). Whereas common side effects of chemotherapy agents include toxicities such as myelosuppression, mucositis, nausea and vomiting, and alopecia—targeted agents' toxicities commonly include vascular, coagulation, dermatologic, immunologic, ocular and pulmonary toxicities (13).

Biotherapy agents are used alone or in combination with chemotherapy agents. Six general categories of biological cancer therapies will be reviewed:

- Monoclonal Antibodies – therapies that signal external cellular pathway targets.
- Protein-Targeted Therapies – therapies that signal internal cellular pathway targets.
- Angiogenesis Inhibitors – therapies that target tumor vasculature and angiogenesis.
- Cytokines – therapies that stimulate a broad-based immune response as opposed to generating a targeted response to a specific tumor antigen.
- Cancer Vaccine Therapies – therapies that signal an individual's own immune system against tumor antigens.
- Radiopharmaceuticals – monoclonal antibody therapies that deliver radioactive molecules to specific cancer cells. These agents will be discussed in the section on radiation therapy.

Monoclonal Antibodies:

This type of therapy targets specific receptors on the outside of tumor cells, which activates pathways on the inside of the cells. These agents are used alone or with other cancer therapies to disrupt cell function and cause cell apoptosis, and also can be used as delivery vehicles of radioactive molecules (e.g., Tositumomab [Bexxar®]) (14).

Table 11 - 4: Possible Side Effects and Nutritional Implications of Monoclonal Antibodies (7,10,14)

Possible Side Effect and Nutritional Implications	
Infusion-related symptoms	Fever, chills, urticaria, flushing, fatigue, headache, dyspnea, hypotension
Gastrointestinal	Nausea, vomiting, diarrhea. Generally mild.
Cardiotoxicity	Dyspnea, peripheral edema, reduced left ventricular function. Increased risk if given in combination with an anthracycline-based regimen.
Myelosuppression	Increased risk if administered with chemotherapy.
Pulmonary toxicity	Increased cough, dyspnea, pulmonary infiltrates, and/or pleural effusions.
Skin Rash and Skin Problems	Rash, facial erythema and hand-foot syndrome.

Table 11 - 6: Protein-Targeted Therapies: Small Molecule Inhibitors (10,14,17)

Target and Mechanism of Action	Agent	Indication
Tyrosine Kinase Inhibitors (TKIs): Inhibits multiple receptor tyrosine kinases, which are involved in tumor growth and angiogenesis and metastasis.	• Erlotinib (Tarceva®) • Gefitinib (Iressa®) • Imatinib (Gleevec®) • Sorafenib (Nexavar®) • Sunitinib (Sutent®)	• Locally advanced or metastatic non-small cell lung cancer or pancreatic cancer • Refractory non-small cell lung cancer • Philadelphia (PH) + CML, GIST, MDS, refractory Ph+ ALL • Renal cell cancer, hepatocellular cancer • GIST, renal cell cancer, pancreatic neuroendocrine tumors
mTOR Inhibitor: *These drugs block angiogenesis by preventing the release of VEGF and PDGF, thus blocking tumor cell proliferation and causing cell death.*	• Temsirolimus (Torisel®) • Everolimus (Affinitor®)	• Renal cell cancer • Renal cell cancer, pancreatic neuroendocrine tumors
Proteasome Inhibitor: *These drugs inhibit the breakdown of intracellular proteins and disrupt the proteasome pathway.*	• Bortezomib (Velcade®)	• Multiple myeloma, mantle cell lymphoma

Molecular targets with signaling effects on the outside of malignant cells and include:

- CD20: B-lymphocyte antigen CD20
- EGFR: epidermal growth factor receptor
- HER-2/neu: human epidermal growth factor receptor 2
- RANKL: receptor activator of nuclear factor kappa-B ligand
- VEGF: vascular endothelial growth factor

Possible side effects of monoclonal antibody therapy are provided in Table 11 – 4.

Table 11- 5: Monoclonal Antibodies: Classification, Mechanisms of Action, Route of Administration and Possible Side Effects provides a comprehensive overview of these agents and is located at end of the chapter.

Protein-Targeted Therapies:
Protein-targeted therapy involves the use of small molecules that are able to penetrate malignant cell membranes to interact with specific areas of the target proteins (16). These agents disrupt cell function, which causes cell apoptosis (cell death). Examples of protein-targeted agents are provided in Table 11 - 6: Protein-Targeted Therapies and Table 11 - 7 summarizes side effects and nutrition implications of these therapies.

Angiogenesis Inhibitors:
Angiogenesis inhibitors hinder the formation of new blood vessels in primary tumors and metastatic tumors, thus preventing their growth, invasion and spread (14,18). This therapy is also known as anti-angiogenesis. Examples of anti-angiogenenic agents are provided in Table 11 - 8: and possible side effects in Table 11 - 9.

Cytokines:
Cytokines stimulate a broad-based immune response. Examples of cytokines are interleukin-2 (IL-2) and interferon-α. Cytokines encourage cell growth, promote cell activation, direct cellular traffic and destroy target cells, including cancer cells (19). They are the chief communication signals of the immune system's T cells to activate a specific immune response to foreign antigens. Examples of cytokines used in biotherapy are presented in Table 11 - 10 and possible side effects are provided in Table 11 - 11.

Cancer Vaccine Therapies:
Unlike targeted therapies, cancer vaccines do not act on a certain pathway in tumor cells (19). Rather, this type of therapy is designed to stimulate an individual's own immune system against abnormal and foreign cells such as cancer cells (16). To date, the Food and Drug Administration (FDA) has approved only one cancer vaccine therapy for use in men with hormone refractory metastatic prostate cancer (e.g., sipuleucel-T [Provenge®]) (20). Refer to Appendix 8 for

possible nutritional implications of this agent. Clinical trials are currently underway for developing treatment vaccines in other types of cancer.

Of note, the FDA has approved two types of vaccines to prevent cancer in healthy people: a vaccine to protect against hepatitis B virus (HBV) which can lead to hepatocellular carcinoma (liver cancer) and vaccines

(Gardasil® and Cervaric®) to protect against human papillomavirus (HPV), which increases one's risk of cervical and oral cancers.

SECTION THREE: HORMONE THERAPY
Principles of Therapy
Hormone therapy, also referred to as hormonal therapy, hormone treatment or endocrine therapy, is used for the treatment of

Table 11 - 7: Possible Side Effects and Nutritional Implications of Protein-Targeted Therapies (7,10,14)

Possible Side Effect and Nutritional Implications	
Skin Rash and Skin Problems	Rash, facial erythema and hand-foot syndrome. Hair depigmentation with Sutent® (causes hair to turn white while on therapy).
Cardiotoxicity	QT prolongation and possible sudden death, monitor patients with previous history of cardiovascular disease; left ventricular dysfunction; hypertension, bleeding; myocardial infarction.
Gastrointestinal	Nausea, vomiting, diarrhea, decreased appetite.

Table 11 - 8: Examples of Angiogenesis Inhibitors (10,12,14,17)

Target	*Agent and Mechanism of Action*	*Indication*
VEGF	• Bevacizumab (Avastin®) • *This drug recognizes and binds to VEGF, thus stopping it from activating the VEGF receptor. This action helps to arrest endothelial cell proliferation and angiogenesis.*	• Metastatic colorectal cancer, non-small cell lung cancer, glioblastoma with progressive disease, metastatic renal cell cancer.
Immunomodulatory Drugs	• Lenalidomide (Revlimid®) • Thalidomide *Mechanism of action is not fully understood. These drugs inhibit pro-inflammatory cytokines (e.g., TNFα, IL-1β, IL-6) and exert anti-angiogenic properties.*	• Multiple myeloma, myelodysplastic syndrome (MDS) • Multiple myeloma, MDS

Table 11 - 9: Possible Side Effects and Nutritional Implications of Angiogenesis Inhibitors (14,17)

Possible Side Effects and Nutritional Implications	
Hypertension	Assess at baseline and monitor blood pressure throughout treatment. If hypertension develops, it is recommended that patients should be managed with oral antihypertensive therapy.
Arterial Thromboembolic Events (ATE) (e.g., myocardial infarction, angina, stroke)	Factors linked to increased risk of ATEs include: • Age > 65 years old • History of angina, stroke or ATEs
Proteinuria	Most patients are asymptomatic. However, proteinuria may occur in up to almost a third of all patients treated with bevacizumab.
Hemorrhage	Possible areas of bleeding include: • Nosebleeds • Hemoptysis • Hematuria • GI bleeding • Vaginal bleeding
GI Perforation:	Can present with abdominal pain, nausea, emesis, constipation, and fever and often occurs within the first 60 days of treatment. Factors linked to increased risk of GI perforation include: • Tumor at anastomotic site • Abdominal carcinomatosis • Bowel obstruction • History of abdominal/pelvic radiation therapy • Recent colonoscopy
Hypothyroidism:	Assess baseline thyroid function. Once therapy begins, monitor for signs and symptoms of hypothyroidism (e.g., increased sensitivity to cold, dry skin, weigh gain, fatigue, myalgias and arthralgias, and depression).

Table 11 - 10: Examples of Cytokines (7,11)

Agent and Mechanism of Action	Indication
• Interleukein-2 or IL-2 (Aldesleukin®) *Stimulates the growth and activity of immune cells (lymphocytes) to kill cancer cells.*	• Metastatic melanoma and metastatic renal cell cancer.
• Interferon-α (Roferon® or Intron A®) *Inhibition of viral replication, and helps to slow the growth of tumor cells or promote their growth into more normal function, and modulation of host immune response.*	• Hairy cell leukemia, malignant melanoma, chronic myeloid lymphoma, AIDS-related Kaposi's Sarcoma, and hepatitis C.

Table 11 - 11: Possible Side Effects and Nutritional Implications of Cytokines (7,11)

Possible Side Effects and Nutritional Implications	
Flu-like symptoms	Fever, chills, headache, arthralgias, myalgias
Constitutional	Fatigue, anorexia
Myelosuppression	Leukopenia, thrombocytopenia, anemia
Gastro-intestinal	Nausea, vomiting, diarrhea
Renal and Cardiotoxicity	Renal insufficiency, capillary leak syndrome

hormone-sensitive cancers (e.g., breast, ovarian, prostate) by the following mechanisms of action:

- Stopping or reducing the body's ability to produce hormones;
- Interfering with or blocking hormone receptors;
- Substituting chemically similar agents for the active hormones that cannot be used by the tumor. (21).

Hormone therapy is categorized by the kind of hormone that is affected and its function, as is indicated in Table 11-12

SECTION FOUR: RADIATION THERAPY

This section provides an overview of the principles and types of radiation therapy available as well as possible side effects including nutrition impact symptoms. These therapies include (22):

- External beam radiation therapy which is the use of ionizing radiation delivered from outside of the body to treat a specific treatment field;
- Brachytherapy or internal radiation therapy which is the temporary or permanent placement of radioactive material precisely placed inside a body cavity, tissue or surface;
- Radiopharmaceutical therapy, which is the use of radioactive substances to systemically treat cancer.

Overview of Radiation Therapy

Radiation therapy is used alone, or in combination with surgery, chemotherapy, biotherapy, and hormonal therapy. In the U.S., approximately 50 to 60 percent of all individuals undergoing cancer treatment receive radiation therapy as a part of their treatment (23). Radiation therapy utilizes high-energy x-rays (ionizing radiation) or other radioactive particles such as electrons, neutrons, protons, beta particles or gamma rays.

Ionizing radiation is used to treat local, regional or systemic disease and other benign conditions (9). The goal of therapy is to eradicate tumor cells while minimizing injury to healthy, normal tissues in a specific area of treatment (24). Ionizing radiation works by damaging the DNA and other cellular components within the cells by causing the following types of interactions (9,24-25):

- Direct:
  - o Physical damage that is caused within the cells by the excitation and ionization of atoms or molecules;
  - o Biological damage that is brought about by damage to critical cellular genetic material.
- Indirect:
  - o Chemical damage that is caused by the formation of highly reactive free radicals within the cells.

While these changes occur to cancer cells as well as normal cells, they prevent cancer cells from reproducing, resulting in cell death. Table 11 – 1 summarizes goals of therapy. Factors radiation oncologists may use to determine which type of radiation therapy is selected and how it will be prescribed for treatment include:

- The type, size, and location of the cancer in the body;
- The proximity of the cancer to normal tissues, structures and organs of the body;
- How far the radiation needs to travel;
- The individual's general health, medical history, age, and performance status;
- Whether or not other types of cancer therapies are indicated such as chemotherapy, biotherapy, and/or surgery. (22)

Types of Radiation Therapy

External Beam Therapy

Megavoltage machines deliver ionizing radiation for treatment via external beam radiation therapy (EBRT), also known as teletherapy. The type of cancer and the tolerance of normal tissues in the treatment field determine the total dose, size, number of fractions and the duration of treatment (23). Dividing doses into multiple fractions helps limit damage to healthy tissue. Side effects experienced occur from radiation damage to the normal cells within the treatment field and are dependent upon the part of the body being treated. Different types of EBRT delivering ionizing radiation directly to cancer cells from a machine outside of the body are outlined in Table 11 - 13.

Table 11 - 12: Categories of Hormonal Agents Used in Cancer Treatment (10,17,21)

Selective Estrogen Receptor Modulators (SERMS) or Antiestrogens: *Nonsteroidal anti-estrogen agents that compete with estrogen for binding to estrogen receptors. Examples of antiestrogen agents include:* • Tamoxifen citrate (Novaldex®) • Toremifene citrate (Fareston®) • Raloxifene (Evista®) *Indications:* Tamoxifen and toremifene are prescribed for breast cancer; Raloxifene is prescribed to treat osteoporosis or for postmenopausal women at risk for breast cancer. *Side Effects and Nutritional Implications:* • Menstrual symptoms: hot flashes, sweating, nausea, vomiting, menstrual irregularities, vaginal dryness • Fluid retention and peripheral edema • Increased risk of endometrial changes and cancer • Thromboembolic complications • Skin changes, rash • Joint ache/pain • Weight gain	Progesterones: *These agents possess anti-estrogenic effects and inhibit the stability, availability, and turnover of estrogen receptors.* • Megestrol acetate (Megace®) *Indications:* Breast, endometrial, renal cell cancers; and as an appetite stimulant in cancer and HIV/AIDS. *Side Effects and Nutritional Implications:* • Weight gain (fluid retention) • Thromboembolic events • Nausea and vomiting • Menstrual bleeding, hot flashes, sweating, and mood change • Hyperglycemia
Aromatase Inhibitors (AIs): *Nonsteroidal and/or steroidal inhibitors of aromatase. AIs block the production of estrogen by inhibiting the conversion of adrenal androgens to estrogens. These agents are primarily used in postmenopausal women because premenopausal women produce too much aromatase for the agents to effectively block. Examples of these agents include:* • Anastrozole (Arimidex®) • Letrozole (Femara®) • Exemestane (Aromasin®) *Indications:* Breast cancer. *Side Effects and Nutritional Implications:* • Hot flashes • Arthralgias • Nausea and vomiting – generally mild • Asthenia • Thromboembolic events • High cholesterol (Letrozole) • Fever, malaise, myalgias • Joint aches/pains	Antiandrogens: *These agents bind to androgen receptors and block the effects of testosterone in androgen-sensitive prostate cancer cells. Examples of antiandrogens include:* • Bicalutamide (Casodex®) • Flutamide (Eulexin®) *Indications:* Prostate cancer. *Side Effects and Nutritional Implications:* • Weight Gain • Hot flashes, fatigue • Decreased libido, impotence • Bone pain Lutenizing hormone-releasing hormone (LHRH) Agonists: *These agents are synthetic proteins similar to naturally-occurring LHRH and they signal the pituitary gland to stop producing luteinizing hormone. This results in the suppression of testosterone to manage the growth and spread of prostate cancer.* • Leuprolide acetate (Lupron®) • Goserelin (Zoladex®) *Indications:* Prostate cancer. *Side Effects and Nutritional Implications:* • Hot flashes, fatigue • Decreased libido, impotence • Bone pain • Gynecomastia • Headache • Muscle weakness

Appendix 8 provides a table outlining possible interactions of chemotherapy, biotherapy and hormone therapy with drugs, nutrients, food, and dietary supplements.

Cancer treatments with curative intent are typically given over the course of several weeks depending upon the type of cancer, and the total dose of radiation to be delivered. Palliative radiation therapy can be delivered in an effort to improve quality of life and manage cancer and cancer-related symptoms such as:

• Treatment given to shrink a metastatic brain or liver lesion that has spread from primary cancer to another area of the body;
• Treatment given to shrink an obstructing tumor near the esophagus to allow for ease of swallowing;
• Treatment given to treat a metastatic bony lesion (e.g., spine, pelvis or rib) to alleviate pain.

The amount of ionizing radiation an individual receives is measured in units called centigray (cGy). Most types of EBRT are given once a day in a single dose or daily fraction up to five days a week. However,

some radiation therapy treatments may be delivered in different ways such as (22):

• Hyperfractionation – smaller doses given more than once a day;
• Hypofractionation – larger doses given once a day or less often to reduce the number of fractions;
• Accelerated fractionation – doses given in larger daily or weekly doses to reduce the number of weeks in a prescribed treatment.

Side Effects

Early side effects of treatment occur during or immediately after completing the course of radiation therapy. Side effects experienced depend upon total dose given, dose per fraction, the overall treatment course and whether or not radiation therapy was combined with other treatment modalities such as chemotherapy or surgery and in what manner given (e.g., concurrent or sequential

Table 11 - 13: Types of EBRT (9,22,26)

Type of Therapy
Three Dimensional Conformal Radiation Therapy (3D-CRT): *Using special computed tomography (CT) scanning and a sophisticated planning system, this type of therapy delivers a prescribed dose of radiation to a precise three-dimensional target area using multi-leaf beam-shaping devices (collimators) or customized blocks in effort to minimize the dose of radiation to the surrounding normal tissue while maximizing dose to cancer cells.*
Intensity Modulated Radiation Therapy (IMRT): *This type of therapy is an advanced form of 3D-CRT which uses computer-controlled, moveable "leaves" to customize the radiation beam by modulating or varying the amount delivered to different parts of the specific area being treated. The goal of therapy is to reduce radiation exposure to surrounding normal tissue while delivering more radiation to cancer cells.*
Image Guided Radiation Therapy (IGRT): *IGRT can be used in conjunction with EBRT, 3D-CRT or IMRT. It utilizes repeated imaging scans, which are taken during the course of a prescribed treatment to help increase the accuracy of therapy to specific targeted tissue. Images taken during treatment are compared to images that were taken during the planning process to account for changes in a patient's position and tumor location.*
Stereotactic Radiosurgery (SRS) and Stereotactic Radiation Therapy (SRT): *SRS and SRT are non-invasive types of therapy that uses image-guided, tumor-targeted and precise patient positioning and/or immobilization (e.g., a head frame or other devices) to deliver high doses of radiation therapy to a small tumor or area. SRS is given in a single dose and SRT treatment is delivered in a fractionated manner over a specific period of time. SRS and SRT are commonly used to treat malignant, metastatic and benign brain tumors, liver and prostate cancers, and other conditions such as arteriovenous malformations (AVMs).*
Total Body Irradiation (TBI): *TBI is a type of treatment where a large dose of radiation is given to the entire body to treat cancer cells that may be present throughout the body. Treatment can consist of a single dose to twice a day fractions over a three-day period depending upon the treatment protocol. TBI is often given in conjunction with high-dose chemotherapy as immunosuppressive treatment for hematological malignancies such as leukemias, myelomas, and lymphomas.*

therapies) (9). Table 11 – 14 outlines nutrition impact symptoms for specific areas of treatment.

Late side effects of treatment can occur months to even years after radiation therapy has been given and are usually a result of damage to the microcirculation within the irradiated area. Effects are more severe when a higher fraction dose is given. Specific late-occurring side effects and nutrition impact symptoms are outlined in Table 11 – 15.

Table 11 - 16 provides possible side effects for individuals receiving total or whole body radiation therapy in preparation for hematopoietic cell transplants for the treatment of malignant (e.g., certain leukemias and lymphomas) and nonmalignant diseases (e.g., aplastic anemia, thalassemia major). The table also highlights nutrition impact symptoms.

Brachytherapy

Brachytherapy is a type of therapeutic radiation therapy that involves the temporary or permanent placement of radioactive material directly into tumors or next to tumors. "Brachy" comes from the Greek word meaning a short distance.

Principles of Therapy

This type of cancer treatment is designed to precisely deliver radiation therapy in an individualized and targeted manner in an effort to spare normal tissue (30). Brachytherapy can be used alone or in combination with EBRT. Radioactive isotopes are sealed inside of tiny pellets or seeds (22) and are then placed within an individual via a variety of specialized applicators such as needles or catheters. Brachytherapy is used to "boost" the delivery of radiation to a tumor and to spare surrounding healthy tissue (9). Methods of brachytherapy cancer treatments are provided in Table 11 - 17 and 18; possible side effects of therapy and nutrition impact symptoms are outlined in Table 11 - 19.

Radiopharmaceutical Therapy

Radiopharmaceuticals are drugs that contain radioisotopes for the systemic treatment of cancer. For the purposes of this chapter, these agents will be grouped into three general categories:

- Radioimmunotherapy Agents
- Radioactive Substances
- Radiopharmaceuticals for the Relief of Metastatic Bone Pain

This section will also include a review of these therapies' mechanism of action, as well as possible side effects and nutrition impact symptoms.

Radioimmunotherapy Agents

Radioimmunotherapy agents are targeted therapies comprised of monoclonal antibodies combined with radioactive substances that deliver radiation therapy directly to cancer cells (10). Action occurs when monoclonal antibodies bind to the CD20 receptor sites on the surface of the cancer cell and the radioisotope kills the cell (7). This type of agent is currently used in the treatment of ß-cell lymphomas; other cancer indications are still under investigation. An example of this type of agent is Ibritumomab and Yttrium 90 (Zevalin®) (10).

Acute side effects and nutrition impact symptoms of radioimmunotherapy include myelosuppression; infusion related reactions; mild nausea and vomiting, diarrhea, decreased appetite; infection; cough, throat irritation and dyspnea; and generalized aches and pains. Possible late side effects include a risk of secondary malignancy (7,10,31).

Radioactive Substances

Another type of radiation therapy utilizing radioactive materials includes radioiodine or iodine 131 for the treatment of certain kinds of thyroid cancer. After part or all of the thyroid gland is removed, iodine 131 is given to destroy the functioning of the thyroid gland,

Table 11 - 14: Possible Acute Side Effects of Site-Specific Radiation Therapy (9,27-28)

Side Effect	TREATMENT FIELD						
	Brain	**Breast**	**Chest**	**Head & Neck**	**Pelvis**	**Rectum**	**Stomach & Abdomen**
Diarrhea					3	3	3
Fatigue	3	3	3	3	3	3	3
Hair Loss*	3	3	3	3	3	3	3
Mouth Changes (Dysgeusia, Oral Mucositis, Xerostomia)							
Nausea & Vomiting	3		3				3
Sexuality & Fertility Changes					3	3	3
Skin Changes* (e.g., Erythema, Pruritis, Moist Desquamation)	3	3	3	3	3	3	3
Throat Changes (e.g., Dysphagia, Odynophagia, Esophagitis)			3	3			
Urinary & Bladder Changes (e.g., Urinary Frequency, Cystitis, Incontinence)					3	3	3
Other Side Effects	Headache, Blurry Vision	Tenderness, Swelling of Irradiated Breast	Cough, Dyspnea	Thick Saliva, Oral Infections, Stiffness of the Jaw, Earaches			

*In the treatment field.

Table 11 - 15: Possible Late Side Effects of Radiation Therapy (9,27-28)

Area Treated	Late Side Effect
Brain	Headache, leukoencephalopathy (e.g., cognitive impairment and changes in memory and attention), dementia
Bone	Damage to osteoblasts, osteopenia
Cardiovascular	Angina upon exertion, pericarditis, cardiac enlargement, congestive heart failure
Esophagus	Esophageal stenosis, fibrosis or necrosis
Gastrointestinal Tract	Diarrhea, malabsorption, chronic enteritis/colitis, intestinal changes (e.g., stricture, ulceration, obstruction, perforation, fistula)
Head and Neck	Trismus, permanent xerostomia, alterations in taste and smell, osteoradionecrosis
Lymphatics	Secondary lymphedema in irradiated area
Pulmonary	Dyspnea, cough, pneumonitis
Sexual Organs	Infertility
Skin	Telangiectasias, pigmentation changes, atrophy, fibrosis
Urinary	Hematuria, cystitis
Other Conditions	Development of secondary malignancies, cataracts (if eye in treatment area)

Table 11 - 16: Possible Side Effects of Total Body Radiation Therapy* (9,24,29)

Organ or Body System	Possible Side Effects
Bone Marrow	*Acute Effects:* anemia, neutropenia, pancytopenia, hemorrhage, infection *Late Effects:* secondary hematological cancers
Brain and Central Nervous System	*Acute Effects:* confusion, meningitis *Late Effects:* cognitive changes, memory loss
Gastrointestinal System	*Acute Effects:* xerostomia, mucositis, esophagitis, nausea, vomiting, diarrhea, electrolyte imbalance, acute graft-vs-host disease *Late Effects:* radiation enteritis, denudation of villi of small intestine, chronic graft-vs-host disease
Skin	*Acute Effects:* generalized erythema, hyperpigmentation *Late Effects:* fibrosis, delayed wound healing, increased risk for basal cell cancers
Other	*Acute Effects:* fatigue, fever, hair thinning or loss *Late Effects:* secondary malignancies, growth and development changes in children and adolescents, osteopenia/osteoporosis, infertility

Used in Combination with Low- or High-Dose Conditioning Chemotherapy.

Table 11 - 17: General Types of Brachytherapy Placement (9,22,24)

Type of Brachytherapy Placement	Type of Cancer	
Interstitial – a radioactive source placed into the tumor.	• Breast • Gynecological • Head and neck	• Lung • Prostate • Rectal
Intracavitary or Contact – a radioactive source placed directly into a surgical or body cavity (e.g., vagina or uterus) near a tumor or an external surface (e.g., skin).	• Gynecological (e.g., cervical and endometrial) • Head and neck	

Table 11 - 18: Type and Source Duration of Brachytherapy (9,22,30)

Type and Source Duration	Description
Temporary – a radioactive source is implanted for a specific duration of time.	*Low Dose Rate or LDR* is a type of brachytherapy that is given in an inpatient setting using a protected, lead-shielded room. Radiation is delivered in a continuous, low-dose radiation manner from a source over several days. The radiation source is held in place by an applicator.
	• An example of LDR therapy is when a tandem and ovoid applicator is used for the treatment of cervical cancer after EBRT has been completed. The duration of time the applicator stays in place is dependent upon each individual's specific cancer, but it generally remains in place 18 to 72 hours.
	Pulsed Dose Rate or PDR is a type of LDR brachytherapy that delivers radiation in short pulses to enhance treatment effectiveness.
	High Dose Rate or HDR is a type of brachytherapy given either in one or several doses separated by at least six hours. In an outpatient setting, radioactive sources are placed remotely through a system of hallow delivery tubes placed into or near a tumor from a HDR after loading machine.
	• A type of HDR for the treatment of breast cancer involves the interstitial placement of multiple catheters into the lumpectomy bed and surrounding margin. Treatment is reduced to five to seven days instead of five to six weeks required for EBRT.
Permanent - *a radioactive source is implanted permanently.*	*Permanent Brachytherapy* uses sealed sources of radiation material (radioactive seeds or pellets), which are inserted and permanently left in the tissue. Over time the radioactivity of the seeds diminishes.
	• An example of this type of therapy is when radioactive seeds containing Iodine-125 or Palladium-103 are permanently placed in the prostate gland for the treatment of prostate cancer.

Table 11 - 19: Possible Acute & Late-Occurring Nutrition Impact Side Effects of Brachytherapy (9,22,30)

Sites of Brachytherapy Treatment	Acute Side Effect	Late-Occurring Side Effect
Breast	No known nutrition-related side effects.	
Gynecological (e.g., uterus, cervix, vagina)	• Nausea • Diarrhea • Discomfort when urinating	• Diarrhea • Bladder irritation
Esophagus	• Esophagitis, dysphagia, odynophagia	• Esophageal stenosis, fibrosis, and/or ulcerations
Prostate	• Discomfort when urinating • Diarrhea • Cramping/bloating • Flatulence • Proctitis	• Urinary stricture • Incontinence • Diarrhea
Tongue	• Mucositis, xerostomia, taste alterations	• Xerostomia, mucosal fibrosis and/or ulceration

Table 11 - 20: Possible Side Effects of Radiopharmaceuticals for Metastatic Bone Pain (9,22,24,33)

Agent	Side Effect
Samarium 153 (Quadramet®) *Indication: for relief of pain for individuals with confirmed osteoblastic bone lesions that enhance on a radionuclide bone scan.*	Acute Side Effects: • Myelosuppression – anemia, thrombocytopenia, neutropenia • Nausea, vomiting • Flushing Late-Occurring Side Effects: • Risk of secondary malignancy
Strontium 89 (Metastron®) *Indication: for the relief of pain for individuals with painful skeletal (bony) metastases.*	Acute Side Effects: • Myelosuppression – anemia, thrombocytopenia, neutropenia • Temporary increase in bone pain • Flushing Late-Occurring Side Effects: • Risk of secondary malignancy
Radium 223 (Xofigo®) *Indication: for the treatment of castration-resistant prostate cancer, symptomatic bone metastases and no known visceral metastatic disease.*	Acute Side Effects: • Myelosuppression – anemia, thrombocytopenia, neutropenia • Nausea, vomiting, diarrhea • Neurological changes – peripheral edema

usually with minimal effect to other parts of the body. Thyroid ablation with radioactive iodine involves a short stay in the hospital and then isolating the individual to prevent radiation exposure to others for a period of time until the radiation dissipates. Acute side effects of radioactive iodine include neck tenderness and swelling, nausea, vomiting, fatigue, salivary gland tenderness and swelling, taste changes, and xerostomia (24). Long-term side effects include an increased risk of secondary malignancies.

Radiopharmaceuticals for the Relief of Metastatic Bone Pain

A method of palliative radiation therapy used for the relief of pain for individuals with symptomatic bone metastases caused by cancer consists of a type of radiopharmaceuticals that can be used with or without other therapies such as bisphophonates, and taxanes-based chemotherapy (32). This type of radiopharmaceutical therapy uses different types of radionuclide agents. These bone-targeted systemic agents bind to osteoblastic areas or skeletal metastatic lesions from the primary cancer (24). Radiation is emitted and it causes the cancer to shrink, thereby relieving pain at the site of metastasis(es). It often

takes one to three weeks after the agent is given before a therapeutic effect is obtained. Examples of these agents include:

- Strontium 89 (Mestastron®)
- Samaruim 153 (Quadramet®)
- Radium 223 (Xofigo®)

Possible side effects of these radiopharmaceuticals and symptoms impacting nutritional status are outlined in Table 11 - 20.

References

1. National Comprehensive Cancer Network (NCCN). *NCCN clinical practice guidelines in oncology (NCCN guidelines).* Available at: http://www.nccn.org/clinical.asp. Accessed June 5, 2013.
2. American College of Surgeons/Commission on Cancer. Cancer Program Standards 2012, Version 1.1: Ensuring Patient-Centered Care Manual. Available at: http://www.facs.org/cancer/coc/programstandards2012.pdf. Accessed July 1, 2013.
3. Academy of Nutrition and Dietetics/Evidence Analysis Library: Oncology Nutrition Evidence-Based Nutrition Practice Guideline. Available at: http://www.adaevidencelibrary.com. Accessed June 6, 2013.

4. Academy of Nutrition and Dietetics. *International Dietetics & Terminology: Reference Manual, Standardized Language for the Nutrition Care Process, 4th edition*. Chicago, IL: Academy of Nutrition and Dietetics; 2013.

5. Academy of Nutrition and Dietetics. *Evidence Analysis Library/Oncology Toolkit: Evidence-Based Nutrition Practice Guideline*. Chicago, IL: Academy of Nutrition and Dietetics; 2010.

6. National Cancer Institute. *NCI Dictionary of Cancer Terms*. Available at: http://www.cancer.gov/dictionary. Accessed June 7, 2013.

7. Polovich M, Whitford JM, Olsen M. *Chemotherapy and Biotherapy Guidelines and Recommendations for Practice, 3rd edition*. Pittsburgh, PA: Oncology Nursing Society, 2009.

8. MD Anderson Cancer Center. Cancer Topics. Available at: http://www.mdanderson.org/patient-and-cancer-information/cancer-information/cancer-topics/prevention-and-screening/chemoprevention/index.html. Accessed June 6, 2013.

9. Iwamoto RR, Haas ML, Gosselin TK. *Oncology Nursing Society's Manual for Radiation Oncology Nursing Practice and Education, 4th edition*. Pittsburgh, PA: Oncology Nursing Society, 2012.

10. Wilkes GM, Barton-Burke, M. *Oncology Nursing Drug Handbook*. Sudbury, MA: Jones and Bartlett, 2012.

11. National Cancer Institute. *Biological therapies*. Available at: http://www.cancer.gov/cancertopics/factsheet/Therapy/biological. Accessed June 18, 2013.

12. National Cancer Institute. *Target Cancer Therapies*. Available at: http://www.cancer.gov/cancertopics/factsheet/Therapy/targeted. Accessed June 8, 2013.

13. Dy GK, Adjei AA. Understanding, recognizing, and managing toxicities of targeted anticancer therapies. *CA Cancer J Clin* 2013; 63: 250-279.

14. Wilkes GM. *Targeted Cancer Therapy: A Handbook for Nurses*. Sudbury, MA: Jones and Bartlett, 2011.

15. Hurdis CA. *N Engl J Med*. 2007;357(1):41

16. National Cancer Institute. *Cancer vaccines*. Available at: http://www.cancer.gov/cancertopics/factsheet/Therapy/cancer-vaccines. Accessed June 18, 2013.

17. Chu E, DeVita VT. *Physicians' Cancer Chemotherapy Drug Manual: 2012*. Burlington, MA: Jones and Bartlett, 2012.

18. National Cancer Institute. *Angiogenesis inhibitors*. Available at: http://www.cancer.gov/cancertopics/factsheet/Therapy/angiogenesis-inhibitors. Accessed June 19, 2013.

19. National Cancer Institute. *Advances in targeted therapies tutorial*. Available at: http://www.cancer.gov/cancertopics/understandingcancer/targetedtherapies/htmlcourse/page2#b. Accessed June 20, 2013.

20. National Institutes of Health. ClinicalTrials.gov: Clinical trials being conducted with spiuleucel-T. Available at: http://www.clinicaltrial.gov/ct2/results?term=sipuleucel%20OR%20sipuleucel-T%20OR%20DN24-02. Accessed June 18, 2013.

21. National Cancer Institute. Hormone therapy. Available at: http://www.cancer.gov/cancertopics/factsheet/Therapy/hormone-therapy. Accessed June 21, 2013.

22. National Cancer Institute. *Radiation therapy for cancer*. Available at: http://www.cancer.gov/cancertopics/factsheet/Therapy/radiation. Accessed July 17, 2013.

23. Halpern MT, Yabroff KR. Prevalence of outpatient cancer treatment in the United States: estimates from the Medical Panel Expenditures Survey (MEPS). *Cancer Invest*. 2008;26(6):647-651.

24. Washington CM, Leaver D. *Principles and Practice of Radiation Therapy, 3rd edition*. St. Louis, MO: Elsevier Health Sciences, 2009.

25. American Society for Radiation Oncology. *Radiation therapy for cancer*. Available at: http://www.rtanswers.org/uploadedFiles/Treatment_Information/Brochures/rtforcancer. Accessed July 15, 2013.

26. Cancer Connection. *Techniques for delivering radiation therapy*. Available at: http://news.cancerconnect.com/techniques-for-delivering-radiation-therapy/. Accessed July 13, 2013.

27. National Cancer Institute. *Radiation Therapy and You*. Available at: http://www.cancer.gov/cancertopics/coping/radiation-therapy-and-you/page8/AllPages/Print. Accessed July 17, 2013.

28. Brown CG. *A Guide to Oncology Symptom Management*. Pittsburgh, PA: Oncology Nursing Society, 2010.

29. Seattle Cancer Care Alliance. *Preparing for transplant*. Available at: http://www.seattlecca.org/client/documents/Preparing_for_Transplant_2011_r2.pdf. Accessed on July 20, 2013.

30. Devin PM. *Brachytherapy: Applications and Techniques*. Philadelphia, PA: LWW, 2007.

31. Chemocare. Radiopharmaceuticals. Available at: http://chemocare.com/chemotherapy/what-is-radiopharmaceuticals.aspx. Accessed August 27, 2013.

32. Sartor O. Overview of samarium 153 Lexidronam in the treatment of painful metastatic bone disease. *Rev Urol* 2004; 6(10): S3-S12.

33. Food and Drug Administration. Xofigo. Available at: http://www.accessdata.fda.gov/drugsatfda_docs/label/2013/203971lbl.pdf. Accessed August 29, 2013.

Table 11 - 3: Chemotherapy: Classification, Mechanism of Action, Route of Administration and Possible Side Effects (7,10,17)

Classification	Mechanism of Action	Medication Name, Route of Administration and Indication	Possible Side Effects and Nutritional Implications
Cell cycle non-specific drugs: active throughout the cell cycle.			
Alkylating Agents	Interferes with DNA bases causing breaks in DNA helix strands, thus preventing DNA replication and transcription of RNA.	Bendamustine (Treanda®) *Route:* IV *Indication:* B-Cell Non Hodgkins Lymphoma (NHL), Chronic Lymphocytic Leukemia (CLL), Mantle Cell Lymphoma	• Myelosuppression • Mild nausea and vomiting, fatigue • Other: Hypersensitivity infusion reactions (fever, chills, pruritis, rash), tumor lysis syndrome.
		Busulfan (Myleran®) *Route:* PO (Busulfex®) *Route:* IV *Indication:* Chronic Myelogenous Leukemia (CML), HCT preparation	• Myelosuppression • Nausea, vomiting, diarrhea, mucositis • Hepatic toxicity • Adrenal insufficiency • Other: pulmonary symptoms (e.g. cough, dyspnea), insomnia, dizziness, anxiety, alopecia
		Carboplatin (Paraplatin®) *Route:* IV *Indication:* bladder, endometrial, germ cell, head and neck, lung, ovarian cancers	• Myelosuppression • Nausea, vomiting • Renal toxicity • Other: Hypersensitivity reaction, mild alopecia, peripheral neuropathy
		Carmustine (BCNU)* *may also be classified as a nitrosourea *Route:* IV *Indication:* Brain cancer, Hodgkins Disease (HD), NHL, multiple myeloma (MM), glioblastoma	• Myelosuppression • Nausea, vomiting • Hepatic toxicity • Renal toxicity • Pulmonary toxicity
		Chlorambucil (Leukeran®) *Route:* PO *Indication:* CLL, HD, NHL	• Nausea, vomiting • Hyperuricemia • Pulmonary toxicity • Other: Skin rash, seizure risk in children
		Cisplatin (Platinol®, CDDP) *Route:* IV *Indication:* bladder, cervical, esophageal, head and neck, lung, NHL, ovarian, prostate, testicular cancers	• Myelosuppression • Nausea, vomiting (acute and delayed), metallic taste • SIADH • Renal toxicity • Hypomagnesmia • Other: Ototoxicity, hypersensitivity infusion reaction, peripheral neuropathy
		Cyclophosphamide (Cytoxan®, CTX) *Route:* IV, PO, IP *Indication:* breast and ovarian cancers, CLL, NHL, HD, MM, mycosis fungoides, neuroblastoma, sarcomas, Wilms' tumors	• Myelosuppression • Nausea, vomiting • Bladder toxicity • Cardiac toxicity • SIADH • Other: Alopecia
		Dacarbazine (DTIC) *Route:* IV *Indication:* HD, malignant melanoma, neuroblastoma, sarcomas	• Myelosuppression • Nausea, vomiting • Other: Flu-like symptoms (e.g. fever, chills), CNS toxicity, photosensitivity
		Ifosfamide (Ifex®) *Route:* IV *Indication:* bladder, cervical, germ cell, head and neck, and lung cancers, HD, NHL, sarcomas *Note:* Mesna and hydration given for urological protection.	• Myelosuppression • Nausea, vomiting, anorexia • Bladder toxicity (e.g. hemorrhagic cystitis, dysuria) • SIADH • Other: Neurotoxicity (e.g. seizure, lethargy), alopecia
		Mechlorethamine (nitrogen mustard) *Route:* IV *Indication:* CLL, CML, HD, NHL, mycosis fungoides	• Myelosuppression • Nausea, vomiting • Hyperuricemia • Other: Pain or inflammation at injection site, alopecia

(Continued)

Table 11 - 3: Chemotherapy: Classification, Mechanism of Action, Route of Administration and Possible Side Effects (7,10,17) *(continued)*

Classification	Mechanism of Action	Medication Name, Route of Administration and Indication	Possible Side Effects and Nutritional Implications
Cell cycle non-specific drugs: active throughout the cell cycle (continued)			
		Melphalan (Alkeran®) *Route:* IV, PO *Indication:* breast and ovarian cancers, multiple myeloma, HCT, polycythemia vera	• Myelosuppression • Nausea, vomiting, mucositis, diarrhea • Other: Hypersensitivity infusion reaction
		Oxaliplatin (Eloxatin®) *Route:* IV *Indication:* colorectal, pancreatic, gastroesophageal cancers	• Myelosuppression • Nausea, vomiting, diarrhea • Neurotoxicity (e.g. peripheral neuropathy, sensitivity to cold, laryngopharyngeal dysesthesia) • Hepatic toxicity • Other: Allergic reaction
		Temozolomide (Temodar®) *Route:* PO *Indication:* astrocytoma, glioblastoma	• Myelosuppression • Nausea, vomiting, fatigue • Headache • Hepatic toxicity • Other: Photosensitivity, rash
		Thiotepa (Thioplex®) *Route:* IV, IM, IT, SC *Indication:* bladder, breast, and ovarian cancers, HD, NHL, sarcoma	• Myelosuppression • Nausea, vomiting, mucositis • Renal toxicity (e.g. hemorrhagic cystitis) • Other: Skin changes (e.g. rash, bronzing of skin)
Cell Cycle: Specific			
Antimetabolites	Interferes with DNA synthesis by acting as false metabolites. They are incorporated into the DNA strand or they block essential enzymes.	Azacitidine (Vidaza®) *Route:* SC, IV *Indication:* Myelodysplastic Syndrome (MDS)	• Myelosuppression • Nausea, vomiting, diarrhea, fatigue • Hypokalemia • Renal toxicity
		Capecitabine (Xeloda®) *Route:* PO *Indication:* colon and metastatic breast cancers	• Myelosuppression • Nausea, vomiting, diarrhea, fatigue • Increased bilirubin • Other: Hand-foot syndrome
		Cytarabine (ARA-C) *Route:* IV, SC, IT, IM *Indication:* Acute Lymphocytic Leukemia (ALL), Acute Myelogenous Leukemia (AML), CML, NHL	• Myelosuppression • Nausea, vomiting, mucositis, anorexia, acute pancreatitis • Neurotoxicity (e.g. lethargy, confusion) • Hepatic toxicity • Pulmonary toxicity • Other: Conjunctivitis, keratitis
		Fludarabine (Fludara®) *Route:* IV *Indication:* CLL, NHL, T-Cell Lymphoma, Hairy Cell Leukemia	• Myelosuppression • Nausea, vomiting, diarrhea • Neurotoxicity • Other: Rash
		Fluorouracil (5-FU) *Route:* IV, topical *Indication:* breast, colorectal, GI, head and neck, pancreatic and ovarian cancers, and hepatoma	• Myelosuppression • Nausea, vomiting, diarrhea, mucositis • Other: Hand-foot syndrome, cardiac toxicity, photosensitivity
		Gemcitabine (Gemzar®) *Route:* IV *Indication:* bladder, breast, ovarian, pancreatic, and lung cancers, NHL, sarcoma	• Myelosuppression • Nausea, vomiting • Pulmonary toxicity • Other: Rash, flu-like symptoms (e.g. fever, chills)
		Mercaptopurine (6-MP) *Route:* PO *Indication:* ALL, AML, CML, NHL	• Myelosuppression • Nausea, vomiting, mucositis, diarrhea • Hepatic toxicity • Hyperuricemia

(Continued)

Table 11 - 3: Chemotherapy: Classification, Mechanism of Action, Route of Administration and Possible Side Effects (7,10,17) *(continued)*

Classification	Mechanism of Action	Medication Name, Route of Administration and Indication	Possible Side Effects and Nutritional Implications
Cell Cycle: Specific (continued)			
		Methotrexate (MTX) *Route:* IM, IV, IT, PO *Indication:* bladder, breast, and head and neck cancers, NHL, CNS lymphoma, ALL, sarcoma	• Myelosuppression • Nausea, mucositis, oral and GI ulcerations • Renal toxicity • Hepatic toxicity • Other: Photosensitivity
		Pemetrexed (Alimta®) *Route:* IV *Indication:* mesothelioma, lung cancer	• Myelosuppression • Nausea, vomiting, diarrhea, fatigue • Other: Rash
		Thioguanine (6-TG) *Route:* PO *Indication:* ALL, AML, CML	• Myelosuppression • Nausea, vomiting, mucositis, diarrhea • Hepatic toxicity • Renal toxicity • Other: Rash
Antitumor Antibiotics	Inhibits cell division by binding to DNA and interfering with RNA synthesis.	Bleomycin (Blenoxane®) *Route:* IV, SC, IM *Indication:* HD, NHL, head and neck cancer, squamous cell cancers of the skin, cervix, vulva and testicular, melanoma	• Pulmonary toxicity • Renal toxicity • Other: Hyperpigmentation, skin and nail changes, hypersensitivity infusion reaction
		Dactinomycin (Actinomycin D) *Route:* IV *Indication:* Ewing sarcoma, rhabdomyosarcoma, Wilm's tumor, testicular cancer	• Myleosuppression • Nausea, vomiting, mucositis, diarrhea, anorexia • Other: Alopecia
		Mitomycin-C (Mutamycin®) *Route:* IV *Indication:* Cancers of the anus, bladder, breast, esophagus, head and neck, lung, pancreas, and stomach	• Myelosuppression • Nausea, vomiting, mucositis, diarrhea, anorexia • Pulmonary toxicity • Renal toxicity • Other: fatigue, alopecia
Antitumor Antibiotics: Anthracyclines		Daunorubicin (Daunomycin®) *Route:* IV *Indication:* ALL, AML	• Myelosuppression • Nausea, vomiting, diarrhea, mucositis, anorexia • Hyperuremia • Other: cardiotoxicity, alopecia, may turn urine red, hyperpigmentation
		Doxorubicin (Adriamycin®) *Route:* IV *Indication:* Cancers of the breast, liver, lung, ovarian, prostate; NHL, HD, MM, ALL, AML; squamous cell of the head and neck	• Myelosuppression • Nausea, vomiting, diarrhea, mucositis, anorexia • Other: cardiotoxicity, hand and foot syndrome, hyperpigmentation, alopecia, red-orange urine
		Doxorubicin liposomal (Doxil®) *Route:* IV *Indication:* AIDS-related Kaposi's Sarcoma, ovarian cancer, MM, sarcoma, hepatocellular carcinoma	• Myelosuppression • Nausea, vomiting, diarrhea, mucositis • Other: cardiotoxicity, hand and foot syndrome, hyperpigmentation, alopecia, red-orange urine, infusion reaction
		Epirubicin (Ellence®) *Route:* IV *Indication:* Breast and gastric cancer	• Myelosuppression • Nausea, vomiting, diarrhea, mucositis • Other: cardiotoxicity, skin rash, alopecia, red-orange urine
		Idarubicin (Idamycin®) *Route:* IV *Indication:* AML, ALL, CML, MDS	• Myelosuppression • Nausea, vomiting, diarrhea, mucositis • Other: cardiotoxicity, alopecia, skin rash, elevation of liver enzymes, red urine

(Continued)

Table 11 - 3: Chemotherapy: Classification, Mechanism of Action, Route of Administration and Possible Side Effects (7,10,17) *(continued)*

Classification	Mechanism of Action	Medication Name, Route of Administration and Indication	Possible Side Effects and Nutritional Implications
Cell Cycle: Specific (continued)			
Epipodophyllo-toxins	Damages the cell prior to mitosis, late S and G2 phases. Inhibits topoisomerase II.	Etoposide (Vepesid®, VP-16) *Route:* IV *Indication:* small cell and non-small cell lung cancer, HD, NHL, gastric cancer, germ cell tumors (testicular)	• Myelosuppression • Nausea, vomiting, diarrhea, mucositis, anorexia • Other: metallic taste during infusion, hypersensitivity reaction, alopecia, orthostatic hypertension
		Teniposide (Vumon®, VM-26) *Route:* IV *Indications:* Childhood ALL	• Myelosuppression • Nausea, vomiting • Other: hypotension, pulmonary toxicity
Taxanes	Active in the mitosis phase of the cell cycle. Anti-microtuble agent, which leads to inhibition of mitosis and cell division.	Paclitaxel (Taxol®) *Route:* IV *Indication:* Bladder, breast, esophageal, head and neck, ovarian, pancreatic, prostate, and small cell and non-small cell lung cancers	• Myelosuppression • Diarrhea, mucositis • Sensory neuropathy • Other: hypersensitivity reaction, alopecia, reversible changes in transaminases, bilirubin, and alkaline phosphatase, arthralgia, myalgia
		Docetaxel (Taxotere®) *Route:* IV *Indication:* Breast, gastric, head and neck, ovarian, prostate, and non small cell lung cancers	• Myelosuppression • Mucositis, diarrhea • Neurotoxicity • Other: fluid retention syndrome, skin and nail changes, hypersensitivity reaction, reversible changes in transaminases, bilirubin, and alkaline phosphatase
		Paclitaxel protein-bound (Abraxane®) *Route:* IV *Indication:* Breast cancer, non small cell lung cancer	• Myelosuppression • Nausea, vomiting, diarrhea, mucositis • Arthralgia, myalgia • Sensory neuropathy • Other: alopecia
Vinca Alkaloids	Binds to protein tubulin and disrupt mitotic spindle formation and prevents cell division in the mitosis phase.	Vincristine (Oncovin®) *Route:* IV *Indication:* ALL, AML, CML, HD, NHL, MM, small cell lung cancer, rhabdomyosarcoma, neuroblastoma, Ewing's sarcoma, Wilms' tumor, brain and thyroid cancers	• Myelosuppression • Sensory neuropathy • Constipation • Other: SIADH, hypersensitivity reactions, jaw pain
		Vinblastine (Velban®) *Route:* IV *Indication:* Breast and testicular cancers, HD, squamous cell head and neck cancer, sarcoma	• Myelosuppression • Mucositis, stomatitis, constipation • Other: hypertension, alopecia, jaw pain
		Vinorelbine (Navelbine®) *Route:* IV *Indication:* Breast, ovarian, and non-small cell lung cancers	• Myelosuppression • Nausea, vomiting, constipation, stomatitis, anorexia • Other: transient elevations in liver function tests

Route of Administration Abbreviations: IM – intramuscular, IP – intrapleural, IT – intrathecal, IV – intravenous, PO – oral, SC – subcutaneous

Table 11 - 5: Monoclonal Antibodies: Classification, Mechanism of Action, Route of Administration and Possible Side Effects (7,10,12,14,17)

Classification	Target	Medication Name, Indication and Route of Administration	Possible Side Effects and Nutritional Implications
Monoclonal Antibodies	CD20	Ibritumomab tiuxetan (Zevalin®) *Indication:* relapsed or refractory B-cell NHL *Route:* IV	• Possible infusion reaction • Myelosuppression • Asthenia • Infections • Nausea, vomiting – generally mild • Cough, dyspnea, sinusitis
	CD20	Rituximab (Rituxan®) *Indication:* B-cell NHL, CLL *Route:* IV	• Possible infusion reaction • Tumor lysis syndrome • Skin reactions • Nausea, vomiting – generally mild • Myelosuppression
	HER2/neu	Pertuzumab (Perjeta™) *Indication:* Metastatic breast cancer *Route:* IV	• Possible infusion reaction • Cardiotoxicity • Fatigue
	HER2/neu	Trastuzumab (Herceptin™) *Indication:* Breast cancer, metastatic gastric cancer *Route:* IV	• Possible infusion reaction • Nausea, vomiting, diarrhea – generally mild • Cardiotoxicity • Myelosuppression – rarely • Pulmonary toxicity
	HER2/neu	Ado-trastuzumab emtansine (Kadcyla™) *Indication:* Metastatic breast cancer *Route:* intravenous	• Possible infusion reaction • Cardiotoxicity • Hepatotoxicity – monitor serum transaminases and bilirubin • Pulmonary toxicity • Thrombocytopenia • Peripheral neuropathy • Constipation
	EGFR	Cetuximab (Erbitux®) *Indication:* Colorectal cancer, head and neck cancer *Route:* intravenous	• Possible infusion reaction • Acneiform skin rash, pruritis • Pulmonary toxicity • Hypomagnesemia • Malaise, asthenia • Nausea, vomiting, diarrhea, anorexia
	EGFR	Panitumumab (Vectibix®) *Indication:* Colorectal cancer *Route:* IV	• Possible infusion reaction • Acneiform skin rash, pruritis • Pulmonary toxicity • Hypomagnesemia • Diarrhea • Malaise
	RANKL	Denosumab (Xgeva®) *Indication:* Bone metastases *Route:* IV	• Nausea, vomiting, diarrhea • Hypocalcaemia • Risk for osteonecrosis of the jaw
	RANKL	Denosumab (Prolia®) *Indication:* Patients with osteoporosis at high risk of fracture *Route:* IV	• Nausea, vomiting, diarrhea • Hypocalcaemia • Risk for osteonecrosis of the jaw

Symptom Management of Cancer Therapies

Laura Elliott, MPH, RD, CSO, LD

Overview

Symptoms associated with cancer treatment can negatively impact a patient's quality of life. Inadequate management of these symptoms can result in a decline in a patient's nutritional status and potentially lead to malnutrition, which has been linked to poorer treatment outcomes. Many patients undergoing treatment report one or more nutrition impact symptoms including anorexia, poor appetite, early satiety, constipation, diarrhea, malabsorption, dysphagia, mucositis, esophagitis, oral candidiasis, xerostomia, thick saliva, taste and smell changes, or fatigue. Effective management of these symptoms can positively affect comfort, weight maintenance, and tolerance of treatment. The most common symptoms are dry mouth, nausea, and constipation, with the most distressing noted to be dry mouth, diarrhea, and stomach pain. Use of the following management strategies can help patients maintain good nutrition status throughout their treatment.

In the tables that follow, Pharmacologic Interventions include brand names of some drugs followed by the drug's generic name in parenthesis.

Anorexia/Poor Appetite/Early Satiety

Anorexia is the loss of appetite or desire to eat.

Early satiety is the feeling of being full after eating or drinking a small amount.

Nutrition Diagnosis: Inadequate energy & nutrient intake related to decreased desire for food and early satiety

Potential Outcomes: Weight loss, nutrient insufficiencies & deficiencies, dehydration, malnutrition

---

Nutrition Interventions for Anorexia

Eat small, frequent meals of calorie dense foods and fluids.

Eat in pleasant surroundings, avoiding stress or conflict at meals.

Eat by the clock rather than waiting for appetite or hunger cues.

View eating as part of treatment.

Consume medical nutrition beverages when eating is too tiring.

Engage in light physical activity to stimulate appetite.

Use easy to prepare and serve foods to preserve energy.

Other considerations:

Evaluate for conditions that may depress appetite (e.g., constipation and depression).

Evaluate use of medications that depress appetite (e.g., medications that manage constipation, nausea, or pain).

Nutrition Interventions for Early Satiety

Choose calorie dense foods or medical nutrition beverages.

Maximize intake when most hungry.

Eat small, frequent meals and snacks.

Eat by the clock rather than waiting for appetite or hunger cues.

Engage in light physical activity to help move food through the GI tract.

Consume liquids between meals, rather than with meals.

Other Considerations:

Evaluate for conditions that may slow gastric emptying (e.g., GERD, diabetes, gastroparesis, obstruction)

Evaluate for use of medications that may slow gastric emptying and influence gastrointestinal function (e.g., opioids, aluminum hydroxide antacids, H2 receptor antagonists, proton pump inhibitors (PPIs), sucralfate, interferon, levadopa)

Pharmacologic Interventions

Antihistimines:
Periactin (1) (cyproheptadine)

Corticosteroids:
Decadron (1) (dexamethasone)
Solu-medrol (2) (methylprednisolone)

Progestational agents:
Provera (2) (medroxyprogesterone acetate)
Megace (3) (megestrol acetate)

Prokinetic agents:
Reglan (4) (metoclopramide)

Antidepressant:
Remeron (5) (mirtazapine); off-label use; should be used with caution and not taken concurrently or after recent use of MAOI medications or diazepam

Constipation

Constipation is a decrease in frequency of bowel movements and/or hard to pass stools that may be due to dehydration, medications, or mechanical changes from anticancer therapy.

Nutrition Diagnosis: Altered GI function related to inadequate food, fluid and/or fiber intake or medications

Potential Outcomes: Infrequent or hard to pass stools, pain, early satiety, nausea, vomiting

Nutrition Interventions

Educate patient on importance of adequate hydration, fiber intake and total food intake on bowel regularity.

Aim for 64 ounces (8 cups) of fluids/day and a slow increase to 25-35 grams of fiber/day as tolerated.

Encourage use of a hot beverage, hot cereal, or high fiber food to stimulate bowel movements.

Incorporate probiotics and/or other supplements that help facilitate bowel movements.

Engage in light activity and/or stretching to improve bowel regularity.

Discuss medications that affect bowel function and encourage appropriate use of stool softeners as needed.

Schedule adequate bathroom time to facilitate bowel movements.

Other Considerations:
Encourage patient to contact doctor if they have had no bowel movement for three days.

Pharmacologic/Non-food Interventions

Bulking agents:
Bran, flaxseed or wheat germ
Citrucel (6) (methylcellulose)
Konsyl (7) (calcium polycarbophil)

Stool surfactants:
Colace (8) (docusate)
Mineral oil

Osmotic laxatives:
MiraLAX (1) (polyethylene glycol)
Lactulose
Milk of Magnesia (9) (magnesium hydroxide)

Stimulant laxative agents:
Carter's Pills (10) (bisacodyl)
Senocot (8) (senna)

Herbals:
Probiotics, slippery elm, aloe juice

Diarrhea

Diarrhea is an increase of three or more stools per day as compared to usual or an increase in liquidity of bowel movements possibly caused by diet; emotional stress; inflammation or irritation of the mucosa of the intestines; certain medications and anticancer treatments such as antibiotics, chemotherapy or radiation therapy to the abdomen and pelvis; lactose intolerance, which may be a preexisting condition or develop as a side effect to treatment; infections; and malabsorption syndrome from disease or anticancer treatment.

Nutrition Diagnosis: Altered GI function related to inability to digest/absorb certain foods, anticancer treatment, and/or medications

Potential Outcomes: Frequent stools, dehydration, electrolyte imbalances, weight loss, fatigue, nutrient insufficiencies & deficiencies, malnutrition

Nutrition Interventions

Identify problem foods or eating habits via a detailed diet and symptom history.

As indicated, encourage a low fat, low fiber, and/or low lactose diet, avoiding gas producing foods, caffeine, and alcohol.

Encourage small, frequent meals.

Consider use of bulking agents, pectin, or soluble fiber foods (applesauce, banana, oatmeal, potatoes, rice) to control diarrhea.

Avoid sorbitol or other sugar-alcohol containing products (e.g., sugarless gum and candy).

Other Considerations:
Consider use of a multivitamin and mineral supplement.

Pharmacologic/Non-food Interventions

Opioid receptor agonist:
Imodium AD (11) (loperamide)
Lomotil (2) (dipheoxylate, atropine)
Sandostatin (12) (octreotide)
camphorated tincture of opium

Anti-inflammatory, anti-diarrheal:
Pepto-Bismol (13) (bismuth subsalicylate)
Kaopectate (14) (attapulgite)

Bile acid sequestrant:
Questran (3) (cholestyramine)

Anticholinergics:
Benadryl (11) (diphenhydramine)

Probiotics

Dysphagia

Dysphagia is pain or difficulty swallowing due to extrinsic compression of the esophagus, mechanical obstruction, neurological dysfunction, oral or esophageal candidiasis, or severe mucositis or esophagitis from chemotherapy or radiation therapy, resulting in a decreased intake.

Nutrition Diagnosis: Inadequate oral intake related to swallowing difficulty

Potential Outcomes: Dehydration, coughing, choking, feeling of "food getting stuck", pain while swallowing, weight loss, nutrient insufficiencies & deficiencies, dehydration, malnutrition

Nutrition Interventions

Use good posture when eating to help prevent aspiration.

Avoid distractions and limit talking while eating.

Encourage double swallows to assure that food clears.

Encourage verbalization after drinks to assure liquids have cleared.

Choose moist foods of a similar texture to help form a cohesive bolus in the mouth.

Consider using thickeners in liquids to slow flow and allow safe swallow.

Avoid use of straws that place food in back of mouth.

Alter textures as needed for safe swallow.

Other Considerations:
Consider Speech and Language Therapist consult.

Pharmacologic/Non-food Interventions

Topical anesthetics:
If patient has functional swallow and experiences pain with swallow, try topical anesthetics, sprays, and lozenges

Xylocaine (15) (lidocaine spray)

Thickeners:
If patient has difficulty with thin liquids, try household or commercial thickeners

Thicken Right (16)

Thicken Up (17)

Thick & Easy (16)

Thick It (18)

Oral Candidiasis

Oral candidiasis may be an opportunistic infection seen as red or white patches in the mouth due to treatment or a depressed immune status, causing taste alterations, sore mouth, and coated tongue.

Nutrition Diagnosis: Inadequate food and beverage intake related to infection, taste alterations, and a sore mouth

Potential Outcomes: Sore mouth and throat, decrease in food intake, weight loss, malnutrition

Nutrition Interventions

Practice good oral hygiene.

Choose soft textured, low acid foods.

Avoid sugar and yeast-derived foods.

Other Considerations:
1 Tbsp. yogurt held in mouth, 5 min. daily

Pharmacologic/Non-food Interventions

Polyenes such as nystatin
Azoles such as Diflucan (2) (fluconazole), Chlorhexidine

Probiotics

Fatigue

Fatigue refers to a lack of energy, tiredness, dizziness, and mental fuzziness possibly caused by anemia, inadequate energy and/or protein intake, weight loss, pain, medications, anticancer treatment, dehydration, and/or sleep disturbances.

Nutrition Diagnosis: Inadequate food and beverage intake or involuntary weight loss related to inadequate energy or protein intake, fatigue, pain, or medications

Potential Outcomes: Poor oral intake, weight loss, weight gain, depression

Nutrition Interventions	Pharmacologic/Non-food Interventions
Review food and fluid intake for adequacy and advise on dietary modifications and need for medical nutrition beverages to promote an adequate energy and nutrient intake.	Blood transfusions Erythropoietin given as Epogen, Procrit (19) (epoetin alpha)
Monitor weight and modify intake plan as needed to stabilize weight or promote weight gain.	
Encourage use of easy to prepare meals, snacks, prepared foods, and energy dense foods.	
Advise patient to keep non-perishable snacks at bedside (e.g., trail mix).	
Consume soft, easy to chew foods.	
Eat small, frequent meals and snacks.	
Eat well when appetite is best, i.e., breakfast.	
Encourage energy saving, limiting "duties or chores" as much as possible.	
Encourage ADL's and light activity.	
Consider physical therapy consult for strengthening.	
Other Considerations:	
Evaluate for anemia as a cause of lack of energy.	
Consider use of a multivitamin and mineral supplement.	

Malabsorption

Malabsorption decreases the ability to digest and absorb nutrients possibly caused by chemotherapy, surgery, medications, medical conditions, or infections. Symptoms may include gas, bloating, gastrointestinal pain, and/or diarrhea.

Nutrition Diagnosis: Altered GI function related to disease process, infection, surgery, medications, chemotherapy, or radiation

Potential Outcomes: Abnormal digestive enzyme studies, cachexia, steatorrhea, weight loss, dehydration, fatigue, nutrient insufficiencies & deficiencies, malnutrition

Nutrition Interventions	Pharmacologic/Non-food Interventions
Conduct a thorough diet and symptom history to determine cause	**To reduce gas:** Gas-X (12) (simethicone) Probiotics
For bloating and gas, avoid cruciferous vegetables and limit swallowed air by avoiding use of straws, carbonated beverages, and chewing gum and by eating slowly and with mouth closed.	**For lactose intolerance:** Lactaid (11) (lactase enzyme) Probiotics
For bloating, cramping, and gas from milk products, eat a low lactose diet and use lactase treated dairy products or lactase pills or drops.	**For gas from beans and legumes and other vegetables:** Beano (6) Probiotics
For gas from beans and legumes, avoid these foods or use Beano drops.	**For diarrhea:** Probiotics *Saccharomyces boulardii* and *Lactobacillus rhamnosus* GG Caution: Bacteremia possible in immuno-compromised hosts.
For chronic diarrhea, try a low insoluble fiber, low fat, low lactose diet.	**For fat malabsorption:**
For bulky, foul smelling stools, eat a low fat diet and use pancreatic enzymes.	Pancreatic enzymes with each meal or snack that contains fat. 4,000 units of lipase per 5-7g of fat or 30,000-40,000 lipase units/meal and 10,000 lipase units/snack, or
For fatty stools, try a low fat diet and pancreatic enzymes.	500 lipase units/kg with meals increasing as tolerated. Do not exceed 2500 lipase units/kg body weight/meal.

Mucositis/Esophagitis

Mucositis/esophagitis is inflammation of the mouth or esophagus usually described as a painful, irritated throat, or the feeling of a lump in the throat. Accompanying symptoms can include indigestion, esophageal reflux, belching, feeling of fullness, and early satiety.

Nutrition Diagnosis: Inadequate energy intake related to disease process or treatment that produces pain when swallowing.

Potential Outcomes: Weight loss, nutrient insufficiencies & deficiencies, malnutrition

Nutrition Interventions

Choose foods lower in acidity and avoid tomato products, citrus juices, and pickled foods.

Choose foods that are less spicy and avoid chili, chili powder, curry, cloves, black pepper, and hot sauces.

Choose foods softer in texture, with added moistness, sauce, or gravy.

Choose cream soups, mashed potatoes, yogurt, eggs, tofu, and pudding.

Serve foods at cool or room temperature.

Prepare smoothies with low acid fruits like melons, bananas, or peaches and add yogurt, milk, or silken tofu.

Avoid alcohol and alcohol containing mouthwashes and tobacco.

For mucositis:

Encourage good oral care.

Sip one Tbsp. honey dissolved in one cup of warm water.

Keep dentures clean and limit their use if they increase irritation.

Avoid carbonated beverages.

Consume ice chips or a frozen ice pop during the administration of a 5-fluorouracil (5-FU) push, and Adriamycin.

For esophagitis:

Recommend patient avoid smoking, chewing tobacco, and drinking alcohol.

Pharmacologic/Non-food Interventions

Anesthetic gels containing lidocaine.

Sore throat gargle made with 3/4 tsp. salt and 1 tsp. baking soda in 4 cups of water. Gargle with 1 cup, 3-4x/day or as directed by physician.

Rinse (orally), swish, and spit with topical analgesic (e.g., viscous lidocaine), anti-inflammatory (diphenhydramine), and a coating agent (Maalox (12)). Use 3-4x/day or as directed by physician.

Glutamine rinses 5 grams 3x/day

Nausea/Vomiting

Nausea and vomiting may be caused by chemotherapy, radiation therapy, immunotherapy, pain, dysgeusia, fatigue, mucous drainage from the mouth and sinuses, flu, constipation, psychological factors, and/or medication such as antibiotics and narcotics.

Nutrition Diagnosis: Inadequate oral food/beverage intake and altered GI function related to disease process or treatment

Potential Outcomes: Dehydration, electrolyte imbalances, weight loss, nutrient insufficiencies & deficiencies

Nutrition Interventions

Eat 5-6 small meals/day.

Limit exposure to food smells by avoiding food preparation areas.

Consider eating cool, light foods with little odor.

Avoid greasy, high fat foods.

Consume liquids between meals, rather than with meals.

Avoid/limit strong smelling lotions, soaps, perfumes, and air fresheners.

Rest with head elevated for 30 minutes after eating.

If nausea medications are prescribed, take as directed. Time meals when nausea medications are working their best.

If taking pain medications, take them with crackers or light food.

Other Considerations:

Consider use of complementary therapies such as ginger tea, ginger-ale, 0.5-1 gram ginger extract, acupressure bracelets, acupuncture, massage, transcutaneous nerve stimulation, distraction strategies, relaxation techniques, or self-hypnosis.

Pharmacologic/Non-food Interventions

For acute nausea and vomiting, consider serotonin antagonists:
Zofran (6) (ondansetron)
Anzemet (20) (dolasetron)
Kytril (21) (granisetron)
Aloxi (22) (palonosetron)

For delayed nausea and vomiting, consider the dopamine antagonists: Phenothiazines such as Compazine (6) (prochlorperazine) or Phenergan (20) (promethazine);

Benzamides such as Reglan (7) (metoclopramide);

Cannabinoids such as Marinol (23) (dronabinol) or Cesamet (24) (nabilone);

Benzodiazapines such as Ativan (25) (lorazepam) or Valium (26) (diazepam);

Corticosteroids such as Decadron (1) (dexamethasone), prednisone

For prevention of chemo-induced vomiting, consider use of:
Decadron (1) (dexamethasone) and Zofran (6) (ondansteron) with a Neurokinin-1 receptor antagonist like Rezonic (6) (casopitant) or Emend (1) (aprepitant);

Also consider use of Reglan (7) (metoclopramide)

Taste and Smell Changes

May be caused by radiation or chemotherapy and be characterized as having little or no sense of taste and smell or heightened sense of metallic, bitter, salty, or sweet tastes. Following treatment, normal taste may take up to a year to return.

Nutrition Diagnosis: Inadequate food and beverage intake related to taste and smell changes

Potential Outcomes: Decreased intake, nutrient insufficiencies & deficiencies, weight loss

Nutrition Interventions

Check mouth for thrush and encourage good oral hygiene.

Suggest rinsing mouth or brushing teeth before eating.

If foods have little or no taste:

Choose fruit marinades for meats, or use lemon, herbs & spices, pickles, or hot sauce to season foods.

If foods have an "off" taste:

Fruity and salty flavors are often well accepted and taste correctly.

Suggest sugar free lemon drops, gum, or mints to improve mouth taste.

For bitter or metallic tastes:

Use spices or seasonings like onion, garlic, or chili powder.

Suck on lemon drops or mints.

Eat using bamboo or plastic silverware or chopsticks.

Flavor water with lemon juice or other fruit flavors.

For too salty, bitter, or acid taste:

Choose foods that are naturally sweet rather than salty or acidic.

Use low sodium products.

Meats taste bitter or strange:

Add fruit based marinade or sweet and sour sauce to meats.

Choose alternative protein sources like eggs, tofu, dairy, or beans.

When smells are bothersome:

Avoid cooking areas during meal prep.

Eat foods that aren't cooked such as smoothies, cold sandwiches, crackers and cheese, or yogurt and fruit.

Avoid use of microwave ovens as they spread food odors.

Use cup with lid and straw to mask food odors.

Pharmacologic/Non-food Interventions

Zinc in form to provide 50 mg elemental zinc.

Zinc Sulfate 220 mg

Zinc Gluconate 71.5 mg

Zinc Glycinate 182 mg

Zinc Aspartate 156 mg

Limit zinc supplementation to no more than 60 days duration due to possible copper deficiency caused by long-term use.

Oral rinse made with 3/4 tsp. salt and 1 tsp. baking soda in 4 cups of water. Rinse mouth with 1 cup 3-4x/day or as directed by physician.

Xerostomia/Thick Saliva

Xerostomia is abnormal dryness of the mouth that causes difficulty eating and talking, taste alterations, and/or thick and ropy saliva.

Nutrition Diagnosis: Inadequate food and beverage intake related to difficulty eating

Potential Outcomes: Decreased oral intake, nutrient insufficiencies & deficiencies, weight loss

Nutrition Interventions

Eat frequent small meals.

Alternate bites and sips at meals.

Add broth, gravies, and sauces to meals and dunk dry foods in liquids.

Sip liquids often throughout the day; aim for 8-10 cups/day.

Chew on carrots or celery.

Swish and spit using club soda or carbonated water.

Use a humidifier at home to moisten air.

Practice good oral hygiene.

Suck on hard candy, frozen grapes, or melon balls.

Avoid alcohol and alcohol containing mouthwashes.

Pharmacologic/Non-food Interventions

Acupuncture

Biotene (6) gel, liquid, spray

BioXtra (27) gel, spray, tablets

Caphosol (28)

Glandosane (29)

Salivart (30)

Xero-Lube (31)

MouthKote (32)

Prevention Therapies:

Ethyol (33) (amifostine)

Salagen (34) (pilocarpine)

Medication References:

1. Merck Whitehouse Station, NJ 08889
2. Pfizer New York, NY 10017
3. Bristol-Myers Squibb New York, NY 10154
4. ANI Pharmaceuticals Baudette, MN 56623
5. Organon Pharmaceuticals, Roseland, NJ 07068
6. GLAXO SMITHKLINE Brentford, UK
7. Konsyl Easton, MD 21601
8. Purdue Pharma LP Stamford, CT 06901
9. Bayer Health Care Pharmaceuticals Wayne, NJ 07470
10. Church & Dwight Co Princeton, NJ 08540
11. McNeil-PPC Skillman, NJ 08558
12. Novartis East Hanover, NJ 07936
13. Proctor and Gamble Cincinnati, OH 45202
14. Chattem Labs Chattanooga, TN 37409
15. Astra Zeneca Wilmington, DE 19850
16. Hormel Austin, MN 55912
17. Nestle Vevey, Switzerland
18. Precision Foods St. Louis, MO 63141
19. LGM Pharma Nashville, TN 37203
20. Sanofi-Aventis Bridgewater, NJ 08807
21. Genentech South San Francisco, CA 94080
22. Helsinn Healthcare Lugano, Switzerland
23. Solvay Pharmaceuticals Marietta, GA 30062
24. Valeant Pharmaceuticals Costa Mesa, CA 92626
25. Biovail Pharmaceuticals, Inc. Bridgewater, NJ 08807
26. Hoffman-LaRoche Basel, Switzerland
27. Lighthouse Health Products Cambridge, Ontario
28. EUSA Pharma Oxford, England
29. Fresenius KABI UK Cheshire, UK
30. Gebauer Company Cleveland, OH 44128
31. Colgate Palmolive Morristown, NJ 07960
32. Parnell Pharmaceuticals San Rafael, CA 94901
33. MedImmune Pharma The Netherlands
34. MGI Pharma Bloomington, MN 55437

Symptom References

Introduction

1. Tong H, Isenring E, Yates P. The prevalence of nutrition impact symptoms and their relationship to quality of life and clinical outcomes in medical oncology patients. *Supportive Care in Cancer*. 2009;17(1):83-90.

Anorexia/Poor Appetite/Early Satiety

1. Cancer and Chemo-Based Lack of Appetite and Early Satiety. Chemocare.com. Accessed 9/27/10 at http://www.chemocare.com/managing/cancer_and_chemobased_lack_of.asp
2. Riechelmann RP, Burman D, Tannock IF, Rodin G, Zimmermann C. Phase II trial of mirtazapine for cancer-related cachexia and anorexia. *Am J Hosp Palliat Care.* 2009;27(2):106-110.
3. Theobald DE, Kirsh KL, Holtsclaw E, Donaghy K, Passik SD. An open-label, crossover trial of mirtazapine (15 and 30 mg) in cancer patients with pain and other distressing symptoms. *J Pain Symptom Manage.* 2002;23(5):442–447. Retrieved from http://www.jpsmjournal.com/article/S0885-3924(02)00381-0/fulltext

Constipation/Diarrhea

1. Elliott L, Levin R, McIver J. Complete Resource Kit for Oncology Nutrition. AND Publications; 2012.
2. Gill C, Eldridge B, Rust D. Nutritional support. In: Gates RA, Fink RM, eds. *Oncology Nursing Secrets.* 2nd ed. Philadelphia, Pa: Hanley & Belfus; 2001:365-384.
3. Grant B. Medical Nutrition Therapy for Cancer. In *Krause's Food and Nutrition Therapy*. 12th ed. Saunders; 2007:959-990.
4. Luthringer S. Nutritional Implications of Radiation Therapy. In: Elliott L, Molseed LL, McCallum PD, Grant B, eds. *The Clinical Guide to Oncology Nutrition*, 2nd ed; 2006:88-93.
5. Beyer P. Medical Nutrition Therapy. Lower Gastrointestinal Tract Disorders. In *Krause's Food and Nutrition Therapy*. 12th ed. Saunders; 2007:673-706.
6. U.S. Department of Agriculture, Agricultural Research Service. 2009. USDA National Nutrient Database for Standard Reference, Release 22. Nutrient Data Laboratory Home Page, Accessed 9/18/2010 at: http://www.ars.usda.gov/ba/bhnrc/ndl

Dysphagia

1. Elliott L, Levin R, McIver J. Complete Resource Kit for Oncology Nutrition. AND Publications; 2012.
2. American Dietetic Association. *National Dysphagia Diet: Standardization for Optimal Care*. Chicago, Ill: American Dietetic Association; 2003.

Fatigue

1. Elliott L, Levin R, McIver J. Complete Resource Kit for Oncology Nutrition. AND Publications; 2012.

Malabsorption

1. MedlinePlus. Bethesda (MD): National Library of Medicine (US). Malabsorption http://www.nlm.nih.gov/medlineplus/ency/article/000299.htm. Updated 8/10/12. Accessed 8/17/12.
2. Francis C. Prebiotic Fibers: Their role in digestive and intestinal health, immune function and mineral absorption. *Oncology Nutrition Connection*. 2008;16(2):7-11.
3. Ross T. Prebiotic Basics: Helping your health from the inside out. *Diabetes Care and Education Newsletter*. 2009.
4. International Food Information Council Foundation. Functional Foods Fact Sheet: Probiotics and Prebiotics. 2009. Food Insight. Published October 15, 2009. Accessed 9/18/2010 at: http://www.foodinsight.org/Resources/Detail.aspx?topic=Functional_Foods_Fact_Sheet_Probiotics_and_Prebiotics
5. American Dietetic Association Evidence Analysis Library, Oncology Nutrition Recommendations, http://www.adaevidencelibrary.com/topic.cfm?cat=3250 Accessed August 21, 2010.
6. Meddles J, Petzel M. Pancreatic Enzymes. ON-Line Oncology Nutrition Dietetic Practice Group Newsletter. Spring 2005, insert.
7. Updated Questions & Answers for Healthcare Professionals and the Public: Use an approved pancreatic enzyme product (PEP). Revised 5/17/12. Accessed 4/12/2013 at: http://www.fda.gov/Drugs/DrugSafety/PostmarketDrugSafetyInformationforPatientsandProviders/ucm204745.htm
8. Damerla V, Gotlieb V, Larson H, Saif MW. Pancreatic Enzyme Supplementation in Pancreatic Cancer. www.Supportiveoncology.net. 2008;6(8):393-396.

Mucositis/Esophagitis

1. Beyer P. Medical Nutrition Therapy for Upper Gastrointestinal Tract Disorders. In *Krause's Food and Nutrition Therapy*. 12th ed. Saunders; 2007:654-672.
2. McCallum PD. Tips for Managing Nutrition Impact Symptoms. In: Elliott, L, Molseed, LL, and McCallum PD, and Grant, B eds. *The Clinical Guide to Oncology Nutrition*, 2nd ed; 2006:241-245.
3. Radler D, Touger-Decker R. Nutrition for Oral and Dental Health. In *Krause's Food and Nutrition Therapy*. 12th ed. St. Louis, MO; Saunders; 2007:647-648.

Nausea/Vomiting

1. Elliott L, Levin R, McIver J. Complete Resource Kit for Oncology Nutrition. AND Publications; 2012.
2. American Cancer Society. Nutrition for the person with cancer during treatment; Nausea. www.cancer.org. Revised 3/15/13. Accessed 4/12/13.

Oral Candidiasis

1. Radler D, Touger-Decker R. Nutrition for Oral and Dental Health. In: Mahan LK, Escott-Stump S, eds. *Krause's Food and Nutrition Therapy*. 12th ed. St.Louis, MO: Saunders; 2007: 636-651.
2. Worthington HV, Clarkson JE, Khalid T, Meyer S, McCabe M. Interventions for treating oral candidiasis for patients with cancer receiving treatment. Cochrane Oral Health Group, School of Dentistry, The University of Manchester, Coupland III Building, Oxford Road, Manchester, UK, M13 9PL. Cochrane Database Syst Rev. 2007;(2):CD001972.

Taste and Smell Changes

1. Halyard MY, et al. Does zinc sulfate prevent therapy-induced taste alterations in head and neck cancer patients? Results of phase III double-blind, placebo-controlled trial from the North Central Cancer Treatment Group (N01C4). *Int J Radiat Oncol Biol Phys*. 2007; 67(5): 1318-22.

Xerostomia/Thick Saliva

1. Radler D, Touger-Decker R. Nutrition for Oral and Dental Health. In *Krause's Food and Nutrition Therapy*. 12th ed. Saunders; 2007: 636-651.

Medications

1. Medication Guide. Accessed at: www.oncologynutriton.org on 6/10/2010.

Nutrition Support in the Oncology Setting

Alison Ryan, MS, RD, CSO, CNSC

Introduction

Nutritional status plays a critical role in the ability to survive cancer and thrive throughout all stages of disease and treatments (1-2). An inability to ingest sufficient oral nutrition for more than short periods can lead to malnutrition, diminish response to cancer treatment and increase the risk of post-operative complications. To prevent malnutrition, specialized nutrition support is employed when the oral feeding route is unavailable or not tolerated. The concern over whether or not nutrition support stimulates tumor growth remains inconclusive (3); these modalities should be limited to patients with clear clinical indications for nutrition support (4-6). Major indicators for nutrition support in the oncology population include mechanical and functional dysfunctions such as dysphagia; gastrointestinal (GI) obstruction; surgery to the head and neck region; the inability to digest and/or absorb complex nutrients and an inability to chew or swallow food and liquids.

Nutrition support can be provided via enteral and parenteral routes (7). This chapter reviews the role of enteral and parenteral nutrition support in the adult oncology population and practice guidelines that promote successful enteral and parenteral nutrition support.

Enteral Nutrition

Enteral nutrition (EN) provides nutrition directly into the GI system, bypassing the oral route. Feeding can be infused via nasogastric and nasoenteric tubes; tubes also can be inserted directly into the stomach and small intestine. Disease-specific, elemental, and standard enteral formulas are available.

Indications for Enteral Nutrition

According to the clinical guidelines of the American Society for Parenteral and Enteral Nutrition (A.S.P.E.N.), patients undergoing major cancer operations do not benefit from routine use of enteral nutrition support. Perioperative nutrition support may be beneficial in moderately or severely malnourished patients if administered for 7-14 days preoperatively, but the potential benefits must be weighed against potential risks and those of delaying the operation. Nutrition support is not an appropriate adjunct to chemotherapy. It is most appropriate in patients receiving active anticancer treatment who are malnourished and who are anticipated to be unable to ingest and/or absorb adequate nutrients for greater than 7-14 days (4). EN is most commonly utilized for the following cancer diagnoses: head and neck, gastric, esophageal and pancreatic cancers.

Benefits of Enteral Nutrition in the Oncology Population

To better maintain GI function EN utilizes the normal physiologic route of nutrition, which also reduces the risk of bacterial translocation when compared with parenteral nutrition (PN) (8). EN formulas may provide soluble and insoluble fibers that can increase stool weight, decrease GI transit time, and reduce the incidence of diarrhea. EN formulas also may contain prebiotic fibers purported to promote the growth of beneficial bacteria in the colon (9).

Compared with PN, EN has a lower prevalence of infectious complications and infectious morbidity, in particular reduced pneumonia and central line infections (10). Other studies have found that EN can reduce hospital length of stay (11) and lower incidence of hyperglycemia (12).

EN is less expensive than PN (12). In a review of critically ill patients, use of EN (versus PN) saved nearly $1,500.00 per patient from reduced incidence of adverse events and $2,500.00 per patient stay because of reduced hospital length of stay. Analysis indicated that shifting 10% of PN fed adult patients in the U.S. to EN would save $35 million annually due to reduced adverse events and another $57 million due to shorter hospital stays (13).

Enteral Nutrition Access

EN can be provided in a variety of ways; access devices are summarized in Table 1.

Most people tolerate being fed into the stomach and do not require duodenal or jejunal feeding access (16). Indications for post-pyloric feedings include gastroparesis, gastric outlet or duodenal obstruction and fistula proximal to the feeding tube location (15).

Tube sizes are described according to French units (F), referring to the outer diameter of the feeding tube. Smaller diameter tubes (5-8 F) are used for standard enteral formulations. Larger (>8F) tubes may be needed for high fiber, viscous, and energy dense formulas. Additionally, larger tubes are preferred for bolus and gravity feeds. Feeding tubes are generally made from polyurethane, latex, or silicone.

Table 1: Enteral Nutrition Feeding Routes and Consideration (14-15)

Enteral Device	Placement	Aspiration Risk	Special Considerations and Notations
Short Term Access (10-15 days)			
Nasogastric/ Orogastric	• Bedside • Intraoperatively	Increased	• Requires radiographic confirmation of catheter tip placement
Nasoduodenal/ Oroduodenal	• Bedside • Intraoperatively • Image-guided • Endoscopic	Increased	• Requires radiographic confirmation of catheter tip placement • Risk of catheter tip migration • Requires infusion pump
Nasojejunal/ Orojejunal	• Bedside • Intraoperatively • Image-guided • Endoscopic	Decreased	• Requires radiographic confirmation of catheter tip placement • Risk of catheter tip migration • Requires infusion pump
Long Term Access (Months to Years)			
PEG Gastrostomy (G-tube)	• Endoscopic • Image-guided	Equivocal	
PEG-J	• Endoscopic • Image-guided	Decreased	• Risk of catheter tip migration and conversion to PEJ • Requires infusion pump
PEJ	• Endoscopic • Image-guided	Decreased	• Requires infusion pump
Jejunostomy (J-tube)	• Surgical	Decreased	• Requires infusion pump

Contraindications for enteral feeding include:

- Bowel obstruction low in GI tract
- Hemodynamically unstable (e.g., low blood pressure, on high dose pressors, mean arterial pressure < 60-70)
- Intractable diarrhea (e.g., rule out C-diff, medication effects, graft-versus host disease of the GI tract)
- Severe active GI bleed
- Ischemic or perforated gut
- High output fistula/ostomy (>500 mL/d)
- Aggressive nutrition intervention not warranted
- Extensive resection of small bowel/significant portion of small bowel not functioning
- Need 100 cm jejunum and 150 cm ileum w/ ileocecal valve for adequate GI absorption of nutrients

Enteral Nutrition Formulations

EN formulations vary in nutrient content, caloric and protein density, macronutrient sources, and water and fiber content. Some contain specialized nutrients (e.g., glutamine, arginine, fish oils, medium chain triglycerides), but data on their routine use are limited (3). Standard formulations, initiated at full strength, are appropriate for the majority of people with cancer. Nearly all formulas are suitable for lactose intolerance and most are gluten-free, but many contain potential food allergens. Labels should be checked thoroughly and often, as manufacturers re-formulate their products regularly. Detailed nutrient analysis, ingredient lists, and clinical indications are available via the Nutrition Care Manual of the Academy of Nutrition and Dietetics (the Academy).

Some patients may require the addition of modular nutrients to enteral feedings. These are most often fiber and protein products, but lipid-and carbohydrate-based products also are used. Modular nutrients are mixed with water and flushed through the feeding tube, which can increase the risk of clogging feeding tubes and contamination. Special attention should be paid to proper sanitation and tube care when utilizing modular nutrients. Table 2 summarizes characteristics of EN formulations.

Tube feedings can be homemade. Recipes have been published in books, journals, and on a variety of websites; a sample recipe is provided at the end of this chapter. Consideration must be given to the nutritional content of the homemade recipe and preparation in terms of tube clogging and food safety. Patients and families should review home tube feeding regimens with an RD.

Most EN formulations provide 70%-85% free water. Additional hydration is needed for normal physiologic function and for patency of feeding tube via water flushes before and after giving medications and every four hours. Fluid needs may increase further when losses are high (e.g. large volume diarrhea) and when certain chemotherapies are given (e.g., Cisplatin). The nutrition assessment should identify total fluid needs of each patient receiving EN.

Initiation and Advancement of Enteral Feedings

The most appropriate feeding method depends on several factors including location of the feeding tube, aspiration risk, GI status and ability of patient or caregiver to handle enteral feeding equipment. There are four primary methods of administration: bolus, intermittent

Table 2: Enteral Nutrition Formulations and Modular Nutrients (17-18)

Enteral Formulation	Characteristics
Standard/Polymeric	Provides general nutritional needs; nutrient density varies from 1-2kcal/mL; protein content varies from 16%-25% of calories; may contain fiber, prebiotics and immune enhancing nutrients such as arginine
Semi-Elemental	For malabsorption, maldigestion, and/or feeding intolerance; nutrient density varies from 1-1.5kcal/mL; some have higher content/ratio of MCT oil; peptide-based protein sources range from 16%-25% of calories; may contain fiber and prebiotics
Elemental/Monomeric	For severely compromised GI; provides 100% free amino acids; are low in fat with higher content/ratio of MCT oil
Disease-Specific	
Diabetic	Reduced carbohydrate content; may provide fiber; may be higher in fat and protein
Renal	Reduced free water, sodium, potassium, phosphorus and calcium Protein content varies from 7%-18% of calories
Trauma/Immune Modulating	May be higher in protein (peptide-based) and calorically dense. May contain arginine, glutamine, EPA, DHA, elevated amounts of vitamin C, vitamin E and beta-carotene
Pulmonary	Nutrient density ~1.5kcal/ml with reduced carbohydrate content Increased lipid content; protein content 16%-18% of calories May provide EPA, GLA and added antioxidants

Abbreviations: MCT=Medium Chain Triglyceride; CKD=Chronic Kidney Disease; ESKD=End Stage Kidney Disease; EPA=Eicosapentaenoic Acid; DHA=Docosahexaenoic Acid; GLA=Gamma Linolenic Acid

Table 3: Administration of Enteral Feeding (14,19)

	Location of Feeding	Delivery Timing	Initiation Rate	Advancement Schedule	Equipment Required
Syringe Bolus	Gastric	~15 minutes	60-120mL first 1-2 feedings	Increase by 60-120mL every 8-12 hours (or every 1-2 feedings)	Catheter Tip Syringe
Intermittent or Gravity Drip	Gastric	~30-35 minutes	60-120mL first 1-2 feedings	Increase by 60-120mL every 8-12 hours (or every 1-2 feedings)	Gravity Bags, Pole
Cyclic	Gastric or Small Intestine	Often a 12-14 hour infusion per day (<24 hours)	10-50mL/hr	Increase by 10-25mL/hr every 8 hours	Infusion Pump with Pole or Backpack
Continuous	Gastric or Small Intestine	20-24 hour infusion	10-50mL/hr	Increase by 10-25mL/hr every 4-24 hours	Infusion Pump with Pole or Backpack

or gravity method, cyclic and continuous. Clinicians also may employ a combination of the methods. Table 3 provides suggestions for the administration of enteral feedings.

Complications

While infectious risks are lower with EN as compared with PN, tube feeding is not without risk. Metabolic aberrations, gastrointestinal intolerance, enteral misconnections, mechanical/tube complications, microbial contamination and drug-nutrient interactions can complicate EN (14).

Metabolic Complications
Refeeding syndrome occurs when malnourished patients are fed full energy needs and/or a high carbohydrate diet. It is potentially life threatening and is characterized by severe electrolyte abnormalities (e.g., hypophosphatemia, hypokalemia, hypomagnesemia) and glucose and fluid shifts which can result in fluid retention, cardiac dysfunction and respiratory failure (20). Conditions increasing risk

of refeeding include chronic malnutrition, prolonged hypocaloric feeding or fasting, NPO greater than 7 days, chronic alcoholism and anorexia nervosa.

Appropriate monitoring and IV replacement of electrolytes with a plan for slow and gradual administration of EN is critical to avoid refeeding syndrome. Once phosphorus, potassium, and magnesium levels have been restored to the normal range, EN should start with 25% of estimated energy needs and advance over 3-5 days to feeding goals (21). The clinician should continue to monitor laboratory values, vital signs and fluid balance until avoidance of refeeding syndrome has been confirmed. Other metabolic complications of EN are summarized in Table 4.

Gastrointestinal Complications

Monitoring of gastric residual volumes (GRV) is one method (though controversial) to prevent aspiration and to assess tolerance to EN. However, the evidence for a clear link between aspiration and GRV is

Table 4: Metabolic Complications and Potential Corrections During EN Therapy (20,22-23)

Condition	Possible Causes	Prevention/Possible Correction
Dehydration	• Inadequate free water administration • Fluid losses (emesis, diarrhea, drains, dialysis) • Concentrated formula	• Increase free water enterally or parenterally • Monitor fluid status/losses; monitor daily weights • Change to 1cal/mL formula
Overhydration	• Excess fluid intake • Refeeding syndrome	• Decrease free water flushes; change to lower free water formula • Monitor fluid status/intake; monitor daily weights
Hyperglycemia	• Insulin resistance or diabetes mellitus • Metabolic stress or sepsis • Steroids	• Change to carbohydrate controlled or fiber-containing formula • Recommend use of or adjust dose of insulin or oral hypoglycemic agents
Hypernatremia	• Inadequate free water • Excess fluid losses (diuresis)	• Increase free water to meet fluid needs • Monitor fluid status, I/O, and daily weights
Hyponatremia	• Water retention/fluid overload • Sodium losses (GI) • Syndrome of inappropriate antidiuretic hormone (SIADH)	• Change to lower free water formula, restrict fluids/free water • Supplement with sodium • Restrict fluids/free water, diuresis
Hypokalemia	• Refeeding syndrome • Excess GI losses • Diuretics/dialysis, insulin therapy • Inadequate intake	• Decrease nutrition delivery to 25% of goal, replace potassium • Replace potassium via IV if severe, via enteral route if hypokalemia is mild • Evaluate need to change EN formula
Hyperphosphatemia	• Kidney insufficiency/failure • Tumor lysis syndrome • Phosphate-containing antacids	• Consider change to lower phosphorus EN formula; recommend phosphate binders • Recommend potential change in medications
Hypophosphatemia	• Refeeding syndrome • Insulin therapy • Phosphate-binding antacids	• Decrease nutrition delivery to 25% of goal, replace phosphorus • Replace phosphorus via IV if severe, via enteral route if mild • Recommend discontinuation or medication adjustments

*EGFR=epidermal growth factor receptor

lacking and checking GRV may be more useful as a screening tool that leads to further medical evaluation instead of simply holding EN. Box 1 provides practice recommendations for monitoring GRV (14). A.S.P.E.N. and the Society for Critical Care Medicine guidelines provide the recommendation to avoid holding EN for gastric residual volumes of less than 500mL in the absence of other signs of intolerance (10).

Other GI complications and possible corrective actions are summarized in Table 5.

Box 1: Suggested Monitoring of Gastric Residual Volumes

1. In the first 48 hours after initiating gastric feeds, check GRV every 4 hours; monitoring may then be decreased to every 6-8 hours in non-critically ill patients

2. If GRV ≤ 250 mL, no change/action is indicated

3. If gastric residuals are ≥250 mL after a second check, consider the use of a promotility agent (e.g., Metaclopramide or Erythromycin)

4. If GRV ≥500 mL, hold EN and perform a physical assessment, GI assessment (assess for abdominal distention, constipation, etc.), evaluate glycemic control, again consider the use of a promotility agent, and consider narcotic alternatives, if able

Mechanical and Microbial Complications

Clogged feeding tubes are fairly common, especially with smaller diameter feeding tubes (<8F) (15). Routine checking of GVRs and monitoring potential interactions between formula and medication may help prevent clogs. Should a feeding tube become clogged, instill 5mL of warm water as near to the clog as possible for 1 minute, then use gentle push-pull motion with a 30-60mL syringe plunger to help dislodge the clog. If unsuccessful, the next step may include use of a commercial declogging device (25).

Medication Interactions

An enteral feeding tube provides a means of medication delivery when the oral route is not available. However, certain medications may interact with the formula or contribute to feeding tube clogs. Liquid suspension formulations should be used when possible. Otherwise, tablets must be crushed thoroughly before mixing with adequate amounts of water to disperse the medication and avoid risk of clogging. Avoid crushing time-release and enterically coated medications as this may significantly increase the rate of absorption or destroy the active ingredients (23). Consultation with a pharmacist or the manufacturer's product guide can help the clinician determine which medications are acceptable to crush. In addition, consult institutional policy regarding holding of EN for medication administration.

Table 5: Gastrointestinal Complications (10,23-24)

Condition	Possible Causes	Prevention/Possible Correction
• High gastric residual volume	• Delayed gastric emptying • Large volume feedings	• Consider addition of prokinetic agents • Consider change to post-pyloric tube • Consider change to concentrated feeding at lower infusion rate
• Aspiration, reflux (GERD)	• Flat head of bed • Incomplete closure of the lower esophageal sphincter • Large volume feeding boluses • Delayed gastric motility	• Elevated head of bed 30°-45° • Use small bore feeding tube • Provide continuous infusion • Consider addition of prokinetic agents
• Nausea, vomiting, abdominal distention, bloating	• Delayed gastric emptying • Rapid infusion of feedings	• Continuous feeding method with low fat and/or isotonic formula • Consider addition of prokinetic agents • Consider change to post-pyloric tube • Minimize use of narcotics, if able • Provide anti-emetics • Initiate feedings at low rate and advance slowly
• Diarrhea	• Medications • Antibiotic-associated diarrhea • Infectious etiology • Bacterial contamination • Fiber-free formula/ high fiber formula • Malabsorption • Steatorrhea	• Evaluate usage of hyperosmolar medications (i.e. sorbitol, magnesium-containing), laxatives, lactulose, etc. • Evaluate usage of antibiotics • Provide anti-diarrheals, if appropriate • Check stool for Clostridium difficile or other infectious pathogens • Observe appropriate hang times, change tubing every 24 hours, utilize closed system in preference to open and powdered, reconstituted formulas • Consider change in fiber content of EN formula • Consider change to elemental or semi-elemental formula • Adjust formula selection to lower fat or higher medium chain triglyceride content; consider adding pancreatic enzymes
• Constipation	• Inadequate fluid intake • Inadequate or excessive fiber provision • Physical inactivity • Medications • GI obstruction, colonic dysmotility, ileus	• Increase free water/fluid intake • Consider change in fiber content of EN formula • Increase activity, if able • Minimize use of narcotics, if able • Recommend addition of stool softeners and/or laxatives • Trial of prune juice • Evaluate and address underlying cause; may need to hold EN

Parenteral Nutrition

Parenteral nutrition (PN) describes the IV infusion of nutrients. It can be a life-saving modality for people with cancer but should not be a routine adjunct to chemotherapy or considered standard to cancer care (4).

Indications for Parenteral Nutrition

There is limited evidence showing that PN can improve outcomes, though it can improve markers of nutritional status. PN is most often indicated in the setting of cancer for preoperative nutrition support in severely malnourished patients and for the following conditions:

- Non-functional or inaccessible GI tract (e.g., bowel rest for ileus and bowel obstruction)
- Severe nausea with vomiting (e.g., radiation enteritis and refractory short bowel syndrome)
- Severe diarrhea or malabsorption
- GI fistula (unless able to feed distal to fistula or if low output fistula)
- Severe acute necrotizing pancreatitis with inability to tolerate EN (26)
- Graft-versus-host disease intolerant to EN support

PN support is significantly more costly than EN support and the risks of providing PN support must be weighed against the benefits. PN is best managed by interdisciplinary nutrition support teams to improve efficacy and safety, reduce complications and maximize cost-effectiveness (27).

Parenteral Nutrition Access

When PN support is indicated, the clinician must establish or recommend intravenous (IV) access. Central IV access via a central venous catheter (CVC) is required for total or central PN. Total or central PN is more commonly used in the oncology setting because most patients have CVCs.

Central IV access positions the distal catheter tip in central vessels (distal vena cava or right atrium). CVCs are either tunneled or non-tunneled. A peripherally inserted central catheter or PICC is an example of a non-tunneled catheter. Broviac®, Hickman®, and Groshong® are a few examples of tunneled catheters. Certain chemotherapeutic regimens may warrant the use of implanted ports. These ports may be utilized as central access for total or central PN infusion, but daily use/access is not generally recommended (28). CVCs must be cared for daily and maintained to avoid central line infections. Two common points of risk for contamination and infection include the insertion site of the catheter and the hub, as this is the direct connection to venous access. In 2011, the Centers for Disease Control and Prevention published guidelines for the prevention of central line associated blood stream infections (29).

To provide peripheral parenteral nutrition (PPN), peripheral IV access is required. PPN is infrequently indicated, as it is appropriate for only short-term duration. It requires a final concentration less than 900 mOsm/L; has a low dextrose concentration (i.e., 5%-10%); requires a large volume to provide significant calories and protein; and increases the risk of thrombophlebitis (28).

Parenteral Nutrition Components

PN provides an admixture of carbohydrate (as dextrose monohydrate), proteins (as amino acids) and fat (as lipid emulsions), with the addition of electrolytes, vitamins and trace elements (see tables 6-9). The exact formulation and distribution of nutrients is based on nutritional requirements and patient tolerance. PN also must provide adequate hydration. If the volume of PN is limited, additional IV fluids must be provided to prevent dehydration.

Dextrose is the primary energy substrate in total or central PN, is available in concentrations from 2.5%-70% and provides 3.4 kcal/g. Dextrose provision should be adequate to support brain function, prevent gluconeogenesis and meet calorie requirements for weight maintenance. Excess dextrose infusion should be avoided to prevent or minimize risks of hyperglycemia and hepatic steatosis.

IV fat emulsions (IVFE) provide additional calories and are a source of essential fatty acids. IVFE are emulsions of safflower and/or soybean oil, egg phospholipid, glycerin, vitamin K and sodium hydroxide. There is potential for allergic reactions; cautious administration and close monitoring is needed in patients at risk for allergic reaction, especially with a soy or egg allergy. A 12-hour hang time limit is recommended for IVFE infused as a separate preparation from dextrose and amino acids (30).

Crystalline amino acid solutions contain both essential and non-essential amino acids and provide 4 kcal/g. Amino acid administration should be adequate to achieve net positive or even nitrogen balance. Parenteral glutamine supplementation may be beneficial in critical illness and in hematopoietic cell transplantation, but product availability is limited in the U.S. and its use is controversial (4,10).

Electrolytes are a critical component of PN solutions and help maintain electrolyte homeostasis and acid-base balance. Table 7

Table 6: Macronutrients in Parenteral Nutrition Solutions (27,31)

	Dextrose	Amino Acids	Lipids/IVFE
Concentration Availability	2.5-70%	3-20%	10%, 20%, 30%
Energy Provision (in kcal/gram)	3.4	4	10 (in 20% & 30%) 11 (in 10%)
Minimal Daily Requirement	100-150 grams	0.8 grams/kg (or individualized based on patient tolerance)	250 mL of 20% IVFE or 500 mL of 10% IVFE twice per week – or 500 mL of 20% IVFE once per week (or 1-2% of total calories as alpha-linoleic acid and 0.5% of total caloric intake as alpha-linolenic acid to prevent EFAD)
Optimal Dosing Range	To meet total daily calorie goals*	0.8-1 gram/kg (if medically stable) 1.2-2 grams/kg (catabolism)	20-30% of calories from fat
Maximum Daily Tolerance	7 grams/kg/day or 5 mg/kg/minute	2.5 grams/kg Individualized, based on patient tolerance	2.5 gram/kg/day or 60% of total calories (if medically stable)
Total Daily Calorie Goals	20-30 kcal/kg (if medically stable) ~15 kcal/kg or 2 mg/kg/minute for refeeding syndrome * Calorie goals are highly variable, and should be based on the patient's individual nutrition goals and tolerance to nutrition therapy. Indirect calorimetry should be performed, when available, and used to determine goal calories.		
Total Daily Fluid Needs	30-40 mL/kg (if medically stable)	Fluid restrictions or limitations may be needed for management of medical conditions such as heart, liver or kidney failure. Consider all sources of fluids, including intravenous fluids and medications.	

Table 7: Standard Parenteral Electrolyte Requirements (27)

Electrolyte	Standard Requirement
Sodium	1-2 mEq/kg
Potassium	1-2 mEq/kg
Acetate	As needed to maintain acid-base balance
Chloride	As needed to maintain acid-base balance
Calcium	10-15 mEq/day
Magnesium	8-20 mEq/day
Phosphorus	20-40 mmol/day

Table 8: Standard Adult Parenteral Vitamin Additives (27)

Vitamin	Daily Requirement	Daily Dose from Available Products
Thiamin (B1)	6 mg	6 mg
Riboflavin (B2)	3.6 mg	3.6 mg
Niacin (B3)	40 mg	40 mg
Folic Acid	600 mcg	600 mcg
Pantothenic Acid	15 mg	15 mg
Pyridoxine (B6)	6 mg	6 mg
Cyanocobalamin (B12)	5 mcg	5 mcg
Biotin	60 mcg	60 mcg
Ascorbic Acid (C)	200 mg	200 mg
Vitamin A	3300 IU	3300 IU
Vitamin D	200 IU	200 IU
Vitamin E	10 IU	10 IU
Vitamin K	150 mcg	0-150 mcg

Table 9: Standard Adult Parenteral Trace Element Additives (33)

Trace Element	Daily Requirement	Daily Dose from Available Products
Chromium	10-15 mcg	4-10 mcg
Copper	0.3-0.5 mg	0.4-1 mg
Iron	Not routinely added	0
Manganese	60-100 mcg	100-800 mcg
Selenium	20-60 mcg	0-60 mcg
Zinc	2.5-5 mg	1-5 mg

provides standard ranges for electrolytes in PN, assuming normal organ function and no excessive losses. Medication related electrolyte abnormalities are common in the oncologic setting; ongoing electrolyte monitoring and PN additive adjustments are imperative.

Vitamins and minerals are added to prevent micronutrient deficiencies and maintain normal physiologic functions. Generally, parenteral vitamin and trace element preparations are adequate to meet needs assuming normal organ and physiologic function with the exception of vitamin D (32). Certain multi-trace element (MTE) products do not contain selenium, presenting a significant risk for selenium deficiency in long-term usage. See Tables 8 and 9 for adult parenteral vitamin and trace element daily requirements. Iron is incompatible with IVFE and should be administered separately from PN or with fat-free PN only.

Select medications that may be compatible with PN include regular insulin and H2 antagonists. Adding these medications to PN saves money and can offer continuous provision of the medication (if 24 hour infusion is provided). A disadvantage may be the inability to discontinue or change the dose without stopping the entire PN infusion.

PN admixtures come in two formats, 2-in-1 and 3-in-1 (or total nutrient admixture/TNA). Two-in-1 formulations provide dextrose and amino acids with electrolytes, vitamins, and minerals; IVFE is administered separately. Three-in-1 includes the IVFE in the admixture (31). A.S.P.E.N. safe practices for ordering PN call for writing orders for total daily dose as opposed to percentages and nutrients per liter (27).

Initiation
Metabolic abnormalities, such as hypokalemia, hypophosphatemia and hyperglycemia should be corrected prior to PN initiation. To avoid significant hyperglycemia and potential refeeding syndrome, it is prudent to initiate total or central PN with 25-50% of goal dextrose, then titrate up as tolerated (34). Patients new to PN are typically started on a continuous or 24 hour infusion. Once tolerance has been established and metabolic derangements corrected, cyclical PN can be considered. Typical cycling times range from 12-16 hours and usually include a one or two hour rate taper to avoid hypoglycemia, though this risk is small (35).

Monitoring
Monitoring lab data, physical exam, weights, and intake and output during PN infusion is critical in assessing a person's tolerance to PN. The PN-savvy RD can proactively monitor and adjust the nutritional plan of care to prevent complications associated with PN infusion. Table 10 provides monitoring guidelines and potential interventions for PN.

Table 10: Suggested Lab and Tolerance Monitoring while on Parenteral Nutrition (36-37)

Parameter	Baseline	Initiation	Stable Patient	Potential Interventions
Na, K, Cl, CO2, BUN, Cr	3	Daily for the first 3 days of PN	1-2 times per week	Adjust additives; adjust fluid and/or protein
Mg, Ca, Phosphorus	3	Daily for the first 3 days of PN	Weekly	Adjust additives
Capillary Glucose	3	Every 6 hours for the first 48 hours, then as needed	As needed	Start dextrose at 25-50% of goal dextrose for refeeding risk or hyperglycemia; provide insulin and/or adjust dextrose
CBC with differential	3		Weekly to monthly	Investigate cause of anemia; adjust hydration
PT, PTT	3		Weekly to monthly	Adjust vitamin K provision
Serum Triglycerides	3	Day one of PN	Weekly to monthly	If TG >400mg/dL, reduce or hold IVFE
ALT, AST, ALP, T bili	3	Day one of PN	Weekly to monthly	First investigate if non-PN related reason for derangement. Cycle PN; decrease dextrose; limit fat to <1gm/kg/day
Weight	3	Daily	2-3 times per week	Adjust fluid and/or calories
Intake and Output	3	Daily	As needed	Adjust fluid/volume
Physical Exam—fluid accumulation, edema, ascites; subcutaneous fat losses; muscle mass losses	3	Daily (for fluid assessment)	Weekly to monthly for fat and muscle losses; as needed for fluid assessment	Adjust fluid/volume; increase calories and/or increase amino acids

Complications

The most common acute complications from PN infusion are derangements in serum levels of blood sugar, potassium, phosphorus and magnesium as well as hypertriglyceridemia and volume/fluid management issues. Additives of potassium, phosphorus and magnesium should be adjusted daily until stable. Subcutaneous insulin may be required to control blood glucose levels (until appropriate amounts of regular human insulin can be added to the PN bag to properly control blood sugar levels).

Box 2: Long-Term Complications from Parenteral Nutrition (34,39-40)

Metabolic
- Endocrinologic: impaired glucose tolerance, hypoglycemia from excess insulin
- Hepatobiliary complications: steatosis, cholestasis, biliary sludge, gallstones
- Renal: azotemia, decrease in glomerular filtration rate, tubular dysfunction
- Metabolic bone disease: osteoporosis, osteomalacia
- Potential Toxicities: manganese, chromium, aluminum, hypertriglyceridemia
- Potential Deficiencies: essential fatty acids, iron, selenium, zinc (with excess GI losses), magnesium, calcium, vitamin D, carnitine, choline

Mechanical
- Catheter occlusion
- Venous thrombosis
- Catheter breakage

Infectious
- Catheter sepsis
- Tunnel infection
- Exit site infections
- Catheter-related bloodstream infection (CRBSI)

Long-term complications from PN infusion include metabolic derangements, nutrient deficiencies or toxicities, organ dysfunction and bone disease (38). See Box 2 for complications of long-term PN. Prevention of and interventions for these long-term complications are described elsewhere in the literature (27).

Transitioning to Oral Nutrition

Oral nutrition should be attempted once safe swallowing is established and the patient can tolerate and metabolize food appropriate for their disease or condition. Oral and/or enteral nutrition should be attempted and re-tried often for patients on long-term PN to prevent gastrointestinal mucosal atrophy and biliary sludge. As oral nutrition increases, EN or PN support may be incrementally decreased. Once a person is meeting ≥75% of their nutritional needs orally, EN/PN may be discontinued.

Nutrition Support in the Home Setting

EN and PN may be provided in the home setting if a patient cannot meet nutritional requirements via an oral route, if there is a clinical indication, and if there is capable patient and/or family support with an appropriate and safe home environment. European and U.S. data show that about 40% of home PN patients have a cancer diagnosis. Retrospective and prospective studies suggest a mean survival time of 53 to 150 days for patients on home PN support (41). And while PN may prolong life in patients with GI obstruction, it also increases complications (42). Required documentation of medical necessity for home nutrition support is extensive. Coordination of care amongst the RD, physician, nursing, speech therapy, and case management is required. Community support, education, and outreach are provided via the Oley Foundation (www.oley.org).

Nutrition Support in Palliative Care and End of Life

Palliative care is meant to improve pain and symptom control and not treat the underlying disease. Nutrition support should be provided when it may improve the quality or length of life. The palliative use of nutrition support therapy in terminally ill cancer patients is addressed in chapter 27.

References

1. Bosaeus I, Daneryd P, Lundholm K. Dietary intake, resting energy expenditure, weight loss and survival in cancer patients. *J Nutr.* 2002 Nov; 132 (11 Suppl): 3465S-3466S.
2. Williams EF, Meguid MM. Nutritional concepts and considerations in head and neck surgery. *Head and Neck.* 1989;11(5):393-9.
3. Bossola M, Pacelli F, Rosa F, Tortorelli A, Doglietto GB. Does Nutrition Support Stimulate Tumor Growth in Humans? *Nutr Clin Pract.* 2011; 26:174-180.
4. August DA, Huhman MB, ASPEN Board of Directors. ASPEN Clinical Guidelines: Nutrition Support Therapy During Adult Anticancer Treatment and in Hematopoietic Cell Transplant. *J Parenter Enteral Nutr.* 2009; 33:472.
5. Bozzetti F, Arends J, Lundholm K, Micklewright A, Zurcher G, Muscaritoli M. E.S.P.E.N. Guidelines on PN: non-surgical oncology. *Clin Nutr.* 2009; 28(4):445-454.
6. Braga M, Ljungqvist O, Soeters P, Fearson K. Weimann A, Bozzetti F. E.S.P.E.N. Guidelines on PN: surgery. *Clin Nutr.* 2009;28(4):378-386.
7. Mercadante S. Parenteral versus enteral nutrition in cancer patients: indications and practice. *Support Care Cancer.*1998;6(2):85-93.
8. Jeejeebhoy KN. Enteral and parenteral nutrition: evidence-based approach. *Proc Nutr Soc.* 2001;60(3):399-402.
9. Mortensen PB, Clausen MR. Short-chain fatty acids in the human colon: relation to gastrointestinal health and disease. *Scand J Gastroenterol.* 2013;31(216):132-148.
10. McClave S, Martindale RD, Vanek VW, et. al. Guidelines for the Provision and Assessment of Nutrition Support Therapy in the Adult Critically Ill Patient. *J Parenter Enteral Nutr.* 2009;33(3):277-316.
11. Peter JV, Moran JL, Phillips-Hughes J. A meta-analysis of treatment outcomes of early enteral versus early parenteral nutrition in hospitalized patients. *Critical Care Medicine.* 2005; 33:213 -220.
12. Huhmann M, August D. Perioperative nutrition support in cancer patients. *Nutr Clin Pract.* 2012;27(5):586-592.
13. Cangelosi MJ, Auerbach HR, Cohen JT. A clinical and economic evaluation of enteral nutrition. *Curr Med Res Opin.* 2011;27(2):413-22.
14. Bankhead R. Enteral Nutrition Practice Recommendations. *J Parenter Enteral Nutr.* 2009;33(2):122-167.
15. Itkin M, DeLegge MH, Fang JC, et al. Multidisciplinary Practical Guidelines for Gastrointestinal Access for Enteral Nutrition and Decompression From the Society of Interventional Radiology and American Gastroenterological Association (AGA) Institute, With Endorsement by Canadian Interventional Radiological Association (CIRA) and Cardiovascular and Interventional Radiological Society of Europe (CIRSE). *Gastroenterology.* 2011;141(2):742-765.
16. Krenitsky J. Gastric versus jejunal feeding: evidence or emotion? *Nutr Issues Practl Gastroenterology.* September 2006;46-65.
17. Cresci G. Enteral Formulations. In: Mueller CM, ed. *The A.S.P.E.N. Adult Nutrition Support Core Curriculum,* 2nd ed. Silver Spring, MD: A.S.P.E.N.; 2012; 185-205.
18. Hegazi RA, Wischmeyer PE. Clinical review: optimizing enteral nutrition for critically ill patients – a simple data driven formula. *Crit Care.* 2011; 15(6):234-244.
19. Parrish C, McCray S. Enteral Feeding: Dispelling Myths. *Nutrition Issues in Practical Gastroenterology.* September 2003.
20. Marinella M. Refeeding Syndrome: an important aspect of supportive oncology. *J Support Oncol.* 2009;7(1):11-16.
21. Kraft MD, Btaiche IF, Sacks GS. Review of the refeeding syndrome. *Nutr Clin Pract.* 2005;20(6):625-633.
22. Parrish C. The refeeding syndrome in 2009: prevention is the key to treatment. *J Support Oncol.* 2009;7(1):20-21.
23. Krzywda EA, Andris DA, Edmiston CE. Parenteral Access Devices. In: Mueller CM, ed. *The A.S.P.E.N. Adult Nutrition Support Core Curriculum,* 2nd ed. Silver Spring, MD: A.S.P.E.N.; 2012; 265-283.
24. Gottschlich MM, et al. *The Adult Nutrition Support Core Curriculum: A Case-Based Approach—The Adult Patient.* Silver Spring, MD. A.S.P.E.N.; 2007.
25. Russell MK. Monitoring Complications of Enteral Feedings. In. Charney P, Malone A. *Academy of Nutrition and Dietetics Pocket Guide to Enteral Nutrition.* 2nd Ed. Chicago, IL. Academy of Nutrition and Dietetics: 2013;155-191.
26. Mirtallo J, Forbes A, McClave S, Jensen G, Waitzberg D, Davies A. International Consensus Guidelines for Nutrition Therapy in Pancreatitis. *J Parenter Enteral Nutr.* 2012;36(3):284-291.
27. Mirtallo J, Canada T, Johnson D, et al. Safe practices for parenteral nutrition. *J Parenter Enteral Nutr.* 2004;28(6):S42-S43.
28. Malone AM, Seres D, Lord L. Complications of Enteral Nutrition. In: Mueller CM, ed. *The A.S.P.E.N. Adult Nutrition Support Core Curriculum,* 2nd ed. Silver Spring, MD: A.S.P.E.N.; 2012; 218-233.
29. O'Grady N, Alexander M, Burns L, et al. Guidelines for the Prevention of Intravascular Catheter-Related Infections. *Clin Infect Dis.* 2011;52(9): 1087-1099 .
30. Centers for Disease Control and Prevention. Guidelines for the prevention of intravascular catheter-related infections. *MMWR* 2002; 51 (No. RR-10):1–28. [Erratum 2002;51:711].
31. Barbara J, Sacks GS. Parenteral Nutrition Formulations. In: Mueller CM, ed. *The A.S.P.E.N. Adult Nutrition Support Core Curriculum,* 2nd ed. Silver Spring, MD: A.S.P.E.N.: 2012; 245-264.
32. Vanek VW, Borum P, Buchman A, et al. Novel Nutrient Task Force, Parenteral Multi-Vitamin and Multi-Trace Element Working Group and American Society for Parenteral and Enteral Nutrition Board of Directors. A.S.P.E.N. Position Paper: Recommendations for Changes in Commercially Available Parenteral Multivitamin and Mulit-Trace Element Products. *Nutr Clin Pract.* 2012;27(4):440-491.
33. Trace Elements [package insert]. New York and Ohio. American Regent. Luitpold Pharmaceuticals, Inc. © 2013.
34. Kumpf VJ. Complications of Parenteral Nutrition. In: Mueller CM, ed. *The A.S.P.E.N. Adult Nutrition Support Core Curriculum,* 2nd ed. Silver Spring, MD: A.S.P.E.N.: 2012;284-297.
35. Nirula R, Yamada K, Waxman K. The effect of abrupt cessation of total parenteral nutrition on serum glucose: a randomized trial. *Am Surg.* 2000;66(9):866-869.
36. Madsen H, Frankel E. The Hitchhiker's Guide to Parenteral Nutrition Management for Adult Patients. *Nutrition Issues in Practical Gastroenterology.* 2006;46-68.
37. Academy of Nutrition and Dietetics Nutrition Care Manual. Parenteral Nutrition Monitoring. Accessed April 2013.
38. Fessler T. Trace Element Monitoring and Therapy for Adult Patients Receiving Long-Term Total Parenteral Nutrition. *Nutrition Issues in Gastroenterology.* March 2005.
39. Ghabril M, Aranda-Michel J, Scolapio J. Metabolic and catheter complications of parenteral nutrition. *Curr Gastroenterol Rep.* 2004; 6(4).327-334.
40. Boncompain-Gérard M, Robert D, Fouque D, Hadj-Aïssa A. Renal function and urinary excretion of electrolytes in patients receiving cyclic parenteral nutrition. *J Parenter Enteral Nutr.* 2000;24(4):234-239.
41. Mackenzie ML, Gramlich L. Home parenteral nutrition in advanced cancer: where are we? *Appl Physiol Nutr Metab.* 2008;33(1):1-11.
42. Chermesh I, Mshiach T, Amit A, et al. Home parenteral nutrition (HTPN) for incurable patients with cancer with gastrointestinal obstruction: do the benefits outweigh the risks? *Med Oncol.* 2011 Mar;28(1):83-88.

BLENDERIZED TUBE FEEDING RECIPES

Note: Patients should be instructed in proper preparation, handling and storage of blenderized tube feeding, as well as proper cleaning of equipment used to prepare the formula to avoid foodborne illness.

CALORIES	1200	1500	1800	2000
INGREDIENTS				
Baby Rice Cereal (Heinz; dry)	¼ cup	¼ cup	1/2 cup	½ cup
Baby Beef (Heinz) 2.5 oz jar	2 Jars	2 Jars	2 Jars	2 Jars
Baby Carrots (Heinz) 4 oz jar	1 Jar	1 Jar	1 Jar	1 Jar
Baby Green Beans (Heinz) 4 oz jar	-	1 Jar	1 Jar	1 Jar
Baby Applesauce (Heinz) 4 oz jar	1 Jar	1 Jar	1 Jar	2 Jars
Baby Chicken (Heinz) 2.5 oz jar	1 Jar	1 Jar	1 Jar	1 Jar
Orange Juice	½ Cup	1 Cup	1 Cup	1 Cup
Whole Milk[1]	2 Cups	2 Cups	2¼ Cups	2¼ Cups
Cream, Half-and-Half	1/3 Cup	¾ Cup	1¼ Cups	1½ Cups
Egg-Cooked[2]	1	1	1	2
Vegetable oil[3]	1 Tbsp	1 Tbsp	1 Tbsp	1 Tbsp
Karo Syrup[4]	2 Tbsp	2 Tbsp	2 Tbsp	2 Tbsp

[1] Substitute lactaid milk if needed
[2] An equivalent amount of pasteurized liquid whole egg can also be used (check label)
[3] Suggest eigher: sunflower, corn or soybean oil (high essential fatty acid content and readily available)
[4] Polycose liquid can be substitute if necessary
Makes 1525 mL total volume

Adapted with permission from the University of Virginia Health System Digestive Health Center (www.ginutrition.virginia.edu)

BLENDERIZED TUBE FEEDING RECIPES *(continued)*

NUTRIENTS	DRIs[1]	CALORIES[3]			
		1200	1500	1800	2000
Kcals	—	1205	1478	1784	1986
Protein (g)	—	58	63	71	79
Total Fat (g)	—	60	72	89	102
Saturated Fat (g)	—	25	32	42	48
Monounsaturated (g)	—	19	22	27	31
Polyunsaturated (g)	—	12	13	14	15
Carbohydrate (g	—	112	151	181	197
Sugar (g)	—	57	79	82	83
Fiber (g) -	—	4	7	7	9
Calcium (mg)	1200	1032	1195	1636	1729
Iron (mg)	10.5	18	19	33	34
Magnesium (mg)	370	199	250	329	344
Sodium (mg)	1500	586	656	744	833
Potassium (mg)	4700	1969	2516	2874	3096
Phosphorus (mg)	700	1019	1152	1491	1643
Zinc (mg)	9.5	8.0	8.8	10.1	11
Vitamin A (RE)	800	1673	1842	1991	2142
Vitamin C (mg)	82	101	149	151	195
Thiamin (mg)	1.1	1.2	1.4	2.2	2.3
Riboflavin (mg)	1.2	2.2	2.5	3.4	3.8
Niacin (mg)	15	17	17	26	27
Pantothenic Acid (mg)	5	4.1	4.8	5.3	6.3
Folate (mcg)	400	112	176	189	215
Vitamin B6 (mg)	1.5	1.0	1.1	1.3	1.4
Vitamin B12 (mcg)	2.4	4.9	5.2	5.8	6.6
Vitamin D (mcg)	10	234	250	294	330
Vitamin E (mg)	15	15	16	16	17
Vitamin K (mcg)	105	49	52	54	80
Water %[2]	—	64	64	64	64

[1]The *average* recommended value for a healthy male or female adult. For more information: http://www.nal.usda.gov/fnic/etext/000105.html
[2]Water may need to be added to thin down the formula ; furthermore, separate water bolus' will be needed to meet hydration needs.
[3]Numbers shaded and in bold print highlight those nutrients that fall below the average DRI's for adults – a Centrum vitamin/mineral supplement (or equivalent) can be crushed and flushed 4-7 days per week as needed to ensure nutrient adequacy of tube feeding.
[4]In some circumstances, additional sodium may need to be added to these mixture

Adapted with permission from the University of Virginia Health System Digestive Health Center (www.ginutrition.virginia.edu)

Nutrition Management of the Surgical Oncology Patient

Maureen Huhmann, DCN, RD, CSO

Introduction:

Various diseases, conditions and medical procedures can greatly impact an individual's ability to ingest and absorb nutrients. For patients with cancer, surgery is utilized as both a palliative and curative intervention; in either case, surgery can have large ramifications on dietary intake and nutrition status. This chapter presents a review of preoperative nutrition planning, postoperative nutrition intervention and long-term needs of surgical oncology patients, with specific attention paid to nutrition consequences of gastrointestinal (GI) surgery.

Surgery and Nutrition Risk

Most surgical procedures have nutritional consequences that can range from mild postoperative nausea to permanent alterations in GI function. In general, surgical intervention to the head and neck, GI tract and abdominal vasculature have the greatest potential for major derangements in nutritional status. The need for surgical resection in these regions also is associated with conditions and symptoms that directly cause or predispose to malnutrition. Compounding this, surgery may increase the risk of malnutrition due to catabolism, nutrient losses and operative trauma, which in combination with anesthesia can cause intestinal dysfunction, impair bowel permeability, alter gut-associated lymphoid tissue and stress the immune system (1).

Nutrition Assessment of the Surgical Patient

Major surgery is linked with deterioration in nutrition status (2-3) that can lead to changes in metabolism, tissue function and body composition (4). As the invasiveness of the procedure increases so can the incidence of complications and severity of protein calorie malnutrition and its consequences (5-6). There is significant correlation between preoperative malnutrition and longer length of hospital stay, postoperative morbidity and mortality (7-11).

Nutrition assessment identifies the presence and extent of malnutrition and the potential metabolic consequences of the anticipated surgical procedure. Accurate nutrition assessment of preoperative patients should include both subjective and objective data (6). Several indices have been explored as indicators of nutrition status in surgical patients, including Subjective Global Assessment, Nutritional Risk Index, and Nutritional Risk Screening (7). Decreased albumin is associated with increased surgical mortality and morbidity, especially sepsis and healing complications (12).

Interactions between malnutrition and the acute phase response limit the accuracy of nutrition indicators such as albumin and prealbumin (6), but they are strong predictors of prognosis within multivariable models. Chapter 3 discusses nutrition screening and assessment of oncology patients.

Preoperative Planning

The nutrition care plan for the pre- and post-operative periods should be determined and discussed with the patient prior to surgery. Research has suggested that enteral tube feeding provided for 10 days prior to surgery can reduce morbidity and mortality in malnourished surgical patients by preserving bowel mucosa and modulating the immune response (6). Early post-operative enteral feeding in patients with moderate or severe preoperative malnutrition can improve surgical outcomes (10-11). Additionally, limited use of postoperative nasogastric tubes for decompression and early oral intake, in combination with limited narcotic analgesia and early mobilization, facilitates faster recovery and earlier discharge (12-13).

Benefits of enteral access in patients with malnutrition usually outweigh the risks of access-related complications (14). However, risks may outweigh benefits in the presence of ascites, peritoneal carcinomatosis, or inoperable bowel obstruction. In the latter situation, tube placement for drainage may assist in the palliation of symptoms.

Preoperative Education

Surgical resection of the head, neck and GI tract is associated with significant postoperative morbidity (15) including weight loss and malnutrition (16). Preoperative education to inform patients of potential postoperative events allows them to play an active role in their recovery, identify signs of complications and anticipate normal physiologic responses to GI surgery that, left untreated, can compromise nutrition status. A postoperative nutrition care plan helps maintain perioperative nutrition status.

Provision of medical nutrition therapy by a registered dietitian (RD)/ registered dietitian nutritionist (RDN) has become commonplace in many settings, including diabetes clinics and doctor's offices. Many insurance companies now require that bariatric surgery patients receive preoperative nutrition education by an RD (17). In fact, this education is associated with improved weight loss and physical activity in these patients postoperatively (18). There are few data on the role of nutrition education in surgical oncology patients. However, studies indicate that preoperative education on expectations and pain management can reduce anxiety (19) and pain (20), and improve outcomes (21).

Postoperative Nutrition Intervention

Following major abdominal surgery, the small bowel regains function almost immediately (22). However, after intestinal resection adaptation of the GI tract may take weeks to even months (22). Most patients resume oral intake within 6–9 days postoperatively (23), though early postoperative feeding (within 24 hours of surgery) can stimulate the return of normal bowel function (11,22).

The American Society for Enteral and Parenteral Nutrition (A.S.P.E.N.) guidelines suggest that nutrition support is indicated only in individuals anticipated to require support for more that 7–10 days unless the patient is malnourished (11). In GI cancer patients, enteral and parenteral postoperative nutrition support has been associated with less morbidity when compared with standard intravenous fluids, with the benefit more pronounced among those receiving enteral nutrition (EN) (23). Jejunal feedings are recommended for the immediate postoperative period in severely malnourished patients and those in whom prolonged inadequate oral intake is expected (24).

Intraoperative placement of feeding tubes has become commonplace during major gastrointestinal procedures (25) and can take the form of a gastrostomy or jejunostomy tube. For patients in whom nutrition support is initiated, support should continue until oral intake is tolerated and consistently meets two thirds to three quarters of their nutrition needs and 1,000 mL fluid for 3 consecutive days (26). When intake reaches 50% of needs, nutrition support should be progressively weaned as oral intake increases (27). Nutrition support of oncology patients is discussed in chapter 13.

Postoperative Management:

Historically, early oral and enteral feeding has been discouraged following major surgery. "Bowel rest" was thought to promote anastomotic healing and prevent nausea. Emerging research contradicts those beliefs; operative trauma can cause intestinal dysfunction (28) but in most patients GI function returns rapidly postoperatively and intraluminal nutrients promote bowel hypertrophy and anastomotic healing (29). In fact, data show that feeding proximal to an anastomosis may make it more resistant to disruption or leak (30). The small intestine regains the ability to absorb nutrients quickly after surgery, even in the absence of peristalsis, and dysmotility can be attenuated if feeding is started within 24 hours postoperatively (31). Unfortunately, the practice of holding oral or EN until bowel sounds return is pervasive (28). Early initiation of EN postoperatively promotes many physiologic benefits including wound healing, gut function and immunity, and reduces length of hospital stay (29-33).

Surgery to the GI tract can be associated with long and short-term complications, the most common of which is altered transit time. Transit may be too fast, too slow, or even occur in the wrong direction (34). Clinical manifestations include dumping syndrome, heartburn, feelings of fullness, pain, meteorism, abdominal distention, dysphagia, constipation, or diarrhea (34). Denervation (35) is one of the many causes of chronic dysmotility, which may cause any or all of these symptoms (33). Strategies for managing nutrition impact symptoms such as dysphagia, constipation, diarrhea and abdominal distention are provided in chapter 12.

Surgeries

The following section addresses nutritional effects of specific surgical procedures.

Head and Neck Surgery (see figures in chapter 21)

The mouth is the initial point of entry to the GI tract. Surgical interventions for head and neck cancer will remove the tumor and a margin of surrounding tissue and can compromise the ability to chew and swallow, thereby impairing the ability to orally ingest nutrients. Depending upon the extent of resection to the oral cavity, tongue and upper airway, patients may experience minor interference with eating to total dependence on EN. For patients who will need postoperative chemoradiotherapy, challenges to oral feeding are compounded by side effects, including mucositis. Chapter 21 provides detailed information on medical nutrition therapy for head and neck cancer and chapter 13 provides additional information on nutrition support of oncology patients.

Peritoneal Surgery

The peritoneum is a thin membrane that lines the inside of the abdomen. Those diagnosed with peritoneal cancer or metastasis present with general GI symptoms including abdominal bloating and cramping, nausea, diarrhea, constipation and anorexia, which can result in unintentional weight loss. The goal of surgical resection is to remove the bulk, if not all of, the disease and to resect surrounding tissue if the disease has spread. Due to the proximity of the peritoneum to the GI system, surgical resections involving the peritoneum have the potential to disrupt normal GI function (36). In addition, peritonitis, or inflammation of the peritoneum, due to intestinal perforation or as a result of surgical intervention, can cause ileus and impair gut absorption.

Perioperative nutrition is necessary to promote wound healing and preserve gut function in patients with peritonitis (36-37). Preoperatively, nutrition impact symptoms should be managed by strategies discussed in chapter 12. It has been suggested that a feeding tube should be placed at the time of surgery in patients with peritoneal infections and resections (36), however parenteral nutrition (PN) is preferred because of the profound ileus that usually accompanies peritonitis. As the peritonitis and ileus resolve, the feeding tube may then be used to initiate EN until an oral diet is tolerated. The extent of surgery dictates post-operative medical nutrition therapy.

Esophageal Surgery (see figures in chapter 19)

The esophagus functions as a conduit for food as it travels from the mouth to the stomach. Dysphagia is the primary preoperative symptom, resulting from esophageal narrowing as the tumor grows. Many patients present with malnutrition due to obstruction and/or side effects associated with neoadjuvant chemoradiotherapy (37).

Surgical options as well as their associated nutritional consequences, including dumping, are discussed in chapter 19; anti-dumping diet recommendations are presented in Appendix 4. The extent of surgery determines the degree of nutrition related symptoms; removal of the lower esophageal sphincter (LES) during surgery contributes to postoperative reflux. In addition, dysmotility of the remaining esophagus and gastric dysmotility occurs secondary to resection of the vagus nerve. This denervation can reduce the ability to experience satiety (38), resulting in overeating and potentially food regurgitation. Adopting a small frequent meal plan limits intake at any one time, helping to prevent overeating episodes.

Approximately 30% of patients experience stricture(s) after esophagectomy (54), which are the result of decreased vascularization and late ischemia in response to a decrease in blood supply to the stomach (38). Strictures often require dilation or stent placement to allow for oral intake. Although dilation is successful in 99% of patients, 50% of patients need to undergo multiple dilations (39). A feeding jejunostomy tube is often placed at the time of esophageal surgery to allow for initiation of EN postoperatively. Data show that intensive nutrition support provided by an RD is associated with weight maintenance and fewer postoperative complications in this population (40).

Stomach Surgery

The stomach is a fist-sized reservoir that stores food until it is sufficiently digested and therefore physiologically ready for entry into the small intestine, where the majority of nutrient absorption occurs. A sphincter muscle at the end of the esophagus controls movement out of the esophagus and into the stomach. Located just past the gastro-esophageal junction, where the esophagus connects to the stomach, the lower esophageal sphincter (LES) relaxes to allow food boluses to enter the stomach. The LES tightens after the bolus passes through to prevent stomach acid and digestive enzymes from refluxing back up and into the esophagus. Food remains in the stomach for a significant time before emptying through the pyloric sphincter into the duodenum. Gastrectomy, the surgical removal of part or all of the stomach, may affect one or both of these sphincters. Removal of the LES can promote acid reflux into the esophagus and occurs in as many as 58% of patients who undergo esophagectomy (41) and 80% of patients who undergo a total gastrectomy (34). Disruption of pyloric function, as occurs with gastrojejunostomy, results in reflux of bile from the small bowel into the residual stomach and even into the esophagus. This is difficult to manage because unlike stomach acid, there are no drugs available to "neutralize" the irritant effects of bile in the esophagus.

Figure 1: The Stomach

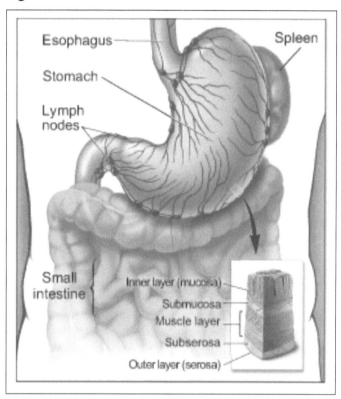

Reprinted with permission
The website of the National Cancer Institute (http://www.cancer.gov).

To varying degrees, gastric resection reduces the capacity of the stomach to hold food and secretions, thereby increasing the risk of unintentional food regurgitation (34). Disruption of the pyloric sphincter and gastrojejunostomy also may lead to dumping syndrome, which is addressed in chapter 19. Untreated, these problems can lead to weight loss, malnutrition, and increased mortality (16).

Gastric acid is important to digestion as well as microbial control in the stomach. Achlorhydria refers to a decrease or cessation of the production of gastric acid. While oral pancreatic enzyme replacement therapy (PERT) can help to compensate for loss of digestive insufficiencies, there is no substitute for the antimicrobial function of gastric acid. Achlorhydria may allow bacterial and fungal overgrowth (42), which can cause pain when eating and lead to suboptimal intake. Chronic gastritis also predisposes to cancer development (43).

The acidic environment of the stomach along with the production of intrinsic factor (IF) assists in the release of vitamin B12 from food and facilitates its absorption in the terminal ileum (44). Loss of IF as a result of proximal gastric resection may result in vitamin B12 malabsorption, which can lead to megaloblastic anemia, and dementia (45). B12 deficiency can develop as early as 1 year after total gastrectomy (46); replacement can be provided via oral, enteral, and parenteral formulations (44-46).

Dysmotility is common following stomach resections and may manifest as delayed or accelerated gastric emptying. Delayed emptying is associated with early satiety, heartburn, dysphagia, aspiration, and pneumonia. Accelerated transit of the hypertonic solutions of the stomach into the small intestine causes dumping syndrome.

Small Bowel Surgery

The small bowel, which is approximately 20 feet long, is the primary site of nutrient absorption. The first and shortest section of the small intestines is the duodenum, which receives pancreatic and bile secretions that facilitate macronutrient absorption. The jejunum is the second section, and comprises about 40% of the small bowel. It transitions to the ileum, the final section and almost 60% of small bowel length. Small bowel resection reduces absorptive surface area, which can alter transit time and contribute to malabsorption and malnutrition. The loss of portions of the jejunum can result in inappropriate secretion of digestive enzymes and accelerate gastric emptying. Significant resection of the lower jejunum and ileum reduces intestinal absorption and may result in short bowel syndrome, usually defined as having less than 30% of normal intestinal length (75 cm in children and 200 cm in adults) (47). Though functional adaptation can occur, significant post-operative loss of small bowel length results in insufficient absorptive surface, which increases the potential for maldigestion and malabsorption and significant nutritional deficiencies.

Gastric acid in the small bowel stimulates release of bicarbonate to neutralize the acid, thereby protecting the function of pancreatic enzymes and bile acid. However, when gastric acid secretion exceeds the amount of bicarbonate available, it deactivates digestive enzymes and deconjugates bile acids, leading to maldigestion, which can cause malabsorption. The presence of

Figure 2: The Parts of the Small Intestines

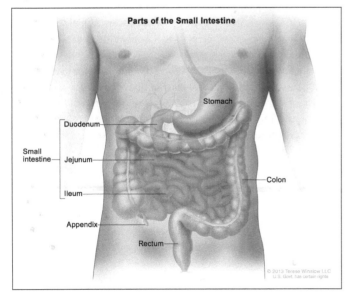

© 2013 Terese Winslow LLC, U.S. Govt. has certain rights

undigested food in the colon can have detrimental effects locally and systemically. Bacteria can ferment undigested carbohydrate and produce D-lactic acid, which can cause metabolic acidosis (48). This is managed with refined carbohydrate restriction (e.g., lactose, fructose, alcohol sugars), antibiotics, and probiotics (48). Several strains of lactobacillus may benefit this population (49-50). Undigested proteins ferment in the colon and can increase ammonia levels. Additionally, massive bowel resection frequently leads to bacterial overgrowth, increasing the risk of bacterial translocation and systemic infection and sepsis (51). Bacterial overgrowth is commonly treated with antibiotics and probiotics (51)

Postoperative anatomy determines absorptive capacity, expected nutrient insufficiencies or deficiencies, and medical nutrition therapy recommendations. However, each case is unique and requires routine monitoring and reassessment. Nutrition recommendations following intestinal surgery are outlined in Appendix 3.

Colon Surgery

The primary digestive function of the colon, a muscular tube that is approximately 15 feet in length, is fluid resorption and electrolyte absorption. Partial and total resections of the colon have, at a minimum, a temporary impact on fluid and electrolyte balance. After resection, the remaining colon undergoes gradual structural and functional adaptation to increase fluid and nutrient absorption. However, this process may take two years or longer (47). Resections of the terminal ileum and colon and creation of an ileostomy and/or colostomy can have permanent effects, possibly requiring regular intravenous fluid replacement. The colon can contain up to 10^{11} or 10^{12} bacterial cells/gram luminal contents, including both beneficial as well as pathogenic bacteria (52). Bacteria in the colon serve a host of functions including synthesis of vitamin K and short-chain fatty acid production as well as defense against pathogenic microorganisms. Following surgery, bacterial overgrowth can occur as the result of impaired intestinal peristalsis or anatomical abnormalities that alter luminal flow (53) and potentially result in translocation of microorganisms, significant morbidity including multisystem organ failure, and even death (54). Perioperative provision of probiotics may decrease postoperative complications (52). Ileocolectomy has been associated with a significant increase in ileal and colonic bacterial counts (55). Bacterial overgrowth in the terminal ileum following ileocecal valve resection can reduce vitamin B12 absorption and result in the need for supplementation.

Decreased transit time frequently occurs with removal of a large section of bowel, ileocecal valve resection, and ileostomy. Postoperative nutrition interventions such as limiting dietary insoluble fiber intake, consuming small, frequent meals, and specific food elimination play a role in palliation of symptoms. Patients with an ileostomy are at an increased risk for dehydration and electrolyte abnormalities (56); there is an increased need for sodium and water to balance increased losses in the stool. Patients are commonly instructed to consume at least 1 liter more fluid than their ostomy output (57). Appendix 3 provides dietary recommendations following intestinal surgery.

Figure 3: The Colon

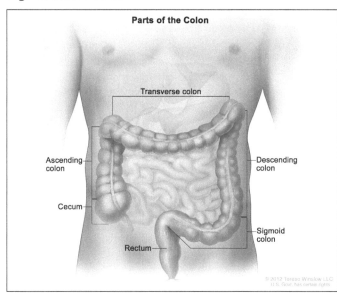

Parts of the Colon

© 2012 Terese Winslow LLC, U.S. Govt. has certain rights

Figure 4: The Liver

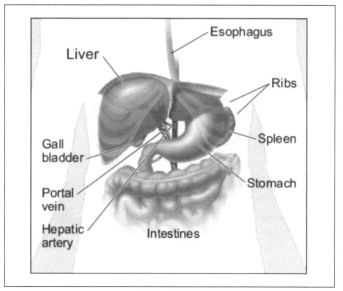

Reprinted with permission
The website of the National Cancer Institute (http://www.cancer.gov)

Pancreatic Surgery (see figures in chapter 24)
The pancreas performs both exocrine and endocrine function. Exocrine functions include production of bicarbonate and pancreatic enzymes, which are important for macronutrient digestion. A complete discussion of pancreatic and bile duct cancer and related medical nutrition therapy is provided in chapter 24. Neuroendocrine tumors of the pancreas such as insulinomas, gastrinomas, glucagonomas and VIPomas can have significant effects on pancreatic endocrine and exocrine function, as summarized in Table 1. Drugs such as octreotide assist in palliation of symptoms from these tumors. Surgery with or without radiotherapy is indicated in bulky or metastatic disease (59). Fortunately, surgery corrects most symptoms of neuroendocrine tumors.

Liver Surgery
The liver is one of the largest organs in the body and is located in the upper right quadrant of the abdomen. The central role of the liver in

nutrient metabolism increases risk of metabolic derangement after liver surgery (61). Preoperative liver disease may cause hypoalbuminemia, hyperglucagonemia, increased energy expenditure, depleted skeletal muscle mass and anorexia (62). Postoperatively, whole-body protein synthesis may be compromised. Reduced synthesis and increased catabolism of serum hepatic protein levels may occur (63) and lead to hypoalbuminemia, resulting in malabsorption due to bowel wall edema as well as fluid retention in the extremities. Postoperative tolerance of the liver resection as well as the liver's ability to regenerate and regain function after liver surgery varies greatly.

Malnutrition postoperatively impacts the return of liver function and regeneration and may increase morbidity and mortality. To promote earlier return of liver function, patients can undergo preoperative portal vein embolization, which induces hepatic hypertrophy and can help preserve functional liver volume (61).

Table 1: Endocrine and Exocrine Effects of Neuroendocrine Tumors (58-60)

Neuroendocrine Tumors	Endocrine and Exocrine Effects	Nutrition Intervention
Insulinomas	Fasting hypoglycemia	• Consume complex carbohydrate-containing food every 2-3 hours
Gastrinomas	Recurrent ulcers, diarrhea, and gastroesophageal reflux	• Primarily treated with medication
		• To limit reflux, avoid alcohol, chocolate, citrus juice, tomato-based products, peppermint, coffee, and onion while also adopting low fat eating habits and consuming smaller volumes of food at mealtime
Glucagonomas	Erythema and diabetes	• Carbohydrate Counting plan
VIPomas	Increased secretion of vasoactive intestinal peptide, Verner-Morrison syndrome, pancreatic cholera or WHDA (watery diarrhea, hypokalemia, and achlorhydria)	• Medications and fluids are usually required to manage losses and limit output • Enteral or parenteral replacement of electrolytes may be needed

Patients with severe postoperative liver dysfunction may develop hepatic encephalopathy. The use of branched chain amino acids (BCAA) to treat hepatic encephalopathy and to improve liver function has been explored (62) but found to be of little benefit (64). When nutrition support is required, standard enteral formula is acceptable for patients with chronic liver disease; use of BCAA should be reserved for patients with severe hepatic encephalopathy (65). Protein restriction is not recommended unless the patient is experiencing mental status changes, when protein intake should be limited to approximately 0.8 g/kg/day.

Long-Term Feeding Issues

Long-term complications can occur after cancer surgery. Upper GI resections can result in abnormal transit, maldigestion and malabsorption, and obstruction, complications that pose significant health risks (66). Rapid intake of food and inadequate mastication after major upper abdominal surgery induces symptoms of heartburn, pain and vomiting (67). Individualized dietary modification and nutrition education is key to recovery (68-70). Table 2 summarizes long-term complications and nutrition interventions.

Conclusion

Surgical intervention in cancer patients can have temporary as well as long term impact on nutrition status. Preoperative planning should be made for postoperative nutrition intervention. Postoperative nutrition intervention may range from alteration in the type and quantity of food to the initiation of EN. Both pre- and postoperative nutrition intervention can help to alleviate many postoperative nutrition issues in the surgical population.

References

1. Cardinale F, Chinellato I, Caimmi S, et al. Perioperative period; immunological modifications. *Int J Immunopathol Pharmacol*. 2011; 24(3Suppl):S3-S12.)
2. Hirano S, Kondo S, Tanaka E, et al. Postoperative bowel function and nutritional status following distal pancreatectomy with en-bloc celiac axis resection. *Dig Surg*. 2010;27(3):212-216.
3. Beaton J, Carey S, Solomon M, Young J. Preoperative and postoperative nutritional status of patients following pelvic exenteration surgery for rectal cancer. *e-SPEN Journal*. 2013.
4. Berstad P, Haugum B, Helgeland M, Bukholm I, Almendingen K. Preoperative body size and composition, habitual diet, and post-operative complications in elective colorectal cancer patients in Norway. *J Hum Nutr Diet*. 2013;26(4):359-368.
5. Hirsch S, de Obaldia N, Petermann M, et al. Nutritional status of surgical patients and the relationship of nutrition to postoperative outcome. *J Am Coll Nutr*. 1992;11(1):21-24.

Table 2: Potential Long-Term Nutrition Issues in Surgical Patients (15,34,38,58,70)

Category	Issue	Manifestation	Nutrition Intervention
Abnormal Transit	Dumping Syndrome	Early: Diarrhea, bloating, nausea, tachycardia immediately – 30 minutes after a meal Late: Hypoglycemic symptoms, dizziness – 90 to 180 minutes after a meal	• Small frequent meals • Separation of solids and fluids at meals • Reduction in simple carbohydrate and concentrated fat intake • Increase in soluble fiber intake
	Reflux Esophagitis	Regurgitation of food and digestive juices causing heartburn, nausea or vomiting	• Small frequent meals • Diet modification (e.g. consume lower fat food, avoid alcohol, consumer smaller volumes per meal or snack) • Use of antacids or sucralfate
	Delayed Gastric Emptying/Gastric Stasis	Early satiety, postprandial fullness, heartburn, dysphagia, aspiration	• Small frequent meals • Diet modification (e.g., consume 5-6 small meals/day, chew food well, avoid fried and greasy foods, moderate fiber intake) • Prokinetic agents
	Pancreaticocibal Asynchrony	Steatorrhea, frequent light greasy stools	• Pancreatic enzyme supplementation at meals and snacks • Supplementation of micronutrients as needed (fat soluble vitamins, calcium, vitamin D)
Malassimilation	Reduced Intake, Impaired absorption, increased losses	Micronutrient deficiencies	• Enteral or parenteral replacement • Pancreatic enzyme supplementation (depending on nutrients malabsorbed)
Obstruction	Stricture, Gastric Outlet Obstruction	Vomiting, Constipation	• Enteral or parenteral nutrition support depending upon extent • Endoscopic balloon dilation or surgical stenting • Promotility agent
Pancreatic Insufficiency	Pancreatic Enzyme Insufficiency	Steatorrhea, bloating	• Pancreatic enzyme replacement

6. Nespoli L, Coppola S, Gianotti L. The role of the enteral route and the composition of feeds in the nutritional support of malnourished surgical patients. *Nutrients.* 2012;4(9):1230-1236.

7. Garth AK, Newsome CM, Simmance N, Crowe TC. Nutritional status, nutrition practices and post-operative complications in patients with gastrointestinal cancer. *J Hum Nutr Diet.* 2010;23(4):393-401.

8. Morgan TM, Tang D, Stratton KL, et al. Preoperative nutritional status is an important predictor of survival in patients undergoing surgery for renal cell carcinoma. *Eur Urol.* 2011;59(6):923-928.

9. Perioperative total parenteral nutrition in surgical patients. The Veterans Affairs Total Parenteral Nutrition Cooperative Study Group. *N Engl J Med.* 1991;325(8):525-532.

10. Klein S, Koretz RL. Nutrition support in patients with cancer: what do the data really show? *Nutr Clin Pract.* 1994;9(3):91-100.

11. August DA, Huhmann MB. A.S.P.E.N. clinical guidelines: nutrition support therapy during adult anticancer treatment and in hematopoietic cell transplantation. *J Parenter Enteral Nutr.* 2009;33(5):472-500.

12. Gustafsson UO, Hausel J, Thorell A, et al. Adherence to the enhanced recovery after surgery protocol and outcomes after colorectal cancer surgery. *Arch Surg.* 2011;146(5):571-577.

13. Gustafsson UO, Ljungqvist O. Perioperative nutritional management in digestive tract surgery. *Curr Opin Clin Nutr Metab Care.* 2011;14(5): 504-509.

14. Gerndt SJ, Orringer MB. Tube jejunostomy as an adjunct to esophagectomy. *Surgery.* 1994;115(2):164-169.

15. Radigan A. Post-Gastrectomy: Managing the nutrition fall-out. *Pract Gastroenterol.* 2004;28(6):63-75.

16. Rey-Ferro M, Castano R, Orozco O, Serna A, Moreno A. Nutritional and immunologic evaluation of patients with gastric cancer before and after surgery. *Nutrition.* 1997;13(10):878-881.

17. Garza SF. Bariatric weight loss surgery: patient education, preparation, and follow-up. *Crit Care Nurs Q.* 2003;26(2):101-104.

18. Nijamkin MP, Campa A, Sosa J, Baum M, Himburg S, Johnson P. Comprehensive nutrition and lifestyle education improves weight loss and physical activity in Hispanic Americans following gastric bypass surgery: a randomized controlled trial. *J Acad Nutr Diet.* 2012;112(3): 382-390.

19. Watt-Watson J, Stevens B, Katz J, Costello J, Reid GJ, David T. Impact of preoperative education on pain outcomes after coronary artery bypass graft surgery. *Pain.* 2004;109(1-2):73-85.

20. Danino AM, Chahraoui K, Frachebois L, et al. Effects of an informational CD-ROM on anxiety and knowledge before aesthetic surgery: a randomised trial. *Br J Plast Surg.* 2005;58(3):379-383.

21. Giraudet-Le Quintrec JS, Coste J, Vastel L, et al. Positive effect of patient education for hip surgery: a randomized trial. *Clin Orthop Relat Res.* 2003 Sep;(414):112-120.

22. Mattei P, Rombeau JL. Review of the pathophysiology and management of postoperative ileus. *World J Surg.* 2006;30(8):1382-1391.

23. Bozzetti F, Gianotti L, Braga M, DiCarlo V, Mariani L. Postoperative complications in gastrointestinal cancer patients: the joint role of the nutritional status and the nutritional support. *Clin Nutr.* 2007;26(6): 698-709.

24. Fearon KC, Luff R. The nutritional management of surgical patients: enhanced recovery after surgery. *Proc Nutr Soc.* 2003;62(4):807-811.

25. Jensen GL, Sporay G, Whitmire S, Taraszewski R, Reed MJ. Intraoperative placement of the nasoenteric feeding tube: a practical alternative? *J Parenter Enteral Nutr.* 1995;19(3):244-247.

26. Thompson CW, Romano M. Initiation, advancement, and transition of enteral feedings In: *Pocket Guide to Enteral Nutrition, 2nd edition.* Charney P, Malone A, eds. Chicago, Ill: Academy of Nutrition and Dietetics; 2012: 88-119.

27. Charney P. Enteral Nutrition: Indications, Options, and Formulations. In: Gottschlich M, ed. *The Science and Practice of Nutrition Support.* Dubuque: Kendall Hunt Publishing; 2001:141-166.

28. Martindale R, McClave S, Taylor B, Lawson C. Perioperative Nutrition: What is the current landscape? *J Parenter Enter Nutr.* 2013;37(5) suppl:5S-20S.

29. Gabor S, Renner H, Matzi V, et al. Early enteral feeding compared with parenteral nutrition after oesophageal or oesophagogastric resection and reconstruction. *Br J Nutr.* 2005;93(4):509-513.

30. Osland E, Yunus RM, Khan S, Memon MA. Early versus traditional postoperative feeding in patients undergoing resectional gastrointestinal surgery: a meta-analysis. *J Parenter Enteral Nutr.* 2011;35(4):473-487.

31. Kalff JC, Turler A, Schwarz NT, et al. Intra-abdominal activation of a local inflammatory response within the human muscularis externa during laparotomy. *Ann Surg.* 2003;237(3):301-315.

32. Wheble GA, Knight WR, Khan OA. Enteral vs total parenteral nutrition following major upper gastrointestinal surgery. *Int J Surg.* 2012;10(4): 194-197.

33. Early enteral nutrition within 24h of colorectal surgery versus later commencement of feeding for postoperative complications. Cochrane Database of Systematic Reviews; 2005. http://gateway.ut.ovid.com. libproxy.umdnj.edu/gw1/ovidweb.cgi. Accessed 2005.

34. Scholmerich J. Postgastrectomy syndromes--diagnosis and treatment. *Best Pract Res Clin Gastroenterol.* 2004;18(5):917-933.

35. Koda K, Saito N, Seike K, Shimizu K, Kosugi C, Miyazaki M. Denervation of the neorectum as a potential cause of defecatory disorder following low anterior resection for rectal cancer. *Dis Colon Rectum.* 2005;48(2):210-217.

36. Genuit T, Napolitano L. Peritonitis and Abdominal Sepsis. 2004; http:// www.emedicine.com/med/topic2737.htm. Accessed 9/15/05.

37. Clavier JB, Antoni D, Atlani D, et al. Baseline nutritional status is prognostic factor after definitive radiochemotherapy for esophageal cancer. *Dis Esoph* 2012. Oct 26. doi: 10.1111/j.1442-2050.2012.01441.x.

38. Lerut TE, van Lanschot JJ. Chronic symptoms after subtotal or partial oesophagectomy: diagnosis and treatment. *Best Pract Res Clin Gastroenterol.* 2004;18(5):901-915.

39. Park JY, Song HY, Kim JH, et al. Benign anastomotic strictures after esophagectomy: long-term effectiveness of balloon dilation and factors affecting recurrence in 155 patients. *Am J Roentgenol.* 2012;198(5): 1208-1213.

40. Ligthart-Melis GC, Weijs PJ, Te Boveldt ND, et al. Dietician-delivered intensive nutritional support is associated with a decrease in severe postoperative complications after surgery in patients with esophageal cancer. *Dis Esophagus.* 2013;26(6):587-593.

41. Shibuya S, Fukudo S, Shineha R, et al. High incidence of reflux esophagitis observed by routine endoscopic examination after gastric pull-up esophagectomy. *World J Surg.* 2003;27(5):580-583.

42. Pereira SP, Gainsborough N, Dowling RH. Drug-induced hypochlorhydria causes high duodenal bacterial counts in the elderly. *Aliment Pharmacol Ther.* 1998;12(1):99-104.

43. Houben GM, Stockbrugger RW. Bacteria in the aetio-pathogenesis of gastric cancer: a review. *Scand J Gastroenterol Suppl.* 1995;212:13-18.

44. Oh R, Brown DL. Vitamin B12 deficiency. *Am Fam Physician.* 2003;67(5):979-986.

45. Malouf M, Grimley EJ, Areosa SA. Folic acid with or without vitamin B12 for cognition and dementia. *Cochrane Database Syst Rev.* 2003(4):CD004514.

46. Adachi S, Kawamoto T, Otsuka M, Todoroki T, Fukao K. Enteral vitamin B12 supplements reverse postgastrectomy B12 deficiency. *Ann Surg.* 2000;232(2):199-201.

47. Weale AR, Edwards AG, Bailey M, Lear PA. Intestinal adaptation after massive intestinal resection. *Postgrad Med J.* 2005;81(953):178-184.

48. Uchida H, Yamamoto H, Kisaki Y, Fujino J, Ishimaru Y, Ikeda H. D-lactic acidosis in short-bowel syndrome managed with antibiotics and probiotics. *J Pediatr Surg.* 2004;39(4):634-636.

49. Gaon D, Garmendia C, Murrielo NO, et al. Effect of Lactobacillus strains (L. casei and L. Acidophillus Strains cerela) on bacterial overgrowth-related chronic diarrhea. *Medicina.* 2002;62(2):159-163.

50. Stotzer PO, Blomberg L, Conway PL, Henriksson A, Abrahamsson H. Probiotic treatment of small intestinal bacterial overgrowth by Lactobacillus fermentum KLD. *Scand J Infect Dis.* 1996;28(6):615-619.

51. Ziegler TR, Evans ME, Fernandez-Estivariz C, Jones DP. Trophic and cytoprotective nutrition for intestinal adaptation, mucosal repair, and barrier function. *Annu Rev Nutr.* 2003;23:229-261.

52. Kinross JM, Markar S, Karthikesalingam A, et al. A meta-analysis of probiotic and synbiotic use in elective surgery: does nutrition modulation of the gut microblome improve clinical outcome? *J Parenter Enteral Nutr.* Mar 2013;37(2):243-253.

53. Husebye E. The pathogenesis of gastrointestinal bacterial overgrowth. *Chemotherapy.* 2005;51(Suppl 1):1-22.

54. Guarner F, Malagelada JR. Gut flora in health and disease. *Lancet.* 2003; 361(9356):512-519.

55. Neut C, Bulois P, Desreumaux P, et al. Changes in the bacterial flora of the neoterminal ileum after ileocolonic resection for Crohn's disease. *Am J Gastroenterol.* 2002;97(4):939-946.

56. Nagle D, Pare T, Keenan E, Marcet K, Tizio S, Poylin V. Ileostomy pathway virtually eliminates readmissions for dehydration in new ostomates. *Dis Colon Rectum.* 2012;55(12):1266-1272.

57. Beyer P. Medical nutrition therapy for lower gastrointestinal tract disorders. In: Maham L, Escott-Stump S, eds. *Krause's Food , Nutrition, and Diet Therapy.* 11th ed. New York: Elsevier; 2004:705-737.

58. Kahl S, Malfertheiner P. Exocrine and endocrine pancreatic insufficiency after pancreatic surgery. *Best Pract Res Clin Gastroenterol.* 2004;18(5): 947-955.

59. Shaib W, Mitchell K, Saif MW. Amelioration of symptoms and reduction of VIP levels after hepatic artery chemoembolization in a patient with sandostatin resistant VIPoma. *Yale J Biol Med.* 2010;83(1):27-33.

60. Igo T, Igarashi H, Jensen RT. Pancreatic neuroendocrine tumors: clinical features, diagnosis and medical treatment advanced. *Best Pract Res Clin Gastrolenrerol.* 2012;26(6):737-753.

61. Schneider PD. Preoperative assessment of liver function. *Surg Clin North Am.* 2004;84(2):355-373.

62. Marchesini G, Marzocchi R, Noia M, Bianchi G. Branched-chain amino acid supplementation in patients with liver diseases. *J Nutr.* 2005; 135(6 Suppl):1596S-1601S.

63. Fuhrman MP, Charney P, Mueller CM. Hepatic proteins and nutrition assessment. *J Am Diet Assoc.* 2004;104(8):1258-1264.

64. Als-Nielson B, Koretz R, Kjaergard L, Gluud C. Branched-chain amino acids for hepatic encephalopathy. *Cochrane Database of Systematic Reviews.* 2005.

65. Poon RT, Fan ST. Perioperative nutritional support in liver surgery. *Nutrition.* 2000;16(1):75-76.

66. McLarty AJ, Deschamps C, Trastek VF, Allen MS, Pairolero PC, Harmsen WS. Esophageal resection for cancer of the esophagus: long-term function and quality of life. *Ann Thorac Surg.* 1997;63(6):1568-1572.

67. Israel A, Sebbag G, Fraser D, Levy I. Nutritional behavior as a predictor of early success after vertical gastroplasty. *Obes Surg.* 2005;15(1):88-94.

68. Chaudhri S, Brown L, Hassan I, Horgan AF. Preoperative intensive, community-based vs. traditional stoma education: a randomized, controlled trial. *Dis Colon Rectum.* 2005;48(3):504-509.

69. Ikeuchi H, Yamamura T, Nakano H, Kosaka T, Shimoyama T, Fukuda Y. Efficacy of nutritional therapy for perforating and non-perforating Crohn's disease. *Hepatogastroenterology.* 2004;51(58):1050-1052.

70. Huhmann M, August D. Surgical Oncology. In: Marion M, Roberts S (eds) *Clinical Nutrition for Oncology Patients.* Boston, MA: Jones and Bartlett; 2009:101-136.

Nutritional Management of the Pediatric Oncology Patient

Danielle Fatemi, MS, RDN, LD
Pamela Sheridan-Neumann, MPH, RDN, LD

Introduction

Good nutrition is essential for the normal growth and development of children. Cancer interrupts growth through a variety of metabolic and treatment effects that reduce appetite and intake. Chemotherapy, radiotherapy and surgery also may promote gastrointestinal side effects that result in nutrient malabsorption, fluid losses and electrolyte imbalances, leaving a child feeling weak and fatigued. A potential consequence of these effects is malnutrition, which can reduce response to treatment, increase infection risk, and compromise quality-of-life. Identifying early signs of malnutrition and providing proactive nutrition intervention may limit the degree and effects of this condition. This chapter reviews pediatric nutrition needs, nutrition risk screening and assessment of the pediatric cancer patient, the effects of malnutrition and the importance of maintaining nutritional status during cancer treatment.

Statistics

Less than 1% of all cancers occur in children; in 2013 about 11,630 pediatric cancer diagnoses are expected in the United States (U.S.) and about 1,310 children are expected to die from cancer (1). The most common childhood cancers (2) are listed in Table 1.

Five-year survival rates of prominent childhood cancers have significantly improved over the past three decades. Surveillance Epidemiology and End Results (SEER) data indicate that five-year survival rate increased from 63% in 1975-1979 to 79% in 1995-1999 (3). Survival is influenced by race (3). SEER data indicate that the five-year survival rate is lower in Hispanic and black children and adolescents (74% and 73%, respectively), compared with 81% of non-Hispanic white children and adolescents (3).

Malnutrition

Cancer and its treatments can lead to a number of adverse effects (4-5) including:
- Anorexia
- Diminished immune response
- Disturbed drug metabolism
- Delayed and compromised wound healing
- Reduced quality of life
- Reduced treatment response
- Reduced survival

Malnutrition also may affect long-term effects of childhood cancer, which include slow or stunted growth and development as well as compromised bone health, eating behaviors and quality of life (6-8). Treatments used for osteosarcoma, acute lymphoblastic leukemia (ALL), retinoblastoma, soft tissue sarcoma, Wilms' tumor and stem cell transplants have been associated with

Table 1: Prevalence of Common Childhood Cancers (2)

Cancer Type	Percent of Childhood Cancers	Origin and Comments
Leukemia	34%	Cancers of bone marrow and blood
Brain and nervous system	27%	Cancers of the brain and spinal cord
Neuroblastoma	7%	Develops in nerve cells in infancy
Wilms tumor	5%	Usually originates in one kidney around age 3 or 4

Lymphoma:
  Hodgkin
  Non-Hodgkin
	
	4%
	4%
		Affects lymph system
		Usually occurs in young adults
		Usually occurs in young children

Rhabdomyosarcoma	3%	Originates in cells that develop into skeletal muscle
Retinoblastoma	3%	Cancer of the eye; usually occurs at age 2, and rarely over age 6

Bone Cancers:
  Osteosarcoma
  Ewing sarcoma
	
	3%
	1%
		Originate where bone is growing fast
		Usually occurs in teens
		Usually occurs in young teens

bone pain, short status, osteoporosis, osteonecrosis and joint stiffness in long term survivors (4,8). A review of 97 survivors of a variety of childhood cancers found reduced bone mineral density and greater risk of fracture after trauma; proposed etiologies included poor nutrition, steroid treatment, radiation dose and altered vitamin D and mineral metabolism (9). Reports show that vitamin D deficiency in children may be as high as 30% to 50% with lower levels seen more often in the U.S. and higher levels seen in Canadian children (10). Given the importance of nutrition and the pivotal role of calcium and vitamin D status in bone health, it is important to implement nutrition intervention to help prevent these consequences.

Children are more susceptible to malnutrition because of their rapid growth, smaller reserves, higher relative needs per weight as compared with adults and greater resting energy expenditure (REE) (11). For the same reasons, they also are more susceptible to protein depletion and are more likely to develop malnutrition during a critical illness (11). Malnutrition has been reported in up to 50% of hospitalized children, including children hospitalized for cancer treatment, but its actual incidence may be underrecognized (12-13). Incidence of malnutrition also may be under-reported because of body composition changes in children with cancer; a large tumor burden, hepatosplenomegaly and ascites can result in a stable weight that masks loss of true body mass (14).

Defining malnutrition in children has proved to be challenging, resulting in a range of definitions (4,12). This lack of consensus has hindered studies examining prevalence and effects of malnutrition, as different criteria result in different outcomes. Historically, malnutrition has been assessed by comparisons to reference data for growth standards, although some clinicians prefer to use weight changes (4). In addition, a new classification scheme for malnutrition has been proposed (12) and the Subjective Global Assessment (SGA) has been modified and validated for use in children (15). Table 2 lists a variety of standards used to diagnose malnutrition.

A multidisciplinary pediatric work group under the auspices of the American Society of Enteral and Parenteral Nutrition (A.S.P.E.N.) (12) proposed a new classification scheme for malnutrition. It considers chronicity, etiology, mechanisms of nutrient imbalance and severity

of malnutrition as well as its impact on outcomes. It primarily utilizes quantifiable and objective measures including anthropometric data. By including etiological details in the definition of malnutrition (e.g., chronic versus acute; illness-related versus behavioral or environmental), the authors propose that interventions will be more specific and likely to promote relevant outcomes. The working group specified five domains as being integral to the evaluation of pediatric malnutrition: anthropometric parameters, growth, chronicity of malnutrition, etiology, and pathogenesis. Table 3 provides this practical scheme to define pediatric malnutrition.

In 2007 Secker and Jeejeebhoy validated the Subjective Global Nutritional Assessment for use in children, using a population of surgical patients. Because the pediatric field interprets SGA as meaning 'small for gestational age', the authors have renamed this tool as the Subjective Global Nutritional Assessment (SGNA) (15). This tool combines clinical judgment with objective criteria to determine a global rating of nutritional status. The authors developed guidelines for performing SGNA and a rating form that was published in 2012 by the Journal of the Academy of Nutrition and Dietetics (18). When completed, the clinician has a score indicative of normal nutrition status, moderate malnutrition or severe malnutrition. The rating form (Figure 1), is used to track data, which can then be used in decision making when determining nutrition interventions.

Cachexia

Cachexia is defined as the loss of both lean and fat mass seen in the context of an illness, including cancer (4,11,13,19-21). While weight loss is the most common symptom, in children the hallmark outcome is growth failure as the result of anorexia, inflammation and altered carbohydrate, fat and protein metabolism. The normal metabolic response to reduced intake is a reduction in protein turnover to help preserve lean body mass. In cachexia, protein turnover accelerates, contributing to muscle breakdown (4,11, 19-21). Nutrition impact symptoms may contribute to weight loss by reducing intake. Chapter 12, *Symptom Management of Cancer Therapies*, provides strategies to limit or control the severity of nutrition impact symptoms that can occur during cancer treatments. However, an increase in energy intake alone does not reverse the underlying metabolic abnormalities of cachexia (4,19-21). A number

Table 2: Select Methods Used to Diagnose Malnutrition in Children

Group or Author	Diagnostic Criteria	Definitions
WHO (16)	Height for age (HFA) z scores between -2 and -3 Height for age (HFA) z scores < -3	Moderate Stunting Severe Stunting
WHO (16)	Weight for height (WFH) z scores between -2 and -3 Weight for height (WFH) z scores < -3	Moderate Wasting Severe Wasting
Waterlow (17)	Uses Weight for age (WFA) to determine mild (80-90% WFA), moderate (70-79% WFA) and severe (<70% WFA) wasting	Wasting
Bauer et al. (4)	Weight Loss >5%	Acute malnutrition
Bauer et al (4)	Height-for-age value (HFA) <5%th percentile	Chronic malnutrition

Table 3: Practical Scheme for Pediatric Malnutrition Definition (12)

Chronicity	Suggested Criteria for Degree of Malnutrition (Anthropometry in Relation to Reference Curves)	Etiology of Energy, Protein, and/or Micronutrient Imbalance	Inflammatory State (CRP, Cytokines)	Pathogenetic Mechanism (Resulting in Nutrition Intake < Requirement)	Outcomes Affected
Acute (<3 months' duration)	Mild malnutrition or at risk of malnutrition (z score <-1)	Illness related Specify disease(s)	Present Usually severe or moderate in acute illness and mild in chronic illness	Starvation (decreased nutrient intake) This may be disease-related food deprivation or behavioral/social (not disease related)	Muscle weakness Include muscle loss Lean body mass depletion
Chronic (3 months or longer)	Moderate (z score between -2 and -3)	Not illness related; behavioral, socioeconomic	Absent Usually in malnutrition that is not related to illness but secondary to starvation from decreased intake/ delivery	Hypermetabolism (increased energy requirement)	Cognitive/developmental delay/deficit
	Severe (z score <-3)			Uncompensated nutrient losses (malabsorption) Inability to assimilate nutrients	Immune dysfunction Others: delayed wound healing, infections, ventilator dependence, longer hospital/ICU stay, etc.

Mehta NM, Corkins MR, Lyman B, et al. *J Parenter Enteral Nutr,* 37(4):460-481, © 2013. American Society for Parenteral and Enteral Nutrition.
Reprinted by Permission of SAGE Publications

Table 4: Energy Need Equations and Recommendations for Normal Weight Children

Energy Need	Description	Males	Females
BMR	Essential physiologic needs	**Indirect Calorimetry** is recommended for overweight children **DRI equation** (27): see equations in Box 1 **WHO** for children 10-18 years (26): REE=12.2 x wt + 746 **Harris Benedict** (26) for ages 10-18 REE= 66.47+13.75 x Wt + 5.0 x Ht - 6.76 x age **Schofield** for children 10-18 years (26) BMR = (Wt only):13.4 x Wt + 693	**Indirect Calorimetry** is recommended for overweight children **DRI equation** (27): see equations in Box 1 **WHO** for children 10-18 years (16): REE = 17.5 x wt + 651 **Harris Benedict** (26) for ages 10-18 REE: 655.10 + 9.56 x Wt + 1.85 x Ht – 4.68 x age **Schofield** for children 10-18 years (26) BMR (Wt only): 17.7 x Wt + 659
Activity Level	Hospitalized Sitting Quietly	1.1-1.2 x BMR	
Growth	Organ maturation and tissue deposition	Highly variable according to age; may be as high as 35% of energy requirements in term neonates	
Other Considerations	Surgery	Immediate post-op needs increase after surgery but that period is short; there is rarely a practical value in using other than usual needs.	

Figure 1: Pediatric SGNA Rating Form

Consider severity and duration of changes, as well as recent progression when rating each item.			
NUTRITION-FOCUSED MEDICAL HISTORY	**SGNA SCORE**		
	Normal	**Moderate**	**Severe**
Appropriateness of Current Height for Age (stunting) a) Height percentile: _____ ☐ ≥ 3rd centile ☐ just below 3rd centile ☐ far below 3rd centile			
b) Appropriate considering mid-parental height[a]?: ☐ yes ☐ no			

c) Serial growth[b]:   ☐ following centiles
            ☐ moving upwards on centiles
            ☐ moving downwards on centiles (gradually or quickly)			

Appropriateness of Current Weight for Height (wasting) Ideal Body Weight = _____ kg Percent Ideal Body Weight: __ __ __ % ☐ >90% ☐ 75-90% ☐ <75%			

Unintentional Changes in Body Weight
a) Serial weight[b]:   ☐ following centiles
            ☐ crossed ≥ 1 centile upwards
            ☐ crossed ≥ 1 centile downwards			

b) Weight loss: ☐ < 5% usual body weight
            ☐ 5-10% usual body weight
            ☐ >10% usual body weight			

c) Change in past 2 weeks: ☐ no change ☐ increased ☐ decreased			

Adequacy of Dietary Intake
a) Intake is: ☐ adequate
            ☐ inadequate - hypocaloric
            ☐ inadequate - starvation (ie, taking little of anything)			

b) Current intake versus usual: ☐ no change ☐ increased ☐ decreased			
c) Duration of change: ☐ < 2 weeks ☐ ≥ 2 weeks			

Gastrointestinal Symptoms
a) ☐ no symptoms
   ☐ one or more symptoms; not daily
   ☐ some or all symptoms; daily			

b) Duration of symptoms: ☐ < 2 weeks ☐ ≥ 2 weeks			

Functional Capacity (nutritionally related)
a) ☐ no impairment, energetic, able to perform age-appropriate activity
   ☐ restricted in physically strenuous activity, but able to perform play and/or
     school activities in a light or sedentary nature; less energy; tired more
     often
   ☐ little or no play or activities, confined to bed or chair > 50% of waking
     time; no energy; sleeps often			

b) Function in past 2 weeks: ☐ no change ☐ increased ☐ decreased			
Metabolic Stress of Disease ☐ no stress ☐ moderate stress ☐ severe stress			

[a]Mid-parental height: Girls: subtract 13 cm from the father's height and average with the mother's height. Boys: add 13 cm to the mother's height and average with the father's height. Thirteen cm is the average difference in height of women and men. For both girls and boys, 8.5 cm on either side of this calculated value (target height) represents the 3rd to 97th percentiles for anticipated adult height. (29)

[b]30% of healthy term infants cross one major percentile and 23% cross two major percentiles during the first 2 years of life, typically towards the 50th percentile rather than away from it. This is normal seeking of the growth channel.

Figure 3. Pediatric Subjective Global Nutritional Assessment (SGNA) rating form. *(continued on next page)*

PHYSICAL EXAM	SGNA SCORE		
	Normal	Moderate	Severe
Loss of subcutaneous fat ☐ no loss in most or all areas ☐ loss in some but not all areas ☐ severe loss in most or all areas			
Muscle Wasting ☐ no wasting in most or all areas ☐ wasting in some but not all areas ☐ severe wasting in most or all areas			
Edema (nutrition-related) ☐ no edema ☐ moderate ☐ severe			

GUIDELINES FOR AGGREGATING ITEMS INTO GLOBAL SCORE

In assigning an overall global score, consider all items in the context of each other. Give the most consideration to changes in weight gain and growth, intake, and physical signs of loss of fat or muscle mass. Use the other items to support or strengthen these ratings. Take recent changes in context with the patient's usual/chronic status. Was the patient starting off in a normal or nutritionally-compromised state?

Normal/Well nourished
This patient is growing and gaining weight normally, has a grossly adequate intake without gastrointestinal symptoms, shows no or few physical signs of wasting, and exhibits normal functional capacity. Normal ratings in most or all categories, or significant, sustained improvement from a questionable or moderately malnourished state. It is possible to rate a patient as well nourished in spite of some reductions in muscle mass, fat stores, weight and intake. This is based on recent improvement in signs that are mild and inconsistent.

Moderately malnourished
This patient has definite signs of a decrease in weight and/or growth, and intake and may or may not have signs of diminished fat stores, muscle mass and functional capacity. This patient is experiencing a downward trend, but started with normal nutritional status. Moderate ratings in most or all categories, with the potential to progress to a severely malnourished state.

Severely malnourished
This patient has progressive malnutrition with a downward trend in most or all categories. There are significant physical signs of malnutrition—loss of fat stores, muscle wasting, weight loss >10%—as well as decreased intake, excessive gastrointestinal losses and/or acute metabolic stress, and definite loss of functional capacity. Severe ratings in most or all categories with little or no sign of improvement.

	Normal	Moderate	Severe
OVERALL SGNA RANKING			

Figure 3. Pediatric Subjective Global Nutritional Assessment (SGNA) rating form. *(continued)*

Reprinted from *J Acad Nutr Diet*, 2012, 112(3), Secker D, Jeejeebhoy KN. How to perform subjective global nutritional assessment in children, 424-431, 2012, with permission from Elsevier

of therapies including use of megestrol acetate and omega-3 fatty acids are being investigated for their effects on cachexia. Megestrol acetate has shown promise in controlling symptoms of cachexia but has had no affect on survival or quality of life (22). A randomized double-blind trial examining effect of a high protein beverage supplemented with omega-3 fatty acids demonstrated an increase in lean body mass and quality of life, but a large multicenter double-blind placebo-controlled trial did not find it successful (23).

Energy Needs

Data regarding energy needs of children with cancer is inconsistent. Energy requirements per kg are significantly greater for children than for adults because of their lower fat reserves and rapid growth rate, but needs for children with cancer may be greater, lower, or similar to needs of healthy children. Energy needs are influenced by diagnosis, stage of disease and treatment status. Most children with leukemia may have near normal REE at diagnosis and during anti-cancer treatment, while those with a large tumor burden or with solid tumors may have higher energy needs (24-25).

Energy is needed to support essential physiologic processes, also known as basal metabolic rate (BMR). Activity level (estimated as 1.1-1.2 x BMR for hospitalized patients), growth, catch-up growth and failure-to-thrive also must be included in a needs estimate (26).

REE is used in place of BMR in equations, though it may be approximately 9% less than BMR and represents baseline needs while asleep (26). Table 4 summarizes common equations and considerations for estimating energy needs of normal weight children and is followed by Box 1, which provides the Estimated Energy Requirements (EER) developed by the Food and Nutrition Board, Institute of Medicine for boys and girls of various age groups.

Recommendation:

Because of research inconsistencies, usual energy needs per age should be assumed, suggesting that the DRIs may be the most appropriate tool for estimating energy needs in normal weight children with cancer.

Box 1: Dietary Reference Intakes for Estimated Energy Requirements (EER) for Children (27)

EER for Ages 0 – 36 months:

Estimated Energy Requirements for ages 0 through 36 months reflect needs for TEE plus energy deposition associated with growth and have been developed by the Food and Nutrition Board of the Institute of Medicine (27):

Age (gender-neutral recommendations)	EER (= TEE + energy deposition)
0-3 months	(89 x weight [kg] − 100) + 175 kcal
4-6 months	(89 x weight [kg] − 100) + 56 kcal
7-12 months	(89 x weight [kg] − 100) + 22 kcal
13-36 months	(89 x weight [kg] − 100) + 20 kcal

EER for Boys Ages 3 – 8 Years:

Estimated Energy Requirements for boys ages 3 through 8 years reflect needs for TEE plus energy deposition associated with growth (21):

Boys ages 3 to 8 years: EER = 88.5 − (61.9 x age [y]) + PA* x (26.7 x weight [kg] + 903 x height [m]) + 20 kcal

*PA = physical activity coefficient for boys:

PA = 1.00 if physical activity level (PAL) is estimated to be ≥ 1.0 < 1.4 (sedentary)

PA = 1.13 if physical activity level (PAL) is estimated to be ≥ 1.4 < 1.6 (low active)

PA = 1.26 if physical activity level (PAL) is estimated to be ≥ 1.6 < 1.9 (active)

PA = 1.42 if physical activity level (PAL) is estimated to be ≥ 1.9 < 2.5 (very active)

EER for Girls Ages 3-8 Years

Estimated Energy Requirements for girls ages 3 through 8 years reflect needs for TEE plus energy deposition associated with growth (21):

Girls: EER = 135.3 − (30.8 x age [y]) + PA* x (10.0 x weight [kg] + 934 x height [m]) + 20 kcal

*PA = physical activity coefficient for girls:

PA = 1.00 if physical activity level (PAL) is estimated to be ≥ 1.0 < 1.4 (sedentary)

PA = 1.16 if physical activity level (PAL) is estimated to be ≥ 1.4 < 1.6 (low active)

PA = 1.31 if physical activity level (PAL) is estimated to be ≥ 1.6 < 1.9 (active)

PA = 1.56 if physical activity level (PAL) is estimated to be ≥ 1.9 < 2.5 (very active)

EER for Boys Ages 9-18 Years:

Estimated Energy Requirements for boys ages 9 through 18 years reflect needs for TEE plus energy deposition associated with growth (21):

Boys ages 9 to 18 years: EER = 88.5 − (61.9 x age [y]) + PA* x (26.7 x weight [kg] + 903 x height [m]) + 25 kcal

*PA = physical activity coefficient for boys:

PA = 1.00 if physical activity level (PAL) is estimated to be ≥ 1.0 < 1.4 (sedentary)

PA = 1.13 if physical activity level (PAL) is estimated to be ≥ 1.4 < 1.6 (low active)

PA = 1.26 if physical activity level (PAL) is estimated to be ≥ 1.6 < 1.9 (active)

PA = 1.42 if physical activity level (PAL) is estimated to be ≥ 1.9 < 2.5 (very active)

EER for Girls Ages 9-18 Years:

Estimated Energy Requirements for girls ages 9 through 18 years reflect needs for TEE plus energy deposition associated with growth (21):

Girls: EER = 135.3− (30.8 x age [y]) + PA* x (10.0 x weight [kg] + 934 x height [m]) + 25 kcal

*PA = physical activity coefficient for girls:

PA = 1.00 if physical activity level (PAL) is estimated to be ≥ 1.0 < 1.4 (sedentary)

PA = 1.16 if physical activity level (PAL) is estimated to be ≥ 1.4 < 1.6 (low active)

PA = 1.31 if physical activity level (PAL) is estimated to be ≥ 1.6 < 1.9 (active)

PA = 1.56 if physical activity level (PAL) is estimated to be ≥ 1.9 < 2.5 (very active)

Overweight Children

For children and adolescents less than 20 years of age, BMI-for-age growth charts developed by the Centers for Disease Control and Prevention (CDC) are used to diagnose overweight and obesity (26,28). BMI-for-age at or above gender-specific 95th percentile reflects obesity and BMI between the 85th and 95th percentile reflects an overweight status (28). The prevalence of overweight and obesity in children and adolescents has increased over the past several decades. According to the CDC, since 1980 obesity prevalence among children and adolescents has almost tripled. Approximately 17% (or 12.5 million) of children and adolescents aged 2-19 years are obese (29). Obesity is a common finding in survivors of ALL, in particular among those who received cranial irradiation. REE in this population is normal and evidence does not suggest an excessive intake. It is assumed that excess weight gain reflects reduced energy expenditure in this population (30).

The 2005 Dietary Reference Intakes for Energy recommend specific equations for weight maintenance in overweight youth ages 3-18 (27). These equations do not include a growth component, and are summarized in Box 2.

Box 2: Dietary Reference Intakes for Estimating Energy Requirements (EER) for Overweight Children (27)

EER for Overweight Boys Ages 3 Through 18 Years:
TEE = 114 − (50.9 × age [y]) + PA* × (19.5 × weight [kg] + 1161.4 × height [m])
*PA is the physical activity coefficient:
PA = 1.00 if PAL is estimated to be ≥ 1.0 < 1.4 (sedentary)
PA = 1.12 if PAL is estimated to be ≥ 1.4 < 1.6 (low active)
PA = 1.24 if PAL is estimated to be ≥ 1.6 < 1.9 (active)
PA = 1.45 if PAL is estimated to be ≥ 1.9 < 2.5 (very active)

EER for Overweight Girls Ages 3 Through 18 Years:
TEE = 389 − (41.2 × age [y]) + PA* × (15.0 × weight [kg] + 701.6 × height [m])
*PA is the physical activity coefficient:
PA = 1.00 if PAL is estimated to be ≥ 1.0 < 1.4 (sedentary)
PA = 1.18 if PAL is estimated to be ≥ 1.4 < 1.6 (low active)
PA = 1.35 if PAL is estimated to be ≥ 1.6 < 1.9 (active)
PA = 1.60 if PAL is estimated to be ≥ 1.9 < 2.5 (very active)

Recommendation:

The above formulas for overweight girls and boys ages 3 to 18 are considered appropriate for baseline needs for overweight children with cancer unless contraindicated by factors found during a nutrition assessment.

Catch-up Growth

The need for catch-up growth is evaluated in a number of ways (31-32):

- Weight-for-stature below 5th percentile on the WHO or CDC clinical growth charts
- Weight or height deficit of more than 2 percentiles from usual percentile channel on the WHO or CDC clinical growth charts
- Weight-for-length less than the 5th percentile or less than 80% of IBW for height per the WHO clinical growth charts
- Body mass index less than 5th percentile on the CDC clinical growth charts

Estimated energy (EE) needs for catch-up growth (kcal/kg/d) = [calories required for age (kcal/kg/d) × ideal weight for age (kg)]/ [actual weight (kg)].

Children with Amputations

The following formula should be used to calculate IBW adjusted for amputation (IBW_{adj}) (27): IBW_{adj} (kg) = Current Weight (kg) x 100/100-% Amputation. For children with amputations who weigh more than 120% of IBW, an adjusted body weight ($A_{dj}BW$) is used in place of IBW_{adj}, as indicated in the following formula: $A_{dj}BW$ (kg) = [(Actual Weight (kg) − IBW_{adj}) x 0.25] + IBW_{adj}

For children with amputations, calculate the IBW using the method above and then adjust this weight for the body part that has been amputated. Table 5 lists amputation sites and the estimated percentage of total body weight contributed by each body part (34).

Table 5: Percentage of Total Body Weight of Various Body Parts (27)

Body Part	Percentage of Total Body Weight
Entire Arm	5
Upper Arm	2.7
Forearm	2.3
Hand	0.7
Entire Leg	16
Upper Leg	10.1
Lower Leg	5.9
Foot	1.5

Protein Needs

The 2005 Dietary Reference Intakes for protein for children (Table 6) were intended for healthy children (27). There is agreement that protein turnover during cancer treatment increases, possibly triggered by inflammation, and promotes a loss of muscle mass. The Children's Oncology Group (COG) states that cancer treatment may increase protein needs by 50% (35). Serum albumin and prealbumin values may indicate depleted protein stores, however these values can be influenced by stress, inflammation, hydration status, and renal and liver function, and should be interpreted cautiously. These levels should be monitored, and when indicated, clinicians should consider alternate tools such as nitrogen balance studies to help assess protein status and the adequacy of protein intake. Protein

Table 6: DRIs for Protein Intake for Children (27)

Age	Adequate Intake (AI)	RDA for boys and girls	RDA for boys	RDA for girls
0-6 months	1.52/g/kg			
7-12 months		1.2 g/kg/d (~ 11 g/d)		
1-3 years		1.05 g/kg/d (~ 13 g/d)		
4-8 years		0.95 g/kg/d (~ 19 g/d)		
9-13 years		0.95 g/kg/d (~ 34 g/d)		
14-18 years			0.85 g/kg/d (~ 52 g/d)	0.85 g/kg/d (~ 46 g/d)

Table 7: Holliday Segar Method for Estimating Fluid Maintenance Needs (35)

Weight (kg)	Fluid Needs
1-10 kg	100 mL/kg (equal to 100 X kg)
11-20 kg	1000 mL for the first 10 kg + 50 mL/kg/day for each additional kg between 11 and 20 kg
>20 kg	1500 mL for the first 20 kg + 20 mL/kg/day for each additional kg over 20 kg

intake should be adjusted as needed to promote anabolism. Table 6 provides DRIs for protein for pediatric age and gender groups.

Fluids

Adequate hydration is essential for good health. Hydration status represents a net balance of intake and output. In cancer patients that balance may be affected by intravenous fluid administration, which increase intake, and losses from fever, vomiting and diarrhea. RDs should routinely assess fluid status by monitoring intake and output records and conditions that influence fluid balance. Thirst is the most common symptom of dehydration. In moderate or severe dehydration heart rate may increase and urine output will decrease. The most common method for estimating fluid maintenance needs in children is the Holliday Segar Method, which is provided in Table 7 (36).

Micronutrient Requirements

Dietary Reference Intakes (DRIs) recommend safe and effective intake ranges (for every age group) for maintaining adequate vitamin and mineral status, and Upper Intake Levels (UL) that identify highest intakes associated with minimal health risk. Insufficient micronutrient intake can impair growth and result in nutrient deficiency-related diseases. The American Academy of Pediatrics (AAP) does not recommend vitamin supplementation for healthy children older than 1 year of age, instead stating that a varied diet is the best source of vitamins. Nevertheless, 34% of almost 11,000 children examined during the 1999-2004 NHANES survey took a multivitamin (MVI) supplement during the previous 30 days (37). AAP does recommend vitamin supplementation for children with chronic disease, eating disorders, malabsorption, liver disease, obese children in weight loss programs and those with food insecurity (38). In general, it is recommended that the DRIs/RDAs be used as a guide for meeting age-appropriate micronutrient needs and that vitamin-mineral supplements (when used) should provide 100% of estimated needs unless a nutrition assessment indicates otherwise.

Calcium and vitamin D may be two micronutrients of concern for pediatric oncology patients because a child's bone health may be compromised during the course of cancer treatment (39). The AAP does recommend that all infants, including those who are exclusively breastfed, consume 400 IU vitamin D daily (40-41). Infant formulas are required to provide from 40 to 100 IU vitamin D per 100 kcal of formula, which provides a minimum of 400 IU per Liter of formula. Most formula-fed infants will ingest this amount or more daily, thus meeting the vitamin D intake goal. Vitamin D content of breast milk is low, so all exclusively breast fed infants should receive 400 IU vitamin D per day from a supplement. The AI and RDA for calcium and vitamin D for children can be found in tables 8 and 9. Unless diagnosed with iron deficiency anemia, iron supplementation is not recommended for children undergoing multiple blood transfusions during treatment.

Table 8: Daily Vitamin D Requirements (RDAs) (40-41)

Age	Vitamin D
1-12 months*	400 IU (10 mcg)
1-13 years	600 IU (15 mcg)
14-18 years	600 IU (15 mcg)

*Adequate Intake (AI)

Cancer Treatments for Children

Chemotherapy, radiation therapy and surgery are associated with numerous nutritional consequences. The following information summarizes some of them. For a complete review of these therapies and their nutritional effects, please refer to Chapter 11.

Chemotherapy Related Consequences

There are numerous nutritional consequences associated with chemotherapeutic agents that can affect metabolism or cell

Table 9: Daily Calcium Requirements (RDAs) (41-42)

Age	Calcium
0-6 months*	200 mg
7-12 months*	260 mg
1-3 years	700 mg
4-8 years	1,000 mg
9-18 years	1,300 mg

*Adequate Intake (AI)

reproduction and result in gastrointestinal (GI) side effects. Adverse effects arising from treatment depend on the drug type, dosage, duration of treatment, rate and mode of drug excretion and individual susceptibility (43).

Radiation Related Consequences

In addition to treating malignant cells, radiation therapy can damage healthy tissue within the irradiated field. Early side effects of radiation therapy are generally related to the specific site being irradiated and may include diarrhea, mucositis, nausea and vomiting (43). Radiation therapy can cause cumulative fatigue (fatigue that increases with time), which also can diminish appetite and overall oral intake. Latent effects (e.g., side effects occurring 3 months or longer after treatment has been completed) vary, depending on the location of the cancer and the age of the child, and can include cognitive impairment, altered bone development and growth, learning and hearing impairment, neuroendocrine problems and secondary malignancies (44). In some instances, side effects of radiation therapy may not manifest for up to 10 years after treatment.

Surgery Related Consequences

Side effects of cancer-related surgery may include postoperative ileus, nausea and vomiting, maldigestion, malabsorption and alterations in substrate metabolism. Surgery also can result in localized effects that may alter the child's ability to consume sufficient oral intake, resulting in inadequate energy, protein, and micronutrient intake (13-14).

Nutrition Risk Screening and Assessment

Nutrition Risk Screening

The purpose of nutrition risk screening is to identify patients at risk of acute malnutrition, nutrient deficiencies, and chronic malnutrition

or stunted growth. Screening should be a quick and efficient process that can be completed by para-professionals as well as professionals. Because few screening tools have been validated in the pediatric population, most tools are institution specific. Many institutions emphasize nutrition screening for all children with cancer at the time of diagnosis and throughout their treatment. Nutrition issues considered important to screening include weight history, presence of current nutrition impact symptoms such as anorexia and nausea, and food security. Pediatric cancer diagnoses with high and low nutritional risk are listed in Table 10.

Nutrition Assessment

Nutrition assessment is significantly more involved and time-consuming than risk screening, and must be conducted by a credentialed nutrition professional (i.e., RD/RDN). It is the process of evaluating anthropometric, dietary, gastrointestinal and medical data as well as functional capacity and metabolic stress to diagnose nutrition problems. Nutrition assessment is ongoing; Table 11 suggests timelines for various conditions.

Evaluations integral to nutrition assessment include (4,12,15,18,45-46):

Medical History

- Review current, acute, past, and chronic health issues. Pay particular attention to gastrointestinal problems including constipation, diarrhea, and indicators for fat malabsorption as well as gastrointestinal symptoms indicative of digestive and absorptive disorders.

Nutrition Focused Physical Examination

- Evaluate overall physical appearance (e.g., cachexia, obesity and hydration status including ascites) as well as signs and symptoms of wasting and nutrient deficiencies.

Biochemical Data

- Though hepatic protein levels are flawed indicators for malnutrition, monitor their serial levels as indicators for healing and recovery. Monitor complete blood counts to help evaluate malnutrition (e.g., low hemoglobin and hematocrit levels may decrease following a period of inadequate protein intake and also are indicative of anemia). Assess iron status via ferritin level, though ferritin also may drop due to inflammation. Evaluate labs relevant to each diagnosis.

Table 10: Pediatric Cancers with High and Low Nutrition Risk (45)

High Risk Pediatric Cancers	Low Risk Pediatric Cancers
Wilms' Tumor (stages III & IV, unfavorable history and relapsed disease)	Acute lymphocytic leukemia with good prognosis
Neuroblastoma (stages III & IV)	Non-metastatic solid tumors
Metastatic solid tumors	Advanced diseases in remission during maintenance treatment
Non-Hodgkin Lymphoma (stages III & IV and relapsed disease)	
Acute Myelogenous leukemia and chronic myelogenous leukemia (newly diagnosed, relapsed)	
Medulloblastoma and other brain tumors	

Table 11: Suggested Pediatric Nutrition Assessment and Reassessment Timelines

Conditions	Assessment/Care Plan	Reassessment
Nutrition support (enteral, parenteral)	Within 24 hours	Minimum one to two times per week with follow-up/intervention as necessary
Hematopoietic Stem Cell Transplant (Initial)		
Weight Loss (3%-5% in past month)		
Weight-For-Length < 10%ile	Within 48 hours	Minimum one time per week
BMI-For-Age <10%ile		
Nothing by mouth (NPO) > 3 days	Within 72 hours	Minimum one time per week
Non-chemotherapy-induced nausea/vomiting/diarrhea		
Mucositis/oral aversion/feeding issues		
Modified Diet		
New Diagnosis		

Anthropometric Measurements

- Evaluate height, weight, mid-upper-arm circumference, mid-upper-arm muscle circumference, and triceps skinfold thickness. Though arm anthropometry is an inexpensive and time-efficient method to assess body composition, it is prone to interpersonal inconsistencies. The institution should have an in-house certification system in place to ensure that RDs are proficient at conducting these measurements.
- Use BMI standards to assess weight.
- Use 2006 WHO charts to assess and track growth of children up to 2 years of age and measured in the supine position for length.
- For children and adolescents use 2000 CDC charts to assess and track growth of children measured via standing height (age 2-20). These charts are recommended over the WHO charts because they do not require transitions between charts as a child ages.
- Use z scores to report anthropometric variables, and obtain z scores from reference and age appropriate growth curves.
- Assess dynamic changes in growth over time and consider a decrease of more than 1 z score problematic.

Dietary Intake Assessment

- Conduct and evaluate a diet history to assess macro- and micronutrient adequacy, adherence to recommended medical nutrition therapy, understanding of recommended therapeutic diets, nutrition support and food safety recommendations. Assess use of functional foods within a diet. Assess use of dietary supplements (e.g., kind, dose, frequency of use) including vitamin, mineral, herbal and botanical supplements.

Medical Tests

- Consider using nitrogen balance studies to assess protein metabolism. Gastrointestinal tests are useful for assessing gastric emptying and steatorrhea though fecal fat tests requiring a high fat diet for three days are usually unnecessary and quite cumbersome and uncomfortable for patients. Other tests relevant to specific diagnoses also are valuable, and are dependent on the diagnosis and medical condition.

Resources for conducting a nutrition assessment:

- 2006 WHO growth charts http://www.who.int/childgrowth/standards/chart_catalogue/en/
- 2000 CDC growth charts http://www.cdc.gov/growthcharts/
- ADA Pocket Guide to Pediatric Nutrition Assessment (2007), available through the Academy of Nutrition and Dietetics, includes information on laboratory assessment, anthropometric assessment and macronutrient and micronutrient requirements.
- 2013 Position of the Academy of Nutrition and Dietetics on Functional Foods
- 2009 Position of the Academy of Nutrition and Dietetics on Nutrient Supplementation
- Natural Medicines Database

Nutrition assessment should be repeated throughout a child's hospital admission to monitor nutritional status, efficacy of nutrition interventions and the need to revise the nutrition care plan.

Integrative Oncology

Many children with cancer are using integrative oncology therapies, sometimes referred to as complementary and alternative medicine (CAM), to reduce symptoms, cope with life-threatening illness and improve overall well-being. Integrative oncology therapies include the use of acupuncture, massage, imagery, energy healing, herbal therapies and nutritional supplements in addition to conventional cancer care. Few studies have examined integrative therapies for safety and efficacy in the pediatric oncology population due to small patient sample sizes and limited reporting of its use (47-48). Health professionals should ask patients and their caretakers in a nonjudgmental way about their use of integrative therapies, and be aware of any potential side effects or interactions with dietary supplements and prescribed drugs. It is also important for RDs/RDNs to counsel patients and their caretakers about the potential benefits and dangers of taking herbal therapies or high dose nutrition supplements. For more information about integrative oncology and dietary supplements, please see Chapters 7 and 8.

Specialized Nutrition Support

Enteral Nutrition

Alternate feeding methods must be considered when a patient is unable to tolerate an oral diet. Enteral nutrition (EN) support has been established as the safest and most effective means of providing alternate nutrition and is preferred to parenteral nutrition (PN) whenever possible (49-50). In addition to being physiologically similar to an oral diet, EN stimulates intestinal mucosa and the immune system, benefits associated with reducing the risk of infection (49-52). When compared with PN, EN is associated with fewer hepatic complications (49-52). Traditional contraindications to EN are similar in adult and pediatric populations and include intractable vomiting and severe diarrhea as well as intestinal obstruction, ischemia, gastrointestinal hemorrhage and peritonitis (11,49-52).

EN has been shown to reverse malnutrition, maintain an acceptable nutritional status and promote growth and development in children with cancer (51). Positive outcomes have been reported for both nasogastric feedings, which are appropriate for up to 3 months, and gastrostomy tube feedings (53-55), which are recommended for children who require enteral support for more than 3 months (53-55). There was concern that neutropenia and thrombocytopenia may increase bleeding risk during tube insertion, but clinical trials have not found these concerns valid (50). Most children with cancer tolerate standard or polymeric formulas, but a full assessment of the individual's medical history is needed to make the appropriate formula choice.

Parenteral Nutrition

PN is indicated when the GI tract cannot be used for a prolonged period (11) and for the following groups (55-57)
- Preterm infants: in the first 3 days of life
- Term infants: in the first 5 days of life
- Children with GI dysfunction due to disease or injury: ≥ 3 days such as intractable vomiting, diarrhea, malabsorption, radiation-induced colitis, post-operative ileus

Short-term use of PN support (less than 7 days) is not generally recommended in any patient population. PN did improve nutrition parameters (e.g., weight, albumin and prealbumin) in a study of children with cancer, but only after 28 days (54). There also is concern that PN may slow the transition to oral intake status/post hematopoietic stem cell transplant, increase infection risk, and increase risk of parenteral nutrition-associated liver disease (PNLD) in pediatric cancer patients (58). If medically feasible, the combined use of PN and EN may alleviate these effects. PNLD is a serious concern of children receiving PN. The use of newly developed intravenous lipid emulsions containing fish oil may reduce the incidence of PNLD. Many of the medications used to treat children with cancer, when combined with PN, can cause biliary dysfunction or steatosis (59). Therefore, having monitoring guidelines regarding the use of PN is invaluable.

When assessing the estimated nutrition needs of overweight and obese children, careful consideration is needed to prevent over- or underfeeding. A.S.P.E.N. has developed guidelines for the nutrition support of hospitalized pediatric patients with obesity (59):
- Body mass index should be used to screen children for obesity.
- Obese pediatric patients may be at increased nutrition risk.
- When possible, energy requirements of obese pediatric patients should be assessed via indirect calorimetry (IC).
- There is no adequate evidence available that justifies use of hypocaloric or hypercaloric feeding during hospitalization of obese children.

Similar to adults, refeeding of previously malnourished patients should proceed cautiously because of the significant risk of diarrhea, vomiting, and circulatory decompensation in the undernourished child. A complete review of nutrition support for the pediatric oncology patient is beyond the scope of this chapter; for more information refer to the A.S.P.E.N. Pediatric Nutrition Support Core Curriculum, which includes the A.S.P.E.N. Pediatric Nutrition Support Handbook, the A.S.P.E.N. Nutrition Support Patient Education Manual and the A.S.P.E.N. Parenteral Nutrition Handbook.

Pediatric Hematopoietic Stem Cell Transplant

Hematopoietic stem cell transplantation (HSCT) is performed to replace defective and diseased bone marrow and to restore immunologic and hematopoietic function. It is a broad treatment category that encompasses transplantation from a variety of sources of hematopoietic stem cells including bone marrow, peripheral blood stem cells and umbilical cord blood. HSCT is a treatment option for children and adolescents with a variety of potentially fatal diseases including both malignant and nonmalignant conditions such as immunodeficiency syndromes, disorders of the bone marrow and inherited metabolic disorders. Table 1 in Chapter 16 outlines these conditions. HSCT offers the only curative option for many of these patients.

There are two types of conditioning regimens: myeloblative and nonmyeloblative. Myloblative regimens include high dose chemotherapy with or without radiation to eliminate disease and ablate bone marrow; nonmyeloblative regimens provide low dose chemotherapy with or without radiation. The HSCT infusion can be autologous, by which the patient receives his or her own cells. Allogenic patients receive cells from another person, related or unrelated. Syngeneic transplant patients receive cells from a genetically identical twin. Donors are selected by multiple factors including human leukocyte antigen (HLA) matching. While full HLA matching is preferred, mismatched donor is appropriate in certain situations. Donor availability and clinical requirements determine the source of cells.

Children undergoing HSCT are at increased risk of malnutrition. Research has shown that greater than 50% of pediatric patients undergoing HSCT were found to have suboptimal nutritional status prior to transplant (61). Suboptimal nutrition prior to HSCT was associated with negative prognostic factors leading to delayed engraftment and post-transplant complications (61). It is essential to closely monitor nutritional status and revise nutrition intervention as needed to assure adequate nutrition support is being provided throughout the transplant process. Nutritional assessment of pediatric patients undergoing HSCT is similar to that of the high risk oncology patient (62). It is critical to assess patient needs, monitor serial anthropometric growth, anticipate nutrition problems, and institute preventative and timely nutrition support (62). The toxicity of the conditioning chemotherapy impacts the integrity of the GI tract causing mucositis, nausea, vomiting, and diarrhea. Symptoms may be further exacerbated by post-transplant complications such as Graft Versus Host Disease (GVHD) of the GI tract and liver, sinusoidal obstructive syndrome (SOS), renal impairment, infections, use of multiple antibiotics, and immunosuppressive medications. Chapter 16 outlines the clinical manifestations and nutritional issues related to GVHD, renal impairment and SOS.

Studies assessing energy requirements for children undergoing HSCT are limited. Based on the current literature, the gold standard for assessing nutritional needs is indirect calorimetry (IC) (63). One study observed decreases in REE following HSCT with an average decrease of 3.4% during each of the first four weeks posttransplant and a trend towards baseline after engraftment (64). PN was provided, and the study proposed that providing an energy intake closer to actual needs might alter body composition changes usually seen in this setting. Results suggested that both groups experienced similar losses of lean body mass and increases in fat mass, as is usually seen after HSCT (65). If unable to use IC, clinical judgment should be used and combined with ongoing nutrition reassessment to monitor for signs of overfeeding and underfeeding. Protein requirements are increased to promote tissue repair and to minimize loss of lean muscle mass. Recommended methods for calculating energy and protein needs for HSCT patients are provided in Table 12. Nutrition support regimens should meet 100% of vitamin and mineral needs (63,66). With increased stool output, zinc status should be monitored and supplementation provided if deficient.

Table 12: Calorie and Protein Requirements for Pediatric HSCT Patients (63,66)

Age	Caloric Needs	Protein Needs (gm/kg/d)
0-12 months	BMR x 1.6-1.8	3
1-6 years	BMR x 1.6-1.8	2.5-3
7-10 years	BMR x 1.4-1.6	2.4
11-14 years	BMR x 1.4-1.6	2
15-18 years	BMR x 1.5-1.6	1.8
>19 years	BEE x 1.5 or 30-35kcal/kg/d	1.5
Post-Engraftment BMR x 1.4-1.6		
BMR: equations in table 4		

Patients undergoing HSCT also are at increased risk for vitamin D deficiency due to the multiple agents that alter bone metabolism. Vitamin D levels should be assessed and supplementation provided as medically indicated (66).

All HSCT patients undergoing an allogeneic transplant should be placed on a neutropenic diet (63); Chapter 16 provides guidelines for this diet. It is also important to follow proper food safety guidelines to minimize any outside sources of bacteria that may cause infection during this process; food safety recommendations also are provided in Chapter 16. In addition to these guidelines, allogeneic transplant patients should avoid all restaurant and fast food until day +100 post-transplant. When excessive diarrhea occurs secondary to complications of HSCT, several dietary modifications, including lactose restrictions, are indicated. Dietary modifications for excessive diarrhea are reviewed in Chapter 16.

The majority of patients undergoing HSCT require nutrition support (63-66). It is important to start the appropriate nutrition intervention as soon as medically feasible to assure adequate nutrition during the post-transplant process. Chapter 16 discusses the relative merits of enteral versus parenteral nutrition for patients undergoing HSCT. Monitoring and evaluating the efficacy of nutrition support in pediatric HSCT patients can be complex. Fluid and electrolyte balance are impacted by multiple factors including type and frequency of nutrition support. Adjustments should be made on a daily basis as needed.

Long-term nutritional issues following HSCT including chronic GVHD, osteoporosis, endocrine complications, iron overload, oral aversion, compromised growth and development are frequent in the pediatric transplant population (67).

References
1. American Cancer Society. What are the key statistics for childhood cancer? http://www.cancer.org/cancer/cancerinchildren/detailedguide/cancer-in-children-key-statistics Last revised 1/18/2013. Accessed 8/20/2013.
2. American Cancer Society. What is cancer in children? http://www.cancer.org/cancer/cancerinchildren/detailedguide/cancer-in-children-types-of-childhood-cancers Last revised 1/18/2013. Accessed 8/20/2013.
3. Batia S. Disparities in cancer outcomes: lessons learned from children with cancer. *Pediatr Blood Cancer*. 2011;56(6):994-1002.
4. Bauer J, Jürgens H, Frühwald MC. Important aspects of nutrition in children with cancer. *Adv Nutr*. 2011;2(2):67-77.
5. Baracos VE, Parsons HA. Metabolism and physiology. In Del Fabbro E, Barabox V, Demark-Wahnefried W, Bowling T, Hopkinson J, Bruera E. *Nutrition and the Cancer Patient*. Oxford University Press; 2010. p7-18.
6. Robison LL. Long-term outcomes of adult survivors of childhood cancer. *Cancer*. 2005;104(11Suppl):2557-2564.
7. Mulrooney DA. Surviving childhood cancer. Cure is not enough. *Mini Med*. 2010;93(10):36-39.
8. National Cancer Institute. Late effects of treatment for childhood cancer. http://www.cancer.gov/cancertopics/pdq/treatment/lateeffects/Patient/page8 Last modified 5/23/2013. Accessed 8/20/2013.
9. Hasseling PB, Hough SF, Neil ED, van Riet FA, Beneke T, Wessels G. Bone mineral density in long-term survivors of childhood cancer. *Int J Cancer*. 1998;11:44-47. http://onlinelibrary.wiley.com/doi/10.1002/%28SICI%291097-0215%281998%2978:11%2B%3C44::AID-IJC13%3E3.0.CO;2-A/pdf Accessed 8-24-2013

10. Wacker M, Holick MF. Vitamin D – effects on skeletal and extraskeletal health and the need for supplementation. *Nutrients*. 2013;5(10):111-148.

11. Prieto MB, Lopez-Herce Cid J. Malnutrition in the critically ill child: the importance of enteral nutrition. *Int J Environ Res Public Health*. 2011;8(11):4353-4366.

12. Mehta NM, Corkins MR, Lyman B, et al. Defining pediatric malnutrition: a paradigm shift toward etiology-related definitions. *J Parenter Enter Nutr*. 2013;37(4):460-481.

13. Pietsch JB, Ford C. Children with cancer: measurements of nutritional status at diagnosis. *Nutr Clin Pract*. 2000;15:185-188.

14. Wieman RA, Balistreri WF. Nutrition Support in Children with Liver Disease. In Baker RD, Davis A., eds. *Pediatric Nutrition Support*. Jones and Bartlet Publishers, Inc., Massachusetts. 2007;459-476.

15. Secker DJ, Jeejeebhoy KN. Subjective global nutritional assessment for children. *Am J Clin Nutr*. 2007;85(4):1083-1089.

16. WHO Multicentre Growth Reference Study Group. WHO child growth standards: length/height-for-age, weight-for-age, weight-for-length, weight-for-height and body mass index-for-age: methods and development. Geneva (Switzerland): World Health Organization; 2006.

17. Waterloo JC. Classification and definition of protein-calorie malnutrition. *Br Med J*. 1972;3(5826):566-569.

18. Secker D, Jeejeebhoy KN. How to perform subjective global nutritional assessment in children. *J Acad Nutr Diet*. 2012;112(3):424-431.

19. Argiles JM, Olivan M, Busquets S, Lopez-Soriano FJ. Optimal management of cancer anorexia-cachexia syndrome. *Cancer Manag Res*. 2010;2:27-38.

20. Sala A, Pencharz P, Barr RD. Children, cancer, and nutrition – a dynamic triangle in review. *Cancer*. 2004;100(4):677-687.

21. Picton SV. Aspects of altered metabolism in children with cancer. *Int J Cancer*. 1998;11:62-64.

22. Lesniak W, Bala M, Jaeschke R, Krzakowski M. Effects of megestrol acetate in patients with cancer anorexia-cachexia syndrome- a systematic review and meta-analysis. *Pol Arch Med Wewn*. 2008;118(11):636-644.

23. Feron KC, Von Meyenfeldt MF, Moses AG, et al. Effect of a protein and energy-dense N-3 fatty acid enriched oral supplement on loss of weight and lean tissue in cancer cachexia: a randomized double blind trial. *Gut*. 2003;52(10):1479-1486.

24. Arends J, Zuercher, Dossett A. Non-surgical oncology – Guidelines on parenteral nutrition, chapter 19. Ger Med Sci. 2009;7:Doc09.

25. Kreyman G, Adoph M, Mueller MJ. Energy expenditure and energy intake – Guidelines on Parenteral Nutrition. *GMS Ger Med Sci*. 2009;7:Doc25 DOI: 10.3205/000084

26. Koletzko B, Goulet O, Hunt J, et al. Energy. *J Pediatr Gastroenterol Nutr*. 2005;41(S2):S5-S11.

27. Food and Nutrition Board. Institute of Medicine. Dietary Reference Intakes for Energy, Carbohydrate, Fiber, Fat, Fatty Acids, Cholesterol, Protein, and Amino Acids (Macronutrients). The National Academies Press. Washington, DC. 2005;107-264. www.nap.edu Accessed 8-22-2013.

28. Centers for Disease Control and Prevention. Use and interpretation of the WHO and CDC growth charts for children from birth to 20 years in the United States. http://www.cdc.gov/nccdphp/dnpa/growthcharts/resources/growthchart.pdf Accessed 8-22-2013

29. Centers for Disease Control and Prevention. Overweight and obesity. http://www.cdc.gov/obesity/childhood/index.html

30. Sklar CA, Mertens AC, Walter, et al. Changes in body mass index and prevalence of overweight in survivors of childhood acute lymphoblastic leukemia: role of cranial irradiation. *Med Pediatr Oncol*. 2000;35(2):91-95.

31. Corrales KM, Utter SL. Growth failure. In: Samour PQ King K. *Handbook of Pediatric Nutrition*, 3rd ed. Sudbury, Mass: Jones and Bartlett Publishers; 2005: 391-406.

32. American Academy of Pediatrics. Failure to thrive (pediatric undernutrition). In: Kleinman RE, ed. *Pediatric Nutrition Handbook*. 5th ed. Elk Grove, Ill: American Academy of Pediatrics; 2004:443-457.

33. Jeong SJ. Nutritional approach to failure to thrive. Kor J Pediatr. Nutritional approach to failure to thrive. *Korean J Pediatr*. 2011;54(7):277-281.

34. Osterkamp LK. Current perspectives on assessment of human body proportions of relevance to amputees. *J Am Diet Assoc*. 1995;95(2):215-218.

35. Nieuwoudt CH. Nutrition and the child with cancer: where do we stand and where do we need to go? *S Afr J Clin Nutr*. 2011;24(3):S23-S26.

36. Meyers RS. Pediatric fluid and electrolyte therapy. *J Pediatr Pharmacol Ther*. 2009;14(4):204-211.

37. Institute of Medicine. Dietary Reference Intakes: Water, Potassium, Sodium, Chloride, and Sulfate. Washington, DC: National Academy Press; 2005.

38. Shaikh U, Byrd RS, Auinger P. Vitamin and mineral supplement use by children and adolescents in the 1999-2004 National Health and Nutrition Examination Survey. *Arch Pediatr Adolesc Med*. 2009. 163(2):150-157.

39. Kleinman RE. Pediatric Nutrition Handbook. 5th ed. Elk Grove Village, IL: American Academy of Pediatrics; 2004.

40. Institute of Medicine, Food and Nutrition Board. Dietary Reference Intakes for Calcium and Vitamin D. Washington, DC: National Academy Press; 2010.

41. Gartner LM, Greer FR. Section on Breastfeeding and Committee on Nutrition. American Academy of Pediatrics. Prevention of rickets and vitamin D deficiency: new guidelines for vitamin D intake. *Pediatrics*. 2003;111(4 Pt 1):908-910

42. Wagner CL, Greer FR. Prevention of rickets and vitamin D deficiency in infants, children, and adolescents. Clinical Report. *Am Acad Pediatrics*. www.pediatrics.org/cgi/doi/10.1542/peds.2008-1862. Accessed 8-20-2013.

43. Sheard NF, Clark NG. Nutrition management of pediatric oncology patients. In: Baker SB, Baker RD, Daved A eds *Pediatric Enteral Nutrition*. New York: Chapman & Hall; 1994:387-398.

44. Barale KV, Charuhas PM. Oncology and marrow transplantation. In: Samour PQ, Helm KK, Lang CE, eds. *Handbook of Pediatric Nutrition*. 2nd ed. Gaithersburg, Md: American Society for Parenteral and Enteral Nutrition; 1999:465-491.

45. Armenian SH, Meadows AT, Bhatia S. Late effects of childhood cancer and its treatment. In: Pizzo PA, Poplack DG, eds. *Principles and Practice of Pediatric Oncology, 6th ed*. Philadelphia, Pa: Lippincott Williams & Wilkins; 2010: 1368-1387.

46. Mosby TT, Barr RB, Pencharz PB. Nutritional assessment of children with cancer. *J Ped Oncol Nursing*. 2009;26(4):186-197.

47. Maqbool A, Olsen IE, Stallings VA. Clinical Assessment of Nutritional Status. In Duggan C, Watkins JB, Walker WA. *Nutrition in Pediatrics*, 4th ed., Ontario, Canada: BC Decker Inc; 2008. 5-14.

48. Post-White J. Complementary and alternative medicine in pediatric oncology. *J Pediatri Oncol Nurs*. 2006;23(5):244-253.

49. Axelrod D, Kazmerski K, Iyer K. Pediatric enteral nutrition. *J Parenter Enteral Nutr*. 2006;30 (1 Suppl):S21-S26.

50. Lloyd DA, Powell-Tuck J. Artificial nutrition: principles and practice of enteral feeding. *Clin Colon Rectal Surg*. 2004;17(2);107-118.

51. Ladas E, Sacks N, Brophy P, Rodgers P. Standards of nutritional care in pediatric oncology: results from a nationwide survey on the standards of practice in pediatric oncology: a Children's Oncology Group (COG) Nutrition Committee. *Pediatr Blood Cancer*. 2006;46(3):339-344.

52. Klawitter B. Pediatric enteral nutrition support. In: Nevin-Folino NL, ed. *Pediatric Manual of Clinical Dietetics*. 2nd ed. Chicago, Ill: American Dietetic Association; 2003:471-493.

53. Barron, MA, Duncan DS, Green GJ, et al. Efficacy and safety of radiologically placed gastrostomy tubes in paediatric hematology/oncology patients. *Med Pediatr Oncol*. 2000;34(3).177-182.

54. Aquino VM, Smyrl ES. Enteral nutrition support by gastrostomy tube in children with cancer. *J Pediatr*. 1995;127(1):58-62.

55. ASPEN Board of Directors and the Clinical Guidelines Task Force. Guidelines for the use of parenteral and enteral nutrition in adult and pediatric patients. *J Parenter Enteral Nutr*. 2002;26(1 Suppl):1Sa-138SA.

56. Charuhas PM, Fosberg KL, Bruemmer B, et al. A double-blind randomized trial comparing outpatient parenteral nutrition with intravenous hydration: effect on resumption with intravenous hydration: effect on resumption of oral intake after marrow transplantation. *J Parenter Enteral Nutr*. 1997;21(3):157-161.

57. Wang TW, Sax HC, Total parenteral nutrition: effects on the small intestine. In: *Clinical Nutrition Parenteral Nutrition*. 3rd ed. Philadelphia, Pa: WB Saunders; 2001:353-365.

58. Christensen ML, Hancock ML, Gattuso J, et al. Parenteral nutrition associated with increased infection rate in children with cancer. *Cancer.* 1993;72(9):2732-2738.

59. Kumpf VJ. Parenteral nutrition-associated liver disease in adult and pediatric patients. *Nutr Clin Pract.* 2006;21(3):279-290.

60. Jesuit C, Dillon C, Compher C, American Society for Parenteral and Enteral Nutrition (A.S.P.E.N.) Board of Directors, Lenders CM. A.S.P.E.N. clinical guidelines: nutrition support of hospitalized pediatric patients with obesity. *J Parenter Enteral Nutr.* 2010;34(1):13-20. http://www. guideline.gov/content.aspx?id=38685

61. White M, Murphy AJ, Hastings Y, et al. Nutritional status and energy expenditure in children pre-bone-marrow-transplant. *Bone Marrow Transplant.* 2005:35(8):775-779

62. Bowman LC, Williams R, Sanders M, Ringwald-Smith K, Baker D, Gajjar A. Algorithm for nutritional support: experience of the Metabolic and Infusion Support Service of St. Jude Children's Research Hospital. *Int J Cancer Suppl.* 1998;11:76-80.

63. Charuhas PM, Lipkin A, et al. Hematopoietic stem cell transplantation. In: Merritt RJ, DeLegge M, Holcomb B, et al, eds. *The A.S.P.E.N. Nutrition Support Practice Manual.* 2nd ed. Silver Spring, MD: American Society for Parenteral and Enteral Nutrition; 2005.

64. Duro D, Bechard LJ, Feldman HA, et al. Weekly measurements accurately represent trends in resting energy expenditure in children undergoing hematopoietic stem cell transplantation. *J Parenter Enteral Nutr.* 2008;32(4):427-432.

65. Sharma TS, Bechard LJ, Feldman HA. Effect of titrated parenteral nutrition on body composition after allogeneic hematopoietic stem cell transplantation in children: a double-blind, randomized, multicenter trial. *Am J Clin Nutr.* 2012;95(2):342-351.

66. Charuhas PM. Nutrition management of oncology and marrow/ hematopoietic stem cell transplantation. In: Amorde-Spalding K, Nieman L, eds. *Pediatric Manual of Clinical Dietetics.* 2nd ed. Update. Chicago, IL: American Dietetic Association; 2008:175-184.

67. Atkinson SA, Halton JM, Bradley C, Wu B, Barr, RD. Bone and mineral abnormalities in childhood acute lymphoblastic leukemia: influence of disease, drugs and nutrition. *Int J Cancer Suppl.* 1998;11:35-39.

Medical Nutrition Therapy for Hematopoietic Cell Transplantation

Paula Charuhas Macris, MS, RD, CSO, FADA

Introduction

Hematopoietic cell transplantation (HCT) is an established therapeutic modality for select hematologic malignancies and solid tumors, as indicated in Table 1 (1). It also is a treatment for certain nonmalignant conditions such as disorders of the bone marrow, immunodeficiency syndromes and inborn errors of metabolism (1).

Table 1: Malignant Diseases Treated by Hematopoietic Cell Transplantation (1)

Hematologic Malignancies Treated with HCT	Acute leukemia Chronic leukemia Lymphoma Hodgkin's disease Myelodysplastic syndrome Multiple myeloma
Solid Tumors Treated With HCT	Advanced stage neuroblastoma Refractory Ewing's sarcoma

Worldwide, over 50,000 transplants are performed each year (2). Survival varies greatly and is dependent upon the malignancy and stage of disease, donor type, graft source, patient age and intensity of conditioning therapy. In recent years, there has been a steady increase in survival rates due to improved techniques in donor matching as well as advances in supportive care and infection control.

The objective of HCT is to replace the malignant or defective marrow in order to restore normal hematopoiesis and immunologic function (3). Treatment consists of a preparative regimen that includes cytotoxic chemotherapy to eradicate the malignant cells; it also may include total body irradiation (TBI).

There are two types of HCT preparative conditioning regimens: myeloablative and nonmyeloablative. Myeloablative regimens utilize both high dose chemotherapy and radiation to eliminate disease and ablate bone marrow. Nonmyeloablative regimens deliver low dose chemotherapy and radiation. An intravenous infusion of autologous (patient's own), syngeneic (genetically identical twin) or allogeneic (from a human leukocyte antigen related or unrelated donor) stem cells follows the preparative regimen. The source of the stem cells may be bone marrow, peripheral blood or umbilical cord blood (1).

After the stem cell infusion, the patient is often neutropenic (decreased number of neutrophils in the blood) and immunosuppressed for a period of two to three weeks until engraftment. Complete immune function does not return for months after transplantation.

Nutrition Assessment

A nutrition assessment should be completed pre-transplant and repeated periodically throughout the transplant course. Assessment involves a comprehensive evaluation that identifies high-risk patients who may require aggressive nutrition intervention. Components of nutrition assessment include a nutrition history, anthropometric assessment and analysis of biochemical indices in addition to a medical history and a review of medical systems.

Nutrition History

The nutrition history includes an assessment of the following oral and gastrointestinal (GI) symptoms: xerostomia, chewing or swallowing difficulties, mucositis or esophagitis, taste alterations, heartburn or reflux, nausea and vomiting, early satiety, anorexia and altered bowel habits. Current dietary modifications and special diets, use of vitamin, mineral and herbal supplements, and food allergies or intolerances should also be evaluated. Stage of eating development and use of infant formulas should be assessed in pediatric patients.

Anthropometry

Baseline measurements, including height and weight, should be obtained to determine body surface area, which is often used to calculate medication dosages and fluid needs. For children <24 months of age, length and occipital frontal circumference should be measured. Baseline anthropometry provides landmark data for serial measurements. The patient's weight history, including pre-illness weight, and weight changes during prior therapy, should be evaluated. Ideal weight should then be determined. For patients >120% ideal weight, an adjusted weight should be calculated (4): Adjusted weight = (Actual weight – ideal weight) (0.25) + ideal weight.

Arm anthropometry may also be obtained during the initial evaluation to assess somatic muscle protein and adipose reserves. Measurements can be useful for assessing changes in body composition (e.g., lean body mass) if they are obtained sequentially and compared over time (5).

Biochemical Indices

Obtain and assess the following chemistries: electrolytes, glucose, renal parameters, liver function enzymes, visceral proteins, blood lipids, ferritin, and 25-OH vitamin D. Information from baseline laboratory values serves as a guide to decisions about changes in the patient's requirements over time, especially if organ function changes (3).

Other Assessment Tools

The assessment should also include a review of the patient's medical history, physical strength and activity level, organ function and level of pain/pain control.

Nutrient and Fluid Requirements

Nutrient and fluid requirements for patients undergoing HCT are outlined in Table 2 (1,3,6).

Nutrition Support

Oral Feedings

Oral feedings are indicated for patients with a functional GI tract. Historically, HCT recipients have been maintained on diets of low microbial content in an attempt to minimize the introduction of pathogenic organisms. While the protective benefits of a low microbial diet for the HCT population have not been established via clinical trials (7), most transplant centers still utilize some type of neutropenic diet to decrease the risk of foodborne infections (8). Until more research has been conducted, elimination of high-risk foods most commonly associated with foodborne illness, as well as safe food handling, is paramount until all immunosuppression therapy has been discontinued (9). Box 1 provides guidelines for limiting food sources of pathogenic organisms. Websites pertinent to food safety for immunosuppressed individuals are shown at the end of this chapter.

Enteral Nutrition

Enteral nutrition is indicated for patients with a functional GI

Table 2: Nutrient Requirements During Hematopoietic Cell Transplantation (1,3,6)

Nutrient	Requirement	Altered Requirements
Calories	Adults: Basal needs x 1.3-1.5 Adolescents and older children: Basal needs x 1.4-1.6 Young children: Basal needs x 1.6-1.8	Increase: Immediate post-transplant period due to metabolic stress induced by the preparative regimen; fever; infections Decrease: Engraftment; absence of metabolic complications
Protein	Adults: 1.5 g/kg/day 15-18 years: 1.8 g/kg/day 11-14 years: 2.0 g/kg/day 7-10 years: 2.4 g/kg/day Birth-6 years: 2.5-3.0 g/kg/day	Increase: Immediate post-transplant period; corticosteroid treatment; CRRT Decrease: Renal or hepatic dysfunction
Carbohydrate	50-60% total energy support	Decrease: Lower dextrose PN concentration with pre-existing diabetes or hyperglycemia Modify oral carbohydrate intake when insulin required
Fat	Minimum dose: 6-8% total calories Maximum dose: 40% total calories	Increase: When providing lower dextrose PN concentrations Decrease: Hyperlipidemia
Fluids	1-10 kg: 100 mL/kg/day 11-20 kg: 1,000 mL + 50 mL for every kg >10/day 21-40 kg: 1,500 mL + 20 mL for every kg >20/day >40 kg: 1,500 mL/m2 body surface area	Increase: Fever; excessive GI losses; hypermetabolism; high-output renal failure; nephrotoxic medications Decrease: Compromised organ function; iatrogenic fluid overload
Vitamins	Parenteral: A.S.P.E.N guidelines Extra vitamin C to promote tissue recovery after cytoreductive therapy: <31 kg: additional 250 mg/day ≥31 kg: additional 500 mg/day Oral: After PN discontinued, oral vitamin-mineral supplement without iron	Decrease: Discontinue extra vitamin C during presence of elevated serum ferritin (>1,000 mcg/L) to decrease oxidative damage from release of free iron RRT: Oral: standard renal vitamin Parenteral: 1/2 dose standard vitamin package + water soluble vitamins; evaluate need for fat soluble vitamin replacement
Trace minerals and electrolytes	Parenteral: A.S.P.E.N. guidelines Oral: After PN discontinued, oral vitamin-mineral supplement without iron	Increase: Calcium during corticosteroid therapy/osteoporosis (Table 5) Zinc with large-volume diarrhea: 1 mg/100 mL stool output Electrolyte needs may be higher with food-drug interactions Decrease: Iron supplementation contraindicated Eliminate copper and manganese from PN in presence of hepatic dysfunction

tract in whom oral intake is inadequate to meet nutrient needs (9). Challenges to enteral feeding in the early post-transplant period have included GI dysfunction associated with regimen-related toxicities, thrombocytopenia, mucositis and esophagitis, neutropenia, lack of enteral access and patient acceptance (10). Vomiting with dislodgement of nasoenteral tubes (11-12), delayed gastric emptying (13) and poor tolerance of rapid advancement of feeds when transitioning from parenteral nutrition (PN) after myeloablative conditioning (14) have been observed. Weight loss due to inadequate energy support (11), decreased body cell mass (15) and electrolyte and mineral deficiencies (16-17) are other reported complications.

Interest in the use of enteral nutrition has increased in the past decade due to the need to decrease cost and the desire to mitigate the risks associated with PN, especially infection (3). Enteral nutrition should be considered in patients who receive nonmyeloablative conditioning regimens or those receiving myeloablative regimens with a lower GI toxicity profile (14). Other conditions where enteral nutrition support may be a viable option include: low risk HCT (autologous or matched related donor), long-term eating problems after engraftment, resolution of conditioning-related mucositis and esophagitis and adequate platelet recovery (as defined by the institution) (3,14).

Both nasoenteric and enterostomy feeding tubes may be used, however, adequate neutrophil and platelet counts are vital before tube placement. A range of enteral formulas are available and the most appropriate will depend on GI tolerance and organ function. Adult and pediatric semi-elemental formulas, renal formulas and concentrated formulas for cases requiring volume restriction may be administered (1,3). The combined use of enteral feedings with PN is an acceptable and cost-effective alternative (18).

Parenteral Nutrition
Candidates for PN during conventional HCT include patients receiving myeloablative conditioning regimens with a high GI toxicity profile, those with refractory gut GVHD and malnourished patients who cannot obtain adequate nutrient support by enteral nutrition alone (3,9). Early studies suggested that PN support during HCT was associated with improved visceral protein status (19), maintenance of body weight (20) and increased disease-free survival in the allogeneic population (21). More recent studies have shown that PN is associated with hyperglycemia and increased risk of bacteremia, which may result in greater morbidity (10,22). To limit these complications, discontinuing the use of PN is recommended once stem cells have engrafted and regimen-related toxicities have resolved (9).

Several studies have examined the role of glutamine supplementation during HCT. Patients maintained on glutamine-enriched PN solutions have been reported to experience decreased hospital stays and reduced incidence of positive blood cultures (23). Conversely, other clinical trials have described significantly higher relapse rates in patients randomized to receive glutamine

Box 1: Diet Guidelines for Immunosuppressed Patients

Immunosuppression increases susceptibility to food borne illness. Diet guidelines for this condition are intended to minimize the introduction of pathogenic organisms into the GI tract by food while maximizing healthy food options. These guidelines should be coupled with evidence-based food safety recommendations to assure proper food preparation and storage in the home and hospital kitchen. High-risk foods identified as *potential* sources of organisms known to cause infection in immunosuppressed patients are restricted.

In general, autologous transplant patients follow the diet during the first three months after HCT. Allogeneic transplant patients should follow the diet until immunosuppressive therapy (e.g., cyclosporine, tacrolimus, prednisone) is discontinued.

Food Restrictions
- Raw and undercooked meat (including game), fish, shellfish, poultry, eggs, sausage and bacon
- Raw tofu, unless pasteurized or asceptically packaged
- Luncheon meats (including salami, bologna, hot dogs, ham) unless heated until steaming
- Refrigerated smoked seafood typically labeled as lox, kippered, nova-style, or smoke or fish jerky (unless contained in a cooked dish); pickled fish
- Unpasteurized milk and raw milk products, nonpasteurized cheese, and unpasteurized yogurt
- Blue-veined cheeses including blue, Gorgonzola, Roquefort, Stilton
- Uncooked soft cheeses including brie, camembert, feta, farmer's
- Mexican-style soft cheese, including queso blanco and queso fresco
- Cheese containing chili peppers or other uncooked vegetables
- Fresh salad dressings (stored in the grocer's refrigerated case) containing raw eggs or contraindicated cheeses
- Unwashed raw and frozen fruits and vegetables and those with visible mold; all raw vegetable sprouts (alfalfa, mung bean, all other)
- Raw or unpasteurized honey
- Unpasteurized commercial fruit and vegetable juices
- Well water must be boiled for 15-20 minutes and consumed within 48 hours

Source: Courtesy of Medical Nutrition Therapy Services, Seattle Cancer Care Alliance, Seattle, Washington.

supplementation (24-25). Current available evidence does not support the role of glutamine supplementation in HCT recipients. Larger, well-designed studies examining the appropriate timing, duration, and long-term effects on outcome are needed before recommendations can be made (3,23). Chapter 13 provides detailed guidelines on managing PN support.

Monitoring Nutrition Support
Daily monitoring of the patient's medical condition, nutritional status, blood chemistries, and treatment-related symptoms is necessary as changes may require modifications in nutrient and fluid support. During the early post-transplant period (from conditioning through the neutropenic phase), weight and total intake and output volumes should be monitored on a daily basis. Oral and intravenous calorie, protein, and fluid intake levels also should be evaluated daily so that appropriate nutrition support can be provided. Monitoring the patient's oral and GI tolerance is necessary when oral feedings or enteral nutrition support is instituted.

Nutritional Considerations During HCT
Oral and GI Complications
Oral and GI manifestations are frequent complications of HCT.

Chapter 12 describes dietary intervention of common nutrition sequelae (e.g., nausea, mucositis and early satiety) of cancer treatments.

Sinusoidal Obstructive Syndrome (SOS)
Sinusoidal obstructive syndrome (SOS), formerly called veno-occlusive disease, may occur as early as 10-20 days after cytoreduction therapy (26). The incidence varies from zero to as high as 50% in some patient populations (26-27). SOS is characterized by toxic injury to the sinusoidal and venular epithelium (3). Clinical symptoms include: insidious weight gain, ascites, right upper quadrant tenderness and painful hepatomegaly; hyperbilirubinemia and renal dysfunction follow (26). Medical nutrition therapy during SOS includes: concentration of PN fluids as well as medication volumes, and reduction of both oral and intravenous sodium to minimize fluid retention. If serum bilirubin increases to > 10 mg/dL, monitor serum triglyceride level (see Chapter 13 for management suggestions for hypertriglyceridemia). During persistent hyperbilirubinemia (serum bilirubin >10 mg/dL), remove biliary excreted trace elements, copper and manganese from PN (1).

Renal Impairment
Renal impairment may be related to chemotherapeutic agents, TBI, nephrotoxic medications (e.g., antibiotics, calcineurin inhibitors), SOS, intravascular volume depletion, and sepsis (1). Nutrition intervention during renal compromise includes: maximize nutrition support within fluid allowance, correct electrolyte imbalances, and maintain sufficient intravascular volume (14). During continuous renal replacement therapy (CRRT), protein and vitamin needs are altered as shown in Table 2 (1,3,6).

Graft-Versus-Host Disease
Graft-versus-host disease (GVHD) is a T-cell mediated immunologic reaction of engrafted lymphoid cells against the host tissues (28). It remains one of the most daunting complications associated with allogeneic HCT, is associated with significant morbidity and even results in mortality (3). The major target organs affected are the skin, liver and GI tract (28). Measures used to prevent or treat GVHD often include multi-drug immunosuppressive therapies, many of which have nutritional implications (see Table 3) (1).

Clinical GI manifestations of GVHD include: nausea, vomiting, anorexia, diarrhea, and abdominal pain. Voluminous, secretory diarrhea and intestinal bleeding occur in advanced disease (28). Intestinal protein losses and fat malabsorption are also characteristic of the mucosal degeneration associated with intestinal GVHD. In addition to immunosuppressive agents, empiric diet guidelines have been developed and emphasize foods low in lactose, fiber, acid, and fat (29); Table 4 summarizes those guidelines. Patients with steatorrhea, pancreatic insufficiency or liver GHVD often benefit from pancreatic enzyme replacement therapy (1).

Infection
Infection is a major source of morbidity and mortality in HCT patients. Treatment includes antibiotic, antiviral and antifungal

Table 3: Therapies Used for Prophylaxis and Treatment of GVHD (1)

Medication//Therapy	Nutritional Implications
Anti-thymocyte Globulin	Nausea and vomiting; diarrhea; stomatitis
Azathioprine	Nausea and vomiting; anorexia; diarrhea; mucosal ulceration; esophagitis; steatorrhea
Beclomethasone Dipropionate	Xerostomia; dysgeusia; nausea
Budesonide	None known
Corticosteroids	Sodium and fluid retention resulting in weight gain or hypertension; hyperphagia; hypokalemia; skeletal muscle catabolism and atrophy; gastric irritation and peptic ulceration; osteoporosis; growth retardation in children; decreased insulin sensitivity and impaired glucose tolerance resulting in hyperglycemia or steroid-induced diabetes; hyperlipidemia
Cyclosporine	Nausea and vomiting; nephrotoxicity; hypomagnesemia; hyperkalemia
Extra Corporeal Photopheresis (ECP)	Intravenous fluid may be necessary to maintain adequate hydration status; monitor calcium status as the citrate anticoagulant can bind calcium and induce hypocalcemia; ECP may not be possible in presence of significant hypertriglyceridemia
Methotrexate	Nausea and vomiting; anorexia; mucositis and esophagitis; diarrhea; renal and hepatic changes
Monoclonal Antibodies	Nausea; hepatotoxicity
Mycophenolate Mofetil	Nausea and vomiting; diarrhea
Pentostatin	Nausea and vomiting; diarrhea; anorexia
Psoralen + Ultraviolet Light	Nausea; hepatotoxicity
Sirolimus	Hypertriglyceridemia
Tacrolimus	Nausea and vomiting; nephrotoxicity; hypomagnesemia; hyperkalemia
Thalidomide	Constipation; nausea; xerostomia
Ursodeoxycholic acid	Nausea and vomiting; diarrhea; dyspepsia

agents, which may induce oral and GI symptoms that impact nutritional status. Intravenous lipids have been implicated as being immunosuppressive; however, lipids provided during HCT have not increased the incidence of bacterial or fungal infections (30).

Long-term Complications and Management
As advances in technology and supportive care measures have improved, the number of long-term HCT survivors continues to increase. With this growth, a greater emphasis is now being placed on treating long-term complications.

Chronic Graft-Versus-Host Disease
Chronic GVHD develops beyond 80-100 days post-transplant, with increased frequency in transplants from nonidentical related and unrelated donors (31). Nutritional implications associated with

Table 4: Graft Versus Host Disease Diet Progression for Gastrointestinal Symptoms

Phase	Clinical Symptoms	Diet	Clinical Symptoms of Diet Intolerance
1. Bowel rest	• GI cramping • Large volume watery diarrhea • Depressed serum albumin • Severely reduced transit time • Small bowel obstruction or diminished bowel sounds • Nausea and vomiting	**Oral:** NPO **IV:** stress energy and protein requirements	
2. Introduction of oral feeding	• Minimal GI cramping • Diarrhea <500 mL/day • Improved transit time • Infrequent nausea and vomiting	**Oral:** isotonic, low-residue, low-lactose fluids **IV:** as for Phase 1	• Increased stool volume or diarrhea • Increased emesis • Increased abdominal cramping
3. Introduction of solids	• Minimal or no GI cramping • Formed stool	**Oral:** allow introduction of solid foods containing minimal lactose, low fiber, low fat, low total acidity, no gastric irritants **IV:** as for Phase 1	As in Phase 2
4. Expansion of diet	• Minimal or no GI cramping • Formed stool	**Oral:** minimal lactose, low fiber, low total acidity, no gastric irritants; if stools indicate fat malabsorption: low fat diet **IV:** as needed to meet nutrition requirements	As in Phase 2
5. Resumption of regular diet	• No GI cramping • Normal stool • Normal transit time • Normal serum albumin	**Oral:** progress to regular diet; acid foods with meals, fiber-containing foods, lactose-containing foods; order of addition will vary, depending on individual tolerances and preferences; patients without steatorrhea should have fat restriction slowly liberalized **IV:** discontinue when oral intake meets nutrient needs	As in Phase 2

chronic GVHD include: weight gain (due to corticosteroid therapy), weight loss, oral sensitivity to spicy or acidic foods, xerostomia, stomatitis, anorexia, reflux symptoms and diarrhea (32). Regular nutrition monitoring is necessary following discharge from transplant centers.

Osteoporosis
Osteoporosis is a recognized complication of HCT with prevalence as high as 50% as early as one year post-transplant (33-34). Risk factors, such as chemotherapy, TBI, and exposure to calcineurin inhibitors and corticosteroids (used for prophylaxis or treatment of GVHD) all impact bone loss (35). Prevention and management of osteoporosis includes calcium and vitamin D supplementation when dietary intake is inadequate. Calcium requirements are summarized in Table 5 (1). Vitamin D needs are typically based on serum levels. Serum 25-OH vitamin D levels <30 ng/mL or those patients treated with corticosteroids are supplemented at a dose of 1,000-5,000 International Units (IU) per day; a higher dose may be necessary with severe deficiency (<20 ng/mL) or malabsorption syndrome (1,35). Bisphosphonate therapy, in conjunction with calcium and vitamin D supplementation, can reverse bone loss (35-36). Regular weight-bearing and muscle strengthening exercises are also recommended (1,35).

Growth and Development Issues
Compromised growth and development (e.g., decreased growth velocity, growth hormone deficiency and delayed pubertal development) are frequent in the pediatric transplant population (37). An annual evaluation with assessment of growth and development is appropriate for children following HCT.

Endocrine Complications
Endocrine problems are common in long-term transplant survivors. The endocrine system is highly susceptible to damage from high-dose chemotherapy and/or TBI resulting in adverse consequences (38). Metabolic syndrome, characterized by hyperlipidemia, insulin resistance and diabetes mellitus, obesity and hypertension, has been reported in both adult and pediatric transplant populations (39-40). Pediatric HCT survivors are more likely to develop diabetes as well as hypertension than the general population and should be monitored throughout adulthood (41-42). Ongoing dietary surveillance is necessary to help identify, prevent, and correct symptoms associated with metabolic syndrome.

Iron Overload
As HCT patients receive a large number of red cell transfusions during their transplant course, iron overload is a frequent long-term problem

(26). Iron supplementation as well as iron-containing multivitamin-mineral supplements should be avoided during and after HCT (1).

Other Late Effects

Secondary malignancies, ocular complications, avascular necrosis, chronic pulmonary effects, thyroid dysfunction, and gonadal hormone insufficiency are among other complications associated with HCT. A detailed review of these late effects has been published (43).

Conclusion

Optimum nutrition management of the highly complex HCT population is vital owing to the multiple adverse oral and GI complications that result from both the disease and treatment. It is essential for RDs to routinely monitor nutrition status throughout HCT treatment and recovery and to provide ongoing intervention, education and counseling so that prevention or early intervention of nutrition-related problems is possible.

Websites pertinent to food safety for immunosuppressed individuals:

www.seattlecca.org/food-safety-guidelines.cfm

www.fda.gov/downloads/Food/ResourcesForYou/Consumers/SelectedHealthTopics/UCM312761.pdf Accessed June 13, 2013.

References

1. Macris PC (ed). Seattle Cancer Care Alliance. *Hematopoietic Stem Cell Transplantation Nutrition Care Criteria.* 3rd edition. Seattle, WA: Seattle Cancer Care Alliance; 2012.
2. Gratwohl A, Baldomero H, Aljurf M, et al. Hematopoietic stem cell transplantation: a global perspective. *JAMA.* 2010;303(16):1617-1624.
3. Lipkin C, Lenssen P, Dickson BJ. Nutrition issues in hematopoietic stem cell transplantation: state of the art. *Nutr Clin Pract.* 2005;20(4):423-439.
4. Renal Dietitians Dietetic Practice Group Adjustment in body weight for obese patients (Appendix B). In Wiggins KL, ed. *Guidelines for Nutrition Care of Renal Patients.* 3rd ed. Chicago, Il: The American Dietetic Association; 2002;113.
5. Rodgers C, Walsh T. Nutritional issues in adolescents after bone marrow transplant: a literature review. *J Pediatr Oncol Nurs.* 2008;25(5):254-264.
6. Task Force for the Revision of Safe Practices for Parenteral Nutrition: Mirtallo J, Canada T, Johnson D, et al. Safe practices for parenteral nutrition. *J Parent Enteral Nutr.* 2004;28(6):S39-S70.
7. Smith LH, Besser SG. Dietary restrictions for patients with neutropenia: a survey of institutional practices. *Oncol Nurs Forum.* 2000;27(3):515-520.
8. Trifilio S, Helenowski I, Giel M, et al. Questioning the role of a neutropenic diet following hematopoietic stem cell transplantation. *Biol Blood Marrow Transplant.* 2012;18(9):1385-1390.
9. August DA, Huhmann MB, and the Society for Parenteral and Enteral Nutrition (A.S.P.E.N.) Board of Directors. A.S.P.E.N. clinical guidelines: Nutrition support therapy during adult anticancer treatment and in hematopoietic cell transplantation. *J Parent Enteral Nutr.* 2009;33(5)472-500.
10. Thompson JL, Duffy J. Nutrition support challenges in hematopoietic stem cell transplant patients. *Nutr Clin Pract.* 2008;23(5):533-546.
11. Sefcick A, Anderton D, Byrne JL, et al. Naso-jejunal feeding in allogeneic bone marrow transplant recipients: results of a pilot study. *Bone Marrow Transplant.* 2001;28(12):1135-1139.
12. Lenssen P, Bruemmer B, Aker SN, et al. Nutrient support in hematopoietic cell transplantation. *J Parent Enteral Nutr.* 2001;25(4):219-228.

Table 5: Calcium Requirements During Corticosteroid Therapy or Osteoporosis (1)

Age (years)	Calcium (mg/day)
7-12 (months)	600
1-3	1,000
4-8	1,200
>9	1,500

13. Eagle DA, Gian V, Lauwers GY, et al. Gastroparesis following bone marrow transplantation. *Bone Marrow Transplant.* 2001;28(1):59-62.
14. Charuhas PM, Lipkin A, Lenssen P, et al. Hematopoietic stem cell transplantation. In: Merritt R (ed). *The A.S.P.E.N. Nutrition Support Practice Manual.* 2nd edition. Silver Spring, MD: American Society for Parenteral and Enteral Nutrition; 2005:187-199.
15. Szeluga DJ, Stuart RK, Brookmeyer R, et al. Nutritional support of bone marrow transplant recipients: a prospective randomized clinical trial comparing total parenteral nutrition to an enteral feeding program. *Cancer Res.* 1987;47(12):3309-3316.
16. Papadopoulou A, MacDonald A, Williams MD, et al. Enteral nutrition after bone marrow transplantation. *Arch Dis Child.* 1997;77(2):131-146.
17. Langdana A, Tully N, Molloy E, et al. Intensive enteral nutrition support in paediatric bone marrow transplantation. *Bone Marrow Transplant.* 2001;27(7):741-746.
18. Mulder POM, Bouman JG, Gietama JA, et al. Hyperalimentation in autologous bone marrow transplantation for solid tumors. Comparison of total parenteral nutrition versus partial parenteral plus enteral nutrition. *Cancer.* 1989;64(10):2045-2052.
19. Uderzo C, Rovelli A, Bonomi M, et al. Total parenteral nutrition and nutritional assessment in leukaemic children undergoing bone marrow transplantation. *Eur J Cancer.* 1991;27(6):758-762.
20. Yokoyama S, Fujimoto T, Mitomi T, et al. Use of total parenteral nutrition in pediatric bone marrow transplantation. *Nutrition.* 1989;5(1):27-30.
21. Weisdorf SA, Lysne J, Wind D, et al. Positive effect of prophylactic total parenteral nutrition on long-term outcome of bone marrow transplantation. *Transplantation.* 1987;43(6):833-838.
22. Fuji S, Kim SW, Mori S, et al. Hyperglycemia during the neutropenic period is associated with a poor outcome in patients undergoing myeloablative allogeneic hematopoietic stem cell transplantation. *Transplantation.* 2007;84(7):814-820.
23. Crowther M, Avenell A, Culligan DJ. Systemic review and meta-analyses of studies of glutamine supplementation in haematopoietic stem cell transplantation. *Bone Marrow Transplant.* 2009;44(7):413-425.
24. Pytlík R, Benes P, Patorkova M, et al. Standard parenteral alanyl-glutamine dipeptide supplementation is not beneficial in autologous transplant patients: a randomized, double-blind, placebo controlled study. *Bone Marrow Transplant.* 2002;30(12):953-961.
25. Sykorova A, Horacek J, Zak P, et al. A randomized, double blind comparative study of prophylactic parenteral nutritional support with or without glutamine in autologous stem cell transplantation for hematological malignancies – three years' follow-up. *Neoplasma.* 2005;52(6)476-482.
26. McDonald GB. Hepatobiliary complications of hematopoietic cell transplantation, 40 years on. *Hepatology.* 2010;51(4):1450-1460.
27. Hogan WJ, Maris M, Storer B, et al. Hepatic injury after nonmyeloablative conditioning followed by allogeneic hematopoietic cell transplantation: a study of 193 patients. *Blood.* 2004;103(1)78-84.
28. Vogelsang GB, Lee L, Bensen-Kennedy DM. Pathogenesis and treatment of graft-versus-host disease after bone marrow transplant. *Ann Rev Med.* 2003;54:29-52.
29. Gauvreau JM, Lenssen P, Cheney CL, et al. Nutritional management of patients with intestinal graft-versus-host disease. *J Am Diet Assoc.* 1981;79(6):673-677.

30. Lenssen P, Bruemmer B, Bowden RA, et al. Intravenous lipid dose and incidence of bacteremia and fungemia in patients undergoing bone marrow transplantation. *Am J Clin Nutr.* 1998;67(5):927-933.

31. Martin PJ, Rizzo JD, Wingard JR, et al. First- and second-line systemic treatment of acute graft-versus-host disease: recommendations of the American Society of Blood and Marrow Transplantation. *Biol Blood Marrow Transplant.* 2012;18(8):1150-1163.

32. Lenssen P, Sherry ME, Cheney CL, et al. Prevalence of nutrition-related problems among long-term survivors of allogeneic marrow transplantation. *J Am Diet Assoc.* 1990;90(6):835-842.

33. Tauchmanova L, Colao A, Lombardi G, et al. Review: Bone loss and its management in long-term survivors from allogeneic stem cell transplantation. *J Clin Endocrinol Metab.* 2007;92(12):4536-4545.

34. Yao S, McCarthy PL, Dunford LM. High prevalence of early-onset osteopenia/osteoporosis after allogeneic stem cell transplantation and improvement after bisphosphonate therapy. *Bone Marrow Transplant.* 2008;41(4):393-398.

35. McClune B, Majhail NS, Flowers MED. Bone loss and avascular necrosis of bone after hematopoietic cell transplantation. *Semin Hematol.* 2012;49(1):59-65.

36. Carpenter PA, Hoffmeister P, Chesnut CH III, et al. Bisphosphonate therapy for reduced bone mineral density in children with chronic graft-versus-host disease. *Biol Blood Marrow Transplant.* 2007;13(6):683-690.

37. Sanders JE. Growth and development after hematopoietic cell transplant in children. *Bone Marrow Transplant.* 2008;41(2):223-227.

38. Dvorak CC, Gracia CR, Sanders JE, et al. NCI, NHLBI/PBMTC first international conference on late effects after pediatric hematopoietic cell transplantation: endocrine challenges - thyroid dysfunction, growth impairment, bone health, & reproductive risks. *Biol Blood Marrow Transplant.* 2011;17(12):1725-1738.

39. Majhail NS, Flowers ME, Ness KK, et al. High prevalence of metabolic syndrome after allogeneic hematopoietic cell transplantation. *Bone Marrow Transplant.* 2009;43(1):49-54.

40. Oudin C, Simeoni MC, Sirvent N, et al. Prevalence and risk factors of the metabolic syndrome in adult survivors of childhood leukemia. *Blood.* 2011;117(17):4442-4448.

41. Hoffmeister PA, Storer BE, Sanders JE. Diabetes mellitus in long-term survivors of pediatric hematopoietic cell transplantation. *J Pediatr Hematol Oncol.* 2004;26;(2):81-90.

42. Hoffmeister PA, Hingorani SR, Storer BE, et al. Hypertension in long-term survivors of pediatric hematopoietic cell transplantation. *Biol Blood Marrow Transplant.* 2010;16(4):515-524.

43. Carpenter PA. Late effects of chronic graft-versus-host disease. *Best Pract Res Clin Haematol.* 2008;21(2):309-331.

Medical Nutrition Therapy for Brain Tumors

Jeannine Mills, MS, RD, CSO, LD

Thanks to Camilo E. Fadul, MD, Associate Professor of Medicine and of Neurology, Geisel School of Medicine, Dartmouth for providing a technical review of this chapter

Overview

The American Brain Tumor Association (ABTA) defines "cancer" as malignant tissue that "can invade and destroy healthy tissue, and tends to spread to distant locations" (1). Cancers that originate in the brain, called primary brain tumors (PBT), however, rarely spread to distant locations (2-3). The Nutrition Care Manual (NCM) of the Academy of Nutrition and Dietetics (the Academy) defines a benign tumor as one that that does not "penetrate or destroy surrounding tissues" yet in the case of a brain tumor the space taken up by a benign tumor enclosed in the skull can lead to deadly increases in pressure inside the skull and destroy and compress the surrounding normal tissue (3-7). A benign tumor in another part of the body may not necessarily infringe on surrounding structures to the point of being life-threatening. Another unique aspect of brain cancer is the fact that a benign, or non-cancerous, brain tumor can be just as deadly as a malignant tumor (2-3). This is also due to the fact that the location of the tumor may be hard to reach, thus increasing risk of damage to other parts of the nervous system during surgical resection (3). In addition, benign brain tumors are treated with the same modalities as malignant ones thereby blurring the distinction between benign and malignant (2). The National Brain Tumor Society may say it best: "Some benign tumors can be as dangerous as malignant ones" if their location is in a "dangerous or inaccessible location, such as the brain stem…conversely, some malignant tumors can be successfully treated" (8). Furthermore, some tumors within the skull but not originating from brains cells, like tumors of the meninges (menigiomas) are also called brain tumors. Therefore, we define brain tumors as "benign" and malignant tumors within the skull.

Brain Tumor Statistics

Based on 2007-2009 data, the lifetime risk for developing cancer of the brain or other part of the nervous system is 0.62% for men and women combined (9). The NCI predicts 23,130 men and women will be diagnosed with brain cancer and 14,080 will die of this disease in 2013 (10). The SEER (Surveillance, Epidemiologoy, and End Results) database indicates that the five-year survival rate following a diagnosis of PBT and central nervous system tumor (including

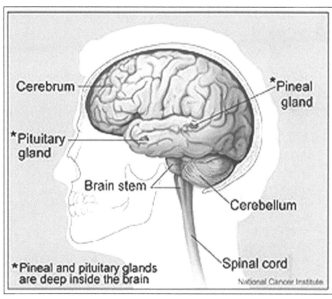

Figure 1: The Brain

Reprinted with permission
The website of the National Cancer Institute (http://www.cancer.gov).

lymphomas, leukemias, tumors of the pituitary and pineal glands, and olfactory tumors of the nasal cavity) is 33.6% for males and 37.0% for females (12).

Characteristics of Primary Brain Tumors

Malignant brain tumors grow rapidly and are invasive to surrounding brain tissue. They can be life-threatening due to their capability of spreading to other parts of the brain and CNS but rarely do they spread beyond brain tissue. Treatment for malignant brain tumors usually requires multiple modalities including surgery, chemotherapy, and radiation therapy (13). Grade I tumors are usually cystic and well defined; their cells are relatively normal in appearance. Grade II tumors are infiltrative but still considered a lower grade. Grades III and IV tumors are higher grades with Grade IV tumors having areas of necrosis. As one would expect, outlook worsens as the grade increases (14-15). Table 1 summarizes common brain tumors and their treatments.

Table 1: Common Primary Brain Tumors and their Treatments (4,8,15-17)

Tumor Type and Grade	Location	Occurrence	Treatment
Astrocytoma cerebrum: Pilocytic Astrocytoma Grade 1	Cerebrum, optic nerve pathways, brain stem, cerebellum	2% of all brain tumors	Surgery and if unable to resect then chemotherapy or radiation therapy
Low Grade Astrocytoma • Grade II	Cerebral hemisphere, brain stem cerebellum	Occur in men and women in their 20's to 50's	Determined by size and location. If unable to resect, then radiation possible. If recurs, then surgery, chemotherapy and/or RT
Anaplastic Astrocytoma • Grade III	Cerebral hemisphere		Surgery and radiation therapy, experimental therapies if tumor continues to grow
Glioblastoma Multiform or Grade IV Astrocytoma		Astrocytes grades II-IV tend to occur in males more than females and most occur in ages 45 and over	Surgery, chemotherapy, radiation therapy
Oligodendroglioma • Grades I-IV		2-4% of all brain tumors, 10-15% of all gliomas. Most common in men and women in their 20s-40s.	Treatment depends on tumor grade. Surgery is standard treatment but can be followed by radiation and chemotherapy for more progressive tumors
Ependymoma • Low grade tumors	i. Supratentorial ii. Infratentorial iii. Myxopapillary		Surgery, radiation sometimes used
Brain Stem Gliomas • Low to high grade	Brain stem	Usually occur in children ages 3-10 years but can occur in adults	Surgery, stereotactic surgery, radiation, and/or chemotherapy
Meningiomas • Grade I is benign • Grade II is also called Atypical Meningioma • Grade III is malignant and is also called Anaplastic Meningioma • Primitive Neuroectodermal Tumors (PNET)	These tumors arise from the meninges which are the membranes covering the brain and spinal cord	Most common in men and women in their 40s and 50s and account for 34% of all primary brain tumors	Surgery, and may involve radiation and/or chemotherapy if the tumor cannot be completely resected Depending on location in brain, some signs of meningioma are dysphagia and loss of taste or smell(13)

Brain Cancer Prevention

According to the American Cancer Society (ACS) "there are no known nutrition risk factors for brain cancer (16). Due to the fact that there have been no identified associations with nutrition and brain tumor prevention, it is not included in current recommendations for diet and physical activity published by the American Cancer Society (ACS) (16). However, there is some evidence to show that in adults a higher antioxidant intake may reduce the risk of developing gliomas (17).

Nutrition Risk Screening and Assessment

Headache is the most common presenting symptom of brain cancer, a symptom that would not trigger a positive nutrition risk screening. In addition, weight loss is rarely a presenting symptom. As a whole, brain tumors are considered low nutrition-risk cancers (18-19). However, medical nutrition therapy (MNT) may be indicated to help manage side-effects of treatment modalities and the tumor itself. Nausea and vomiting frequently occur in cancers located in the brain stem; they also may be caused by the physical location of the tumor in the brain and well as treatments. The nutrition-related effects of the presence of a PBT usually resolve after the tumor has been resected unless surgery is not successful, leading to persistent and worsening symptoms (e.g., nausea, dysphagia, and persistent

cognitive decline). However, chemotherapy and/or radiation therapy also may trigger nausea and vomiting, thus impacting the nutritional well being of the patient. Effects of cancer therapies are thoroughly reviewed in chapter 11 and strategies to manage nutrition impact symptoms (NIS) of cancer therapies are provided in chapter 12.

Primary and metastatic brain tumors occasionally may cause SIADH as a result of an increase in intracranial pressure or from the effects of intracranial disease on the brain. When this occurs it may be important to restrict water intake and provide hypertonic saline if sodium level is exceedingly low (20).

Pretreatment factors such as normal nutrition status and a high Karnofsky Performance Score (KPS) can enable a person to handle brain tumor treatment more successfully (21); the most significant factors associated with longer survival are KPS and age (22). Thus it is important to address any signs of nausea and eating difficulties when they arise in order to maintain an acceptable nutritional status. Pretreatment hyperglycemia is associated with decreased survival as seen in a study that followed patients after surgical resection for malignant astrocytomas (23).

Goals for Nutritional Care of the patient with PBT.

Nutritional goals should be aligned with:

1. Controlling physical symptoms that contribute to nutritional decline from the tumor itself, treatment modalities and NIS;
2. Caregiver support to include helping families cope with day to day living;
3. End of life care.

Abnormal swallowing can occur, and has been associated with reduced coordination and alertness in cases of advanced brain cancer. In a study that examined prevalence and effects of swallowing dysfunction in PBT, swallowing difficulties were more severe than reported by degree of dysphagia, raising the concern for silent aspiration (24). Swallowing evaluation by a speech and language pathologist (SLP) can evaluate this risk. Results of this evaluation may require modifications in food textures, and in some cases consideration of a feeding tube. Chapter 12 provides suggestions for managing NIS, including dysphagia.

Treatment

Nutritional care of the patient undergoing treatment for PBT involves management of NIS including dysphagia, constipation, fatigue, low or increased appetite, xerostomia, hyperglycemia, dysgeusia and ageusia. Chemotherapy, radiation therapy, anti-seizure medications, and intermittent or prolonged use of steroids can impact the nutritional status of the patient with PBT. Drug nutrient interactions should also be considered when caring for the patient with brain tumor. Table 2 summarizes adverse effects of treatments used to treat PBT.

Corticosteroid Treatment

Glucocorticoids have long been used as a brain cancer treatment to reduce brain swelling and risk of encephalopathy (26). These drugs also may reduce disease and treatment related nausea. Side effects of corticosteroids are well described and include excessive weight gain with cushionoid appearance, truncal obesity, hyperglycemia, immunosuppression and muscle weakness. This class of drugs also reduces bone mineralization and can lead to osteoporosis. Dexamethasone and phenytoin are commonly prescribed together; if enteral nutrition support is involved in care it is important to check for interactions between enteral formulas and phenytoin. Depending upon the patient's disease status and length of time these medications are given, nutrition intervention may be indicated for hyperglycemia and obesity. The RD also may need to educate the patient on calcium and vitamin D needs and bone health.

Caregiver support

The burden of PBT includes poor long-term survival, cognitive impairment, seizures, paralysis and permanent neurological damage, causing considerable burden on patients and caregivers alike. Role changes within the family may include taking on new responsibilities in feeding, shopping, and caring for children. The RD may be instrumental in providing caregiver guidance on cooking and shopping and community resources for food provisions, which may alleviate added stress.

Table 2: Adverse Effects of Medications Used to treat PBTs (25)

Brand name	Purpose	Adverse Effects
Keppra®	Antiepileptic	Diarrhea, dizziness, fatigue, headache, loss of appetite
Depakote®	Antiepileptic	Diarrhea, headache, loss of appetite or increased appetite, constipation, loss of bladder control, weight gain or weight loss
Topamax®	Antiepileptic	Altered taste, diarrhea or constipation, joint or muscle aches, headache, indigestion, tremors, decreased appetite, nausea
Dilantin®	Antiepileptic	Constipation, excessive hair growth on face or body, difficulty sleeping, nausea
Tegretol®	Antiepileptic	Increased sweating, nausea, clumsiness or unsteadiness, diarrhea or constipation, headache
Trileptal®	Antiepileptic	Stomach upset, tremors, insomnia, constipation or diarrhea, decreased appetite, nervous, headahce
Neurontin®	Antiepileptic	Dizziness, fatigue, nausea, slurred speech, fatigue, tremors, weight gain, constipation, difficulty walking or controlling muscles
Dexamethasone®	Corticosteroid, treats inflammation	Headache, nausea, vomiting, skin problems-acne, thin and shiny skin, weight gain
Temodar®	Chemotherapy	Nausea, taste changes, difficulty sleeping, dry skin, hair loss, headache, loss of appetite Take ondansetron one hour prior to Temodar®; do not eat for 2 hours prior to taking Temodar®
Avastin®	Monoclonal antibody	Constipation, diarrhea, dry skin, headache, loss of appetite, nausea, vomiting
PCV Procarbazine (generic) Lomustine (generic) Vincristine (generic)	Chemotherapy	Follow low tyramine diet when on procarbazine Constipation, diarrhea, dark skin color, hair loss, dizziness, dry mouth Hair loss, decreased appetite, nausea, vomiting Diarrhea, hair loss, jaw pain, decreased appetite
Camptosar®	Chemotherapy	Constipation, hair loss, headache, decreased appetite, nausea, vomiting, stomach upset
Radiation Therapy		Xerostomia, taste changes, loss of appetite, fatigue

Dealing with patient depression and other negative emotions can be as challenging for the care provider as the physical care of the patient (27). In addition, adverse emotions can have detrimental effects on appetite and consequently lead to weight loss. Cognitive decline with PBT may be linked to tumor progression as much as it is to treatment modality. Managing challenging neurocognitive changes including memory loss, impaired reasoning and processing, attention deficits, and problems with the ability to sequence or perform multiple tasks at one time can be difficult. There may be impulsive behavior of patients with frontal lobe lesions in which some patients may overeat simply due to repetitive desire to eat the same foods each day in same and often larger volumes (22,27).

Novel Nutritional Treatment Modalities

Both the Ketogenic Diet (KGD) and short-term calorie restriction target energy metabolism, angiogenesis, and inflammation through the IGF-1 signaling. This in turn reduces the availability of glucose and glutamine. Some patients turn to alternative cancer treatment and diets such as the Budwig Diet; this diet is addressed in chapter 8.

The Ketogenic Diet

Researchers are keenly interested in the use of a ketogenic diet in the treatment of brain cancer (28-34). Under normal circumstances brain cells prefer glucose as their main energy source. If glucose is not available, normal brain cells can easily shift to ketones for energy (28-34). Malignant brain cells are unable to shift to ketones for energy; they rely solely on glucose in order to live. This is thought to be at least partially due to dysfunctional mitochondria in the malignant cells (30). With this principle in mind, in 1995 Nebling and colleagues published a landmark study that employed the use of the ketogenic diet in two human subjects who had unresectable high grade gliomas and had each already undergone extensive radiation and chemotherapy. The objective of the study was to cut off the food supply to the malignant cells to slow or halt further growth. The ketogenic diet was successful in long-term management of the tumors for these two subjects (31). In 2010 a published case report from Zuccoli and colleagues revealed the success of a 65-year-old female with glioblastoma who began consuming a ketogenic diet prior to standard treatment. She continued the diet throughout the treatment period. Ten weeks after the diet was stopped an MRI confirmed a recurrence of the tumor (34). Further animal studies have continued to show success with a ketogenic diet in controlling gliomas in mice (30-31).

There are some researchers who firmly believe that treatment of PBT should predominately take on a metabolic approach by targeting both glucose and glutamine. Seyfried and associates maintain that the ketogenic diet "can represent a viable non-toxic option for the management of malignant brain cancer" (34). Unfortunately, it may be difficult for patients to adhere to the diet and compliance can be an issue. Maintaining ketones in ranges needed to target angiogenesis and control tumor growth can be challenging. Schmidt and associates evaluated the safety and feasibility of the ketogenic diet in advanced cancer patients (35). The most frequent side effects were constipation, vomiting, decreased energy, and hunger. They did not study the effect of the diet on the disease itself. Limitations of this study included patients with advanced disease. There is a need for well-designed, large and randomized studies to judge effects of KGD on quality of life and cancer progression before we can confidently recommend this diet for PBT patients.

Calorie Restriction

Short-term starvation (STS) studies have shown protection in some models from chemotoxicity. Increased efficacy of chemotherapeutic agents has been demonstrated in mouse models including neuroblastoma and GBM. Caloric restriction may have a role in decreasing circulating IGF-1 and may protect against cancer. In research involving mice it has been shown that a calorie-restricted diet can reduce the tumor grade by slowing tumor growth, decreasing tumor density, and decreasing angiogenesis and the ability for the tumor to invade surrounding tissue (36). While a calorie-restricted diet may lead to ketosis the mechanisms for effecting tumor growth with a calorie-restricted diet are thought to be related to "protective mechanisms" induced by the effect of mild hunger on the immune system (37). Long term calorie restriction has no significant effect on IGF-1 and may exacerbate weight loss (38).

End of Life Care

Both physical and neurological symptoms at end of life require recognition and intervention by a multidisciplinary team. A systematic review retrospectively examined the records (2005-2011) of patients with malignant PBT and described the psychosocial and supportive needs of patients and their care providers during the last weeks of life (23).

- Drowsiness and loss of consciousness occurred in 85-90%
- Weakness 62-80%
- Seizures 30-56%
- Headaches 53-62%
- Fatigue 25-67%
- Dysphagia 10-79%

End of life decisions regarding tube feedings occurred in 13% of patients and hydration needs were addressed in 87% of patients in the study (28). RDs can be an integral member on the team in guiding patients and their families through these difficult decisions.

Conclusion

Medical Nutrition Therapy should be individualized for each patient depending on the location of the tumor and any physiological effects that interfere with nutrition risk or status, the patient's nutrition status or medical comorbidities prior to diagnosis, and any nutrition-related treatment side effects. Scientific evidence for any particular nutrients or phytochemicals for the prevention of a brain tumor have yet to be determined. There has been research for the use of the ketogenic diet or a combination of a low calorie ketogenic diet as well as calorie restriction to manage malignant brain tumors but the evidence is limited and further studies are warranted. Supportive care is essential for patients with PBT and their caregivers. Exceptional care involves the resourcefulness and compassion of the multidisciplinary team, which should include an RD.

References

1. American Brain Tumor Association. *Dictionary for Brain Tumor Patients, 4th ed.* Des Plaines, IL: American Brain Tumor Association; 2002.
2. Black P. Brain Tumor Society. Brain tumor facts and statistics 2006. http://www.tbts.org. Accessed July 18, 2006.
3. Brain and Spinal Cord Tumors in Adult. What are brain and spinal cord tumors? http://www.cancer.org/Cancer/BrainCNSTumorsinAdults/DetailedGuide/brain-and-spinal-cord-tumors-in-adults-what-is-cancer. Last Medical Review May 9,2011. Accessed May 5, 2012.
4. Oncology General Guidelines. Nutrition Care Manual. Academy of Nutrition and Dietetics. http://nutritioncaremanual.org/content.cfm?ncm_content_id=83960. Accessed April 23, 2012.
5. Rees JH. Diagnosis and treatment in neuro-oncology: an oncological perspective. *Br J Radiol.* 2011;84(Spec Issue 2):S082-S089.
6. Giglio P, Gilbert MR. Neurologic complications of cancer and its treatment. *Curr Oncol Rep.* 2010:12(1):50-59.
7. Brain tumor primary adults. PubMed, National Center for Biotechnology Information. http://www.ncbi.nlm.nih.gov/pubmedhealth/?report=printable. Last reviewed December 1, 2011. Accessed June 6, 2012.
8. Brain Tumor Information:Tumor Types. National Brain Tumor Society. http://braintumor.org/patients-family-friends/about-brain-tumors/tumor-types/?print=1&searchTxt=cancer. 2011. Accessed June 9, 2012.
9. SEER Stat Fact Sheets: Brain and Other Nervous System. Surveillance Epidemiology and End Results. http://seer.cancer.gov/statfacts/html/brain.html. Accessed May 29, 2013.
10. National Cancer Institute. What You Need to Know About Brain Tumors. http://www.cancer.gov/cancertopics/wyntk/brain/page1/AllPages. Posted 4/29/2009. Accessed 9/15/2103.
11. American Cancer Society. American Cancer Society Facts and Figures 2013. Atlanta: American Cancer Society; 2013 http://www.cancer.org/research/cancerfactsfigures/cancerfactsfigures/cancer-facts-figures-2013 Accessed 8/20/2013.
12. National Cancer Institute. Surveillance, Epidemiology, and End Results (SEER). http://seer.cancer.gov/statfacts/html/brain.html. 2013. Accessed 9/15/2013.
13. American Association of Neuroscience Nurses. Guide to the Care of the Patient with Craniotomy Post-Brain Tumor Resection. http://www.aann.org/pdf/cpg/aanncraniotomy.pdf. 2006. Accessed April 26, 2012.
14. Tatter SB. The new WHO Classification of Tumors affecting the Central Nervous System. Neurosurgical Services Massachusetts General Hospital. http://neurosurgery.mgh.harvard.edu/newwhobt.htm. Accessed May 25, 2012.
15. Classification of Brain Tumors. American Association of Neurological Surgeons. Available at http://www.aans.org/en/Media/Fact%20Sheets/Classification%20of%20Brain%20Tumors.aspx. Accessed July 1, 2012.
16. ACS Guidelines on Nutrition and Physical Activity for Cancer Prevention. Diet and activity factors that affect risks for certain cancers. http://www.cancer.org/healthy/eathealthygetactive/acsguidelinesonnutritionphysicalactivityforcancerprevention/acs-guidelines-on-nutrition-and-physical-activity-for-cancer-prevention-dietand-activity.Last Revised 8/20/2012. Accessed 7/12/2013
17. Tedeschi-Blok N, Lee M, Sison JD, et al. Inverse association of antioxidant and phytoestrogen nutrient intake with glioma in the San Francisco Bay Area: A case-control study. *BMC Cancer.* 2006;6:148. http://www.biomedcentral.com/147-2407/6/148. Accessed December 25, 2007.
18. Ravasco P, Monteiro-Grillo I, Camilo ME. Does nutrition influence quality of life in cancer patients undergoing radiotherapy? *Radiother Oncol.* 2003;67(2):213-220.
19. Grant B, Byron J. Nutritional implications in chemotherapy. In: Elliott L, Molseed L, McCallum PD, eds., with Grant B, technical ed. *Medical Nutrition Therapy in Oncology.* 2nd ed. Chicago, IL: American Dietetic Association; 2006:72-87.
20. Zietse R, van der Lubbe N, Hoorn EJ. Current and future treatment options in SIADH. *Clin Kid J.* 2009;2(3):iii12-iii19.
21. Bauer JD, Capra S. Nutrition intervention improves outcomes in patients with cancer cachexia receiving chemotherapy: A pilot study. *Support Care Cancer.* 2005;13(4):270-274.
22. Schubart JR, Kinzie MB, Farace E. Caring for the brain tumor patient: Family caregiver burden and unmet needs. *Neuro Oncol.* 2008; 10(10):61-72.
23. McGirt MJ. Persistent outpatient hyperglycemia is independently associated with decreased survival after primary resection of malignant brain astromcytomas. *Neurosurgery.* 2008;23(2):286-291.
24. Newton HB, Newton C, Pearl D, Davidson T. Swallowing assessment in primary brain tumor patients with dysphagia. *Neurology.* 1994;44(10): 1927-1932.
25. Clinical Pharmacology. Elsevier DecisionSupport. www.clinical pharmacology-ip.com. Accessed 8/20/2013.
26. Dietrich J, Rao K, Pastorino S, Kesan S. Corticosteroids in brain cancer patients: benefits and pitfalls. *Expert Rev Clin Pharmacol.* 2011;4(2): 233-242.
27. Ford E, Catt S, Chalmers A, Fallowfield L. Systemic review of supportive care needs in patients with primary malignant brain tumors. *Neuro Oncol.* 2012;14(4): 392-404.
28. Zhou W, Mukherjee P, Kiebish, MA, et al. The calorie restricted ketogenic diet, an effective alternative therapy for malignant brain cancer. *Nutr Metabol.* 2007:22(4):5.
29. Maurer GD, Brucker DP, Bahr O, et al. Differential utilization of ketone bodies by neurons and glioma cell lines: a rationale for ketogenic diet as experimental glioma therapy. *BMC Cancer.* 2011;Jul 26; 11:315. http://www.ncbi.nlm.nih.gov/pubmed/21791085. Accessed July 1, 2012.
30. Seyfried BT, Kiebish M, Marsh J, Mukherjee P. Targeting energy metabolism in brain cancer through calorie restriction and the ketogenic diet. *J Cancer Res Ther.* 2009;5Suppl1:S7-S15.
31. Nebeling LC, Miraldi F, Shurin SB, Lerner E. Effects of a ketogenic diet on tumor metabolism and nutritional status in pediatric oncology patients: two case reports. *J Am Coll Nutr.* 1995;14(2):202–208.
32. Zuccoli G, Marcello N, Pisanello A, et al. Metabolic management of glioblastoma multiforme using standard therapy together with a restricted ketogenic diet: Case Report. *Nutr Metab (Lond).* 2010;22;7:33. Published on-line April 22, 2010. http://www.ncbi.nlm.nih.gov/pmc/articles/PMC2874558?report. Accessed July 7, 2012.
33. Seyfried T, Kiebish M, Marsh J, Shelton LM. Metabolic management of brain cancer. *Biochimica et Biophysica Acta.* 2011;1807(6):577-594.
34. Seyfried T, Marsh J, Shelton LM. Is the restricted ketogenic diet a viable alternative to the standard of care for managing malignant brain cancer? *Epilepsy Res.* 2012;100(3):310-326.
35. Schmidt M, Pfetzer N, Schwab M. Effects of a ketogenic diet on the quality of life in 16 patients with advanced cancer: A pilot trial. *Nutr Metab.* 2011; 27(8):854. doi: 10.1186/1743-7075-8-54.
36. Mukherjee P, El-Abbadi MM, Kasperzyk JL, et al. Dietary restriction reduces angiogenesis and growth in an orthotopic mouse brain tumour model [abstract]. *Br J Cancer.* 2002;20;86(10):1615-21. http://www.ncbi.nlm.nih.gov/pubmed/12085212. Accessed July 7, 2012. PMID: 12085212.
37. Kouda K, Lki M. Beneficial effects of mild stress (hormetic effects): dietary restriction and health [abstract]. *J Physiol Anthropol.* 2010;29 (4):127-32. http://www.ncbi.nlm.nih.gov/pubmed/2068325. Accessed July 7, 2012. PMID: 20686325.
38. Brandhorst S, Wei M, Hwang S, Morgan TE. Short-term calorie and protein restriction provide partial protection from chemotoxicity but do not delay glioma progression. *Exp Gerontol.* 2013;48(10):1120-1128.

Medical Nutrition Therapy for Breast Cancer

Vicky Newman, MS, RD

Overview

Breast cancer is the most frequently diagnosed cancer in women after skin cancer (1-3) and the second leading cause of cancer death in women, exceeded only by lung cancer (3). Current data suggest that one in every eight women will be diagnosed with breast cancer during her lifespan (1). Men also develop breast cancer, but this disease is 100 times more common among women than men (1). National Cancer Institute (NCI) estimates suggest that 232,340 women will be diagnosed with breast cancer and 39,620 women will die from this disease in 2013 (3). The decline in incidence of female breast cancer seen between 2000 and 2003 has been attributed to fewer women using menopausal hormone therapy (1). Since 2003, breast cancer incidence rates have been stable (1).

Death rates for breast cancer have steadily decreased in women since 1989, with larger decreases in women younger than 50 than in those 50 years and older (2-3). The five-year relative survival rate for female breast cancer patients has improved from 63% in the early 1960s to an average of 90% today (1,4). Breast cancer survivors now account for almost a quarter (22%) of all cancer survivors and 40% of female cancer survivors in the United States (U.S.) (1,5).

While the majority of breast cancers originate in cells lining milk ducts and in breast lobules (i.e., glands that produce milk), breast cancer is a heterogeneous disease. Menopausal status and the presence or absence of estrogen receptors (ER), progesterone receptors (PR), and human epidermal growth factor receptor-2 (HER-2) result in unique biological characteristics that influence cancer treatment, progression and prognosis (6-7). When prescribing the most effective treatment(s) for breast cancer, oncologists consider receptor status as well as breast cancer stage and pathology reports.

Risk Factors for Breast Cancer

Besides being female, increasing age is the most important risk factor for breast cancer. Approximately 12% of invasive breast cancers are found in women younger than 45, while 65%-70% are found in women age 55 and older (1,6,8-9). Potentially modifiable risk factors include weight gain after age 18, being overweight or obese (for postmenopausal breast cancer), and use of combined estrogen and progestin hormone therapy (1). Epidemiological studies commonly suggest that alcohol intake increases risk of breast cancer (9-11), but data addressing the effect of alcohol intake on breast cancer survival is equivocal. There was no significant association between alcohol intake and breast cancer-specific survival among women with invasive breast cancer enrolled in the Swedish Mammography Cohort (12), and other studies suggest an inverse association or no association between pre-and post-diagnosis alcohol intake and all-cause mortality (13-15).

The benefit of physical activity in reducing breast cancer risk is evident for post-menopausal and the most active pre-menopausal women (16). Breast cancer survivors who are physically active are less likely to die from breast cancer than women who are inactive (17-20). Two large studies, The Nurses' Health Study (21) and the Collaborative Women's Longevity Study (22) found that those reporting an activity level of at least 3 metabolic equivalent task (MET) hours per week had significantly lower risk of death from all causes and from breast cancer. The After Breast Cancer Pooling Project, which combined data measuring physical activity of a large number of breast cancer survivors 23 months after diagnosis, found that breast cancer mortality was reduced by 25%, and all-cause mortality by 27%, in women engaging in > 10 MET hours per week of physical activity when compared with women who were less physically active (23). Brisk walking at a rate of 4 miles/hour (15 minute mile) for 2.5 hours/week (or for 30 minutes 5 days/week) is roughly equivalent to 10 MET hours/week. More information on MET values for various activities is available (24-25).

Beneficial effects of physical activity may be augmented by healthy eating, as prospective observation of a multi-ethnic cohort of women with breast cancer found that independent of obesity, survivors engaging in any recreational physical activity and consuming better quality diets had significantly lower all-cause mortality and reduced risk of death from breast cancer after six years of follow-up (26). Longer survival after receiving a breast cancer diagnosis has also been reported in physically active women with high vegetable-fruit intake regardless of obesity status (20).

Other breast cancer risk factors include very dense breast tissue, high bone mineral density, biopsy-confirmed hyperplasia and never having children or having a first child after age 30 (1,4,6). Several breast cancer susceptibility genes have now been identified, including BRCA1 and BRCA2. Up to eighty percent of women with an inherited mutation in BRCA1 or BRCA2 will develop breast cancer, and usually bilateral breast cancer, sometime during their lives, compared with about 12% of women in the general population (27-29).

Staging:

Once breast cancer is diagnosed, physical examination, biopsy and imaging tests determine the clinical stage, while pathologic staging also considers post-operative findings. The American Joint Committee on Cancer (AJCC) has developed a system of staging cancers according to the size of the tumor (T), whether the cancer has spread to the lymph nodes (N), and whether the cancer has metastasized (M) (30). This system is discussed in chapter 1. Clinicians can access the complete AJCC staging system for breast cancer on both The American Cancer Society website (31) and the National Cancer Institute website (32).

Treatment and Treatment Challenges

Breast-conserving surgery (lumpectomy) followed by local radiation therapy has replaced mastectomy as the preferred surgical approach for treating early-stage breast cancer. Combination chemotherapy is a standard of care in the adjuvant treatment of operable breast cancer. The goal of this systemic therapy is to eradicate cancer cells that may have spread beyond the breast. Neoadjuvant chemotherapy, or chemotherapy given before surgery to reduce the size of the tumor and to increase the chance of breast-conserving surgery, is also an option.

In addition to surgery, radiation and chemotherapy, hormonal therapy with selective estrogen receptor modulators (SERMs) and aromatase inhibitors is now considered standard treatment for women with estrogen receptor-positive (ER+) breast cancer, both as adjuvant therapy and in the treatment of advanced disease. SERMs (e.g., tamoxifen and raloxifene or fluvestrant) decrease growth of estrogen-sensitive cells by binding to the estrogen receptor, while aromatase inhibitors (including anastrozole, exemestane and letrozole) block estrogen production. The Breast Cancer Prevention Trial randomly assigned over 13,000 women to either tamoxifen or a placebo for five years. After seven years of follow-up, tamoxifen reduced risk of developing invasive breast cancer by about 50 percent in high-risk postmenopausal women (33). A subsequent large randomized trial, the Study of Tamoxifen and Raloxifene, also sponsored by NCI, found that taking raloxifene for five years was as effective as tamoxifen in reducing risk of invasive breast cancer in postmenopausal women (34). Tamoxifen and raloxifene also are used to reduce breast cancer risk among those at high risk of this disease. The monoclonal antibody trastuzumab is an accepted treatment for breast cancers that overproduce the human epidermal growth factor receptor 2 (HER2) protein (1).

Table 1 outlines tumor variants according to hormone status and over-expression of human epidermal growth factor protein-2 (HER2) and potential benefits of hormone-based therapy. Traditional treatments such as surgery, chemotherapy and radiation are also used in the treatment of these cancers but are not addressed in this table.

Table 1: Molecular Variants of Hormone-Receptive Cancers (35-37)

Molecular Variant	Prevalence and Biology	Therapies Used to Treat Hormone-Dependent Cancers

ER+ (Estrogen Receptor positive)	• Approximately two-thirds of breast cancers are estrogen receptor positive.
	• Estrogen stimulates growth of ER+ breast cancers.
		• ER and/or PR positive tumors are responsive to endocrine therapies to various degrees. They include:
		  – Selective estrogen-receptor response modulators (SERMs) such as tamoxifen prevent estrogen from binding to receptors.
		  – Aromatase inhibitors stop estrogen production in post-menopausal women. They are not used before menopause.
		  – Estrogen-receptor downregulators (ERDs) block effects of estrogen in breast tissue.
		  – Luteinizing hormone-releasing hormone agents (LHRHs) such as Lupron Depot and Zoladex shut down the ovaries so they do not produce estrogen. They are given via injection.
		• Breast cancers with combined positive and negative receptor status do not respond as well to hormone treatments but other treatments, including chemotherapy, are available.

PR + (Progesterone Receptor positive)	• Approximately two-thirds of ER+ breast cancers are also PR+. • Progesterone stimulates growth of PR+ breast cancers.	
ER+/PR-; ER-/PR+; ER-/PR- cancers can reflect combinations of estrogen and progesterone receptor status	• Approximately 10% of breast cancers are ER+/PR-; 5% are ER-/PR+; and 20% are ER-/PR-.	
HER2 positive Human Epidermal Growth Factor Receptor-2	• Approximately 20% of breast cancers are HER-2 positive. • These breast cancers contain large amounts of a protein (HER2/neu) that promotes cancer growth. HER2 positive breast cancers are fast growing and aggressive.	• Monoclonal antibodies such as herceptin are used to treat HER-2 positive cancers.
Triple negative breast cancer (TNBC) is negative for estrogen, progesterone, and HER2 receptors.	• Approximately 15-20% of breast cancers are triple negative. • Most breast cancers caused by the BRCA1 gene are triple negative. • Triple negative breast cancer is more common among young and African American women.	• Hormone therapy is generally ineffective against TNBC but other treatments including chemotherapy are available. • TNBCs have poorer prognosis than other breast cancers.

Aromatase inhibitors (but not selective estrogen-response modulators such as tamoxifen) are associated with bone loss (36), so it is recommended that patients prescribed these drugs consume adequate calcium and vitamin D or vitamin D supplements when deficient (38). In addition, data suggest that vitamin D may have anti-inflammatory activity, inhibit biological activity of estrogen, and promote apoptosis, each of which may be protective against breast cancer (39). The Dietary Reference Intake for calcium for women is 1,000 mg/day for ages 19-50 and 1,200 mg/day for those 51 years and older, while the recommended intake of vitamin D is 600 IU/day for adults ages 19-70 years and 800 IU/day for adults 71 years and older (40). For every 100 IU of vitamin D3 consumed, serum 25(OH)D level increases approximately 1.0 ng/mL (40). Though vitamin D supplementation is indicated in cases of deficiency, the U.S. Preventive Services Task Force (USPSTF) states that daily supplementation with ≤400 IU vitamin D3 and ≤1000 mg calcium has no effect on fracture incidence in community-dwelling postmenopausal women, and that there is inadequate evidence to make a recommendation on the effect of higher supplemental doses of vitamin D and calcium on fracture incidence (41).

Given the risk to bone health in this population and the importance of enhancing quality of life in cancer survivors, it is essential for RDs to educate and counsel breast cancer survivors taking aromatase inhibitors on medical nutrition therapy that promotes bone strength. Recommendations include consuming recommended amounts of calcium and vitamin D within the survivor's preferred or recommended diet (i.e., vegetarian diet, vegan diet, lactose restricted diet, etc.), consuming dietary components that enhance calcium absorption and engaging in lifestyle factors such as weight-bearing activities that promote bone strength. Researchers have not yet reached consensus on ideal vitamin D levels for optimal health (42). According to the Office of Dietary Supplements (ODS) of the National Institutes of Health (NIH), a target 25(OH)D level > 20 ng/mL (1 nmol/L = 0.4 ng/mL) is adequate for bone health (43). While ODS cautions that 25(OH)D levels should remain <50 ng/mL (43), it has also been suggested that the optimal 25(OH)D level for prevention of breast cancer is 40-60 ng/mL (39).

Chemotherapy can result in a number of nutrition impact symptoms including decreased appetite, nausea, vomiting, fatigue, emotional changes, constipation, diarrhea, mucositis and taste changes that can lead to involuntary weight loss and nutritional insufficiencies. Table 2 outlines common nutrition impact symptoms associated with chemotherapy agents used to treat breast cancer (44-49). Radiation also results in a number of side effects (50-51), but its longest lasting symptom is fatigue, which can make it difficult to prepare meals and eat at regular intervals. Strategies to resolve or mitigate these challenges are outlined in Chapter 12.

Table 2: Nutrition Impact Symptoms Associated with Commonly Used Chemotherapy, Biologic, and Endocrine Therapy Agents (42-47)

Agent generic name (Trade Name)	Classification	Hair Loss	Nausea / Vomiting	Constipation / Diarrhea	Peripheral Neuropathy/Diarrhea	Myelo-suppression	Miscellaneous
CHEMOTHERAPY AGENTS							
Capecitabine (Xeloda®)	Antimetabolite		X	D		X	Palmar-plantar syndrome, Mucositis, Increased bilirubin, Fatigue, Ocular toxicity (eye irritation, decreased vision, corneal deposits
Carboplatin (Paraplatin®)	Platinum alkylating agent	X	X		X	X	Skin rash, Hypersensitivity reaction, Pulmonary toxicity (late effects), Dyslipidemia (late effect), Reproductive late effects: Gonadal dysfunction, oligomenorrhea, amenorrhea, premature menopause, infertility, Ocular toxicity (rare cases of blurred vision, eye pain, maculopathy, and optical neuropathy with transient cortical blindness in patients with impaired kidney function)
Cyclophosphamide (Cytoxan®)	Alkylating agent	X	X		X	X	Acute hemorrhagic cystitis (bleeding in the urinary bladder), Late effects: bladder fibrosis, dysfunctional voiding vesicoureteral reflux, hydronephrosis, hemorrhagic cystitis, Cardiomyopathy with high-dose therapy, Paronychia [painful inflammation around fingernails and toenails], Hyperpigmentation, Pulmonary toxicity (late effects), Secondary malignancy (late effects), Reproductive late effects: Gonadal dysfunction, oligomenorrhea, amenorrhea, premature menopause, infertility, Ocular toxicity (reversible blurred vision; keratoconjunctivitis sicca)
Docetaxel (Taxotere®)	Microtubule inhibitor	X	X		X	X	Hypersensitivity reaction, Fluid retention, Skin and nail changes (skin rash; nail shedding; grooves in nail plate), Palmar-plantar syndrome, Hyperpigmentation, Mucositis, Paresthesia, Ocular toxicity (epiphora [blocked tear duct results in watery eyes], narrowing of tear ducts)

(Continued)

Table 2: Nutrition Impact Symptoms Associated with Commonly Used Chemotherapy, Biologic, and Endocrine Therapy Agents (42-47) *(continued)*

Agent generic name (Trade Name)	Classification	Hair Loss	Nausea / Vomiting	Constipation / Diarrhea	Peripheral Neuropathy Diarrhea	Myelo-suppression	Miscellaneous
CHEMOTHERAPY AGENTS *(continued)*							
Doxorubicin (Adriamycin®)	Antineoplastic anthracycline	X	X			X	Red discoloration of urine, Mucositis, Photosensitivity, Hyperpigmentation, Palmar-plantar syndrome, Paronychia [painful inflammation around fingernails and toenails], Nail shedding; grooves in nail plate, Fibrosis, Obstruction, Enteritis, adhesions, ulcers (late effects), Radiation recall, Cardiac toxicity, Ocular toxicity (conjunctivitis, increased tear production <u>*Do not exceed a lifetime cumulative dose of 550mg/m2 (450mg/m2 if you have had prior chest irradiation or simultaneous cyclophosphamide treatment*</u>
Epirubicin (Elience®)	Antineoplastic anthracycline	X	X	D		X	Red discoloration of urine, Mucositis, Cardiac toxicity, Esophagitis, Amenorrhea, Premature menopause
Fluorouracil (5-FU)	antimetabolite	X	X	D		X	Anorexia, Mucositis, Palmar-plantar syndrome, Increased tear production, Photosensitivity, Darkening of the veins, Hyperpigmentation, Blistering; Dry skin, Cardiac toxicity (rare), Ocular toxicity (25% - 35% report ocular effects, which may include inflammation of cornea and/or conjunctiva, cicatricial exropion (scar tissue turns eyelid inward), ankyloblepharon (eyelids fuse at the margin), blepharospasm (eye spasms), blurred vision, photophobia, nystagmus, eye pain, and circumorbital edema)
Gemcitabine (Gemzar®)	Antimetabolite		X			X	Fever, Flu-like symptoms, Rash, Perianal pruritus, Lung toxicity with longer infusion times, Trichomegaly [increased hair growth of eyelashes and eyebrows]
Ixabepilone (Ixempra®)	Microtubule inhibitor or "epothilone B analog"	X	X	D	X	X	Fatigue; musculoskeletal pain, Peripheral neuropathy [frequently cited as reason to discontinue treatment], Altered taste sensation, Dizziness; insomnia; cognitive impairment, Headache; syncope; cerebral hemorrhage; poor coordination, Coagulopathy [thrombosis; embolism; hemorrhage; hypovolemic shock], Pulmonary toxicity [cough, pneumonitis, hypoxia, pulmonary edema]
Methotrexate (MTX)	Antimetabolite		X			X	Mucositis, Oral or gastrointestinal ulceration, Paronychia [painful inflammation around fingernails and toenails], Renal toxicity, Photosensitivity, Liver toxicity, Neurotoxicity with high dose therapy, Ocular toxicity (blepharitis [inflammation of eyelids at lash follicles], conjunctival hyperemia, increased tear production, periorbital edema, photophobia, eye pain)
Paclitaxel (Taxol®)	Microtubule inhibitor	X		D	X	X	Hypersensitivity reaction, Facial flushing, Hyperpigmentation, Skin rash, Myalgia, Mucositis, Ocular toxicity (scintillating scotomas ["shooting lights"] occurs in 20% of cases)
Paclitaxel albumin-stabilized nanoparticle formulation (Abraxane®) (albumin-bound)	Microtubule inhibitor	X	X	D	X	X	Myalgia, Arthralgia, Mucositis
Vinorelbine (Navelbine®)	Microtubule inhibitor, vinca alkaloid	X	X		X	X	Neurotoxicity, Pulmonary toxicity (late effects), Musculoskeletal late effects: osteopenia, osteoporosis, avascular necrosis, muscle weakness
BIOLOGIC THERAPIES							
Aromatase Inhibitors							
Anastrozole (Arimidex®)	Selective nonsteroidal aromatase inhibitor		X	C or D			Hot flashes, Vaginal dryness, Osteoporosis, Bone and Joint pain (commonly reported), Mild swelling of arms and legs, Dry skin, rash and scaling, Flulike syndrome [fever; malaise; myalgia], Arthralgia [morning stiffness of joints]headaches [mild], Decreased energy; weakness

(Continued)

Table 2: Nutrition Impact Symptoms Associated with Commonly Used Chemotherapy, Biologic, and Endocrine Therapy Agents (42-47) *(continued)*

Agent generic name (Trade Name)	Classification	Hair Loss	Nausea / Vomiting	Constipation / Diarrhea	Peripheral Neuropathy Diarrhea	Myelo-suppression	Miscellaneous
BIOLOGIC THERAPIES							
Aromatase Inhibitors *(continued)*							
Exemestane (Aromasin®)	Irreversible steroidal aromatase inactivator		X				Hot flashes; increased sweating, Increased appetite; weight gain, Depression; insomnia, Headache, Fatigue, Pain [unspecified]
Letrozole (Femara®)	Competitive nonsteroidal aromatase inhibitor		X				Hot flashes, Myalgia and arthralgia, Headache [mild], Fatigue [mild]
Estrogen Receptor Antagonist or Downregulator							
Fulvestrant (Faslodex®)	Estrogen receptor antagonist		X				Arthralgia, Hot flashes, Anorexia; abdominal pain, Headache [mild] flulike syndrome [fever, malaise, myalgia]
Luteinizing Hormone-Releasing Hormone Agents (LHRHs)							
Leuprolide (Lupron®)			X	C or D			Hot flashes, Breast enlargement or tenderness, Diabetes, Emotional lability, Headaches, Vaginal dryness, Dizziness, Fatigue
Goserelin (Zoladex®)			X	C			Hot flashes, Headache, Fatigue, Breast pain, Vaginitis, Emotional labillity, Breast changes, Sweating, Acne,
Selective Estrogen Receptor Modulators							
Tamoxifen (Nolvadex®)	Nonsteroidal antiestrogen		X	C or D			Hot flashes, Vaginal discharge; vaginal dryness, Mood swings, Dry skin; rash; scaling, Flulike syndrome [fever, malaise, myalgia], Arthralgia [morning joint stiffness], Headaches, Fatigue; weakness, Increased risk for deep vein thrombosis (blood clot), Ocular toxicity (cataracts; decreased color vision [increased with doses greater than 20mg/day]; retinal toxicity; corneal opacities; retinopathy; vision loss that may be irreversible), Increased risk for endometrial cancer and uterine sarcoma (late effects)
Monoclonal Antibodies							
Bevaclzumab (Avastin®)	Monoclonal antibody		X	C		X	Asthenia, Pain, Abdominal pain, Fatigue, Headache, Anorexia, Dyspepsia, Dizziness, Leukopenia, Neutropenia, Thrombocytopeia
Pertuzumab (Perjeta®)	Monoclonal antibody		X	C		X	Embryo-fetal toxicity, Left ventricular dysfunction, Alopecia, Neutropenia, Fatigue, Leukopenia, Asthenia
Lapatinib (Tykerb®)	Tyrosine kinase inhibitor- acts on the epidermal growth factor receptors (EGFR) HER-1 and HER-2		X	D			Diarrhea may be severe enough to require fluid/electrolyte replacement, Palmar plantar syndrome, Fatigue, Stomatitis; dyspepsia; mucositis, Dyspnea [shortness of breath], Pain in back and extremities, Insomnia, Liver toxicity – may be severe and require dose reduction, Cardiac toxicity [decreased left ventricular ejection fraction; prolonged Q-T interval]
Trastuzumab (Herceptin®)	Anti-human HER2 monoclonal antibody						Flu-like symptoms are common; Cardiac toxicity is less common but can occur

Table compiled by Lori Johnson, RN, MSN, OCN, Clinical Nurse Educator, Moores UCSD Cancer Center, lJJohnson@ucsd.edu.

Lymphedema

Even with the increased use of sentinel lymph node dissection, lymphedema remains a concern among breast cancer survivors. However, aerobic physical activity and resistance training appear to be both safe and effective in reducing the incidence of lymphedema among survivors at high risk of this condition, and in improving the symptoms and severity of lymphedema for those in whom the condition was preexisting (52). Because obesity is a major risk factor for lymphedema, weight management is recommended for survivors who are overweight or obese (52-54).

Nutritional Status and Breast Cancer

When compared with other malignancies, women with breast cancer are less likely to present with weight loss or malnutrition. A review of malnutrition among different cancers found that overall prevalence was 30.9%, but was seen in only 18% of those with breast cancer, even though 44% had metastatic disease (55).

The serious implications of weight loss and malnutrition on cancer treatment and outcome are widely recognized for most cancers (56); being overweight and obese conveys equally deleterious effects on those with breast cancer (52-53). However, weight management efforts in this group need to be balanced against the risk of sarcopenia (57). Cancer patients in every weight category are likely to have depleted muscle mass, which is associated with poorer performance status and decreased survival (58).

Nutritional Needs of Breast Cancer Survivors

The 2012 American Cancer Society (ACS) Nutrition and Physical Activity Guidelines for Cancer Survivors state that intentional weight loss during treatment, at rates up to a two-pound per week weight loss, may not be contraindicated for those who are overweight or obese (52). This recommendation may appear to contradict the long-held view that weight loss during cancer treatment negatively impacts treatment outcome, but it reflects strong evidence that weight gain and being overweight or obese increases risk of breast cancer recurrence and mortality.

Evidence has established a strong link between obesity and risk of post-menopausal breast cancer (59-61). In addition, being overweight or obese as well as gaining weight post-treatment may result in poorer outcomes (61-62), and many women gain weight during treatment for breast cancer. While there is no direct evidence from randomized trials that intentional weight loss (in overweight breast cancer survivors) after diagnosis improves outcomes, interpretation of available epidemiologic evidence collectively leans toward a beneficial effect of gradual, intended weight loss while preserving lean body mass for obese/overweight patients with breast cancer.

RDs are challenged to implement nutrition interventions, both during and after treatment for breast cancer, which help maintain lean body mass while promoting a gradual loss of excess fat stores. Limiting the rate of any weight loss to recommended safe amounts is one way to achieve this goal. Encouraging regular moderate physical activity as tolerated is also desirable. In addition, to discourage disease recurrence it is also important to promote a biological environment unfriendly to the growth of breast cancer (e.g., one that reduces inflammation). The ACS (52) and the World Cancer Research Fund/American Institute for Cancer Research (WCRF/AICR) (63) each provide evidence-based nutrition information for cancer survivors; their general recommendations are outlined in Appendix 1. Routine nutrition reassessment is essential so the RD can modify the nutrition care plan according to current nutrition needs of each breast cancer survivor.

There are a variety of formulas in use for estimating energy needs for cancer survivors that are reviewed in chapter 4. Unless nutrition assessment indicates otherwise, the energy intake goal for normal-weight breast-cancer survivors in active treatment is approximately 25-30 kcal/kg/day (64). While low-fat diets providing generous amounts of fruits and vegetables are often recommended, the high prevalence of metabolic syndrome in those breast cancer patients with central obesity is increasing interest in diets that reduce glucose and insulin levels (65). This approach may place equal or more attention on controlling refined carbohydrate intake and possibly total carbohydrate intake as long as the overall

macronutrient distribution meets nutrient needs. Protein needs of cancer (including breast cancer) patients with normal renal function range from 1.0 to 1.5 g/kg, based on stress level (66). Baseline nutrient and electrolyte needs are assumed to be consistent with recommendations of the Institute of Medicine of the National Academies (67), but should be monitored throughout treatment and modified as indicated by ongoing nutrition reassessment.

Medical Nutrition Therapy for Breast Cancer Treatment and Healthy Survivorship:

1. Promote a gradual loss of excess fat stores while preserving lean body mass: Provide energy, protein, micronutrient and fluid needs as indicated by nutrition assessment, allowing a gradual rate and level of weight loss consistent with accepted standards (i.e. loss of body weight <5% over one-month; <7.5% over 3 months; <10% over a six-month period) (68).

2. Enhance quality of life during cancer treatment: Counsel patients on strategies to manage nutrition impact symptoms (NIS) of treatments, including chemotherapy and radiation therapy, monitor NIS, and modify the nutrition plan as indicated to improve symptom management. See Chapter 12 for specific counseling points for managing NIS.

3. Promote post-operative recovery: Following any surgery the RD should promote wound healing nutrition practices, including adequate energy, protein, and micronutrient intake, with an emphasis on nutrients integral to wound healing.

4. Promote post-treatment recovery and healthy survivorship: As soon as treatment status and recovery from treatment allows, MNT should transition to a survivorship plan that promotes a healthy weight range and intake of foods and nutrients found to be protective against breast cancer recurrence, as recommended by ACS and AICR.

Health Enhancing Strategies for Breast Cancer

Comprehensive approaches that involve diet and behavior modification combined with increased aerobic and strength training exercise have shown promise in either preventing weight gain or promoting weight loss, reducing biomarkers associated with inflammation and co-morbidities, and improving lifestyle behaviors, functional status, and quality of life in this patient population (69). However, only 20% to 30% of breast cancer survivors are physically active (52) and approximately 50% are overweight or obese (70). Regular moderate physical activity helps to reduce several key biological indicators of cancer risk, including sex hormone levels, insulin resistance, and inflammation. Physical activity can also help strengthen the immune system, which plays an important role in controlling the growth and spread of cancer cells.

Diet Composition

Researchers are actively investigating the effects of diet on breast cancer survival. Diet quality in breast cancer survivors was assessed by four standardized scores (Healthy Eating Index, Diet Quality Index-Revised, Recommended Food Score, and the Alternate Mediterranean Diet Score) and compared to survival statistics to examine the effect of healthy eating on survivorship among females who had been treated for invasive Stage I-III breast cancer. The only significant association found was between a higher Alternate Mediterranean Diet Score and lower risk of non-breast cancer death in women with low physical activity (71).

Two large randomized controlled trials (RCTs) have tested whether diet modification after the diagnosis of early-stage breast cancer affects cancer outcomes. The Women's Intervention Nutrition Study (WINS) tested a low-fat diet ($\leq$ 15% of energy) in 2,437 postmenopausal women with early-stage breast cancer. On average the women in the intervention arm decreased fat intake to 20% of energy at year 1, which resulted in a 24% reduction in new breast cancer events (72). The Women's Healthy Eating and Living (WHEL) Study examined the effect of a diet very high in vegetables, fruit, and fiber and low in fat (20% of energy intake) on cancer outcomes in 3,088 pre- and postmenopausal breast cancer survivors who were followed for an average of 7.3 years (20). Recurrence-free survival did not differ between the two study arms. However, serum estrogens at baseline were independently associated with poor prognosis, and a protective effect of the diet was observed in the subgroup of women who did not report hot flashes at enrollment (73). These findings suggest that reproductive hormonal status may influence whether a high-vegetable, fruit, and fiber diet affects prognosis. In addition, longitudinal exposure to carotenoids was associated with breast cancer-free survival regardless of study group assignment (74). Thus, diet before the diagnosis of cancer and over the long-term may be as important as short-term dietary change post-diagnosis (72). Interest in controlling refined and perhaps total carbohydrate intake in this population is increasing, but the ideal diet composition for promoting desirable glucose, insulin, triglyceride, HDL, leptin and adeinopectin levels has not yet been identified (65).

Fatty Acids

While inverse associations have been found between fat intake and breast cancer recurrence and/or survival, these associations typically disappear with energy-adjustment (72). However, emerging research in nutrigenomics indicates that the type and amount of dietary fatty acids ingested likely play a role in breast cancer risk and progression. For example, women with certain polymorphisms in genes involved in fat metabolism who consume $\geq$ 17.4 g/d of linoleic acid (LA) may have a higher risk of breast cancer (75). Women ingesting an 1800 calorie/day diet and following the current American Heart Association (AHA) recommendation (LA Intake up to 10% calories) would exceed this LA intake.

The omega-3 fatty acids eicosapentaneoic acid (EPA) and docosahexaenoic acid (DHA) inhibit the proliferation of breast cancer cells in vitro and reduce the initiation and progression of these tumors in laboratory animals (76-77). While the association between self-reported dietary intake of fish, total omega-3 PUFA, EPA, and DHA intake and breast cancer risk in cohort studies has been mixed, studies that analyzed blood biomarkers of these fatty acids have reported an inverse association, though this association

may not be causal (78). A recent analysis of more than 35,000 postmenopausal women reported a reduced risk of ductal breast cancer in those using fish oil supplements (79). And an examination of data from the WHEL study suggested that EPA and DHA intake from marine sources (though not from fish oil supplements) reduced additional breast cancer events and all-cause mortality. The association was not linear; analysis suggested that EPA/DHA intake greater than 73 mg/d (from marine foods) reduced risk of additional breast cancer events by 25% (78).

This research supports recommendations of the 2010 Dietary Guidelines for Americans to consume $\geq$ 8 ounces of fish per week (80). For those considering omega-3 fat supplements (e.g. fish oil supplements), the FDA considers an omega-3 fat intake up to 3 grams per day within Generally Regarded As Safe (GRAS) standards (81). The AHA states that omega-3 fat intake up to 4 grams daily may be appropriate (e.g., for cholesterol lowering) but a health care provider should supervise intake greater than 3 grams to avoid potential side effects such as excessive bleeding (82).

Fiber and Lignans

A systematic review and meta-analysis of prospective studies reported an inverse association between dietary fiber intake ($\geq$ 25 g/day) and breast cancer risk (83). When comparing women who ate the most fiber to those who ate the least, women who consumed the highest amounts of fiber had a 7% lower risk of breast cancer.

Several cellular and animal studies suggest that lignans, whose biologic structure is similar to estrogen, may reduce tumor growth and help prevent metastasis (84). A case-control study found that women in the highest, as compared with the lowest, tertile of total lignan intake had a significantly lower breast cancer risk regardless of menopausal status; premenopausal women in the highest tertile also showed a reduced risk for developing invasive disease (84). Lignans are widely available in whole grains, seeds, nuts, legumes, fruit, and vegetables; flaxseeds are a particularly rich source.

Soyfood

Soy is a rich source of isoflavone phytochemicals, which have weak estrogenic activity and may protect against hormone-dependent cancers, especially when ingested during childhood or adolescence (85-86). For the breast cancer survivor, current evidence suggests no adverse effects on recurrence or survival from consuming soy and soyfoods, and there is the potential for these foods to exert a positive synergistic effect with tamoxifen. The Life After Cancer Epidemiology (LACE) Study and the WHEL Study noted a trend towards an improved prognosis in those consuming soy (87-88). Consuming two to three servings of soyfood per day is likely acceptable, based on usual intake in Asia and amounts of soy consumed in epidemiological studies and clinical trials. With one serving of traditional soyfood providing approximately 35 mg isoflavones (89), this recommendation would provide a maximum daily isoflavone intake of approximately 100 mg, which is close to the upper intake range in Asia (88). RDs generally recommend consuming traditional soyfoods (soybeans, tofu, tempeh), rather than products made with isolated soy protein or isoflavone supplements. This is because soy foods provide a wider variety of nutrients and other bioactive compounds, many of which have synergistic, anticancer effects.

Green Tea

Green tea is a rich source of antioxidant flavonoids, including the catechin epigallocatechin-3-gallate (EGCG), believed to be responsible for most of the health benefits associated with this beverage (90). Though findings from studies examining associations between tea intake and total cancer risk have been inconsistent, several studies have demonstrated that green tea has a protective effect against breast cancer and can also inhibit cancer cell growth and invasion. A recent meta-analysis encompassing 5617 cases of breast cancer showed that green tea consumption of greater than 3 cups daily was inversely associated with breast cancer recurrence (91). While more research is needed, unsweetened green tea appears to be a good beverage choice for breast cancer survivors.

Summary

Breast cancer is responsible for significant morbidity and mortality. Extensive research suggests that diet and nutrition, through habits that balance energy intake with output and provide a variety of anticancer nutrients and other protective biological compounds, can help prevent risk and recurrence of breast cancer. RDs are charged with providing evidence-based nutrition interventions to support prevention, treatment, recovery, and survivorship of this disease. Table 3 provides some practical tips breast cancer survivors should consider to reduce risk of recurrence or progression.

Table 3: Tips to Reduce Breast Cancer Risk and Progression (8,61,77,88-91)

- **Maintain a healthy weight (BMI greater than 18.4 and less than 25)**

- **Enjoy a physically active lifestyle**
  - Move more (>10,000 steps daily)
  - Exert yourself (30-60 minutes moderate activity daily)
  - Preserve muscle mass with strength training (>2 times/week)

- **Eat plenty of vegetables and fruits (BIG color & STRONG flavor best)**
  - Vegetables (4-5 servings/day)
  - Fruits (2-3 servings/day)

- **Choose carbohydrates wisely**
  - Best sources are non-starchy vegetables, beans/legumes, fruits, whole grains
  - Eat more beans/legumes (>3-4 servings/week)
  - Limit refined carbohydrates (sugars, other sweeteners, and foods made with white flour)

- **Focus on healthy fats**
  - Choose healthy fats obtained from whole foods (including nuts, seeds, avocados, fish)
  - Limit or avoid fried foods, savory snack foods, fast foods
  - Limit or avoid salad dressings, mayonnaise
  - Limit or avoid red meat (less than 11 oz/week) and consume little, if any, processed or deli meat

- **Select beverages carefully**
  - Water is your best bet
  - Avoid sweetened beverages
  - Limit fruit juice & alcoholic beverages (≤ 1/day)

References

1. American Cancer Society. Cancer Facts & Figures 2013. http://www.cancer.org/research/cancerfactsfigures/cancerfactsfigures/cancer-facts-figures-2013. Atlanta: American Cancer Society. 2013. Last Revised 2/22/13. Accessed 4/17/13.
2. Howlader N, Noone AM, Krapcho M, Neyman N, Aminou R, Altekruse SF, et al. (eds). *SEER Cancer Statistics Review, 1975-2009 (Vintage 2009 Populations)*, National Cancer Institute. Bethesda, MD, http://seer.cancer.gov/csr/1975_2009_pops09/ Accessed 10/18/12
3. American Cancer Society. What are the key statistics about breast cancer? http://www.cancer.org/cancer/breastcancer/detailedguide/breast-cancer-key-statistics. Atlanta: American Cancer Society 2013. Last revised 2/26/13. Accessed 4/20/13.
4. American Cancer Society. Cancer Treatment and Survivorship Facts & Figures. 2012-2013. Atlanta: American Cancer Society 2012. Copyright 2012. http://www.cancer.org/acs/groups/content/@epidemiologysurveilance/documents/document/acspc-033876.pdf Accessed 9/10/12.
5. Knobf MT, Coviello J. Lifestyle interventions for cardiovascular risk reduction in women with breast cancer. *Curr Cardiol Rev.* 2011;7(4): 250-257.
6. National Cancer Institute, (2012). What you need to know about breast cancer: Treatment. Retrieved from http://www.cancer.gov/cancertopics/wyntk/breast/page7. Accessed 6/28/13.
7. Chen J-Q, Russo J. ERα negative and triple negative breast cancer: molecular features and potential therapeutic approaches. *Biochem Biophys Acta.* 2009. 1796(2):162-175.
8. American Cancer Society. What are the risk factors for breast cancer? http://www.cancer.org/Cancer/BreastCancer/DetailedGuide/breast-cancer-risk-factors (Accessed 7/10/12)
9. Thomson CA. Diet and breast cancer: understanding risks and benefits. *Nutr Clin Pract.* 2012;27(5):636-650.
10. Smith-Warner SA, Spiegelman D, Yaun S-S, van den Brandt PA, Folsom AR, Goldbohm RA, et al.. Alcohol and breast cancer in women. *JAMA.* 1998;279 (7:535–540
11. Chen WY, Rosner B, Hankinson SE, Colditz GA, Willett WC. Moderate alcohol consumption during adult life, drinking patterns, and breast cancer risk. *JAMA.* 2011;306(17):1884-1890.
12. Harris HR, Bergkvist L, Wolk A. Alcohol intake and mortality among women with invasive breast cancer. *Br J Cancer.* 2012;106(3):592-595.
13. Beasley J, Newcomb P, Trentham-Dietz A, Hampton J, Bersch A, Passarelli M, et al. Post-diagnosis dietary factors and survival after invasive breast cancer. *Breast Cancer Res Treat.* 2010;128(1):229-236.
14. Flatt SW, Thomson CA, Gold EB, Natarajan L, Rock CL, Al-Delaimy WK, Patterson RE, Saquib N, Caan BJ, Pierce JP. Low to moderate alcohol intake is not associated with increased mortality after breast cancer. *Cancer Epidemiol Biomarkers Prev.* 2010;19(3):681-688.
15. Newcomb PA, Kampman E, Trentham-Dietz A, et al. Alcohol consumption before and after breast cancer diagnosis: associations with survival from breast cancer, cardiovascular disease, and other causes. *J Clin Oncol.* 2013;31(16):1939-1946.
16. Bertram LA, Stefanick ML, Saquib N, Natarajan L, Patterson RE, Bardwell W, et al. Physical activity, additional breast cancer events, and mortality among early-stage breast cancer survivors: findings from the WHEL study. *Cancer Causes Control.* 2011;22(3):427-435.
17. Emaus A, Veierod MB, Tretli S, et al. Metabolic profile, physical activity, and mortality in breast cancer patients. *Breast Cancer Res Treat.* 2010;121(3):651–660.
18. Friedenreich CM, Gregory J, Kopciuk KA, Mackey JR, Courneya KS. Prospective cohort study of lifetime physical activity and breast cancer survival. *Int J Cancer.* 2009;124(8):1954-1962.
19. Patterson RE, Cadmus LA, Emond JA, et al. Physical activity, diet, adiposity and female breast cancer prognosis: a review of the epidemiologic literature. *Maturitas.* 2010;66(1):5-15.

20. Pierce JP, Stefanick ML, Flatt SW, Natarajan L, Sternfeld B, Madlensky L, et al. Greater survival after breast cancer in physically active women with high vegetable-fruit intake regardless of obesity. *J Clin Oncol*. 2007;25: 2345-2351.

21. Holmes MD, Chen WY, Feskanich D, Kroenke CH, Colditz GA. Physical activity and survival after breast cancer diagnosis. *JAMA*. 2005;293(20): 2479–2486

22. Holick CN, Newcomb PA, Trentham-Dietz A, et al. Physical activity and survival after diagnosis of invasive breast cancer. *Cancer Epidemiol Biomarkers Prev*. 2008;17(2):379–386.

23. Beasley JM, Kwan ML, Chen WY, Weltzien EK, Korenke CH, Lu W, et al. Meeting the physical activity guidelines and survival after breast cancer: findings from the after breast cancer pooling project. *Breast Cancer Res Treat*. 2012;131(2):637-643.

24. Ainsworth BE, Haskell WL, Herrmann SD, Meckes N, Bassett Jr DR, Tudor-Locke C, et al. 2011 Compendium of Physical Activities: a second update of codes and MET values. *Medicine and Science in Sports and Exercise*. 2011;43(8):1575-1581.

25. Ainsworth BE, Haskell WL, Herrmann SD, Meckes N, Bassett Jr DR, Tudor-Locke C, et al. The Compendium of Physical Activities Tracking Guide. Healthy Lifestyles Research Center, College of Nursing & Health Innovation, Arizona State University. Retrieved [date] from the World Wide Web. https://sites.google.com/site/compendiumofphysicalactivities/

26. George SM, Irwin ML, Smith AW, Newhouser ML, Reedy J, McTiernan A, et al. Post diagnosis diet quality, the combination of diet quality and recreational physical activity, and prognosis after early-stage breast cancer. *Cancer Causes Control*. 2011;22(4):589-598.

27. National Cancer Institute. BRCA1 and BRCA2: Cancer Risk and Genetic Testing. http://www.cancer.gov/cancertopics/factsheet/Risk/BRCA. Accessed 1/28/13

28. American Cancer Society. Breast Cancer: Early Detection. Breast Cancer Risk Factors You Cannot Change. Last Revised 2/6/13. Accessed 4/29/13. http://www.cancer.org/cancer/breastcancer/moreinformation/breastcancerearlydetection/breast-cancer-early-detection-risk-factors-you-cannot-change

29. Watts KJ, Meiser B, Mitchel G, Kirk J, Saunders C, Peate M, et al. How should we discuss genetic testing with women newly diagnosed with breast cancer? Design and implementation of a randomized controlled trial of two models of delivering education about treatment-focused genetic testing to younger women newly diagnosed with breast cancer. *BMC Cancer*. 2012;12:320. Published online 2012 doi: 10.1186/1471-2407-12-320.

30. Breast. In: Edge SB, Byrd DR, Compton CC, et al., eds.: AJCC Cancer Staging Manual. 7th ed. New York, NY: Springer, 2010, pp 347-76.

31. American Cancer Society. How is breast cancer staged? Revised 2/26/13. Accessed 4/20/13. http://www.cancer.org/cancer/breastcancer/detailedguide/breast-cancer-staging from *AJCC: Breast. In: Edge SB, Byrd DR, Compton CC, et al., eds.: AJCC Cancer Staging Manual. 7th ed. New York, NY: Springer, 2010, pp 347-76.*

32. National Cancer Institute. Stage information for breast cancer. http://www.cancer.gov/cancertopics/pdq/treatment/breast/health professional/page3.

33. Fisher B, Costantino JP, Wickerham DL, Cecchini RS, Cronin WM, Robidoux A, et al. Tamoxifen for Prevention of Breast Cancer: Current Status of the National Surgical Adjuvant Breast and Bowel Project P-1 Study. *J Natl Ca Inst*. 2005;97(22):1652-1662.

34. Vogel VG, Costantino JP, Wickerham DL, Cronin WM, Cecchini RS, Atkins JN, et al. Effects of tamoxifen vs raloxifene on the risk of developing invasive breast cancer and other disease outcomes: the NSABP Study of Tamoxifen and Raloxifene (STAR) P–2 trial. *JAMA*. 2006; 295(23): 2727–2741.

35. National Cancer Institute. Breast Cancer Treatment. Last modified 4/4/13. Accessed 4/26/13. http://www.cancer.gov/cancertopics/pdq/treatment/breast/healthprofessional/page6.

36. Hadji P, Body JJ, Aapro MS, Brufsky A, Coleman RE, Guise T, et al. Practical guidance for the management of aromatase inhibitor-associated bone loss. *Ann Oncol*. 2008;19(8):1407-1416.

37. Robertson L, Hanson H, Seal S, Warren-Perry M, Hughes D, Howell I. BRCA1 testing should be offered to individuals with triple negative breast cancer diagnosed below 50 years. *Br J Cancer*. 2012;106(6): 1234-1238.

38. Peppone LJ, Huston AJ, Reid ME. The effect of various vitamin D supplementation regimens in breast cancer patients. *Breast Cancer Res Treat*. 2011;127(1):171-177.

39. Shao T, Klein P, Grossbard ML. Vitamin D and breast cancer. *Oncologist*. 2012;17(1):36-45

40. Committee to Review Dietary Reference Intakes for Vitamin D and Calcium, Food and Nutrition Board, Institute of Medicine. Dietary Reference Intakes for Calcium and Vitamin D. Washington, DC: National Academy Press, 2010.

41. U.S. Preventive Services Task Force. *Vitamin D and Calcium Supplementation to Prevent Fractures in Adults: Clinical Summary of USPSTF Recommendation*. AHRQ Publication No. 12-05163-EF-2. February 2013. http://www.uspreventiveservicestaskforce.org/uspstf12/vitamind/vitdsumm.htm Accessed April 20, 2013.

42. Weishaar T, Vergili JM. Vitamin D status is a biological determination of health disparities. *J Academy Nutr Dietetics*. 2013;113(5):643-651

43. Office of Dietary Supplements. Dietary Supplement Fact Sheet: Vitamin D. Reviewed June 24, 2011. http://ods.od.nih.gov/factsheets/VitaminD-HealthProfessional/ Accessed 4/16/13.

44. Ixempra (ixabepilone) for injection package insert. Princeton, NJ: Bristol-Myers Squibb company; 2011 Oct. Cited in Clinical Pharmacology, (2012). Retrieved from http://www.clinicalpharmacology-ip.com/Forms/Monograph/monograph.aspx?cpnum=3577&sec=monadve.

45. National Cancer Institute, (2012). Drugs approved for breast cancer. Retrieved from http://www.cancer.gov/cancertopics/druginfo/breastcancer.

46. National Comprehensive Cancer Network, (2012). NCCN clinical practice guidelines in oncology: breast cancer. Version 3.2012. Retrieved from http://www.nccn.org/professionals/physician_gls/pdf/breast.pdf.

47. Oncology Nursing Society, (2009). *Chemotherapy and biotherapy guidelines and recommendations for practice*. Pittsburgh, PA: ONS Publishing Division. ISBM: 978-1-890504-81-6.

48. Newton, S. Hickey M, Marrs J. *Oncology nursing advisor: A comprehensive guide to clinical practice*. St. Louis, MO: Mosby Elsevier. 2009. ISBN: 978-0-323-04597-1.

49. Prescher-Hughes DS and Alkhoudairy CJ. *Clinical practice protocols in oncology nursing*. Sudbury, MA: Jones and Bartlett Publishers. 2007.

50. American Cancer Society, (2012). *Radiation therapy for breast cancer*. Retrieved from http://www.cancer.org/cancer/breastcancer/detailedguide/breast-cancer-treating-radiation.

51. Constantine C, Parhar P, Lymberis S, Fenton-Kerimian M, Han SC, Rosenstein, BS, et al. Feasibility of accelerated whole-breast radiation in the treatment of patients with ductal carcinoma in situ of the breast. *Clinical Breast Cancer*. 2008;8(3). doi: 10.3816/CBC.2008.n.031.

52. Rock CL, Doyle C, Demark-Wahnefried W, Meyerhardt J, Courneya KS, Schwartz AL, et al. Nutrition and physical activity guidelines for cancer survivors. *CA Cancer J Clin*. 2012;62(4):243-274.

53. Demark-Wahnefried W, Campbell KL, Hayes SC. Weight management and its role in breast cancer rehabilitation. *Cancer*. 2012;118(8 suppl): 2277-2287.

54. McNeely ML, Peddle C, Yurick JL, et al. Conservative and dietary interventions for cancer-related lymphedema-A systemic review and meta-analysis. *Cancer*. 2011;117:1136-48.

55. Pressoir M, Desne S, Berchery D, Rossignol G, Poiree B, Meslier M, et al. Prevalence, risk factors and clinical implications of malnutrition in French Comprehensive Cancer Centres. *Br J Cancer*. 2010;102(6):966-971.

56. Norman K, Pichard C, Lochs H, Pirlich M. Prognostic impact of disease-related malnutrition. *Clin Nutr*. 2008;27(1):5-15.

57. Prado CM, Baracos VE, McCargar LJ, et al. Sarcopenia as a determinant of chemotherapy toxicity and time to tumor progression in metastatic breast cancer patients receiving capecitabine treatment. *Clin Cancer Res*. 2009;15:2920–2926.

58. Santarpia L, Contaldo F, Pasanisi F. Nutrition screening and early treatment of malnutrition in cancer patients. *J Cachexia Sarcopenia Muscle*. 2011;2(1):27-35.

59. Ahn J, Schatzkin A, Lacey JV Jr, et al. Adiposity, adult weight change, and postmenopausal breast cancer risk. *Arch Intern Med*. 2007;167:2091-2102.

60. Eliassen AH, Colditz GA, Rosner B, Willett WC, Hankinson SE. Adult weight change and risk of postmenopausal breast cancer. *JAMA*. 2006;296:(2) 193-201.

61. Harvie M, Howell A, Vierkant RA, et al. Association of gain and loss of weight before and after menopause with risk of postmenopausal breast cancer in the Iowa women's health study. *Cancer Epidemiol Biomarkers Prev*. 2005;14(3):656-661.

62. Majed B, Moreau T, Asselain B. Curie Institute Breast Cancer Group. Overweight, obesity and breast cancer prognosis: optimal body size indicator cut-points. *Breast Cancer Res Treat*. 2009;115(1):193–203.

63. Food, nutrition, physical activity, and the prevention of cancer: a global perspective. Washington DC: World Cancer Research Fund/American Institute for Cancer Research; 2007.

64. Hurst JD and Gallagher AL. Energy, macronutrient, micronutrient, and fluid requirements In *The Clinical Guide to Oncology Nutrition*, 2nd edition. Editors: Elliott L, Molseed LL, McCallum PD. American Dietetic Association: p 54-71.

65. Champ C, Volek JS, Siglin J, Jin L, Simone NL. Weight gain, metabolic syndrome, and breast cancer recurrence: are dietary recommendations supported by the data? *Int J Breast Cancer*. 2012;2012:506868. doi: 10.1155/2012/506868.

66. Russell M and Malone AM. Nutrient requirements In *ADA Pocket Guide to Nutrition Assessment*, 2nd ed, Editors Charney P and Malone AM. American Dietetic Association, 2009.p 167-191.

67. Dietary Reference Intakes (DRIs): Elements. Food and Nutrition Board, Institute of Medicine, National Academies. http://www.iom.edu/ Activities/Nutrition/SummaryDRIs/~/media/Files/Activity%20Files/ Nutrition/DRIs/New%20Material/6_%20Elements%20Summary.pdf Accessed November 5, 2012.

68. Lefton J, Malone AM. Anthropometric Assessment. In *ADA Pocket Guide to Nutrition Assessment*, 2nd ed, Editors Charney P and Malone AM. American Dietetic Association, 2009.p 154-166.

69. Campbell KL, Van Patten CL, Neil SE, et al. Feasibility of a lifestyle intervention on body weight and serum biomarkers in breast cancer survivors with overweight and obesity. *J Acad Nutr Diet*. 2012;112(4): 559-567.

70. Nechuta SJ, Caan BJ, Chen WY. The after breast cancer pooling project: rationale, methodology, and breast cancer survivor characteristics. *Cancer Causes Control*. 2011;22(9):1319-1331.

71. Kim EH, Willett WC, Fung T, Rosner B, Holmes MD. Diet quality indices and postmenopausal breast cancer survival. *Nutr Cancer*. 2011;63(3);381-388.

72. Robien K, Demark-Wahnefried W, Rock CL. Evidence-based nutrition guidelines for cancer survivors: Current guidelines, knowledge gaps, and future research directions. *J Am Diet Assoc*. 2011;111(3):368-375.

73. Gold EB, Pierce JP, Natarajan L, Stefanick ML, Laughlin GA, Caan BJ, et al. Dietary pattern influences breast cancer prognosis in women without hot flashes: the women's healthy eating and living trial. *J Clin Oncol*. 2009;27(3):352-9. doi: 10.1200/JCO.2008.16.1067. Epub 2008 Dec 15.

74. Rock CL, Natarajan L, Pu M, et al. Women's Healthy Eating & Living Group. Longitudinal biological exposure to carotenoids is associated with breast cancer-free survival in the Women's Healthy Eating and Living Study. *Cancer Epidemiol Biomarkers Prev*. 2009;18(2):486-494.

75. Simopoulos AP. Genetic variants in the metabolism of omega-6 and omega-3 fatty acids: their role in the determination of nutritional requirements and chronic disease risk. *Exper Biol Med*. 2010;235(7): 785-795.

76. Spencer L, Mann, C, Metcalfe M, Webb M, Pollard C, Spencer D, et al. The effect of omega-3 FAs on tumour angiogenesis and their therapeutic potential. *Eur J Cancer*. 2009;45(12):2077-86.

77. Bougnoux P, Hajjaji N, Maheo K, Couet C, Chevalier S. Fatty acids and breast cancer: sensitization to treatments and prevention of metastatic re-growth. *Prog Lipid Res*. 2010;49(1):76-86.

78. Patterson RE, Flatt SW, Newman VA, et al. Marine fatty acid intake is associated with breast cancer prognosis. *J Nutr* 2011;141(2):201-206. Epub 2010 Dec 22.

79. Brasky TM, Lampe JW, Potter JD, Patterson RE, White E. Specialty supplements and breast cancer risk in the VITamins and Lifestyle (VITAL) Cohort. *Cancer Epidemiol Biomarkers Prev* 2010;19(7):1696-708.

80. U.S. Department of Agriculture and U.S. Department of Health and Human Services. Dietary Guidelines for Americans, 2010. 7th Edition, Washington, DC: U.S. Government Printing Office, December 2010.

81. Department of Health and Human Services, US Food and Drug Administration. Substances affirmed as generally recognized as safe: menhaden oil. *Federal Register*. June 5, 1997. Vol. 62, No. 108: pp 30751–30757. 21 CFR Part 184 [Docket No. 86G-0289].

82. Kris-Etherton PM, Harris WS, Appel LJ; American Heart Association. Nutrition Committee. Fish consumption, fish oil, omega-3 fatty acids, and cardiovascular disease. *Circulation*. 2002;106:2753.

83. Aune D, Chan DSM, Greenwood DC, Vieira AR, Rosenblatt DAN, Vieira R, et al. Dietary fiber and breast cancer risk: a systematic review and meta-analysis of prospective studies. *Ann Oncology*. 2012 doi:10.1093/ annonc/mdr589.

84. McCann SE, Hootman KC, Weaver AM, Thompson LU, Morrison C, Hwang H, et al. Dietary intakes of total and specific lignans are associated with clinical breast tumor characteristics. *J Nutr*. 2012;142(1):91-98.

85. Kushi LH, Doyle C, McCullough M, et al. American Cancer Society guidelines on nutrition and physical activity for cancer prevention. *CA Cancer J Clin*. 2012;62(1):30-67.

86. Messina M. Insights gained from 20 years of soy research. *J Nutr*. 2010;140:2289S-2295S.

87. Caan BJ, Natarajan L, Parker B, et al. Soy food consumption and breast cancer prognosis. *Cancer Epidemiol Biomarkers Prev*, 2011;20(5):854-858.

88. Messina M. Expert Interview with Mark Messina, PhD: soyfood and breast cancer. *Oncology Nutrition Connection*. 2010;19(1):3-6.

89. NDSR, 2010, University of Minnesota, Nutrition Data System for Research (includes data from USDA Database for the Isoflavone Content of Selected Foods, Release 2.0, September 2008.

90. Trujillo E and Ross S. Tea and cancer prevention. National Cancer Institute, Division of Cancer Prevention. Accessed 5/29/13.

91. Johnson R, Bryant S, Huntley AL. Green tea and green tea catechin extracts: An overview of the clinical evidence. *Maturitas*. 2012;73(4): 280-287.

92. Newman VA. Fighting cancer with food and activity. J Calif Dental Hygien Assoc 2012 (Summer);27(2):25-27.

93. National Cancer Institute. www.cancer.gov/cancertopics/factsheeet/risk/ obesity (accessed 6/28/13).

94. U.S. Department of health and Human Services. www.healthlgov/ paguidelines (accessed 6/28/13)

95. Tudor-Locke C, Bassett Dr Jr. How many steps/day are enough? Preliminary pedometer indices for public health. *Sports Med*. 2004; 34(1):1-8.

Medical Nutrition Therapy for Esophageal Cancer

Maureen Leser, MS, RD, CSO, LD

Definition and Prevalence

Esophageal cancer (EC) ranks as the eighth most common cancer in the world, and its incidence is rising in the United States (U.S.) (1). EC is three to four times more common in men than women, and in the U.S. the median age at diagnosis is 67 years (2-5). In 2013, 17,990 new cases of esophageal cancer and 15,210 deaths from this disease are expected. Five-year survival for all cases of EC is 19%, but survival almost doubles when diagnosed at an early or localized stage (2-5).

Most esophageal cancers originate from two types of cells found in the esophagus. Squamous cell carcinomas (SCC) arise in the upper two-thirds of the esophagus from squamous cells, which usually

Figure 1: The Esophagus

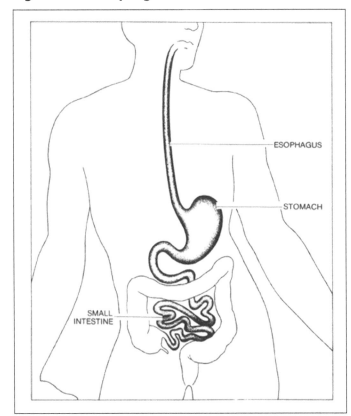

Reprinted with permission
The website of the National Cancer Institute (http://www.cancer.gov).

populate the esophagus. Adenocarcinomas of the esophagus (AE) arise from columnar epithelial cells commonly found in the lower third of the esophagus (1-3). Historically, SCC accounted for the majority of EC cases, but over the past several decades incidence of AE in the U.S. has dramatically increased; total EC cases are now equally split between SCC and AE (1). Esophageal tumors generally originate in the inner layers of the esophagus and spread inward and outward through the esophageal wall before metastasizing to other organs.

Anatomy

The esophagus is a 10-13 inch long hollow, muscular tube that allows food to pass from the throat to the stomach (3,5). Sphincter muscles at both ends of the esophagus control movement of food into and out of this tube. The upper esophageal sphincter (UES) relaxes when it senses the need to swallow a food bolus. Just past the gastro-esophageal junction, where the esophagus connects to the stomach, the lower esophageal sphincter (LES) relaxes to allow food boluses to enter the stomach. The LES tightens after the bolus passes through, thus preventing stomach acid and digestive enzymes from moving up and into the esophagus.

Risk Factors

Smoking and alcohol are primary risk factors for SCC; carcinogens from tobacco smoke and chronic irritation from alcohol will damage squamous cells and potentially promote carcinogenesis (1,3,6). Infections from Helicobacter Pylori and Human Papillomavirus (HPV) also are risk factors for SCC (7-8). In South America, an important risk factor for SCC is the beverage mate, which is an herbal infusion usually sipped at scalding temperatures through a metal straw (9). Less common risk factors for SCC include Tylosis A, a rare familial disease characterized by skin thickening that carries an almost 50% lifetime risk of developing this disease (10). Esophageal achalasia, an esophageal motility disorder that results in an unusually strong LES and retention of food in the esophagus, also increases risk of SCC (10).

AE is predominately diagnosed in the lower third of the esophagus and the gastro-esophageal junction (1,3,5). Gastro-esophageal reflux disease (GERD) is a primary risk factor for AE because reflux sends gastric acids, which damage esophageal tissue, back up and into the esophagus (11-15). GERD also increases the risk of Barrett's Esophagus (BE) by 3-5 fold (11-15). BE, which is characterized by inflamed tissue in the lower esophagus, may be an intermediate stage between GERD and AE, and is associated with a 30-60 fold increased risk of AE (11-15). GERD and BE are more often diagnosed in obese individuals, which may explain why obesity is also associated with an increased risk of AE (15).

GERD is commonly managed with proton-pump inhibitors, H-2 antagonists, and prokinetic agents; patients with GERD also may benefit from wearing looser clothing and not lying down after eating (16). Because GERD is over twice as common in obese individuals as compared with those with BMIs in the normal range, weight management for obesity is also recommended for this condition (15). Research trials have not examined efficacy of specific dietary modifications, but those diagnosed with GERD are commonly advised to avoid alcohol, chocolate, citrus juice, tomato-based products, peppermint, coffee, and onion while also adopting low fat eating habits and consuming smaller volumes of food at mealtime (15).

Researchers are actively examining associations between various dietary intake patterns and cancer risk; some evidence suggests that dietary patterns emphasizing plant foods may decrease EC risk, in particular when compared with intake patterns that emphasize animal products (17-18).

Symptoms and Staging
Symptoms of EC rarely occur when the disease is localized. As the cancer grows, swallowing becomes difficult (dysphagia), and heartburn-like pain often occurs. Additional symptoms include hoarseness, coughing, anorexia, and weight loss (3). When reported to a medical doctor (MD), symptoms suggestive of esophageal cancer trigger a diagnostic workup that begins with a physical examination followed by biochemical tests and radiographic studies. Barium swallows, endoscopic ultrasounds, PET scans, chest and/or abdominal CTs, MRIs, and biopsies are among tests performed (3). When EC is diagnosed, results from diagnostic tests are used to stage EC. The American Joint Committee on Cancer (AJCC) has developed a widely used staging system based on Tumor size, extent of lymph Node involvement, and Metastasis (19). The National Cancer

Table 1: Nutrition Related Effects of Esophageal Cancer TreatmentsΔ (23-25)

Agent Generic name (Brand Name)	Anorexia	Nausea / Vomiting	Diarrhea	Constipation	Mucositis	Altered Taste	Myelo-suppression
Chemotherapies:							
Capecitabine (Xeloda®)		3	3				3
Carboplatin (Paraplatin®)		3					3
Cisplatin (Platinol, CDDP®)		3	3			3	3
Docetaxel (Taxotere®)		3	3		3		3
Doxorubicin (Adriamycin®)	3	3	3		3		3
Epirubicin (Ellence®)		3	3		3		3
Fluorouracil (5-FU)*		3	3		3		3
Irinotecan (Camptosar®)	3	3	3				3
Methotrexate**		3			3		3
Mitomycin (mytamycin®)	3	3	3		3		3
Oxaliplatin*** (Eloxatin®)		3	3				3
Paclitaxel (Taxol®)		3	3		3		3
Topotecan (Hycamtin®)	3	3	3		3		3
Vinorelbine (Navelbine®)	3	3		3			3
Radiation Therapy to the esophagus	Common symptoms include anorexia, fatigue, dysphagia, odynophagia, and heartburn						
Targeted Therapies:							
Cetuximab (Erbitux®);	3	3	3				
Trastuzumab (Herceptin™)		3	3				3
Bevacizumab (Avastin®)			3		3		

Δ Refer to chapter 11 for details about cancer treatments.

* Suck on ice chips pre/post IV bolus to reduce mucositis
** Avoid vitamin supplements providing folic acid (drug limits bio-physiology of folic acid)
*** Avoid all cold foods when taking this drug

Institute also has described stages of esophageal cancer; their system uses Roman numerals I (early stage esophageal cancer), II, III, and IV (advanced esophageal cancer) (3).

Treatments

Treatments for EC include esophageal dilation to temporarily relieve obstruction, chemotherapy, radiation therapy, combined chemo-radiation, targeted therapy, and surgery (3,20). For those diagnosed with metastatic disease, Karnofsky performance scores and ECOG performance scores influence treatment options. When Karnofsky performance score is ≥60% or ECOG performance score is ≤2, chemotherapy along with supportive care is indicated (21-22). When performance status scores do not meet these standards, treatment may be limited to best supportive care. See Appendix 2 for a summary of performance status assessment methods.

Table 1 outlines nutrition impact symptoms associated with common chemotherapy agents, radiation therapy, and targeted therapies used to treat EC. Please see Chapter 11 for a full discussion of types of cancer therapies and their full range of side effects and Chapter 12 for strategies to manage nutrition impact symptoms.

Surgery:

EC patients eligible for surgery commonly undergo one of two operations: esophagectomy or esophagogastrectomy (3,20,26).

Esophagectomy involves surgical removal of cancerous tissue within the esophagus, nearby lymph nodes, and possibly part of the stomach. The remaining part of the esophagus is then connected to the stomach.

Esophagogastrectomy involves surgical removal of the cancerous tissue within the esophagus, nearby lymph nodes, and the top portion of the stomach. The remaining stomach is then pulled up and connected to the remaining portion of the esophagus. On occasion the surgeon uses a small section of the colon to reconnect the esophagus to the stomach. This surgery is often required when esophageal cancer has advanced and spread to the upper portion of the stomach.

Figure 2: Anatomical Changes in Esophagectomy

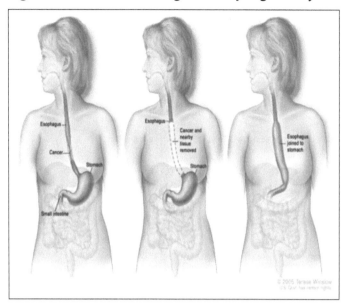

© 2005 Terese Winslow, U.S. Govt. has certain rights

Dumping Syndrome After Esophagectomy or Esophagogastrectomy:

By altering digestive anatomy, esophagectomy and esophagogastrectomy surgeries affect digestion and absorption. Both procedures can speed up gastric emptying, allowing incompletely digested and hyperosmolar chyme to enter the small intestine (SI) (24-25). When fluids rush to the SI to normalize osmolarity, the high fluid volume, along with hormonal and vasomotor changes, result in bloating, abdominal cramps, nausea, and dumping. Symptoms often increase after eating foods high in sugar (24-25) and diminish or resolve when medical nutrition therapy is implemented. Table 2 summarizes the timing, symptoms, and general nutrition management recommendations for the two type of dumping; see Appendix 4 for Anti-Dumping dietary guidelines.

Table 2: Anti-Dumping Diet

	Timing	Symptoms	Medical Nutrition Therapy for Dumping Syndrome: (24-25)
Early Dumping (75% of cases)	10-30 minutes post-prandial	Epigastric fullness, nausea, vomiting, abdominal cramps, bloating, diarrhea, Lightheadedness, diaphoresis, desire to lie down, borborygmi, pallor, palpitations	An Anti-Dumping diet should limit foods high in concentrated sugars. Foods high in soluble fiber may help reduce symptoms. Lactose-free foods may be better tolerated than foods with lactose. Small amounts (e.g. < 1 tablespoon per meal) of butter, oil, or margarine can be added to food for energy but fried and greasy foods should be avoided. Drink liquids 30 minutes before or after meals, but not during meals. Eat 5-6 small meals daily and avoid eating large portions. Eating slowly and chewing food into very small pieces or until liquefied may also help manage this condition.
Late Dumping (25% of cases)	1-3 hours post-prandial	Hunger, perspiration, tremors, difficulty concentrating	

In Western countries, approximately 50% of patients with esophageal cancer are ineligible for surgery because of comorbidities or being diagnosed at an advanced stage (26). In these cases, esophageal stent insertion and/or laser ablation may provide palliation (26). Ablation is intended to shrink the size of the tumor, allowing soft or pureed foods and/or liquids to pass through to the stomach while stent insertion is intended to create a bypass through the esophagus. The primary goal of each treatment is to relieve symptoms of dysphagia. In this setting, the RD will continue to provide appropriate nutrition interventions for nutrition impact symptoms.

Malnutrition and Esophageal Cancer

Inadequate energy intake and weight loss (together) are now considered sufficient diagnostic criteria for malnutrition (27). Incidence of malnutrition in cancer ranges from 15%-80% (28) with increased prevalence occurring in gastrointestinal cancers. Pre-operatively, malnutrition may make someone ineligible for surgery. Post-operatively, malnutrition increases morbidity and mortality. It can delay wound healing and increases risk of post-operative infections and dehiscence of surgical anastomosis (29-30). Malnutrition increases the risk of chemotherapy and radiation treatment breaks and incomplete treatment, each of which is associated with reduced response rates to radio- and chemotherapy, shorter periods of remission, and increased mortality (31-33). All of these factors are potentially significant for those diagnosed with esophageal cancer, which has a 78.9% prevalence of malnutrition (32). In addition, up to 90% of EC patients lose ≥5% of body weight while 16% lose >15% of body weight after surgery (34).

Energy and Nutrient Requirements of Esophageal Cancer Patients

There is general agreement that energy expenditure (EE) is increased in cancer patients (35-37), though emerging research suggests that EE may vary according to diagnosis (38). There is limited research on energy needs specific to esophageal cancer. Reviews of energy expenditure in malnourished gastrointestinal

cancer patients found that most were normometabolic (38) and that EE in malnourished and well-nourished EC patients were similar (39), though REE may be reduced by up to 30% in starvation (40). A small study estimated energy needs (based on resting energy expenditure (REE) + Activity Factors) of EC patients at between 30-35 kcal/kg (41), consistent with usual recommendations for nutrition repletion in oncology patients (42).

Protein needs of cancer patients with normal renal function range from 1.0 to 1.6 g/kg, based on stress level (42). Other baseline nutrient (43-44), electrolyte, and fluid needs (42) are assumed to be consistent with Dietary Reference Intakes (DRIs) or as indicated from a nutrition assessment. Table 3 summarizes estimated nutrient needs for the esophageal cancer patient.

Nutrition Risk Screening and Assessment of the Esophageal Cancer Patient

Most EC cases present with involuntary weight loss (47) and patients are at high risk of poor intake during treatment, criteria that should trigger a positive nutrition risk screening (48) and nutrition assessment. The Evidence Analysis Library (EAL) of the Academy of Nutrition and Dietetics recommends pre-treatment evaluation and weekly visits for six weeks during chemoradiation treatment for esophageal cancer (49).

Dysphagia is the most common presenting nutrition impact symptom of EC, and occurs when a tumor mass grows into the esophageal tube. Worldwide, over 70% of patients diagnosed with EC present with weight loss and dysphagia (47). Once treatment begins, additional symptoms further contribute to difficulty eating and weight loss.

Enteral Nutrition

Even when combined with supportive medications such as antiemetics, oral diet may not sustain nutritional status throughout chemoradiation treatment. To meet nutritional needs, EC patients

Table 3: Estimated Nutrient Requirements for Esophageal Cancer (42-46)

Nutrient	Estimated Nutrient Needs
Energy (42)	30-35 kcal/kg or as determined during a nutrition assessment
Protein, assuming normal renal function (42)	1.0-1.2g/kg if weight is stable and patient is non-stressed; 1.2-1.6g/kg if patient is stressed and has been losing weight and lean body mass
Vitamins (43)	100% of DRI or adjusted per specific needs (e.g., RD to advise patient if antioxidant supplements should be avoided during treatment)
Minerals (44)	100% of DRI or adjusted per specific needs (e.g., some chemo drugs increase renal loss of magnesium, thus increasing needs)
Electrolytes (45)	100% of DRI or adjusted per specific needs (e.g., electrolyte losses may increase needs)
Fluid (46)	Body Surface Area Method: 1500 mL/m^2 Daily water requirements based on body weight = (< 10 kg: 100 mL/kg; 11-20 kg: 1000 mL + 50 mL/kg for each kg > 10 kg; >20 kg: 1500 mL+ 20 mL/kg for each kg>20 kg) Findings from nutrition assessment may indicate a different need (e.g., increased need when fluid losses increase due to diarrhea)

undergoing treatment may require enteral nutrition (EN) via a Jejunostomy (J) tube.

The EAL of the Academy states that EN has been shown to maintain weight during chemoradiation therapy but not to improve tolerance to treatment or survival (50). A best evidence topic in surgery concluded that early EN provided no clinical benefit when compared with a no-feeding strategy because of morbidity associated with enteral catheters, but authors acknowledged that studies reviewed had limitations including small numbers and heterogeneous treatment of control groups (51). In a review of 463 patients who underwent an esophagogastrectomy for EC and received enteral feeds, authors concluded that feeding jejunostomy was effective at meeting nutrition goals (achieved by POD 3 in 88% of the group), safe, economic, and well tolerated (52). Another review states that it is important to establish an enteral feeding route for esophagectomy patients because of the prevalence of mortality (5-10%) and morbidity (30-40%) associated with this operation and because 50% of patients experiencing complications do not tolerate an oral diet for 30+ days after surgery (53). Until this debate is resolved by additional research, many medical centers will continue to utilize EN for their EC patients because of the prevalence of malnutrition and eating difficulty experienced in this population. Nutrition support is addressed in Chapter 13; issues specific to the EC population are noted here.

- Jejunostomy tube feedings are preferred to gastric feedings because they allow early post-operative feeding beyond the anastomosis and do not interfere with post-operative gastric healing (54).
- Full strength, isotonic EN polymeric formulas are generally well tolerated when infused into the jejunum (55). Clinicians may test tolerance of an energy dense feeding (e.g., 1.5 versus 1.0 kcal/mL) to provide more nutrition in a smaller volume. Use of energy dense formulas require more frequent tube flushes.
- Semi-elemental or elemental formulas should usually be reserved for selected individuals with significant small bowel dysfunction or malabsorption.
- Fiber containing formulas may decrease the risk of bacterial overgrowth. To decrease risk of tube blockages when infusing fiber-containing formula, do not administer medications via the tube (56) and flush the tube at every scheduled interval (57).
- A small study by Ryan et al. demonstrated that EN formulas supplemented with omega-3 fats helped preserve lean body mass in esophagectomy patients (58), but additional evidence is needed before this practice can be widely recommended.

Conclusion:

EC and its treatments pose significant nutritional problems. RDs provide proactive, evidence-based nutrition care individualized to meet each patient's unique needs throughout the continuum of disease. Such care is integral to successful EC treatment and recovery.

References

1. Melhado RE, Alderson D, Tucker O. The changing face of esophageal cancer. *Cancers*. 2010;2:1379-1404; doi:10.3390/cancers2031379.
2. American Cancer Society: Cancer Facts and Figures 2013. Atlanta, Ga: American Cancer Society, 2013. http://www.cancer.org/research/cancerfactsfigures/cancerfactsfigures/cancer-facts-figures-2013. Accessed June 5, 2013.
3. National Cancer Institute. What you need to know about cancer of the esophagus. http://www.cancer.gov/cancertopics/wyntk/esophagus Revised April 2013. Accessed June 4, 2013.
4. National Cancer Institute. Surveillance Epidemiology and End Results. SEER Stat Fact Sheets: Esophagus. http://seer.cancer.gov/statfacts/html/esoph.html Accessed March 5, 2012.
5. American Cancer Society. Esophagus Cancer. http://www.cancer.org/Cancer/EsophagusCancer/DetailedGuide. Revised January 18, 2013. Accessed June 1, 2013.
6. Kamangar F, Chow WH, Abnet CC, Dawsey SM. Environmental causes of esophageal cancer. *Gastroenterol Clin North Am*. 2009;38(1):27-57, vii.
7. Ye W, Held M, Lagergren J, et al.: Helicobacter pylori infection and gastric atrophy: risk of adenocarcinoma and squamous-cell carcinoma of the esophagus and adenocarcinoma of the gastric cardia. *J Natl Cancer Inst*. 2004;96(5):388-96.
8. Syrjanen KJ, HPV infections and oesophageal cancer. *J Clin Pathol*. 2002;55(10):721-718.
9. Islami F, Boffetta P, Ren J, et al. High-temperature beverages and foods and esophageal cancer risk – a systematic review. *Int J Cancer*. 2009;125(3):491-524.
10. American Cancer Society. Risk factors for cancer of the esophagus. http://www.cancer.org/cancer/esophaguscancer/overviewguide/esophagus-cancer-overview-what-causes Accessed November 5, 2012.
11. Lagergren J, Bergström R, Lindgren A, et al. Symptomatic gastroesophageal reflux as a risk factor for esophageal adenocarcinoma. *N Engl J Med*. 1999;340 (11): 825-831.
12. Kubo A, Corley DA, Jensen CD, et al. Dietary factors and the risks of esophageal adenocarcinoma and Barrett's Esophagus. *Nutr Res Rev*. 2010;23(2):230-246.
13. Milind R and Attwood SE. Natural history of Barrett's esophagus. *World J Gastroenterol*. 2012;18(27):3483–3491.
14. Cossentino MJ, Wong RK. Barrett's esophagus and risk of esophageal adenocarcinoma. *Semin Gastrointest Dis* 2003;14(3):128-135.
15. Fenti D, Scaioli E, Baldi F, et al. Body weight, lifestyle, dietary habits and gastroesophageal reflux disease. *World J Gastroenterol*. 2009;15(14): 1690-1701.
16. Nwokediuko SC. Current trends in the management of gastroesophageal reflux disease: a review. *Gastroenterol*. 2012; 2012:391631. Published online 2012 July 11. doi: 10.5402/2012/391631
17. Bravi F, Edefonti V, Randi G, et al. Dietary patterns and the risk of esophageal cancer. *Annals of Oncology*. 2012;23(3):765-770.
18. Li WQ, Park Y, Wu JW, et al. Index-based dietary patterns and risk of esophageal and gastric cancer in a large cohort study. *Clin Gastroenterol Hepatol*. 2013 Apr 13. pii: S1542-3565(13)00463-1. doi: 10.1016/j.cgh.2013.03.023. [Epub ahead of print]
19. American Joint Committee on Cancer. *AJCC Cancer Staging Manual*. 6th ed. New York, NY: Springer; 2002.
20. National Cancer Institute. Esophageal Cancer Treatment; Treatment Option Overview (PDQ ®). http://www.cancer.gov/cancertopics/pdq/treatment/esophageal/HealthProfessional/page4 Accessed November 5, 2012.
21. Karnofsky D, Abelmann W, Craver L, Burchenal J. The use of nitrogen mustard in the palliative treatment of cancer. *Cancer*. 1948;1:634–656
22. Oken MM, Creech RH, Tormey, DC, et al. Toxicity and response criteria of the Eastern Cooperative Oncology Group. *Am J Clin Oncol* 1982;5(6): 649-655.
23. Ilson DH. Esophageal cancer chemotherapy: recent advances. *Gastrointest Cancer Res*. 2008;2(2):85-92.
24. Ukleja A. Dumping syndrome In: Nutrition issues in Gastroenterology, series #35. Parris CR, editor. *Practical Gastroenterology*. 2006;32-46

25. Tack J, Arts J, Caenepeel P, De Wulf D, Bisschops R. Pathophysiology, diagnosis and management of postoperative dumping syndrome. *Nat Rev Gastroenterol Hepatol.* 2009.6(10):583-590.

26. Kari RC, Schreiber R, Boulware D, et al. Factors affecting morbidity, mortality, and survival in patients undergoing Ivor Lewis esophagogastrectomy. *Ann Surg.* 2000;231(5):635-643.

27. White JV, Guenter P, Jensen G, et al. Consensus statement of the Academy of Nutrition and Dietetics/American Society for Parenteral and Enteral Nutrition: characteristics recommended for the identification and documentation of adult malnutrition (undernutrition). *J Acad Nutr Diet.* 2012;112(5):730-738.

28. Bozzetti F, Mariani L, Salvatore LV. The nutritional risk in oncology: a study of 1,453 cancer outpatients. *Support Care Cancer.* 2012;29(8):1919-1928.

29. Chambrier C and Sztark F. French clinical guidelines on perioperative nutrition. Update of the 1994 consensus conference on perioperative artificial nutrition for elective surgery in adults. *J Vasc Surg.* 2012. Oct 26. pii: S1878-7886(12)00077-X. doi: 10.1016/j.jviscsurg.2012.06.006.

30. Bozzetti F, Gianotti L, Braga M, Carlo VD, Mariani L. Postoperative complications in gastrointestinal cancer patients: the joint role of the nutritional status and the nutritional support. *Clin Nutr.* 2007;26(6): 698-709.

31. Aviles A, Yañez J, López T, et al. Malnutrition as an adverse prognostic factor in patients with diffuse large cell lymphoma. *Arch Med Res.* 1995;26(1):31–34

32. Baker LA, Gout BS, Crowe TC. Hospital malnutrition: prevalence, identification and impact on patients and the healthcare system. *Int J Environ Res Public Health.* 2011;8(2):514-527.

33. Santaparia L, Contaldo F, Pasanisi F. Nutrition screening and early treatment of malnutrition in cancer patients. *J Cachexia Sarcopenia Muscle.* 2011;2(1):27-35.

34. Bower MR, Martin RC. Nutritional management during neoadjuvant therapy for esophageal cancer. *J Surg Oncol.* 2009;100(1):82-87

35. Cao D-x, Zhang B, Quan Y, et al. Resting energy expenditure and body composition in patients with newly detected cancer. *Clin Nutr.* 2010;29(1):72-77.

36. Khor SM and Mohd Baidi B. Assessing the resting energy expenditure of cancer patients in the Penang general hospital. *Mal J Nutr.* 2011;17(1): 43-53.

37. Jatoi A, Daly BD, Hughes V, et al. The prognostic effect of increased resting energy expenditure prior to treatment for lung cancer. *Lung Cancer.* 1999;23(2):153-158.

38. Dempsey DT, Feurer ID, Knox LS, et al. Energy expenditure in malnourished gastrointestinal cancer patients. *Cancer.* 1984.53(6): 1265-1273.

39. Thomson SR, Hirshberg A, Haffejee AA, et al. Resting metabolic rate of esophageal carcinoma patients: a model for energy expenditure measurement in a homogenous cancer population. *J Parenter Enteral Nutr.* 1990;14(2):119-121.

40. Buchman AL, Letter to the Editor: Resting Energy Expenditure in Patients with esophageal carcinoma. *J Parenter Enteral Nutr.* 1990;14(3):550.

41. Okamoto H, Ssaki M, Johtatsu T, et al. Resting energy expenditure and nutritional status in patients undergoing transthoracic esophagectomy for esophageal cancer. *J Clin Biochem Nutr.* 2011;49(3):169-173.

42. Hurst JD and Gallagher AL. Energy, macronutrient, micronutrient, and fluid requirements In: *The Clinical Guide to Oncology Nutrition, 2nd edition.* Editors: Elliott L, Molseed LL, McCallum PD. American Dietetic Association: p 54-71.

43. Dietary Reference Intakes (DRIs): Recommended Dietary Allowances and Adequate Intakes, Vitamins. Food and Nutrition Board, Institute of Medicine, National Academies. http://www.iom.edu/Activities/Nutrition/ SummaryDRIs/~/media/Files/Activity%20Files/Nutrition/DRIs/New%20 Material/2_%20RDA%20and%20AI%20Values_Vitamin%20and%20 Elements.pdf Accessed November 5, 2012.

44. Dietary Reference Intakes (DRIs): Elements. Food and Nutrition Board, Institute of Medicine, National Academies. http://www.iom.edu/ Activities/Nutrition/SummaryDRIs/~/media/Files/Activity%20Files/ Nutrition/DRIs/New%20Material/6_%20Elements%20Summary.pdf Accessed November 5, 2012.

45. Dietary Reference Intakes (DRIs): Electrolytes and Water. http://www.iom. edu/Activities/Nutrition/SummaryDRIs/~/media/Files/Activity%20Files/ Nutrition/DRIs/New%20Material/9_Electrolytes_Water%20Summary.pdf Food and Nutrition Board, Institute of Medicine, National Academies. Accessed November 5, 2012.

46. Russell M and Malone AM. Nutrient requirements In *ADA Pocket Guide to Nutrition Assessment,* 2nd ed, Editors Charney P and Malone AM. American Dietetic Association,2009.p 167-191.

47. Lopes AB and Fagundes RB. Esophageal squamous cell carcinoma-precursor lesions and early diagnosis. *World J Gastrointest Endosc.* 2012;16;4(1):9-16.

48. Charney P and Marian M. Nutrition Screening and Nutrition Assessment. In *ADA Pocket Guide to Nutrition Assessment,* 2nd ed, Editors Charney P and Malone AM. American Dietetic Association, 2009. p 1-19.

49. Evidence Analysis Library. Academy of Nutrition and Dietetics Oncology (Onc) Esophageal Cancer: Chemoradiation and Medical Nutrition Therapy (MNT). Accessed November 6, 2012.

50. Evidence Analysis Library. Academy of Nutrition and Dietetics Oncology (Onc) Esophageal Cancer: Chemoradiation and Use of Enteral Nutrition. Accessed November 6, 2012.

51. Wheble GA, Benson RA, Khan OA. Is routine postoperative enteral feeding after oesophagectomy worthwhile? *Interact Cardiovasc Thorac Surg.* 2012;15(4):709-712.

52. Wani ML, Ahangar AG, Lone GN, et al. Feeding jejunostomy: does the benefit overweight the risk (a retrospective study from a single centre). *Int J Surg.* 2010;8(5):387-390.

53. Couper G, Jejunostomy after oesophagectomy: a review of evidence and current practice. *Proc Nutr Soc.* 2011;79(3):316-320.

54. Gupta V, Benefits versus risks: a prospective audit. Feeding jejunostomy during esophagectomy. *World J Surg.* 2009;33(7):1432-1538.

55. Kudsk KA, Jacobs DO. Nutrition. In: *Surgery: Basic Science and Clinical Evidence,* second edition. Ed, Norton JA, Barie PS, Bollinter R, et al. Springer Science+Business Media, LLC, 2008. p 111-138.

56. Collier P, Kudsk KA, Gezer J, Brown RO. Fiber-containing formula and needle catheter jejunostomies: a clinical evaluation. *Nutr Clin Pract.* 1994;9(3):101-103.

57. Boullata J, Brantley S, Corkins M, et al. Enteral Nutrition Practice Recommendations Task Force. Enteral Nutrition Practice Recommendations. Academy of Enteral and Parenteral Nutrition http:// www.ismp.org/tools/articles/ASPEN.pdf Accessed November 7, 2012

58. Ryan AM, Reynolds JV, Healy L, et al. Enteral nutrition enriched with eicosapentaenoic acid (EPA) preserves lean body mass following esophageal cancer surgery: Results of a double-blinded randomized controlled trial. *Ann Surg.* 2009;249(3):355-363.

Nutrition Management for Cancers of the Gastrointestinal Tract

Colleen Gill, MS, RD, CSO

Introduction

The gastrointestinal (GI) tract processes food to provide energy and nutrients for life. It also is an essential component of the immune system and helps manage fluid and electrolyte status. The unique anatomy of these essentially hollow organs digests food, converts macronutrients to micronutrients, and absorbs micronutrients. Digestion begins in the mouth, which prepares food to travel down the esophagus to the stomach. Along the way, nutrients are sent to the liver for further processing or storage and the gallbladder provides bile, which is essential for fat digestion and absorption. The final steps of digestion occur in the colon, which reabsorbs fluid, electrolytes and some minerals while preparing wastes for excretion.

This chapter provides an overview of the prevalence, survival, risk factors, signs and symptoms, treatments and nutritional management for the following GI cancers: stomach, colorectal, liver, gallbladder, and anus. Cancers of the head and neck, esophageal cancer, and pancreas and bile duct cancers are discussed in their own chapters and will not be addressed here. In addition, Chapter 14 provides a review of nutrition management strategies for patients undergoing surgeries involving the GI tract.

Possible Alterations in Nutrient Absorption

The oncology registered dietitian nutritionist (RDN) plays an essential role on the oncology team caring for individuals with cancers of the GI tract. A thorough understanding of normal gut function and possible alterations as result of a cancer and its treatment is essential for optimizing nutritional status, quality of life, and treatment outcomes. Across the diversity of GI cancers, one similarity is clear; early symptoms are often vague and diagnoses are frequently delayed until cancers are well advanced, thus placing patients at nutritional risk. In addition, the subsequent treatment of GI cancers can further impact the very structures involved in digestion and absorption of the nutrients. Specifically, surgical intervention can permanently alter the geography of the GI tract, while systemic (e.g., chemotherapy and biotherapy) and/or site-

Figure 1: Sites of Nutrient Absorption in the Gastrointestinal Tract

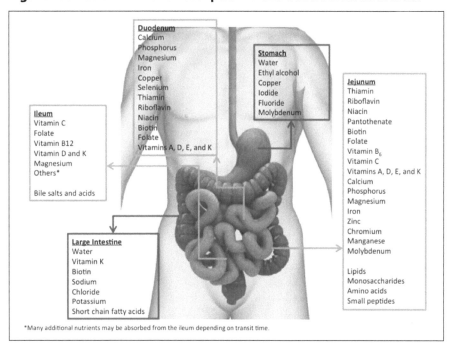

*Many additional nutrients may be absorbed from the ileum depending on transit time.

specific (e.g., radiation therapy) treatment modalities disproportionally impact the rapidly dividing cells that comprise the digestive system.

Macro- and micronutrients are digested and absorbed across the GI mucosa. Figure 1 is included to highlight the specific sites of nutrient absorption along the GI tract that may be impacted by the presence of cancer and prescribed treatment regimen.

Energy and Nutrient Requirements for Patients with Cancers of the GI Tract

As stated throughout the chapters of this book, it is generally agreed that cancer patients have increased energy expenditure (EE), although current evidence implies that EE differs depending upon their cancer diagnosis (1). The Academy of Nutrition and Dietetics' Evidence Analysis Library and chapter 4 outlines in detail evidence-based recommendations for precisely measuring resting metabolic rate and the nutrient needs of healthy to critically ill individuals (2). The information in Table 1 provides clinicians with additional information.

Table 1: Energy and Protein Needs in GI Cancer (3-9)

Nutrient	Estimated Nutrient Needs (per day as determined by nutrition assessment)
Nutrient needs for cancers of the stomach, colon, rectum, gallbladder and anus are similar to those of other cancers patients, as outlined in Chapter 4. Energy and protein needs in liver cancer are provided below	
Liver Disease *(including patients with ascites, cirrhosis or encephalopathy)*	
Energy	• 25-40 kcal/kg based on dry weight or determined ideal body weight for patients with ascites* • 35-40 kcal/kg for patients with stable cirrhosis • 25-35 kcal/kg for patients without encephalopathy • 35 kcal/kg for patients with acute encephalopathy • 30-40 kcal/kg for stable patients that are malnourished
Protein, assuming normal renal function	• 1.0-1.5 gm/kg for all patients, except those with encephalopathy • 0.6-0.8 gm/kg for patients with acute encephalopathy
*Estimated fluid excess in patients with ascites	• Mild ascites: 3-5 kg • Moderate ascites: 7-9 kg • Severe ascites: 14-15 kg

Gastric (Stomach) Cancer

Definition, Prevalence and Survival

The stomach is a fist-sized muscular organ that receives food via the esophagus, expanding in size to accommodate the volume. The stomach is comprised of two sections. The upper section is referred to as the proximal stomach (containing the cardia which is closest to the esophagus, the fundus, and the body). The lower section is known as the distal stomach (containing the antrum and the pylorus, which is the closest part of the stomach to the duodenum). Acid secreted by cells in the gastric wall helps break down food, releases vitamin B12 from food and provides protection against bacterial contamination. Food is blended and liquefied in the stomach; after particles of food are reduced to <1 – 2 mm in size, the resulting soup, called chyme, is emptied out of the stomach gradually, through the pyloric sphincter and into the duodenum, which is the first section of the small intestines. The contents of the stomach and duodenum trigger feedback mechanisms that control appetite and also affect the pace of stomach emptying into the small bowel. Refer to Chapter 14 for additional information regarding the function of the stomach prior to and after surgical resection.

Gastric cancer is the seventh leading cause of death in the United States (U.S.), although incidence has declined over the past 50 years (10). In Asia and developing countries incidence has not declined, prevalence is greater than in the U.S., and lack of refrigeration is considered a major risk factor. Approximately 22,000 Americans are diagnosed with gastric cancer each year and almost 11,000 will die as result of their disease (10). Stage at diagnosis has a significant impact on survival, with five-year U.S. survival rates >70% at Stage 1, falling to 4% at stage IV. Overall five-year survival is 28%, worsening with age > 60 and when tumors are > 5 cm or poorly differentiated (10).

The majority (90% to 95%) of gastric cancers are adenocarcinomas, but etiology and treatment are determined by location (11). Inflammatory changes related to infection with Helicobacter pylori (H. pylori) is believed to be the leading cause of gastric cancers,

especially in the distal stomach. Genetic variations in the host and bacteria along with environmental factors also impact the risk of developing precancerous lesions. Hereditary cancer syndromes also are linked to the development of gastric cancer (10). These include Lynch Syndrome, familial adenomatous polyposis (FAP), Li-Fraumeni Syndrome, and BRAC1 and BRAC2 mutations (10). Cancers of the gastro-esophageal junction (GEJ) and proximal (cardia) stomach share risk factors with esophageal cancer and are treated similarly. Gastric cancers most frequently metastasize to liver, lung or bone.

Other rarer forms of gastric tumors include lymphomas, leiomyosarcoma, and GI stromal tumors (GIST), and are not detailed here. These cancers also interfere with stomach function, and have side effects and treatment regimens similar to those described in

Table 2: Risk Factors for Gastric Cancers (10-17)

Location of Gastric Cancer	Risk Factors
Cardia/GEJ	• Being overweight or obese • Gastroesophageal Reflux Disease (GERD)
Both Cardia/Non-cardia	• Heavy alcohol intake • Smoking, use of tobacco products • Lack of physical activity
Non-cardia	• Chronic H. pylori infection • Hypochlorhydria • Atrophic gastritis • Autoimmune disorders resulting in pernicious anemia • Prior stomach surgeries including gastric bypass • History of childhood malnutrition • Salted and smoked foods (e.g. meats and fish, and pickled vegetables) • High heme iron intake from meats • High intake of grilled and processed meats • Low intake of fruits and vegetables, in particular those providing beta-carotene and vitamin C

Table 3 Nutrition Related Effects of GI Cancer Treatments Δ (19-24)

Agent Generic name (Brand Name)	Cancer Site	Anorexia	Nausea / Vomiting	Diarrhea	Consti-pation	Mucositis	Altered Taste	Myelo-suppression
Chemotherapy Agent:								
Capecitabine (Xeloda®)	G, C, GB		3	3				3
Carboplatin (Paraplatin®)	G		3					3
Cisplatin (Platinol, CDDP®)	G, C, H, GB, A		3	3			3	3
Docetaxel (Taxotere®)	G		3	3		3		3
Doxorubicin (Adriamycin®)	G, H	3	3	3		3		3
Epirubicin (Ellence®)	G		3	3		3		3
Fluorouracil (5-FU)*	G, C, H, GB, A		3	3		3		3
Gemcitabine (Gemzar®)	GB		3			3		3
Irinotecan (Camptosar®)	G, C	3	3	3				3
Mitomycin (mytamycin®)	G, A	3	3	3		3		3
Oxaliplatin*** (Eloxatin®)	G, C, GB		3	3				3
Paclitaxel (Taxol®)	G		3	3		3		3
Ziv-albercept (Zaltrap®)	C	3		3		3		3
Radiation therapy to the abdomen (stomach, liver, gallbladder)	Common side effects of external beam radiation therapy to the abdomen include: abdominal pain and discomfort, nausea, vomiting, urinary and bladder changes, diarrhea, changes in appetite, anorexia, and fatigue.							
Radiation therapy to the pelvis (small intestine, colon, rectum)	Common side effects of external beam radiation therapy to the pelvis include: diarrhea, bowel gas and bloating, urinary and bladder changes, proctitis, changes in appetite, anorexia, and fatigue.							
Biotherapy:								
Bevacizumab (Avastin®)	C, GB	3	3	3	3	3		3
Cetuximab (Erbitux®)	C, GB	3	3	3				
Panitumumab (Vectibix®)	C	3	3	3		3		3
Sorafenib (Nexavar®)	H	3	3	3				
Regorafenib (Stivarga®)	C	3	3	3		3		3
Trastuzumab (Herceptin®)	G, GB		3	3				3

Δ Refer to chapter 11 for details about cancer treatments.
A – Anal Carcinoma
C – Colorectal Cancer
G – Gastric Cancer
GB – Gallbladder Cancer

H – Hepatocellular (Liver) Cancer
* Suck on ice chips pre/post IV bolus to reduce mucositis
*** Avoid all cold foods when taking this drug

this chapter. Their nutritional management is also similar. About 3% of all gastric cancers are Carcinoid tumors which will be discussed later in the chapter.

Risk Factors

Gastric cancer is more common in men than women (10) and there is higher incidence of gastric cancer in minorities, specifically Hispanic Americans, African Americans, and Asian Americans (10). Risk factors according to the site are outlined in Table 2.

Signs and Symptoms

Early satiety (feeling full or bloated after eating), heartburn or indigestion, abdominal pain and discomfort, nausea, vomiting with or without blood, anorexia and unintended weight loss are common symptoms of gastric cancer. Because these symptoms are associated with a variety of other conditions, they are sometimes initially ignored. These symptoms can lead to reduced food intake, which may partially explain why malnutrition and weight loss occurs in >70% of people diagnosed with gastric cancer. Additional symptoms include unexplained anemia related to impaired iron absorption and gastroesophageal reflux disease (GERD).

When gastric cancer is suspected the diagnostic workup usually begins with an upper endoscopy with biopsy, HER2/neu testing, and when confirmed imaging studies may include endoscopic ultrasound (EUS), computed tomography (CT) and positron emission tomography (PET) scans (18).

Treatment

Treatment for gastric cancer includes chemotherapy, biotherapy, radiation therapy and surgery. Common treatment regimens include two or more of these treatment modalities. Factors determining choice of regimen take into consideration the size, location, and stage of disease, and the individual's age and general health. Most importantly, oncologists base treatment decisions on evidence-based guidelines outlined in the *National Comprehensive Cancer Network (NCCN) Clinical Practice Guidelines in Oncology* for gastric cancer (18).

Each treatment modality is associated with unique side effects, which are often intensified when therapies are combined. Chapter 11 provides an extensive review of cancer treatments including chemotherapy, biotherapy and radiation therapy, and possible side effects associated with these modalities. Treatment regimens can result in nutrition impact symptoms (NIS) such as anorexia, nausea, vomiting and gastric pain (among other symptoms), which can lead to extremely limited intake and rapid, unintended weight loss. Medical and nutrition management of NIS (see chapter 12 for management strategies) are initially preferred to enteral nutrition.

Systemic (e.g. chemotherapy and biotherapy) and/or site-specific radiation therapy, if indicated, are given either preoperatively, perioperatively (pre and post surgery) or postoperatively. Table 3 outlines commonly experienced NIS of gastric cancer treatments.

Nutrition Management

Surgical resections of gastric tumors can be partial or total, and may be curative or palliative. Types of partial gastrectomies include: Billroth I (gastroduodenostomy), Billroth II (gastrojejunostomy), partial gastric resection, and Rouex-en-Y procedure. Recovery can be extended, thus feeding tubes are often placed at the time of surgery for nutrition support during the transition to oral feedings. The following gastric cancer nutrition matrix (see Table 4) outlines nutrition management strategies for various surgeries and symptoms experienced. Although not stated in literature, many oncologists and surgeons often prefer to avoid pre-operative gastrostomy tube feeding placement in patients with favorable prognoses because of potential complications for the pending

Table 4: Medical Nutrition Therapy (MNT) Matrix for Gastric Cancer Surgery (25-28)

Possible Nutrition-Related Complications	Nutrition Management Suggestions
Gastrectomy (Partial or total)	**Pre-op Nutrition Intervention:** • Small, frequent meals and intake of soft, easy-to-digest foods and fluids, as tolerated. **Post-op Nutrition Intervention:** • Small, frequent feedings of ice or water are initiated first on post-op day 1 and 2. Once tolerated, initiate small, frequent meals comprised of soft, easy-to-digest foods and fluids. Food should be chewed thoroughly. • Initially limit refined carbohydrate foods and lactose. • Avoid greasy and fried foods and initially limit total fat intake by choosing low fat foods. • Include a protein source with each meal. • Separate solids from fluids; wait 30 to 60 minutes before or after eating solids before consuming fluids. • As oral diet tolerance is established, the diet is liberalized. When jejunal tube feedings are used for nutrition support: • Continuous feedings (pump) are indicated. • Fiber-free 1.0 standard formula, over 8 – 20 hours, advancing as tolerated. • Begin with small volumes of full strength formula (~20-30 cc/hour) and advance as tolerated. • Refer to Chapter 13 for a complete discussion of enteral nutrition support and Chapter 14 for preoperative and postoperative nutritional management.
Gastroesophageal reflux disease	• Small, frequent (5-6 meals/day) intake of food. • Elevate head at least 30 degrees while sleeping.
Dumping Syndrome	• Follow anti-dumping diet and recommendations described in Chapter 19 and Appendix 4. • Eat 5 – 6 small meals daily and avoid large portions. • Limit foods high in concentrated sugars. • Drink liquids 30 minutes before or after meals.
Osteoporosis risk and interventions	Gastrectomy increases the risk of osteoporosis: • Recommend DEXA scanning every 2 years for individuals with low BMI, significant weight loss, other risk factors. • Monitor serum vitamin D levels (goal > 20 ng/mL). • Encourage total calcium intake of 1500 mg/day. When calcium supplements are needed choose calcium citrate, divide doses (≤ 500 mg/dose) and separate from iron-rich foods or oxalates. • Recommend smoking cessation, limiting alcoholic beverage intake and increased weight bearing exercise.
Vitamin/mineral Malabsorption	Risk of nutritional anemias may be increased due to possible malabsorption of iron, folate, and vitamin B12: • Monitor serum iron status. Review strategies to maximize iron absorption. Iron supplementation may be indicated. • Monitor serum Vitamin B12. Vitamin B12 supplementation may be indicated. • Monitor serum folate via RBC and folate level. Folic acid supplementation may be indicated.
	Note: Appendices 3-5 provide dietary recommendations for various GI surgeries

gastrectomy. Additional information on gastric surgeries is available in chapter 14.

Colorectal Cancer (CRC)
Definition, Prevalence and Survival
The colon, or large bowel, is a muscular tube that stretches from the ileum to the rectum and is responsible for maintaining hydration and conserving electrolytes by reabsorbing fluid and salts. Transit through the small bowel can take one to four hours, but transit through the colon may take 10 times as long, slowing significantly as a side effect of many medications, including narcotics. The walls of the colon contract with waves of peristalsis to move the stool along, reducing its volume as fluid is reabsorbed. It is then stored in the sigmoid colon until evacuation into the rectum, typically one to two times a day. The rectum is an eight-inch reservoir with sphincters that relax on signals from the nervous system, followed by contractions to expel stool. The colon is home to bacteria that can have beneficial effects through production of short chain fatty acids that support colon health. Unfortunately, the colon also can be infected with harmful types of bacteria, such as clostridium difficile (c. diff.) and escherichia coli (e. coli).

The vast majority of CRC develop over a multi-year transition from a 5% subset of adenomatous polyps. Disruption of gatekeeper/growth regulatory genes, particularly APC, accounts for 85% of CRC. Another 15% result from changes in the caretaker genes that maintain genetic stability (29).

Ten-fold global variations reflect environmental influences, increasing rapidly where a Western lifestyle is adopted. In the U.S., it is the third most common cancer, with a 5% lifetime risk that is 30% higher in males. Fortunately, a 57% compliance with colonoscopy screening has led to a 2.7% annual decline in incidence, although with significant ethnic disparities that are multi-factorial and influenced by access to health care (30).

In 2013, over 102,000 cases of colon cancer and 40,000 new cases of rectal cancer are expected while almost 51,000 people are expected to die from colon cancer and rectal cancer combined (29).

Inflammatory bowel disease (IBD) increases risk, varying with extent and duration, and will also increase side effects of treatment. Familial adenomatous polyposis (FAP) accounts for 1% of CRC, and hereditary non-polyposis colon cancer (HNPCC) known as Lynch Syndrome accounts for 2%-4% of diagnoses. Another 20% of cases of CRC are linked to a positive family history. Diagnosis at early, treatable stages has improved five-year survival to > 65%, 90% if localized, but only 12% when there are distant metastases (30).

When disease recurs after treatment, it is typically within three years and most often in the liver, where resection of isolated metastases may still be curative.

Risk Factors
Table 5 lists risk factors associated with the development of colorectal polyps and CRC. The colon's direct contact with food and

Table 5: Risk Factors for CRC (29-30)

Risk Factors
- Being over age 50
- Presence of adenoma polyps in the colon
- Inherited syndromes (e.g. HNPCC, FAP, Peutz-Jeghers syndrome, MUTYH-associated polyposis)
- Race and ethnicity (e.g. African Americans, Ashkenazi Jews)
- Type II diabetes mellitus
- Overweight and obesity, especially abdominal obesity
- Smoking, use of tobacco products
- Heavy alcohol use
- Physical inactivity
- History of ulcerative colitis or Crohn's disease
- Intake of polyaromatic hydrocarbons (PAH) and heterocyclic amines (HCA) formed as result of grilling at high temperatures over extended times
- Diets high in red meats and processed meats
- Low serum Vitamin D levels and low calcium intake

carcinogens accounts for strong associations with nutrition and lifestyle factors and offers opportunities for prevention along the continuum of carcinogenesis.

Signs and Symptoms
A change in bowel habits (e.g., having diarrhea, constipation, or a narrowing of the stool) is the most common symptom of CRC (29, 30). Additional symptoms include: heme-positive stools or unexplained anemia, abdominal pain or bloating, nausea and vomiting, finding blood in the stool (bright red or very dark), unintended weight loss and fatigue.

Symptoms suggestive of CRC trigger a diagnostic workup that includes a colonoscopy and a biopsy of suspicious areas. When confirmed, additional tests such as carcinoembryonic antigen (CEA), CT scans, PET scans, and endorectal ultrasounds or pelvic magnetic resonance imaging (MRI) scans are routinely performed (31-32). Staging depends on these findings as well as pathology reports. The American Joint Committee on Cancer (AJCC) has developed a widely used TNM classification system, based on *Tumor* size, extent of lymph *Node* involvement, and *Metastasis* (33). The National Cancer Institute (NCI) also has described stages of colorectal cancer; their system uses Roman numerals I (early stage, when the tumor has grown into the inner wall but not through the wall), II, III, and IV (advanced stage, when the cancer has spread to other parts of the body such as the liver or lungs) (29).

Treatment
Surgery is the primary curative therapy for both colon and rectal tumors and is also used palliatively to relieve obstruction. After removing the diseased area, the surgeon will reconnect the healthy parts. Occasionally, the surgeon cannot reconnect remaining parts of the colon, and in a surgery called a colostomy, creates a stoma

Figure 2: Surgery for CRC

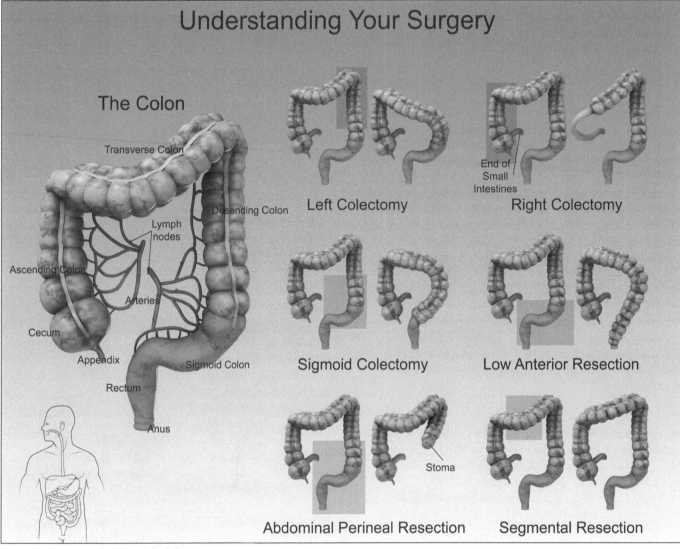

Reprinted with permission by Christine Eberle Barron

(opening in the abdominal wall) through which the upper end of the intestine is attached (while the other end is surgically closed). A bag fits over the opening to collect waste material. Depending upon the location of the stoma and the amount of colon removed, absorption is altered. Sometimes the ostomy can be reversed to a normal anatomy; other times the ostomy is permanent. Diet tolerance, fluid and electrolyte status, and complications such as "pouchitis" depend on several factors including the extent of colon excised.

Commonly performed surgical interventions for the treatment of CRC are illustrated in Figure 2. These surgeries include: polypectomy and local exicision, colectomy, low anterior resection, abdominal perineal resection (APR), proctectomy with colo-anal anastomosis, ileostomy, and colostomy. Chapter 14 provides additional information on surgeries for CRC.

Other treatment modalities for CRC include chemotherapy, biotherapy (targeted therapy) and radiation therapy. If indicated, these can be given either as adjuvant or neoadjuvant therapies depending on the size, location, stage of the disease and the individual's age and general health. Oncologists base treatment decisions on evidence-based guidelines as outlined in the *NCCN Clinical Practice Guidelines in Oncology* for colon and rectal cancer (31-32).

Nutrition Management

As seen with gastric cancer, CRC treatment regimens are associated with side effects, which are often intensified when therapies are combined. Refer to Chapter 11 for an extensive review of cancer treatments including chemotherapy, biotherapy, and radiation therapy, and possible side effects associated with these modalities. Commonly experienced symptoms of combined modality treatment include mucositis, diarrhea, nausea, vomiting, and fatigue (among others), which can lead to changes in appetite and unintended weight loss. Table 3 outlines NIS of specific CRC treatment regimens. Depending upon the agents prescribed and if given in combination,

Table 6: Diet and Lifestyle Recommendations for CRC survivors (31-62)

Diet and Lifestyle Recommendations

- Avoid consuming a Western dietary pattern (e.g. large amounts of fatty meat, processed foods, refined carbohydrates, and alcohol). Limit consumption of red and processed meats.
- Eat a wide variety of vegetables, fruits, legumes and whole grains. Include non-fat or low fat dairy foods, fish and poultry in the diet.
- Increase fiber intake; maximum benefit is derived from mixed sources (e.g., soluble and insoluble fibers).
- If alcohol is used, limit intake.
- Maintain a healthy weight.
- Engage in regular physical activity.
- Dietary supplements are not associated with benefit in survival, with the exception of calcium. Supplementation of calcium should be recommended only at levels to achieve adequacy by supplementing dietary intake.
- Sufficient levels of serum vitamin D is moderately protective and may have benefit in survivorship.
- Folic acid supplementation remains controversial with a possible U-shaped effect, or dual role (i.e. preventive if used before any cancer has formed and harmful if used after a cancer has formed).

NIS will vary greatly. Additional management strategies for NIS are outlined in Chapter 12.

After surgery, the majority of individuals will ultimately be able to tolerate most foods, but initially should modify diet to allow the body time to adapt to its new anatomy. If the small bowel is functioning normally, most nutrients will be absorbed by the time chyme reaches the colon. Dietary modifications then focus on measures to slow movement of chyme through the remaining colon and retain as much fluid and electrolytes as possible.

Refer to Appendix 5 for dietary recommendations for ostomies. These recommendations apply to the early post-operative period (usually the first six to eight weeks). If this diet is well tolerated and output meets guidelines (in volume and consistency), other foods can be gradually added to the diet. Many people are eventually able to tolerate most foods.

Table 6 provides diet and lifestyle recommendations for CRC survivors for reducing risk of cancer recurrence.

Table 7 outlines nutrition management suggestions for specific CRC treatments and possible side effects.

Table 7: Medical Nutrition Therapy Matrix for CRC (63-66)

Possible Nutrition-Related Complications	Nutrition Management Suggestions

Small bowel resections	• Depending upon the extent of the remaining GI tract, the transition to a more normal food intake may take weeks to months. Of note, some patients may never tolerate normal concentration or volumes of food. Enteral or parenteral nutrition may need to be considered to maintain adequate fluid and nutrition status.
	• Small, frequent, mini meals (6/day) are usually better tolerated than fewer, larger feedings.
	• Fluid and electrolytes should be provided in small, frequent amounts. Consider use of oral rehydration solutions when fluid losses result in dehydration and /or fluid losses routinely exceed fluid intake.
	• If terminal ileum has been resected:
	  o Monitor serum Vitamin B12 levels.
	  o Monitor for diarrhea; addition of bile acid sequestrants may be indicated.
	  o Because of losses, fat soluble vitamins A, D, E, K, and calcium, zinc, and magnesium may need to be supplemented.

Colectomy with reanastomosis	• Encourage intake of small, more frequent meals. • Monitor fluid and electrolyte status. • Advise dietary interventions (e.g. low fiber diet) to slow transit time, if indicated.
Colostomy and ileostomy	• Assess and manage possible fluid and electrolyte imbalances. If indicated, increase fluid intake, (e.g. electrolyte solutions, sports drinks, broth and vegetable juices) to cover losses of sodium and potassium. • Patients should be encouraged to drink at least 1 L more than their output daily and increase fluid intake as necessary. • Assess stool consistency and odor. Provide dietary strategies, as needed.
Ileal Pouch: "J-pouch" (folds of the ileum are joined together to make a small pouch which is connected to the ileum and rectum)	• Monitor for pouchitis (inflammation/infection of the surgically constructed pouch) o Acute pouchitis is easily treated with antibiotics but can be difficult to manage if chronic. • Educate regarding dietary interventions (e.g.,limit caffeine, avoid lactose in lactose-deficient patients, limit fructose and sorbitol). Stress adequate fluid and electrolyte intake due to increase in intestinal losses. • Reinforce anti-diarrheal medication use.
Pelvic radiation therapy	• Refer to Table 3 for possible side effects and chapter 12 for strategies to manage NIS
Chemotherapy and biotherapy	• Refer to Table 3 for possible side effects and see chapter 12 for strategies to manage NIS.
Possible vitamin and mineral malabsorption	• Monitor serum vitamin D levels, supplementing to maintain normal levels • Encourage a calcium-rich diet, supplement as needed to promote total intake of DRI. • Vitamin B12 supplementation, if ileum is resected. • Folate supplementation may be indicated because of low fresh vegetable and fruit intake.
	Note: Appendices 3-5 provide specific dietary recommendations for GI surgeries

Hepatocellular Cancer (HCC)

Definition, Prevalence and Survival

The liver is the largest organ in the body, and the only one with regenerative properties. It is essential for survival through its roles in processing and storing nutrients, including glycogen, and in production of cholesterol and proteins such as albumin and clotting factors. It assists digestion of fats through secretion of bile. All blood circulating from the stomach and bowel flows through the liver where carcinogens and drugs are detoxified. Waste products are secreted into bile and excreted in stool or into the blood and excreted in urine.

HCC accounts for the majority of primary liver cancers, with > 80% multifocal, arising in cirrhotic livers typically related to hepatitis with or without alcohol abuse. The rapid cellular proliferation associated with the liver repair process increases risk of genetic changes and cancer. The liver is also a common site of metastases from other primary cancers.

Most cases of HCC (85%) occur in developing countries, including Asia (67) and are linked to endemic levels of hepatitis B (HBV) which directly alters liver DNA and confers a lifetime risk of liver cancer of 10 – 25% (67-68). In the U.S., HCC is associated with cirrhosis from chronic hepatitis C (HCV), alcohol abuse and/or nonalcoholic fatty

Table 8: Risk Factors for HCC (68-82)

- Gender (HCC is more common in men)
- Hepatitis B (HBV) and Hepatitis C (HVC) infection
- Heavy alcohol use
- Aflatoxin
- Hemochromatosis
- Inherited metabolic diseases
- Cirrhosis
- Obesity
- Type II Diabetes mellitus
- Anabolic steroids
- Environmental exposure (e.g. drinking water contaminated with arsenic)

liver disease (NAFLD). U.S. rates of 4.5/100,000 (66-67) are highest in non-white and immigrant populations. Males have three times the incidence of females, possibly due to androgen stimulation and relative exposure to toxins and hepatitis. Liver cancer is the sixth most common cancer worldwide, and the third leading cause of death from cancer.

Overall five-year survival is 15%, worsening with degree of cirrhosis. Those receiving a liver transplant have a survival rate of 50%-60%,

Table 9: Treatment Options for HCC (80-83)

Treatment Options
Surgery • Is dependent upon whether the patient has potentially resectable, transplantable, or operable disease. Other factors considered include: age, performance status, and general health. • Types of surgery include: partial hepatectomy and liver transplant. • Side effects of liver surgery include: bleeding, blood clots, infection, diarrhea, pain, fatigue, and damage to the remaining liver or rejection of the transplanted organ.
Ablation • Involves the use of a small probe (that transmits high energy radio waves, heat or cold) or alcohol injected via a needle directly into the tumor to kill cancer cells; is best suited for tumors < 3 cm across. • An option for patients not eligible for liver surgery or transplant. • Types of ablation include: radiofrequency ablation, cryoablation, percutaneous ethanol ablation, and microwave. • Common side effects include: abdominal pain, infection in the liver, bleeding, nausea, vomiting, and fatigue. • Please refer to Chapter 14 for additional information regarding the nutritional management and consequences for patients undergoing liver surgeries.
Embolization • Involves injecting a substance (chemotherapy or radioactive beads) to block or reduce blood flow to the tumor. • An option for patients not eligible for liver surgery or transplant and for patients with tumors larger than 3 cm across. • Side effects commonly experienced include: abdominal pain, nausea, vomiting, infection and inflammation in the liver, fever and fatigue.
Chemotherapy • Is usually palliative; agents often used include Doxorubicin, 5-FU and Cisplatin. • Hepatic artery infusion of agents limits side effects but requires a catheter placement. • Refer to Chapter 11 for anticipated side effects and NIS of chemotherapy agents.
Biotherapy (Targeted therapy) • Refer to Table 3 for Sorafenib and its anticipated NIS. • Other side effects of Sorafenib therapy may include: rash, bleeding problems, hand-foot syndrome, and fatigue.
Radiation therapy • Refer to Table 3 for anticipated nutrition impact symptoms of external beam therapy to the abdomen. • Radioembolization uses radioactive microspheres and injects them into hepatic artery. Side effects of this type of therapy include: abdominal pain, nausea, inflammation, infection in the liver, blood clots, and fever.

though few qualify for transplant and their cancer often recurs due to underlying risk factors (67). Approximately 27% of cases are resectable, but only 5% are surgical candidates.

Risk Factors
Table 8 lists risk factors associated with increased risk for developing HCC.

Signs and Symptoms
Signs and symptoms of HCC usually do not manifest until the later stages of the disease. Symptoms can include: nausea, vomiting, an enlarged liver, pain in the abdomen, a swollen abdomen, itching, yellow colored skin and eyes (jaundice), worsening of existing cirrhosis or hepatitis, loss of appetite, early satiety, fatigue and unintended weight loss. Some liver tumors secrete hormones and can cause hypercalcemia, hypoglycemia, and erythrocytosis (i.e., facial redness and flushing) (80-81).

Symptoms suggestive of HCC trigger a diagnostic workup that may include liver imaging studies (e.g. ultrasound, MRI, CT scan), biopsy of suspicious area(s) and laboratory studies (e.g. liver function tests, alpha fetoprotein, bilirubin, and prothrombin time) (80-81). When HCC is confirmed, additional tests such as a hepatitis panel, a complete history and physical and a chest CT scan are usually performed (82).

Treatment
Treatment options for patients with HCC are outlined in Table 9. These options include surgery, ablation, embolization, chemotherapy, biotherapy (targeted therapy), and radiation therapy. Oncologists base treatment decisions on evidence-based guidelines outlined in the *NCCN Clinical Practice Guidelines in Oncology* for hepatobiliary cancer (82). Other factors considered include: the size, location and number of tumor(s) in the liver; how well the liver is functioning; if cirrhosis is present or not; possible side effects of treatment and whether the cancer has spread outside the liver (80).

Gallbladder Cancer (GBC)
Definition, Prevalence, and Survival (see Figure 3)
The gallbladder is a small, pear shaped organ that sits beneath the liver, collecting and storing bile that flows from the liver via bile ducts. When food enters the duodenum, the secretion of cholecystokinin (CCK) causes gallbladder contractions, releasing alkaline bile into the duodenum via the common bile duct. The alkaline bile helps neutralize acid from the stomach and also emulsifies fats, assisting enzymes in breaking down fat for absorption. Gallstones can develop in the duct, blocking flow and causing inflammation and pain when the gallbladder is stimulated to contract after eating.

Gallbladder cancer (GBC) is the most common of biliary tract tumors and is the leading cause of cancer mortality in certain ethnic groups and geographical areas. It is linked to a genetic susceptibility, with chronic irritation and inflammation due to stones or chronic

Figure 3: The Gallbladder

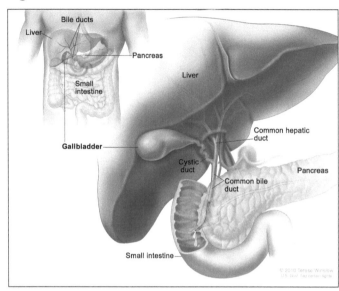

© 2010 Terese Winslow, U.S. Govt. has certain rights

infection leading to dysplasia (83-87). GBC affects women at two to three times the rate of men and its incidence increases with age. Estimated cases of GBC for 2013 include over 10,000 new cases diagnosed and over 3,200 deaths (84). It is the leading cause of cancer mortality in Chilean and North Indian women, with high incidence rates in East Asia and Central Europe as well.

Survival rates are poor, with a mean survival of six months and a five-year survival rate of 5%. Initially vague abdominal symptoms are associated with advanced disease at diagnosis. Poor prognosis is in part related to anatomic issues that include a gallbladder wall of < 3 mm and close adjacent structures contributing to ease of local metastatic spread. Diagnosis at early stages has much better prognosis, but is relatively rare, typically incidental to a cholecystectomy.

Risk Factors
No specific food is convincingly tied to GBC, but there were limited indications that peppers/capsicums may increase risk (83-86). Smoking and drinking increased risk in men. Risk factors for GBC are outlined in Table 10.

Table 10: Risk Factors for GBC (31, 84-86)

- Gallstones
- Obesity
- Female gender
- Ethnicity and race (e.g. highest in Mexican Americans and Native Americans)
- Diabetes
- Biliary abnormalities
- Parasitic infection (e.g. salmonella)
- Industrial and environmental chemicals

Table 11: Treatment Options for GBC (83-88)

Treatment Options
Surgery   • Two types of surgeries are typically undertaken for treatment of GBC: potentially curative or palliative surgery.   • Potentially curative surgery is performed to resect the cancer.   • Palliative surgery is performed to relieve pain and/or prolong life.   • Side effects of surgery include: bleeding, pain, infection, and complications from anesthesia.
Chemotherapy   • Refer to Table 3 for specific agents and associated NIS.
Biotherapy (Targeted therapy)   • Refer to Table 3 for specific agents and associated NIS.
Radiation therapy   • Refer to Table 3 for anticipated side effects of external beam radiation therapy to the abdomen.
Palliative care   • Bile duct stents help to reduce jaundice-related symptoms, but they often re-occlude and require revision. Of note, jaundice often indicates a poorer prognosis.   • Biliary bypass can be performed to allow bile to drain from the liver and gallbladder that has been blocked by cancer.   • Proactive pain management.

Signs and Symptoms

Common symptoms of GBC include a vague abdominal pain, nausea, vomiting, fever, taste changes, anorexia, and jaundice due to bile duct compression (84).

Treatment

Treatment options for patients with GBC are outlined in Table 11. These options include surgery, chemotherapy, biotherapy (targeted therapy), radiation therapy, and palliative care because of its usually advanced stage at diagnosis. Oncologists base treatment decisions on evidence-based guidelines outlined in the *NCCN Clinical Practice Guidelines in Oncology* for hepatobiliary cancer (82). Other factors considered include: the type and stage of the cancer, possible side effects of treatment, age, and general health (86).

Nutrition Management

As seen with other cancers presented in this chapter, GBC treatment regimens are associated with side effects which are often intensified when therapies are combined. Refer to Chapter 11 for additional information pertaining to chemotherapy, biotherapy, and radiation therapy, and possible side effects associated with these treatment modalities. GBC treatment regimens can result in nutrition impact symptoms such as mucositis, diarrhea, nausea, vomiting, and fatigue (among other symptoms), which can lead to changes in appetite and unintended weight loss.

Anal Cancers

Definition, Prevalence and Survival

The anus is the opening at the end of the GI tract. The anal canal is about an inch and a half long tube that connects the rectum to the anus and is surrounded by a sphincter that keeps stool or feces from leaking out. The point in the anal canal that meets the outside of the skin at the anus is referred to as the anal verge. Stool is comprised of the waste matter that remains after the colon has absorbed water and liquid from digested food. Stool is stored in the rectum and from

there passes through the anal canal and anus to outside of the body once the anal sphincter relaxes during a bowel movement.

Invasive anal cancers include squamous cell carcinomas and are the most prevalent anal cancers in the U.S. Squamous cells line the anal margin and most of the anal canal. Another type of anal cancer is adenocarcinomas; these cancers typically develop in the cells that line the upper part of the anal canal adjacent to the rectum. These cancers are treated the same way as rectal cancer. Other less common types of anal cancers are malignant melanomas, cloacogenic carcinoma, and basal cell carcinomas.

Anal cancer is uncommon in the U.S., accounting for only 4% of all cancers of the lower GI tract (89). However, new cases are on the rise and its incidence is linked to certain sexual practices (e.g. anal intercourse, multiple partners). Approximately 7,060 Americans will be diagnosed with anal cancer in 2013 and 880 will die as result of their disease (89). Stage at diagnosis for squamous cell-type carcinomas has a significant impact on survival, with five-year U.S. survival rates of >70% at Stage 1, decreasing to 21% at stage IV (89).

Risk Factors

Risk factors for anal cancer are outlined in Table 12.

Signs and Symptoms

More than half of all people diagnosed with anal cancer experience bleeding. Other common side effects of anal cancer include: rectal bleeding or itching, pain in the anal area, change in stool diameter, abnormal anal discharge, and swollen lymph nodes in the groin.

Procedures used to diagnosis anal cancer include digital rectal examination, anoscopy, rigid proctosigmoidoscopy, biopsy, and HIV and HPV testing, if indicated (90). Other diagnostic measures include inguinal lymph node evaluation, and gynecological examination and cervical screening for women. Imaging studies include

Table 12: Risk Factors for Anal Cancer (89)

> • Human papilloma virus (HPV) infection
>
> • Human immunodeficiency virus (HIV) infection
>
> • Multiple sexual partners
>
> • Smoking
>
> • Individuals with immunosuppression (e.g. post organ transplant)
>
> • Race (more common in African Americans)
>
> • Gender (more common in women than men)
>
> • History of other cancers or cervical dysplasia (e.g. cervix, vagina, or vulva) which are also linked to HPV infection

ultrasound; CT scans of chest, abdomen and pelvis to evaluate extent of disease; MRI; and PET scan.

Treatment and Nutritional Implications

Treatment for anal cancer includes chemotherapy, radiation therapy, and surgery. Common treatment regimens often include one or more of these treatment modalities. Factors determining choice of regimen take into consideration the size, location, and stage of disease, and the individual's age and general health. Oncologists base treatment decisions on evidence-based guidelines outlined in the *NCCN Clinical Practice Guidelines in Oncology* for anal cancer (90). Each treatment modality is associated with unique side effects as outlined below and can be intensified when therapies are combined.

Chemotherapy agents commonly prescribed to treat anal carcinomas are Mitomycin and 5-FU used in combination or Cisplatin and 5-FU. Chemotherapy can result in NIS such as oral mucositis, nausea, vomiting, and diarrhea, which can lead to loss of appetite and unintended weight loss.

External beam radiation therapy is directed to the inguinal lymph nodes, pelvis, anus and perineum. Side effects of radiation therapy include skin changes, temporary anal irritation and pain, nausea, vomiting, diarrhea, discomfort while having bowel movements, and fatigue. Women may experience side effects to their vagina including irritation, discomfort and pain. Long term side effects of radiation therapy may result in scar tissue forming in the anal canal and anus, chronic radiation-induced proctitis, and weakened bones in the pelvis and hip (89, 91).

Surgical interventions for anal cancers consist of local resection of the anal tumor and surrounding area or an abdominoperineal resection (APR) ,which is a more extensive procedure that removes the anus, anal sphincter, surrounding tissue, and lymph nodes. Because the anus is removed an ostomy (colostomy) is created to evacuate stool. See Appendix 5 regarding nutrition and ostomies.

Conclusion

Gastrointestinal cancers pose challenges to both patients and clinicians. Evidence-based medical nutrition therapy is essential for improving the functional status and quality of life of patients with these cancers.

References

1. Dempsy DT, Feurer ID, Knox LS, et al. Energy expenditure in malnourished gastrointestinal cancer patients.*Cancer.* 1984;53(6):1265-1273.
2. Academy of Nutrition and Dietetics/Evidence Analysis Library. Available at: http://www.adaevidencelibrary.com. Accessed: September 16, 2013.
3. Russell M. Malone AM. Nutrient requirements In: Charney P, Malone AM (eds). *ADA Pocket Guide to Nutrition Assessment, 2nd edition.* Chicago, IL: Academy of Nutrition and Dietetics, 2009:167-191.
4. Hurst JD, Gallagher AL. Energy, macronutrient, micronutrient, and fluid requirements In: Elliott L, Molseed LL, McCallum PD, Grant BL (eds). *The Clinical Guide to Oncology Nutrition, 2nd edition.* Chicago, IL: Academy of Nutrition and Dietetics. 2006:55-71.
5. Gottschlich MM, ED. *The ASPEN nutrition core curriculum: a case-based approach-the adult patient.* Silver Spring, MD: American Society for Parenteral and Enteral Nutrition; 2007:649-675.
6. Cheung K, Lee SS, Raman M. Prevalence and mechanisms of malnutrition in patients with advanced liver disease, and nutrition management strategies. *Clin Gastroenterol Hepatol* 2012;10(2):117-125.
7. Plauth M, Cabré E, Riggio O, et al. ESPEN guidelines on enteral nutrition: liver disease. *Clin Nutr* 2006;25(2):285-294.
8. Delich PC, Siepler JK, Parker P. Liver disease. In: Gottshlich MM, ed. The ASPEN nutrition support core curriculum: a case-based approach-the adult patient. Silver Spring, MD: American Society for Parenteral and Enteral Nutrition, 2007:540-557.
9. Krenitsky J. Nutrition for patients with hepatic failure. In: Nutrition issues in gastroenterology, series #6. *Practical Gastroenterology* 2003;(6):23-42.
10. American Cancer Society. *Stomach Cancer.* Available at: http://www.cancer.org/cancer/stomachcancer/detailedguide/stomach-cancer-key-statistics. Accessed September 13, 2013.
11. Gonzalez CA, Agudo A. Carcinogenesis, prevention and early detection of gastric cancer: where we are and where we should go. *Int J Cancer.* 2012;130(4):745-753.
12. Liu C, Russell RM. Nutrition and gastric cancer risk: an update. *Nutrition Reviews.* 2008;66(5):237-249.
13. Yang P, Zhou Y, Chen B, et al. Overweight, obesity and gastric cancer risk: results from a meta-analysis of cohort studies. *Eur J Cancer.* 2009;45(16): 2867-2873.
14. Duell EJ, Travier N, Lujan-Barroso L, et al. Alcohol consumption and gastric cancer risk in the European Prospective Investigation into Cancer and Nutrition (EPIC) cohort. *Am J Clin Nutr.* 2011;94(5):1266-1275.
15. Ward MH, Cross AJ, Abnet CC, Sinha R, Markin RS, Weisenburger DD. Heme iron from meat and risk of adenocarcinoma of the esophagus and stomach. *Eur J Cancer Prev.* 2012;21(2):134-138.
16. Wu CY, Wu MS, Kuo KN, Wang CB, Chen YJ, Lin JT. Effective reduction of gastric cancer risk with regular use of nonsteroidal anti-inflammatory drugs in Helicobacter pylori-infected patients. *J Clin Oncology.* 2010; 28(18):2952-2957.
17. National Cancer Institute. *What you need to know about stomach cancer™.* Available at: http://www.cancer.gov/cancertopics/wyntk/stomach/page1. Accessed September 13, 2013.
18. National Comprehensive Cancer Network. *NCCN Guidelines: Gastric Cancer, Version 2.2013.* Available at: http://www.nccn.org/professionals/physician_gls/pdf/gastric.pdf. Accessed September 13, 2013.
19. Polovich M, Whitford JM, Kelleher LO. *Chemotherapy and biotherapy guidelines and recommendations for practice.* 3rd ed. Pittsburgh, PA: Oncology Nursing Society; 2009.
20. Chemocare. *Drug information.* Available at: http://chemocare.com/chemotherapy/drug-info/default.aspx. Accessed September 14, 2013.
21. Chu E, DeVita VT. Physicians' Cancer Chemotherapy Drug Manual 2012. Burlington, MA: 2012.
22. Wilkes GM, Barton-Burke M. Oncology Nursing Drug Handbook 2012. Burlington, MA: 2012.
23. Iwamoto RR, Hass ML, Gosselin TK. Manual for Radiation Oncology Nursing Practice and Education, 4th edition. Pittsburg, PA: Oncology Nursing Society: 2012.
24. National Cancer Institute. *Radiation therapy for cancer.* Available at: http://www.cancer.gov/cancertopics/factsheet/Therapy/radiation. Accessed September 13, 2013b.

25. Tack J, Arts J, Caenepeel, P, De Wulf D, Bisschops R. Pathophysiology, diagnosis and management of postoperative dumping. *Nat Rev Gastroenterol Hepatol*. 2009;6(10):583-590.

26. Ukleja A. Dumping syndrome In: Nutrition issues in Gastroenterology, series #35. Parrish CR, editor. *Practical Gastroenterology*. 2006;32-46.

27. Krenitsky JS, Decher N. Chapter 28: Medical nutrition therapy for upper gastrointestinal tract disorders *In Krause's Food in the Nutrition Care Process, 13th edition*. Editors: Mahan LK, Escott-Stump S, Raymond JL. St. Louis, MO: Elsevier: p 592-609.

28. Carey S. Bone health after major upper gastrointestinal surgery In: Nutrition issues in gastroenterology, series #115. Parris CR, editor. *Practical Gastroenterology*. 2013;46-55.

29. National Cancer Institute. *What you need to know about colon and rectal cancer™*. Available at: http://www.cancer.gov/cancertopics/types/colon-and-rectal. Accessed September 13, 2013.

30. American Cancer Society. *Colorectal Cancer*. Available at: http://www.cancer.org/cancer/colonandrectalcancer/detailedguide/colonandrectal-cancer-key-statistics. Accessed September 13, 2013.

31. National Comprehensive Cancer Network. *NCCN Guidelines: Colon Cancer, Version 1.2014*. Available at: http://www.nccn.org/professionals/physician_gls/pdf/colon.pdf. Accessed September 13, 2013.

32. National Comprehensive Cancer Network. *NCCN Guidelines: Rectal Cancer, Version 4.2013*. Available at: http://www.nccn.org/professionals/physician_gls/pdf/rectal.pdf. Accessed September 13, 2013.

33. American Joint Committee on Cancer. *What is cancer staging?* Available at: http://cancerstaging.org/references-tools/Pages/What-is-Cancer-Staging.aspx. Accessed September 14, 2013.

34. World Cancer Research Fund / American Institute for Cancer Research. Food, Nutrition, Physical Activity, and the Prevention of Cancer: A Global Perspective. 2007.

35. World, World Cancer Research Fund / American Institute for Cancer Research. Continuous Update Project Report Summary. Food, Nutrition, Physical Activity, and the Prevention of Colorectal Cancer. 2011.

36. Vargas AJ, Thompson PA. Diet and nutrient factors in colorectal cancer risk. *Nutr Clin Pract*. 2012;27(5):613-623.

37. Chan DS, Lau R, Aune D, et al. Red and processed meat and colorectal cancer incidence: meta-analysis of prospective studies. *PloS one*. 2011;6(6):e20456.

38. Gorham ED, Garland CF, Garland FC, et al. Optimal vitamin D status for colorectal cancer prevention: a quantitative meta analysis. *Am J Prev Med*. 2007;32(3):210-216.

39. Boyle T, Keegel T, Bull F, Heyworth J, Fritschi L. Physical Activity and Risks of Proximal and Distal Colon Cancers: A Systematic Review and Meta-analysis. *J Natl Cancer Inst*. 2012;104(20):1548-1561.

40. Courneya KS, Booth CM, Gill S, et al. The Colon Health and Life-Long Exercise Change trial: a randomized trial of the National Cancer Institute of Canada Clinical Trials Group. *Current Oncology*. 2008;15(6):279-285.

41. Aune D, Chan DS, Lau R, et al. Dietary fibre, whole grains, and risk of colorectal cancer: systematic review and dose-response meta-analysis of prospective studies. *BMJ*. 2011;343:d6617.

42. Aune D, Chan DS, Lau R, et al. Carbohydrates, glycemic index, glycemic load, and colorectal cancer risk: a systematic review and meta-analysis of cohort studies. *Cancer Causes & Control*. 2012;23(4):521-535.

43. Song Y, Manson JE, Lee IM, et al. Effect of combined folic Acid, vitamin b6, and vitamin B12 on colorectal adenoma. *J Natl Cancer Inst*. Oct 2012;104(20):1562-1575.

44. Rock CL, Doyle C, Demark-Wahnefried W, et al. Nutrition and physical activity guidelines for cancer survivors. *CA: A Cancer Journal for Clinicians*. 2012;62(4):243-274.

45. Fung TT, Hu FB, Wu K, Chiuve SE, Fuchs CS, Giovannucci E. The Mediterranean and Dietary Approaches to Stop Hypertension (DASH) diets and colorectal cancer. *Am J Clin Nutr*. 2010;92(6):1429-1435.

46. Haydon AM, Macinnis RJ, English DR, Giles GG. Effect of physical activity and body size on survival after diagnosis with colorectal cancer. *Gut*. 2006;55(1):62-67.

47. Macdonald RS, Wagner K. Influence of Dietary Phytochemicals and Microbiota on Colon Cancer Risk. *J Agric Food Chem*. 2012;60(27):6728–6735.

48. Ng K, Meyerhardt JA, Chan JA, et al. Multivitamin use is not associated with cancer recurrence or survival in patients with stage III colon cancer: findings from CALGB 89803. *J Clin Oncol*. 2010;28(28):4354-4363.

49. Giovannucci E, Stampfer MJ, Colditz GA, et al. Multivitamin use, folate, and colon cancer in women in the Nurses' Health Study. *Ann Int Med*. 1998;129(7):517-524.

50. Gaziano JM, Sesso HD, Christen WG, et al. Multivitamins in the Prevention of Cancer in Men: The Physicians' Health Study II Randomized Controlled Trial. *JAMA*. 2012;308(18):E1-E10.

51. Papaioannou D, Cooper KL, Carroll C, et al. Antioxidants in the chemoprevention of colorectal cancer and colorectal adenomas in the general population: a systematic review and meta-analysis. *Colorectal Dis*. 2011;13(10):1085-1099.

52. Carroll C, Cooper K, Papaioannou D, Hind D, Pilgrim H, Tappenden P. Supplemental calcium in the chemoprevention of colorectal cancer: a systematic review and meta-analysis. *Clin Ther*. 2010;32(5):789-803.

53. Giovannucci E. Epidemiological evidence for vitamin D and colorectal cancer. *J Bone Min Res*. 2007;22 Suppl 2:V81-85.

54. Wactawski-Wende J, Kotchen JM, Anderson GL, et al. Calcium plus vitamin D supplementation and the risk of colorectal cancer. *N Engl J Med*. 2006;354(7):684-696.

55. Ng K, Wolpin BM, Meyerhardt JA, et al. Prospective study of predictors of vitamin D status and survival in patients with colorectal cancer. *Br J Cancer*. 2009;101(6):916-923.

56. Gibson TM, Weinstein SJ, Pfeiffer RM, et al. Pre- and postfortification intake of folate and risk of colorectal cancer in a large prospective cohort study in the United States. *Am J Clin Nutr*. 2011;94(4):1053-1062.

57. Stevens VL, McCullough ML, Sun J, Jacobs EJ, Campbell PT, Gapstur SM. High levels of folate from supplements and fortification are not associated with increased risk of colorectal cancer. *Gastroenterol*. 2011;141(1):98-105, 105 e101.

58. Figueiredo JC, Mott LA, Giovannucci E, et al. Folic acid and prevention of colorectal adenomas: a combined analysis of randomized clinical trials. *Int J Cancer*. 2011;129(1):192-203.

59. Mason JB, Dickstein A, Jacques PF, et al. A temporal association between folic acid fortification and an increase in colorectal cancer rates may be illuminating important biological principles: a hypothesis. *Ca Epidemiol Biomarkers Prev*. 2007;16(7):1325-1329.

60. Cole BF, Baron JA, Sandler RS, et al. Folic acid for the prevention of colorectal adenomas: a randomized clinical trial. *JAMA*. 2007;297(21):2351-2359.

61. Carroll C, Cooper K, Papaioannou D, et al. Meta-analysis: folic acid in the chemoprevention of colorectal adenomas and colorectal cancer. *Aliment Pharmacol Ther*. 2010;31(7):708-718.

62. Huncharek, M, Muscat J, Kupelnick B. Colorectal cancer risk and the dietary intake of calcium, vitamin D, and dairy products: a meta-analysis of 26,335 cases from 60 observational studies. *Nutr Cancer*. 2009;61(1):47-69.

63. Parrish CR, Quatrara B. The art of reinfusing intestinal secretions. *J Support Oncol*. 2010;8(2):92-96.

64. Decher N, Krenitsky JS. Chapter 29: Medical nutrition therapy for lower gastrointestinal tract disorders *In Krause's Food in the Nutrition Care Process, 13th edition*. Editors: Mahan LK, Escott-Stump S, Raymond JL. Elsevvier: p 610-644.

65. Mimura T, Rizzello F, Helwig U, et al. Once daily high dose probiotic therapy (VSL#3) for maintaining remission in recurrent or refractory pouchitis. *Gut*. 2004;53(1):108-114.

66. Jemal A, Bray F, Center MM, Ferlay J, Ward E, Forman D. Global cancer statistics. *CA: A Cancer Journal for Clinicians*. 2011;61(2):69-90.

67. El-Serag HB. Hepatocellular carcinoma. *N Engl J Med*. 2011;365(12):1118-1127.

68. El-Serag HB, Engels EA, Landgren O, et al. Risk of hepatobiliary and pancreatic cancers after hepatitis C virus infection: A population-based study of U.S. veterans. *Hepatology*. 2009;49(1):116-123.

69. Giovannucci E, Harlan DM, Archer MC, et al. Diabetes and cancer: a consensus report. *CA: A Cancer Journal for Clinicians*. Jul-Aug 2010;60(4):207-221.

70. Deugnier Y. Iron and liver cancer. *Alcohol*. Jun 2003;30(2):145-150.

71. Ascha MS, Hanouneh IA, Lopez R, Tamimi TA, Feldstein AF, Zein NN. The incidence and risk factors of hepatocellular carcinoma in patients with nonalcoholic steatohepatitis. *Hepatology*. 2010;51(6):1972-1978.

72. Schlesinger S, Aleksandrova K, Pischon T, et al. Abdominal obesity, weight gain during adulthood and risk of liver and biliary tract cancer in a European cohort. *Int J Cancer*. 2013;132(3):645-657.

73. Wang C, Wang X, Gong G, et al. Increased risk of hepatocellular carcinoma in patients with diabetes mellitus: a systematic review and meta-analysis of cohort studies. *Int J Cancer*. 2012;130(7):1639-1648.

74. Wang P, Kang D, Cao W, Wang Y, Liu Z. Diabetes mellitus and risk of hepatocellular carcinoma: a systematic review and meta-analysis. *Diabetes Metab Res Rev. 2013*;28(2):109-122.

75. Welzel TM, Graubard BI, Zeuzem S, El-Serag HB, Davila JA, McGlynn KA. Metabolic syndrome increases the risk of primary liver cancer in the United States: a study in the SEER-Medicare database. *Hepatology*. 2011;54(2):463-471.

76. Zhang ZJ, Zheng ZJ, Shi R, Su Q, Jiang Q, Kip KE. Metformin for liver cancer prevention in patients with type 2 diabetes: a systematic review and meta-analysis. *J Clin Endocrinol Metab*. 2012;97(7):2347-2353.

77. Schwartz JM, Carithers RL. Epidemiology and etiologic associations of hepatocellular carcinoma. In: Basow D, ed. *UpToDate*. Waltham, MA: UpToDate; 2012.

78. Liu Y, Chang CC, Marsh GM, Wu F. Population attributable risk of aflatoxin-related liver cancer: Systematic review and meta-analysis. *Eur J Cancer*. 2012;48(14):2125-2136.

79. Freedman ND, Cross AJ, McGlynn KA, et al. Association of meat and fat intake with liver disease and hepatocellular carcinoma in the NIH-AARP cohort. *J Natl Cancer Inst*. 2010;102(17):1354-1365.

80. American Cancer Society. *Liver Cancer*. Available at: http://www.cancer.org/cancer/livercancer/detailedguide/liver-cancer-key-statistics. Accessed September 14, 2013.

81. National Cancer Institute. *What you need to know about liver cancer*™. Available at: http://www.cancer.gov/cancertopics/types/liver. Accessed September 14, 2013.

82. National Comprehensive Cancer Network. *NCCN Guidelines: Hepatobiliary Cancer, Version 4.2013*. Available at: http://www.nccn.org/professionals/physician_gls/pdf/hepatobiliary.pdf. Accessed September 14, 2013.

83. Gatto M, Bragazzi MC, Semeraro R, et al. Cholangiocarcinoma: update and future perspectives. *Dig Liv Dis*. 2010;42(4):253-260.

84. National Cancer Institute. *What you need to know about gallbladder*™. Available at: http://www.cancer.gov/cancertopics/types/gallbladder. Accessed September 14, 2013.

85. Ren HB, Yu T, Liu C, Li YQ. Diabetes mellitus and increased risk of biliary tract cancer: systematic review and meta-analysis. *Cancer Causes Control*. 2011;22(6):837-847.

86. American Cancer Society. *Gallbladder Cancer*. Available at: http://www.cancer.org/cancer/gallbladdercancer/detailedguide/gallbladder-cancer-key-statistics. Accessed September 14, 2013.

87. Mehrotra B. Treatment of advanced, unresectable gallbladder cancer. In: Basow D, ed. *UpToDate*. Waltham, MA: UpToDate; 2012.

88. Valle J, Wasan H, Palmer DH, et al. Cisplatin plus gemcitabine versus gemcitabine for biliary tract cancer. *N Engl J Med*. 2010;362(14): 1273-1281.

89. American Cancer Society. *Anal Cancer*. Available at: http://www.cancer.org/cancer/analcancer/detailedguide/anal-cancer-key-statistics. Accessed September 15, 2013.

90. National Comprehensive Cancer Network. *NCCN Guidelines: Anal Cancer, Version 1.2014*. Available at: http://www.nccn.org/professionals/physician_gls/pdf/anal.pdf. Accessed September 15, 2013.

91. National Cancer Institute. PDQ: health professionals – anal cancer. Available at: http://www.cancer.gov/cancertopics/pdq/treatment/anal/HealthProfessional. Accessed September 15, 2013f.

Medical Nutrition Therapy for Head and Neck Cancer

Andreea Nguyen, MS, RD, CSO, LD, CNSC
Eric Nadler, MD, MPP

Introduction

Malignant tumors that arise in the oral cavity, nasal cavity, sinuses, lips, salivary glands, throat and larynx are classified as head and neck cancers (HNC). Most originate in the layering of the mucosal surfaces. Under the microscope, normal mucosal cells present as scales (squamous), and approximately 90% of head and neck cancers are called squamous cell carcinomas. The other ten percent of head and neck cancers include adenocarcinoma, melanoma, adenoid cystic carcinoma and thyroid cancers that are found in the head and neck region.

Statistics, Symptoms, and Risk Factors

According to the National Cancer Institute (NCI), HNC accounts for 3 percent of all cancer cases in the United States (U.S.). In 2013, an estimated 41,380 cases of HNC and 7,890 deaths from HNC are expected (1-3). Symptoms may include a lump or sore that does not heal, a sore throat that does not go away, difficulty swallowing, and a change or hoarseness in the voice (1).

The most important risk factors for HNC are alcohol and tobacco use, particularly for cancers of the oral cavity, oropharynx, hypopharynx and larynx. An exception is salivary cancer, for which risk factors include older age, radiation exposure and workplace exposure to toxins such as asbestos. Infection with human papilloma virus (HPV) is an important and increasing risk factor for oropharyngeal cancer. According to the Centers for Disease Control and Prevention (CDC), more than 2,370 new cases of HPV-associated oropharyngeal cancers are diagnosed in women and nearly 9,360 are diagnosed in men each year in the U.S. (2).

Location of Head and Neck Cancers

Figure 1 provides an overview of the locations of HNC described by the area in which it originates, as follows:

Oral cavity includes the lips, front two thirds of the tongue, gingiva, buccal mucosa, floor of the mouth, hard palate and small area behind the wisdom teeth.

Salivary glands include parotid glands (found in front and just below each ear), sublingual glands (found under the tongue in the floor of the mouth) and submandibular glands (found below the jawbone).

Figure 1: Overview of the Head and Neck

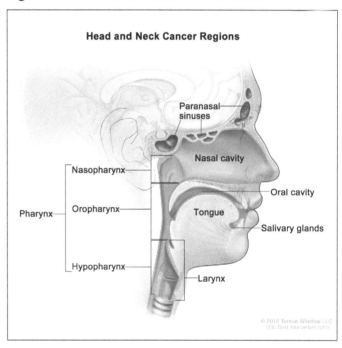

© 2012 Terese Winslow LLC, U.S. Govt. has certain rights

Paranasal sinuses are small spaces in the bone of the head surrounding the nose and the nasal cavity.

Pharynx, a hollow tube starting behind the nose leading to the esophagus, is divided into the nasopharynx (upper part of the pharynx), oropharynx (middle part of the pharynx including the soft palate, the base of tongue, and the tonsils), and hypopharynx (lower portion of the pharynx).

Larynx includes the vocal cords and the epiglottis.

Lymph nodes (not pictured) in the upper part of the neck: Squamous cancer cells appearing only in the lymph nodes of the upper part of the neck are referred to as metastatic squamous cell carcinoma with unknown primary.

Treatment

HNC management has become increasingly complex. The specific site of disease as well as disease stage and pathologic findings guide the appropriate surgical procedure, radiation targets, dose and fractionation, and indications for chemotherapy. Single-modality treatment with surgery or radiotherapy is generally recommended for the approximately 30%-40% of patients who present with early stage disease (stage I or stage II primary small tumors with no primary nodal involvement). The two modalities result in similar survival rates in these individuals. In contrast, combined modality therapy, in particular chemoradiation (CRT), is generally recommended for the approximately 60% of patients diagnosed with locally or regionally advanced disease (usually stage III or IV tumors), which may include underlying structures and/or metastasis to regional nodes (4-7).

Surgery

The goal of surgery is to remove the tumor with a margin of healthy tissue. If the cancer has spread, the neck lymph nodes may need to be removed as well. Surgical intervention can cause swallowing difficulties, dependent on the degree and site of the resection. For example, resection of the floor of the mouth or base of tongue places a patient at greater risk of requiring supplemental feeding and ongoing intervention by a speech and language pathologist (SLP) to maintain speech and swallowing function. Side effects of the surgery may include swelling, pain, and/or structural deformities, such as loss of teeth, hemiglossectomy (i.e., removal of part of the tongue), soft palate fistula, or tracheostomy, making it difficult to chew or swallow and potentially limiting nutrient intake.

Radiation

Radiation therapy acts by directing x-rays to cancerous regions, causing damage to cell DNA so cells cannot replicate. Rapidly dividing cells, such as those lining the oral mucosa, are the most susceptible to radiation damage. As a result, side effects may include mucositis, odynophagia, thick saliva, xerostomia, trismus, pharyngeal fibrosis and decreased appetite as a result of dysgeusia. Radiation therapy also can exacerbate tooth decay; pre-existing damaged teeth may need to be removed prior to treatment.

Intensity-modulated radiation therapy (IMRT) is an advanced form of radiation therapy allowing more precise cancer targeting while reducing the dose to normal tissues. IMRT is now widely used in HNC as it reduces long-term toxicity in oropharyngeal, paranasal sinus and nasopharyngeal cancers by reducing the dose to one or more major structures including salivary glands, temporal lobes, mandible, auditory and optic structures (6).

In the setting of CRT, most studies have used conventional fractionation at 2.0 Gy per fraction to 70 Gy or more in 7 weeks with single-agent Cisplatin given every 3 weeks at 100 mg/m^2 (6). Other fraction sizes (i.e., 1.8 Gy, conventional), other dosing schedules of Cisplatin, other single agents, multiagent chemotherapy, and altered fractionation with chemotherapy have been evaluated alone or in combination (6). Radiation has a cumulative effect, meaning that each day is worse than the day before with the above-mentioned side effects occurring between 10-15 fractionations and intensifying through the remainder of the treatment.

Table 1: Nutritional Implications of Chemotherapeutic Agents Commonly Used in the Treatment of Head and Neck Cancer

Medication	Potential Side Effects with Nutritional Implications
Bleomycin (Blenoxane®)	• Nausea, vomiting, poor appetite, weight loss and mouth sores*
Cisplatin (Platinol®, CDDP)	• Nausea, vomiting, and kidney toxicity** • Peripheral neuropathy, loss of appetite, taste changes, metallic taste*
Cetuximab (Erbitux®)	• Low magnesium level** • Nausea, vomiting, diarrhea, constipation*
Carboplatin (Paraplatin®)	• Nausea, vomiting, taste changes** • Diarrhea, constipation, mouth sores*
Docetaxel (Taxotere®)	• Nausea, diarrhea, mouth sores** • Vomiting*
Gemcitabine (Gemzar®)	• Mild nausea, vomiting, poor appetite** • Diarrhea, mouth sores*
Ifosfamide (Ifex®)	• Nausea, vomiting, poor appetite**
Methotrexate (MTX)	• Mouth sores, nausea, vomiting, poor appetite** • Diarrhea*
Paclitaxel (Taxol®)	• Mild nausea and vomiting, diarrhea, mouth sores**
Fluorouracil (5FU)	• Diarrhea, nausea and possible vomiting, poor appetite, taste changes, metallic taste**

Incidence of symptoms occurring in 10-29% of patients, and **incidence of symptoms occurring in greater than 30%** according to the following source: Chemotherapy Drugs – Chemocare. Chemotherapy Drugs and Drugs Often Used During Chemotherapy. http://www.chemocare.com/chemotherapy/drug-info/default.aspx. Accessed December 28, 2012 (11). Brand names are listed in parentheses.

Chemotherapy

The standard therapy for patients with locally advanced disease remains concurrent Cisplatin and radiation treatment (6). Over the past ten years, multiple studies have attempted to improve upon this combined treatment. Evidence suggests that induction chemotherapy (given prior to combined chemo-radiation treatment) with Fluorouracil and Cisplatin improves locoregional treatment for head and neck squamous-cell carcinoma (8). Additional research suggests that adding Docetaxel to the Fluorouracil and Cisplatin induction regimen can improve the response to treatment, significantly reduce the risk of disease progression and extend survival (9-10). Further, multiple options can be used for the radiation-based portion of the treatment given after induction chemotherapy. Radiation alone, radiation plus Cetuximab or weekly Carboplatin are among the options (6). Researchers continue to evaluate the best combinations and schedule for chemotherapy and radiation treatments in HNC.

Chemotherapy treatments can result in adverse events; Table 1 provides a list of commonly used chemotherapy drugs in HNC and their nutrition related side effects.

Currently, outside of clinical trials, oncologists must first consider whether induction chemotherapy is warranted before determining which particular drug (if any) should be combined with radiation. Many factors influence this decision, including patient age, clinical involvement of primary tumor and local-regional lymph nodes, amount of mucosal surface to be irradiated and associated co-morbidities of the patient.

In an effort to improve the understanding of the nutritional side effects of HNC treatment, as well as codify nutrition intervention throughout the treatment, four distinct nutritional phases have been identified (see Figure 2) that form the pyramid experienced by HNC patients receiving concurrent CRT. As outlined in Figure 2, these phases, beginning pre treatment and ending post treatment, provide an estimated rather than a definite timeline as each patient's response to treatment and side effects can be different. Among variables that influence treatment course are the location of the tumor and the amount of area being radiated, which is usually directly proportional to the severity of treatment-induced toxicities. These nutritional phases provide a better understanding and picture of the nutritional effects of HNC treatment, as well as nutrition interventions that support nutritional status throughout treatment. Table 2 outlines grades of toxicities that may be experienced during CRT.

Nutritional Challenges

HNC patients commonly experience a diminished oral intake as well as painful and impaired chewing and swallowing due to local symptoms, which may occur before diagnosis and/or as a result of cancer treatment. They may also present with pre-existing nutritional deficiencies associated with excessive alcohol consumption and/or tobacco use as well as decreased appetite and

Table 2: The World Health Organization Oral Toxicity Scale (14)

Grade 0	No change over baseline
Grade 1	Soreness +/- erythema
Grade 2	Erythema, ulcers and patient can swallow solid food
Grade 3	Ulcers with extensive erythema; patient cannot swallow solid food
Grade 4	Mucositis so severe that oral alimentation is not possible; patient needs alternative method of feeding

cachexia resulting from the malignancy (12). In fact, patients with HNC experience one of the highest rates of malnutrition among all cancer diagnoses with 25-50% of these patients at risk for malnutrition prior to starting treatment (13). Furthermore cancer treatment itself can result in significant toxicities such as dysphagia, odynophagia, dysgeusia, stomatitis, xerostomia, and nausea and vomiting, each of which can contribute to inadequate intake and thereby compromise nutritional status (15). Since maintaining desirable nutritional goals (16) throughout CRT via an oral diet alone is very difficult, alternative methods of nutrition support (particularly enteral feeding through a Gastrostomy or G-tube) are often necessary (13,17).

Nutritional goals for head and neck cancer (16)

- Weight maintenance during and after treatment
- Weight maintenance post treatment until the patient is able to consume solid food
- Successful, break free completion of treatment
- Minimal, if any, weight loss in overweight or obese patients until patient is fully recovered from treatment and is able to eat without difficulties
- Weight maintenance during transitional feedings from enteral nutrition support

Currently, the use of prophylactic G-tube placement is controversial. The literature identifies risk factors associated with potential need for a feeding tube in HNC patients, including stage IV tumors, primary pharyngeal tumors, combined surgery and radiotherapy, and preoperative weight loss of more than ten pounds (18). In addition, G-tube placement is a potential preventive measure for malnutrition identified as unintentional weight loss combined with an inability to consume an oral diet because of disease and treatment-related symptoms (19), each of which are seen in the HNC population. The prophylactic placement of a G-tube, rather than reactive placement after significant weight loss and an extended period of inadequate food and fluid intake, has many benefits, including less weight loss. This is important because weight loss was the strongest independent predictor of shortened survival in a series of HNC patients treated with multiple modalities (20). Undernutrition in HNC patients is associated with poor treatment outcomes, including morbidity, infections, cancer recurrence, mortality, and poor quality of life (20). Poor nutrition contributes to a

Figure 2: Summary of Four Nutritional Phases of CRT treatment for HNC

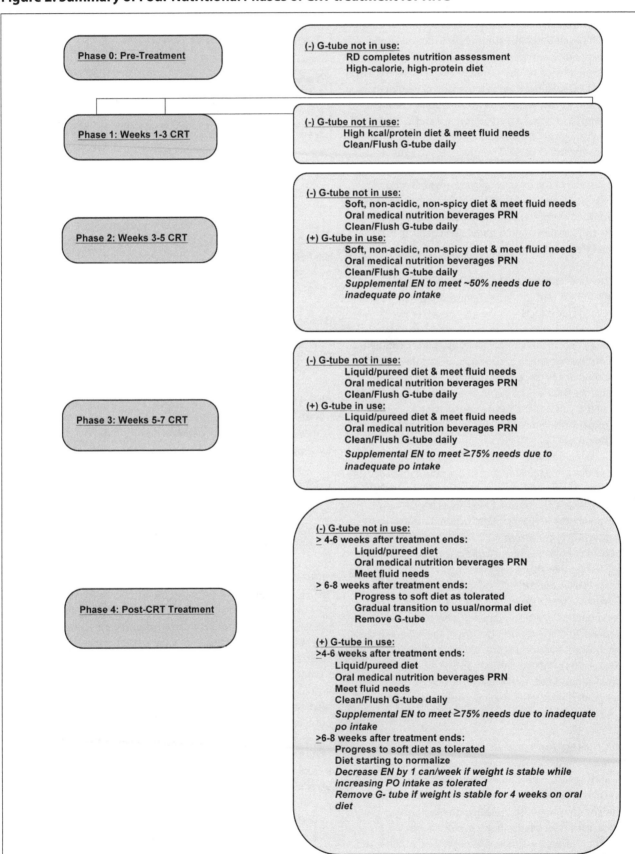

series of complications, including a compromised immune system, which can lead to unhindered tumor growth, treatment delays or interruptions which are associated with poorer outcomes, and loss of muscle mass, which jeopardizes respiratory function and impairs patient mobility and performance status (20-21). Medical personnel must be aware that unintentional weight loss is an important predictor of malnutrition in the HNC population, even in those patients whose BMI is not suggestive of malnutrition (21), and that benefits of prophylactic G-tube feeding include fewer hospital admissions for dehydration or malnutrition, less treatment interruptions and/or delays, and better quality of life during treatment (15,17,22-23). Therefore, it is important to stress weight maintenance in all patients treated for HNC.

Many patients hesitate to accept the idea of having a feeding tube placed, as it can be a foreign and frightening concept. To alleviate this, discussions should address a feeding tube as a "life jacket" in case there is ever a need for alternative access to food, water or medication administration, and reassure patients that a G-tube is usually temporary and discontinued as soon as it is medically warranted. No one can better explain and understand what it is like to go through this treatment other than a cancer survivor; encouraging patients to attend local support groups can be a great way to connect and learn from others whose intake has been improved via tube feedings.

While common concerns associated with G-tube placement include long-term dependence on enteral feedings and persistent dysphagia from nonuse of the muscles involved with swallowing and subsequent decreased quality of life, Osborne et al (24) showed that HNC patients with G-tubes generally have a positive or neutral experience. To further mitigate these risks, the nutrition plan developed by the registered dietitian (RD) should guide tube feeding administration, weaning, and timely G-tube removal and a Speech Language Pathologist (SLP) should direct interventions that maintain swallowing function.

Table 3 provides an outline of RD nutrition care practice for CRT for HNC patients. Specific tips for the various phases are provided below, but for detailed information about nutrition assessment, nutrition support, and dietary supplements the reader should refer to chapters 3,13 and 8, respectively.

Phase 0: Pre-Treatment

A comprehensive nutrition assessment (25) is integral to phase 0 and includes but is not limited to estimation of energy, protein and fluid needs, diet and weight history, and a discussion regarding use of integrative therapies including types and doses of dietary supplements taken. This will provide the RD with information important to developing a safe and effective nutrition care plan that will help the patient achieve nutritional goals (16), manage nutrition impact symptoms and minimize potential adverse effects of integrative therapies (25).

RDs should provide patients with educational handouts, including recipes that highlight coping mechanisms for anticipated side effects of each patient's treatment regimen. It is important for patients to understand that "food is medicine" and essential for nourishment. At this time the medical team also should consider arrangements for a prophylactic G-tube after thoroughly discussing its use and purpose with the patient and/or family member(s). When supplemental vitamins and minerals are indicated, it is important to follow Dietary Reference Intake (DRI) guidelines, as excess amounts of these nutrients (in particular antioxidants) may potentially interfere with treatment (13).

Phase 1: Weeks 1-3- of CRT

Once treatment starts, nutrition intervention continues to focus on a diet providing recommended energy and protein intake, as tolerated. Most patients tolerate and accept such a diet for the first three weeks of CRT, defined here as Phase 1. However, use of medical nutrition beverages and/or alternative nutrition support may be indicated in those patients with advanced cancers and/or who have had pretreatment weight loss as discussed in Phase 2. When a G-tube is present, its integrity and function are confirmed and healing of the G-tube site is routinely checked.

Phase 2: Weeks 3-5 of CRT

As treatment progresses from weeks 3 through 5, side effects such as dysphagia, odynophagia, xerostomia, dysgeusia, thick oral secretions, and grade 1 and 2 oral mucositis start to impede the patient's oral fluid and food intake. Table 3 provides a number of oral diet recommendations for maintaining nutrition status during phase 2 and managing dry mouth. Artificial saliva sprays and oral lubricants also may be useful for managing dry mouth, as are chewing sugar free gum and use of alcohol free mouth rinses.

Managing copious mouth/throat secretions, often described as being stringy or ropey, is a major problem for patients with high-grade mucositis. The mucus causes queasiness and gagging, which further complicates efforts to maintain adequate hydration and nutrition. While folklore suggests using meat tenderizer, pineapple or kiwi to break these thick secretions, in the literature the following strategies are found to be useful (26):

- Regular rinses with salt and soda solution (1 L water with ½ teaspoon baking soda and ½ teaspoon salt)
- Caphosol up to 10 times per day during treatment and 2-3 weeks after treatment
- Scopolamine transdermal patch may be an effective drying agent
- Elevation of the head of the patient's bed to at least 30 degrees will help reduce edema and protect the airway
- A cool mist vaporizer may lubricate and mobilize secretions
- Lorazepam may help block a cycle of repeated gagging and associated nausea
- A portable suction machine may help clear secretions
- Increased fluid intake can help thin secretions

Table 3: Head and Neck Cancer: RD Nutrition Practice Summary for Chemoradiation Therapy (CRT)

Phase/ Timeframe	Nutrition Framework	Oral Diet	Tube Feeding	Energy, Protein, and Fluid Needs
0 Pretreatment (2 weeks prior to CRT)	• RD will complete a nutrition assessment, determine nutrition diagnoses and develop a nutrition plan based on evidence-based nutrition interventions. • RD will counsel patient on a 5-6 small meal/day plan that meets recommended energy, protein, & micronutrient needs. • RD will educate patient on prophylactic enteral nutrition (EN) (e.g., potential need for EN, formula options, EN regimen). • RD will educate patient on oral hygiene regimen.	• Provide high kcal/high protein diet, potentially including medical nutrition beverages. • Vitamin/mineral intake should be close to 100% of DRIs; avoid vitamin/mineral supplements unless nutrition diagnosis indicates a need.	• Consider prophylactic G-tube placement.	**Energy** • Normometabolic: 25-30 kcal/kg/day • Hypermetabolic or goal of weight gain: 30-35 kcal/kg/day • Obese: 21-25 kcal/kg/day **Protein** • Nonstressed: 1-1.5 g protein/kg • Hypermetabolic or protein-losing enteropathy: 1.5-2.5 g protein/kg **Fluid** • 30-35 ml/kg • Fluid needs may be greater in cases of excess fluid loss (e.g., vomiting, diarrhea, losses via fistulas). • All recommendations will be adjusted per concurrent medical status and needs.
1 Weeks 1-3 of CRT	• During routine nutrition reassessments the RD will monitor tolerance of oral diet and reassess weight, hydration status and overall nutrition needs. • RD will assess patient for mucositis, dysguesia, dysphagia & xerostomia (e.g., using WHO Oral Toxicity Scale to assess for mucositis). • Based on results of nutrition reassessment, RD will revise nutrition plan as needed (e.g., oral diet modifications, fluid needs and sources, etc.). • RD will advise patient on use of oral medical nutrition beverages and will reinforce oral hygiene regimen recommendations.	• Same as Phase 0	• Clean/flush G-tube daily (w/ 60 mL free water twice per day – Phases 1 - 4).	• If indicated, adjust from Phase 0 recommendations per weight status (and change), protein status and hydration status.
2 Weeks 3-5 of CRT	• Same as Phase 1 unless nutrition reassessment indicates need for revisions (e.g., oral diet modifications, EN adjustments, changes in EN infusion rates, fluid needs and sources, etc.). If PO intake falls below 50% of estimated needs, start EN.	• Provide high kcal/ high protein soft diet as tolerated; non-acidic, non-fibrous, non-spicy foods; and avoid hot and ice cold liquids. • Incorporate oral medical nutrition beverages as needed (Phases 2 – 4). • Total (i.e., between oral diet and EN) vitamin/mineral intake should be close to 100% of DRIs; avoid vitamin/mineral supplements unless nutrition diagnosis indicates a need (Phases 2 – 4).	• If PO intake falls below 50% of estimated needs, initiate EN to meet approximately 50% energy needs. • Provide recommendations on appropriate tube feeding formula and infusion schedule.	• Adjust from Phase 0 recommendations per weight status (and change), protein status and hydration status.
3 Weeks 5-7 of CRT	• Same as Phase 1 unless nutrition reassessment indicates need for revisions (e.g., oral diet modifications, EN adjustments, changes in EN infusion rates, fluid needs and sources, etc.).	• Provide liquid/pureed diet; non-acidic, non-fibrous, non-spicy foods; and avoid hot and ice cold liquids. • Incorporate oral medical nutrition beverages as needed (Phases 2 – 4). • Total (i.e., between oral diet and EN) vitamin/mineral intake should be close to 100% of DRIs; avoid vitamin/mineral supplements unless nutrition diagnosis indicates a need (Phases 2 – 4).	• Follow RD recommendations on appropriate EN formula and infusion schedule; implement changes in EN plan based on results of nutrition reassessment (Phases 3 – 4). • EN regimen usually increased to ≥75% estimated energy needs.	• Adjust from Phase 0 recommendations per weight status (and change), protein status and hydration status.
4 Post-treatment	• Same as Phase 3	• Provide liquid/pureed diet; non-acidic, non-fibrous, non-spicy foods; and avoid hot and ice cold liquids. • Incorporate oral medical nutrition beverages as needed (Phases 2 – 4). • Total (i.e., between oral diet and EN) vitamin/mineral intake should be close to 100% of DRIs; avoid vitamin/mineral supplements unless nutrition diagnosis indicates a need (Phases 2 – 4). • Slowly advance to soft foods as tolerated.	• EN usually provides ≥75% estimated needs for the first 4-6 weeks post treatment. • ~ 6-8 weeks post treatment, decrease EN by 1 can every week if weight is stable, oral diet is tolerated and oral intake improves. • Remove feeding tube if weight is stable and EN has not been used for 4 weeks.	• Adjust from Phase 0 recommendations per weight status (and change), protein status and hydration status.

EN via a G-tube is indicated when oral intake is inadequate (i.e., patient is unable to consume >50% of estimated energy and nutrient needs) and weight loss occurs despite oral nutrition interventions. Health insurance policies and regulations need to be researched to determine insurance coverage for tube feedings and supporting documentation required to obtain insurance coverage. During phase 2 EN may provide between 25-50% of estimated needs or more, depending on the patient's oral intake and tolerance.

The RD should counsel the patient and family on:
- type of feeding method best tolerated by the patient (e.g., bolus, gravity or pump)
- feeding schedule (e.g., intermittent, nighttime, continuous)
- type of EN formula (e.g., standard formula providing 1.0 kcal/ml, energy-dense providing >1.5 kcal/ml, elemental, low fat and/or low-fiber formula)

There is a paucity of data identifying the optimal method of tube feeding administration. Typically, patients are started on bolus, transitioned to gravity if not tolerating bolus, and further changed to pump if gravity feeds are not tolerated. The risk with this methodology is that patients may be losing weight during this transition process. Research to determine the optimal delivery method to maximize tolerance and quickest transition to goal needs is ongoing.

Phase 3 (weeks 5-7 of CRT)
As treatment continues and patients enter Phase 3, they often experience grade 3 or 4 oral mucositis. Available medications may not completely alleviate these symptoms, and as a result few patients can meet their energy and fluid needs via an oral diet, even after food textures have been modified (i.e., use of pureed foods or extremely soft casseroles, cream based soups or other liquid foods or fluids) and medical nutrition beverages provided. More often than not, patients are dependent on their feeding tubes for nutrition; at this treatment phase EN frequently provides as much as 75% of estimated energy, protein, and nutrient needs.

Even though EN via G-tube can be life saving during this treatment, it is important to recognize and overcome challenges encountered. These include selecting the most appropriate type of tube feeding formula, establishing an efficient and effective method of tube feeding administration, and managing scheduling conflicts. Disease-induced gastroparesis, side-effects of chemotherapy, and medications (i.e., narcotics, calcium-channel blockers, antiemetics, and some antidepressants) may make it difficult to tolerate high fat and high fiber tube feeding formulas when administered via gastric route (27). RDs must monitor tolerance of energy-dense tube feeding formulas (often used to meet high energy demands) since their higher fat or osmolality may induce gastrointestinal discomfort and intolerance. The method of tube feeding administration also may influence tolerance of the EN regimen at goal. A slower, more constant infusion, as seen with changing from bolus to gravity or gravity to pump, may improve tube feeding tolerance in cases of

nausea, vomiting, or early satiety. Medications may improve tolerance, such as initiating a promotility agent to facilitate gastric emptying and implementing a bowel regimen in cases of constipation. Gravity or pump assisted tube feeding also can be helpful in situations where a patient's schedule does not allow enough time to infuse a high volume of formula and water via the bolus method every couple of hours between daily trips to treatment and medical appointments

Phase 4 (Post-Treatment)
Chemoradiation-induced nutrition impact symptoms persist for weeks after the conclusion of active treatment. Patients continue to require modified foods and/or be dependent on EN for the first four to six weeks after treatment ends. After this initial post-treatment phase, which occasionally may last longer than six weeks, side effects will subside slowly. The feeding plan will be liberalized as indicated by symptoms and the SLP should continue to assess the swallowing mechanism and share findings with the RD. Approximately six to eight weeks post treatment, side effects continue to resolve and oral diet continues to transition to a normal variety of textures and amounts. The patient will be weaned off of EN if it was provided. When weight is stable, EN is typically decreased by 240 mL formula per week, while concurrently increasing oral intake. This process continues until the patient is completely weaned from EN. The G-tube should be removed when the patient has not used it for nutrition, hydration or medication and the weight is stable for approximately one month.

There is concern that EN dependence can linger despite improvement in oral mucositis and/or normal swallowing function. Lack of taste, dry mouth, and perhaps a lower motivation level or the "convenience" of using the G-tube rather than eating can play a role in prolonged use of EN post treatment. This reinforces the need of ongoing and close monitoring of nutritional status for months after the treatment has been completed. To help patients successfully transition from EN to an oral diet, weekly follow-ups are common and include a weight check, physical examination, laboratory monitoring and nutrition reassessment.

Conclusions
HNC patients are a complex population with a wide array of nutritional challenges. The role of the RD within the multidisciplinary team is imperative, as the nutritional status of these patients is tenuous throughout CRT. Maximizing a patient's nutritional status, as reflected by interventions that limit weight loss and preserve lean body mass, improves treatment outcomes by preventing treatment delays and unplanned hospitalizations. Defining unique nutritional phases of CRT can serve as both a treatment algorithm for the RD and an educational tool for the patient. Tracking a patient through the nutritional phases of CRT helps the RD provide timely, safe, appropriate, and effective nutrition intervention. Finally, and most importantly, a multidisciplinary team approach, effective symptom management, and early and ongoing intervention by the RD are vital to optimize quality of life and clinical outcomes in HNC patients.

References

1. National Cancer Institute. Oral Cancer Prevention PDQ. Incidence and Mortality. http://www.cancer.gov/cancertopics/pdq/prevention/oral/HealthProfessional/Page2#Section_159 Revised 2/15/13. Accessed April 28, 2013.

2. Centers for Disease Control and Prevention. Human Papillomavirus (HPV) – Associated Cancers. http://www.cdc.gov/cancer/hpv/statistics/headneck.htm. Accessed November 11, 2012.

3. SEER Training Modules, *Module Name*. U. S. National Institutes of Health, National Cancer Institute. Accessed June 25, 2012. <*http://training.seer.cancer.gov/*>.

4. Forastier AA, Goepfert H, Maor M, et al. Concurrent chemotherapy and radiotherapy for organ preservation in advanced laryngeal cancer. *N Engl J Med*. 2003; 349(22):2091-2098.

5. Adelstein DJ, Lavertu P, Saxton JP, et al. Mature results of a phase III randomized trial comparing concurrent chemoradiotherapy with radiation therapy alone in patients with stage III and IV squamous cell carcinoma of the head and neck. *Cancer*. 2000; 88(4):876-883.

6. National Comprehensive Cancer Network (NCCN). NCCN guidelines for treatment of cancer by site. http://www.nccn.org/professionals/physician_gls/pdf/head-and-neck.pdf. Accessed November 16, 2012.

7. Denis F, Garaud P, Bardet E, et al. Final results of the 94-01 French head and neck oncology and radiotherapy group randomized trial comparing radiotherapy alone with concomitant radiochemotherapy in advanced-stage oropharynx carcinoma. *J Clin Oncol*. 2004;22(1):69-67.

8. Pignon JP, Bourhis J, Domenge C, Designe L. Chemotherapy added to locoregional treatment for had and neck squamous-cell carcinoma: three meta-analysis of updated individual data. *Lancet*. 2000; 355(9208): 949-955.

9. Vermorken JB, Remenar E, van Herpen C, et al. Cisplatin, fluorouracil, and docetaxel in unresectable head and neck cancer. *N Engl J Med*. 2007;357(17):1695-1704.

10. Posner MR, Hershock DM, Blajman CR, et al. Cisplatin and Fluorouracil alone or with Docetaxel in head and neck cancer. *N Engl J Med*. 2007; 357(17):1705-1715.

11. Chemotherapy Drugs – Chemocare. Chemotherapy Drugs and Drugs Often Used During Chemotherapy. http://www.chemocare.com/chemotherapy/drug-info/default.aspx. Accessed December 28, 2012.

12. Rabinovitch R, Grant B, Berkey BA, et al. Impact of nutrition support on treatment outcome in patients with locally advanced head and neck squamous cell cancer treated with definitive radiotherapy: A secondary analysis of RTOG trial 90-03. *Head and Neck*. 2005; 28(4):287-296.

13. Isering E. Esophageal and Head and Neck Cancer. In: Marian M, Roberts S, eds. *Clinical Nutrition for Oncology Patients*. Sudbury, MA: Jones & Barlett; 2010: 165-185.

14. World Health Organization. Handbook for reporting results of cancer treatment. Geneva, Switzerland: World Health Organization; 1979:15-22.

15. Lee JH, Machtay M, Unger LD, et al. Prophylactic gastrostomy tubes in patients undergoing intensive irradiation for cancer of the head and neck. *Arch Otolaryngol Head Neck Surg*. 1998;124(8):871-875.

16. 2010 American Dietetic Association *Oncology Toolkit*. Medical Nutrition Therapy Summary Page for Oncology Nutrition: Head and Neck Cancer.

17. Chang JH, Gosling T, Larsen J, et al. Prophylactic gastrostomy tubes for patients receiving radical radiotherapy for head and neck cancers: A retrospective review. *J Med Imaging and Radiat Oncol*. 2009;53(5): 494-495.

18. Gardine RL, Kokal WA, Beatty JD, et al. Predicting the need for prolonged enteral supplementation in the patient with head and neck cancer. *Am J Surg*. 1988;156(1):63-65.

19. White J, Guenter P, Jensen G, Malone,A, Schofield M. Consensus Statement: Academy of Nutrition and Dietetics and American Society for Parenteral and Enteral Nutrition: Characteristics recommended for the identification and documentation of adult malnutrition (undernutrition). *J Parenter Enteral Nutr*. 2012;36:275.

20. Locher JL, Bonner JA, Carroll WR et al. Prophylactic percutaneous endoscopic gastrostomy tube placement in treatment of head and neck cancer: A comprehensive review and call for evidence-based medicine. *J Parenter Enteral Nutr*. 2011;35(3):365-374.

21. Loh KW, Gerritsen A, Borel Rinkes IHM, et al. Unintentional weight loss is the most important indicator of malnutrition among surgical cancer patients. *Neth J Med*. 2012;70(8)365-369.

22. Piquet MA, Ozsahin M, Larpin I, et al. Early nutrition intervention in oropharyngeal cancer patients undergoing radiotherapy. *Support Care Cancer*. 2002;10(6):502-504.

23. Fietkau R. Principles of feeding cancer patients via enteral or parenteral nutrition during radiotherapy. *Strahlenther Onkol*. 1988;174(3):47-51.

24. Osborne JB, Collin LA, Posluns EC, Stokes EJ, Vandenbussche KA. The experience of head and neck cancer patients with a percutaneous endoscopic gastrostomy tube at a canadian cancer center. *Nutr Clin Pract*. 2012; 27(5):661-668.

25. Charney P, Cranganu A. Nutrition Screening and Assessment in Oncology. In: Marian M, Roberts S, eds. *Clinical Nutrition for Oncology Patients*. Sudbury, MA: Jones & Bartlett; 2010:21-43.

26. Rosenthal DI, Trotti A. Strategies for managing radiation-induced mucositis in head and neck cancer. *Semin Radiat Oncol*. 2009;19(1):29-34.

27. Marian M. Medical nutrition therapies in head and neck cancers. *Support Line*. 2010;32:16-23.

Medical Nutrition Therapy for Lung Cancer

Maureen Leser, MS, RD, CSO, LD

Background

Almost unheard of during the early decades of the 20th century, lung cancer rates among men increased from 4.9 per 100,000 in 1930 to 75.6 per 100,000 in 1990 (1), parallel to increases in smoking prevalence. As smoking rates have fallen over the past several decades (to 24.7% of the adult population in 1997), rates of lung cancer have also decreased (1-2). Nevertheless, lung cancer remains the leading cause of cancer-related death in the United States (U.S.), and tobacco use accounts for 87% of lung cancer deaths (3). Two or three out of every 100 men and one or two of every 100 women who are over 60 years of age will be diagnosed with lung cancer over the next ten years (4). Lung cancer cases of never smokers (i.e., an adult who has smoked fewer than 100 cigarettes in a lifetime) are attributed to a variety of predominantly environmental risks including secondhand smoke and exposure to radon gas. If considered a unique disease, never-smoker cases would rank seventh among causes of cancer mortality in the U.S. (5). In the U.S. in 2013, the National Cancer Institute predicted 228,190 new cases and 159,480 deaths from lung cancer (6). The five-year survival rate for lung cancer is a dismal 15.7%, mainly because this disease is usually diagnosed after it has spread. When diagnosed locally the five-year survival is 49%, rather than 16% when diagnosed regionally and 2% when diagnosed with distant metastasis (7). Lung cancer in never-smokers has approximately a 30% greater survival rate than cases in smokers.

Types of Lung Cancer

Small cell and non-small cell lung cancers are the predominant types of lung cancer diagnosed (8-9).

Figure 1: The Lung

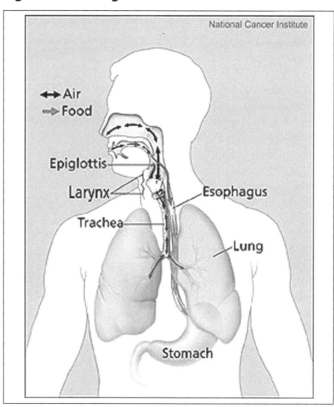

Reprinted with permission
The website of the National Cancer Institute (http/www.cancer.gov)

Table: Risk Factors, Prevalence and Survival of Lung Cancers (8-10)

Criteria	Small Cell Lung Caner (SCLC)	Non-small Cell Lung Cancer (NSCLC)
General Information	Includes oat cell cancer	The most common type of lung cancer; includes squamous cell carcinoma, adenocarcinoma and large cell carcinoma
Prevalence	~15% of total cases	~70%-85% of total cases
Risk Factors	Cigarette smoking; second-hand smoking; radon gas exposure; asbestos exposure; excessive alcohol intake; exposure to arsenic, chromium and nickel (usually through a workplace)	Cigarette Smoking; nonsmoking women chronically exposed to cooking fumes generated from burning wood or frying fat at high temperatures
Symptoms	Cough, dyspnea, involuntary weight loss, debility, bone pain, neurologic compromise, hoarseness	Cough, bloody cough, persistent cough, shortness of breath, chest pain, wheezing, hoarseness, involuntary weight loss

Health Disparities: Men are at greater risk of lung cancer than women because of their higher rate of smoking, but smoking has increased among women since the mid 1980s. Black men have higher rates of lung cancer than white men.

Diagnosis and Staging

Imaging tests for lung cancer include CT scans, which are used to visualize the size of a lung tumor and whether it has spread. PET scans and MRIs are often used to determine whether lung cancer has spread to the brain or spine and bone scans will determine whether the cancer has spread to bone (7).

The American Joint Committee on Cancer (AJCC) has developed a widely used staging system based on *Tumor* size, extent of lymph *Node* involvement, and *Metastasis* (11). The National Cancer Institute also has described stages of lung cancer. Information on the NCI system can be accessed at http://www.cancer.gov/cancertopics/wyntk/lung/page6 (7). In both systems, early stages reflect localized disease. As regional lymph nodes and tissue become involved, a higher stage is diagnosed. The highest stages reflect disease within the lung, in lymph nodes and regional tissue, and distant metastasis.

Treatments

Primary treatments for lung cancer include surgery, radiation therapy, chemotherapy and targeted therapy. Surgical options include a lobectomy (removal of an affected lobe), pneumonectomy (removal of an entire lung) and a wedge resection (removal of a section of a lung). Lobectomies are associated with better outcomes than wedge resection, but eligibility for extensive surgery may be limited by performance status, which is influenced by nutritional status.

Radiation, chemotherapy and targeted therapy also are used to treat lung cancer. Common chemotherapy agents used include Carboplatin, Cisplatin, Docetaxel, Etoposide, Gemcitabine, Irinotecan, Methotrexate, Pemetrexed, Vinblastine and Vinorelbine, while targeted therapy agents include Cetuximab, Trastuzumab and Bevacizumab. Both chemotherapy and targeted therapy agents can result in a variety of nutrition impact symptoms (NIS) including anorexia, nausea/vomiting, diarrhea/constipation, mucositis and altered taste. Chapter 11 discusses the mechanism of action and side effects of each agent; chapter 12 provides nutrition interventions to manage these effects.

Nutrition Risk Screening and Assessment

The consequences of malnutrition have been well documented and include reduced absorption of drugs used in cancer treatment, reduced response to treatment and slower post-operative recovery. In the lung cancer population almost 60% have lost significant weight when diagnosed (12), suggesting that the diagnosis alone should trigger a positive nutrition risk screening and a nutrition assessment.

In this population evidence has found that weight loss can shorten survival (13-14). Weight loss greater than 5% has been associated with lower Karnofsky performance status and quality of life (15). Malnourished lung cancer patients with hypoalbuminemia experience more toxicity during chemotherapy treatment than those without malnutrition (16). In particular hypoalbuminemia may increase the severity of toxicity in agents that bind with albumin (e.g., Cisplatin and Paclitaxel).

Epidemiologic studies have found an inverse association between BMI and lung cancer risk. An interesting finding in data from the state of Florida, which is home to 6% of all lung cancer patients in the U.S., is that those who are obese when diagnosed live longer than those who have experienced weight loss (17). In patients who have lost weight and in those who are obese, nutrition intervention to manage chemotherapy-induced NIS is important for limiting their effects on intake and nutritional status; experience suggests these symptoms should be addressed as early as possible in the treatment process.

The high prevalence of weight loss and malnutrition in patients with lung cancer has been partially attributed to being diagnosed at late stages. Metabolic factors also may contribute to this observation. A small study (n=19) suggested that weight losing lung cancer patients experience an increased rate of gluconeogenesis, which is an energy consuming process (18). In addition, approximately 50% of those with lung cancer also present with congestive obstructive pulmonary disease (COPD), which is associated with weight loss, muscle wasting, and a change in muscle fiber that is more susceptible to fatigue (19). Potential causes of muscle atrophy include lower rates of protein synthesis and increased rates of protein degradation. In addition, basal metabolism may be increased due to systemic inflammation and increased work required for breathing (19). Just as excess weight is associated with longer survival in lung cancer patients, weight gain in underweight COPD patients is associated with longer survival (20); these observations support the importance of interventions to maintain weight in overweight lung cancer patients and to increase or stabilize weight in those who are losing weight. It can be difficult to achieve a greater intake in some patients diagnosed with lung cancer, and there is inadequate evidence to determine which intervention may achieve the desired results (e.g., oral intake, use of medical nutrition beverages, enteral support). In addition, current evidence is unable to distinguish between failure to provide intervention versus failure of the intervention itself (20).

Levels of branched chain amino acids (BCAA) are reduced In those with low muscle mass and in COPD patients. Lung cancer patients over the age of 70 with compromised pulmonary function, who have a higher operative mortality than those with adequate pulmonary function, were assigned to receive 6.2 grams of BCAA daily along with physical exercise prior to surgery versus conventional treatment. In addition to BCAA supplementation, RDs optimized diet therapy for subjects in the intervention arm. Postoperative complication rates after lobectomy in the CVPR (conventional) and CHPR (intervention) groups were 48.3% and 28.6%. Study weaknesses include small numbers (29 subjects in the intervention group and 21 subjects in the conventional treatment group) and lack of randomization. Prospective, randomized studies are needed to confirm the benefit of this intervention (21).

Nutrition Needs in Lung Cancer

A nutrition assessment will identify individual nutrition needs; however, the high rate of weight loss and malnutrition in the lung cancer population suggests a need for energy repletion and thus energy needs of 30-35 kcal/kg/day, see Chapter 4. Protein needs are 1.2-1.5 g/kg/day, see Chapter 4.

Evidence suggests there is no benefit for consuming more than the Dietary Reference Intake (DRI) for micronutrients, and high intakes may be harmful. Providing high doses of beta-carotene increased the number of lung cancer cases in some studies (22-25). Conversely, greater intake of food high in carotenoids may help prevent lung cancer (26). Selenium supplementation has been found to be beneficial only among those with lower selenium status (27).

Nutritional Considerations of Older Cancer Patients with Lung Cancer

The average age when diagnosed with lung cancer is 70 years. Older patients experience more fatigue and experience more toxicity from treatments than younger patients (28-29), thus early intervention is essential. In addition, clinicians need to pay particular attention to dentition, food access, reliance on prepared foods, and the ability to independently complete activities of daily living. These factors help determine the amount of assistance the patient may need to consume the recommended diet.

CIPN and Glutamine

Cisplatin, Vinorelbine, Docetaxel and Paclitaxel, commonly used in lung cancer treatment, pose a risk of peripheral neuropathy, which is among the most disabling effects of chemotherapy. Over 20 clinical trials have concluded that up to 30 grams per day of oral glutamine supplementation is safe and reduces toxic effects of treatment but this evidence has been rated as limited/weak (30). Nevertheless, the positive results suggest a need for additional well-designed trials. Western diets usually provide <10 grams of glutamine daily, thus supplements are required for a greater intake. Powdered glutamine supplements are preferred because they are well-absorbed and less expensive than the liquid form (30). Because this treatment shows promise it is important for clinicians to follow results of future studies on this therapy (30).

Nutrition Intervention in Advanced Lung Cancer

Advanced cancers include those that are not curable and that have metastasized (31). These cancers are usually associated with NIS that impair quality of life. Palliative care, which aims to relieve and reduce symptoms while sustaining well-being and improving quality of life (32), is often recommended over curative care in advanced cases. Palliative goals focus on maintaining adequate hydration and managing NIS. Many advanced stage survivors have cancer-induced cachexia, which results in systemic inflammation and associated muscle proteolysis and lipolysis (33). There is general agreement that adequate nutrition intake may not reverse the metabolic changes seen in cachexia, but it is reasonable to promote as high an intake as possible and comfortable for the patient because there is no research

that contraindicates this approach; it may slow the rate of weight loss and provide comfort to the patient and family. Chapter 12 provides a strong foundation for managing NIS in this population, and experienced RDs often can help the patient significantly improve intake. Provision of enteral nutrition support in this setting remains controversial. It may be possible to increase energy and nutrient intake over that consumed orally, but has not been shown to impact cancer survival (34). In addition, A.S.P.E.N. states that nutrition support is rarely indicated in palliative cases (33). Chapter 27, *Nutrition Management of Oncology Patients in Palliative and Hospice Settings*, provides guidelines for the use of nutritional support in advanced cancer patients. When contraindicated, it is still essential for the RD to provide nutrition intervention that will help the patient consume as much food and liquids as desired via the oral route.

Conclusion

Lung cancer is frequently diagnosed at late stages; those diagnosed commonly present with weight loss; obese lung cancer patients survive longer than those who are losing weight; and lung cancer treatments result in NIS that compromise intake. For these reasons lung cancer should trigger a positive nutrition risk screening. All lung cancer patients should receive nutrition intervention from an RD with the goal of reducing the severity of NIS, improving oral intake, and stabilizing weight.

References

1. Centers for Disease Control and Prevention. Lung Cancer Awareness. http://www.cdc.gov/cancer/dcpc/resources/features/lungcancer/ Last updated June 25, 2013. Accessed 8/31/2013.
2. Centers for Disease Control and Prevention. Ch 2. A Historical Review of Efforts to Reduce Smoking in the United States. In *Reducing Tobacco Use. A Report of the Surgeon General*. 2000. http://www.cdc.gov/tobacco/data_statistics/sgr/2000/complete_report/pdfs/chapter2.pdf Accessed 8/20/2013.
3. American Cancer Society. Tobacco-Related Cancers Fact Sheet. http://www.cancer.org/cancer/cancercauses/tobaccocancer/tobacco-related-cancer-fact-sheet. Last Reviewed 11/09/2012 Accessed 8/20/2012.
4. Cataldo JK, Dubey S, Prochaska JJ. Smoking cessation: an integral part of lung cancer treatment. *Oncology*. 2010;78(5-6):289-301.
5. Thun MJ, Hannan LM, Adams-Campbell LL, et al. Lung cancer occurrence in never-smokers: an analysis of 13 cohorts and 22 cancer registry studies. 2008; PLoS Med 5(9): e185. doi:10.1371/journal.pmed.0050185.
6. National Cancer Institute. Surveillance Epidemiology and End Results. SEER Stat Fact Sheets: Lung and Bronchus. http://seer.cancer.gov/statfacts/html/lungb.html. Posted to the SEER website 2013. Accessed 8/20/2013.
7. National Cancer Institute. What You Need To Know About Lung Cancer. http://www.cancer.gov/cancertopics/wyntk/lung/page1/AllPages. Posted 9/17/2012. Accessed 7/18/2013.
8. International Agency for Research on Cancer Cancer: Causes, Occurrence and Control. IARC: Lyon; 1990.
9. Peto R, Darby S, Deo H, Silcocks P, Whitley E, Doll R. Smoking, smoking cessation, and lung cancer in the UK since 1950: combination of national statistics with two case-control studies. *BMJ*. 2000;321(7257):323–329.
10. Kalemkerian GP, Akerley W, Bogner P, et al. Small cell lung cancer. Clinical practice guidelines in oncology. *J Natl Compr Canc Netw*. 2013;11(1): 78-98.
11. American Joint Committee on Cancer. *AJCC Cancer Staging Manual*. 6th ed. New York, NY: Springer; 2002.
12. Bruera E. (1997). ABC of palliative care. Anorexia, cachexia, and nutrition. *BMJ*. 1997;315(7117):1219–1222.

13. Jatoi A, Yingwei Q, Kendall G, et al. The cancer anorexia/weight loss syndrome: exploring associations with single nucleotide polymorphisms (SNPs) of inflammatory cytokines in patients with non-small cell lung cancer. *Support Care Cancer*. 2010;18(10):1299-1304.

14. Ross PJ, Ashley S, Norton A, et al. Do patients with weight loss have a worse outcome when undergoing chemotherapy for lung cancer? *Br J Cancer*. 2004;90:1905-1911.

15. Scott HR, McMillan DC, Brown DJ, Forrest LM, McArdle CS, Milroy R. A prospective study of the impact of weight loss and the systemic inflammatory response on quality of life in patients with inoperable on-small cell lung cancer. *Lung Cancer*. 2003;40(3):295-299.

16. Arrieta O, Ortega RMM, Villanueva-Rodriguez G, et al. Association of nutritional status and serum albumin levels with development of toxicity in patients with advanced non-small cell lung cancer treated with paclitaxel-cisplatin chemotherapy: a prospective study. *BMC Cancer*. 2010; 10: 50. doi: 10.1186/1471-2407-10-50.

17. Yang R, Cheung MC, Pedrosa FE, Byrne MM, Koniaris LG, Zimmers TA. Obesity and weight loss at presentation of lung cancer are associated with opposite effects on survival. *J Surg Res*. 2011;170(1):e75-e83.

18. Leij-Halfwerk S, Dagnelie PC, van den Berg JWO, Wattimena JDL, Hordijk-Luijk CH, Wilson JHP. Weight loss and elevated gluconeogenesis from alanine in lung cancer patients. *Am J Clin Nutr*. 2000;71(20):583-589.

19. Wüst RC, Degens H. Factors contributing to muscle wasting and dysfunction in COPD patients. *Int J Chron Obstruct Pulm Dis*. 2007; 2(3):289-300.

20. Schols AMWJ. Nutritional and metabolic modulation in chronic obstructive pulmonary disease management. *Eur Resp J*. 2003;22(46): 81s-86s.

21. Harada H, Yamashita Y, Misumi K, et al. Multidisciplinary team-based approach for comprehensive preoperative pulmonary rehabilitation including intensive nutritional support for lung cancer patients. PLoS One. 2013; 8(3): e59566.

22. Hennekens CH, Buring JE, Manson JE, et al. Lack of effect of long-term supplementation with beta carotene on the incidence of malignant neoplasms and cardiovascular disease. *N Eng J Med*. 1996;334:1145-1149. DOI: 10.1056/NEJM199605023341801.

23. Willett WC, Stampfer MJ. What vitamins should I be taking, doctor? *N Engl J Med*. 2001;345(25):1819-1824.

24. The Alpha-Tocopherol, Beta Carotene Cancer Prevention (ATBC) Study Group. The effect of vitamin E and beta carotene on the incidence of lung cancer and other cancers in male smokers. *N Engl J Med*. 1994;330:1029-1035. DOI: 10.1056/NEJM199404143301501.

25. World Cancer Research Fund/American Institute for Cancer Research. Food, Nutrition, Physical Activity, and the Prevention of Cancer: a Global Perspective. Washington DC: AICR (2007).

26. Omenn GS, Goodman GE, Thornquist MD, et al. Effects of a combination of beta carotene and vitamin A on lung cancer and cardiovascular disease. *N Engl J Med*. 1996;334(18):1150-1155.

27. Fritz H, Kennedy D, Fergusson D. Selenium and lung cancer: a systematic review and meta analysis. PLoS ONE 6(11): e26259. doi:10.1371/journal. pone.0026259

28. Butt Z, Rao AV, Lai JS, Abernethy AP, Rosenbloom SK, Cella D. Age-associated differences in fatigue among patients with cancer. *J Pain Symptom Manage*. 2010;40(2):217-223.

29. Hurria A, Togawa K, Mohile SG. Predicting chemotherapy toxicity in older adults with cancer; a prospective multicenter study. *J Clin Oncol*. 2011;29(25):3457-3465.

30. Hall D, Gilmore A, Carson JA. Can oral glutamine supplementation reduce peripheral neuropathy in chemotherapy patients? *Oncology Nutrition Connection*. 2012;20(4):3-9.

31. American Cancer Society. What is advanced cancer? http://www.cancer. org/treatment/understandingyourdiagnosis/advancedcancer/advanced-cancer-what-is. Reviewed 7/17/2012. Accessed 7/20/2013.

32. Kirkova J, Walsh D, Rybicki L, et al. Symptom severity and distress in advanced cancer. *Palliat Med*. 2010;24(3):330-339.

33. Gullett NP, Mazurak V, Hebbar G, Ziegler TR. Nutritional interventions for cancer-induced cachexia. *Curr Prob Cancer*. 2011;35(2):58-90.

34. Kotler D. Cachexia. *Ann Intern Med*. 2000;133(8):622-634.

Medical Nutrition Therapy for Ovarian Cancer

Tricia Cox, RD, CSO, LD, CNSC

Introduction

The ovaries are two almond shaped reproductive organs located on each side of the pelvis. They secrete the female hormones estrogen and progesterone, and in women of reproductive age release monthly eggs (1-3). After menopause ovaries stop releasing eggs and secrete smaller volumes of hormones. Ovarian cancer is the fifth leading cause of cancer death among women and the most lethal of gynecological cancers (1-3).

There are three main types of cells in the ovaries. Epithelial cells cover the ovary; germ cells are located inside the ovary and develop into eggs released into the fallopian tubes during reproductive years; and stromal cells produce female hormones. Tumors can originate from any of these cells, but occur most commonly in epithelial cells. Recent findings suggest that a range of molecularly distinct cancers also may grow in ovaries including a high-grade serous ovarian cancer originating in the distal fallopian tube (1).

Symptoms of early stage (I/II) ovarian cancer are vague and often ignored; approximately 70% of cases are diagnosed at an advanced stage. Symptoms of advanced ovarian cancer include stomach and pelvic pain or pressure, early satiety, involuntary weight loss and abdominal swelling.

Prevalence and Prognosis

In 2013, the National Cancer Institute predicted that 22,240 women will be diagnosed with ovarian cancer and 14,230 will die from this disease (4). Lifetime risk of ovarian cancer is about 1 in 72. Prognosis has not significantly improved since platinum based chemotherapies were introduced 30 years ago (5). Five-year survival rate is approximately 94% for stage IA ovarian cancer; 66% for Stage II cancer, 34% for stage II, and 18% for stage IV. Successful surgery is important; complete resection is associated with a five-year greater survival when compared with post-operative presence of residual tumor (6).

Risk factors for ovarian cancer include:
- Age: Ovarian cancer risk increases with age (1). Half of all ovarian cancers are diagnosed in women over the age of 63.
- Height and Body Mass Index (BMI): A higher height and a BMI ≥30 increases ovarian cancer risk (7).
- Reproductive history: Giving birth, taking oral contraceptives for greater than five years, breastfeeding and tubal ligation reduce ovarian cancer risk (8).

Figure 1: The Ovaries

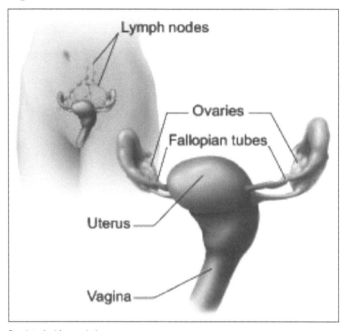

Reprinted with permission
The website of the National Cancer Institute (http://www.cancer.gov)

- Family history: From 5-15% of ovarian cancers are genetically determined (1,9-10).
- Genetic Mutations: BRCA1, BRCA2, and RAD51C mutations increase the risk of high-grade serous ovarian cancers. Prophylactic bilateral salpingo-oophorectomy may reduce risk in carriers of these mutations by 80% (5,10).

Nutrition and Ovarian Cancer Prevention

Data from the Nurses Health Study found no clear associations between methionine, vitamin B6, or multivitamin use and ovarian cancer risk overall or by FRalpha tumor status (11). Data also found that increased hip circumference was associated with a lower ovarian cancer risk in postmenopausal women (7). The lack of association found between BMI and ovarian cancer risk in this study contradicts other research (12). Neither individual food groups nor dietary quality has been associated with ovarian cancer risk (13).

Diagnosis and Staging

The diagnostic workup for ovarian cancer includes a physical examination, pelvic exam (though not a pap smear), blood test for CA-125 (which is found on the surface of ovarian cancer cells), an ultrasound, laparotomy or laparoscopy, and biopsy (1). CT scans, barium enema x-ray, and colonoscopy are performed to check for metastatic disease. Ovarian cancer can be staged according to the American Joint Committee on Cancer (AJCC) TNM System, which describes the extent of the primary Tumor (T), the absence or presence of metastasis to nearby lymph Nodes (N), and the absence or presence of distant Metastasis (M) (14). The National Cancer Institute (NCI) also has published a staging system and is provided below (3).

Table 1: NCI Staging System for Ovarian Cancer

Stage	Criteria
I	Cancer cells are found in one or both ovaries
II	Cancer cells have spread from either or both ovaries to other tissues in the pelvis.
III	Cancer cells have spread outside the pelvis or to regional lymph nodes
IV	Cancer cells have spread to organs such as the liver or lungs

Ovarian Cancer Treatment

Depending upon the stage when diagnosed, ovarian cancer is primarily treated with surgery and chemotherapy; radiation therapy also may be used. Targeted therapies in ovarian cancer are rarely incorporated in standard therapy regimens.

Surgery

Surgical resection of the primary tumor and microscopically visible masses is recommended in all cases. Complete resection significantly improves survival (6), though it may be difficult to achieve in advanced cases. Intestinal surgery may be needed in 30%-50% of advanced cases (6). Surgery to the abdominal region may require postoperative medical nutrition therapy, depending on resulting anatomy and gastrointestinal function, and is addressed in the section on nutrition assessment.

Chemotherapy

Platinum-based chemotherapy, usually provided in three to six treatment cycles, is considered the standard of care following surgery for ovarian cancer. Platinum-based regimens may be combined with Carboplatin and Paclitaxel. In advanced cases, Taxane chemotherapy is combined with platinum-based treatment (6). Chemotherapy may be infused intravenously or through the abdominal cavity, referred to as intraperitoneal chemotherapy. Radiation therapy is not considered standard treatment for ovarian cancer, but when provided, radiation beams may be directed at the entire pelvic region, resulting in significant nutrition impact. Table 2 summarizes nutrition impact symptoms (NIS) of common treatments used for ovarian cancer.

Intraperitoneal (IP) chemotherapy has been associated with longer survival (1-3), but also more severe gastrointestinal side effects and NIS.

Table 2: Common Nutrition Impact Symptoms of Select Ovarian Cancer Therapies* (15)

Treatments	Nausea & Vomiting	Anorexia	Mucositis & Stomatitis	Diarrhea	Myelo-suppression
Chemotherapy					
Altretamine (Hexalen®)	3	3		3	3
Capecitabine (Xeloda®)	3			3	
Carpoplatin (Paraplatin®)	3				3
Cisplatin (Platinol®)	3				3
Cyclophosphamide (Cytoxan®)	3				3
Etoposide (VP-16)	3	3	3	3	3
Gemcitabine (Gemzar®)	3				3
Ifosfamide (Ifex®)	3	3			3
Irinotecan (CPT-11, Camptosar®)	3	3	3	3	3
Doxorubicin liposomal (Doxil®)	3		3	3	3
Melphalan	3		3	3	3
Paclitaxel (Taxol®)			3	3	3
Pemetrexed (Alimta®)	3			3	3
Topotecan	3	3	3	3	3
Vinorelbine (Navelbine®)	3	3	3		3
Radiation	Diarrhea and Fatigue				

• Other nutrition impact symptoms also may occur, though not as commonly. In addition, common symptoms such as nausea may lead to a reduced intake even when anorexia is not a primary side effect of the chemotherapy agent.

A retrospective study examining associations between BMI and survival in advanced ovarian cancer found that loss of body weight during chemotherapy was a significant indicator for poor overall survival (16). Cancer-related weight loss results in a loss of skeletal muscle as well as fat stores (17). In a group of ovarian cancer patients, consuming amino acids (40 grams essential and nonessential amino acids dissolved in a flavored distilled water beverage) showed an anabolic effect (17).

McGough et al (18) found that more than 70% of patients who receive pelvic radiation develop acute gastrointestinal symptoms, particularly severe diarrhea. One randomized controlled trial found that one to two teaspoons of psyillium fiber in the form of Metamucil taken daily during treatment was effective in reducing incidence and severity of diarrhea (19). A double-blind and placebo-controlled trial assessed the affects of VSL#3, a probiotic containing four strains of lactobacillus, three strains of Bifidobacterium and one strain of streptococcus thermophilus versus a placebo in patients undergoing pelvic radiation (20). In this study 32% of the intervention group developed radiation enteritis versus 52% of the control group; the control group had three times more bowel movements per day as compared with the intervention group. Other reviews have not found that elemental diets, probiotic supplementation or low fat diets help prevent or treat radiation-induced diarrhea. No trials have evaluated the effects of soluble fiber on radiation-induced diarrhea, but there is biologic plausibility for this intervention.

Nutrition Screening and Assessment of Patients with Ovarian Cancer

The close proximity of the ovaries to gastrointestinal and urinary systems can lead to many nutrition-related problems as ovarian cancer spreads. Because of this, as well as the frequency of malnutrition and gastrointestinal symptoms seen in this population, the diagnosis of ovarian cancer alone should trigger a positive nutrition risk screening. Malnutrition is seen in up to 80% of patients with gastrointestinal cancers (21), including metastatic ovarian cancer. The aggressiveness of ovarian cancer treatment is associated with significant morbidity that further contributes to the risk of malnutrition. Laky et al. utilized the subjective global assessment (SGA) and patient generated-subjective global assessment (PG-SGA) to assess the nutritional status of 194 patients with gynecological cancer and found that 24% were classified as malnourished; 67% of those patients had ovarian cancer (22). In another study, although the PG-SGA is considered most appropriate for identifying malnutrition, the prognostic nutritional index (PNI) was more likely to identify malnutrition in gynecologic cancers (23).

Weight loss is diagnostic for malnutrition, but ascites, which skews weight, is a common finding in patients with ovarian cancer. Nutrition assessment of weight status should consider this phenomena; conducting a nutrition-focused physical assessment will help clarify the fluid status.

Surgery is the most important treatment for ovarian cancer. Poor nutritional status has been associated with increased postoperative morbidity and mortality in surgical patients (24). Albumin and prealbumin are two markers that have been linked with outcomes in this population; among 235 patients undergoing surgery for ovarian cancer, low serum albumin was associated with poor survival. Higher serum albumin (>10G/L) increased survival from a median of 4.8 months to a median of 43.2 months, independent of age and stage of disease (25). Of 108 patients who underwent surgery for ovarian cancer, lower prealbumin levels increased the risk of postoperative complications (26). Eighty-eight patients with prealbumin levels <18mg/dL were more likely to experience blood loss, unplanned ICU visits, hospital readmission, gastrointestinal injury and greater (> 14 days) length of stay than those with higher prealbumin levels. Twenty-four patients with prealbumin levels <10mg/dL were at even greater risk of these complications, and post-operative mortality was seen only in this group of 24. Whether these complications could be reduced in this population by pre-operative or early post-operative nutrition intervention or nutrition support has not been explored.

According to American Society for Parenteral and Enteral Nutrition guidelines for adults undergoing anticancer treatment, preoperative nutrition support (e.g., enteral (EN) or parenteral (PN) support) is recommended for patients who are already malnourished (27). In cases of moderate to severe malnutrition, nutrition support may be beneficial when provided seven to fourteen days prior to surgery (27). However, other studies have seen benefit in as little as one to three days prior to surgery (28).

Early postoperative oral intake is recognized as safe and decreases length of hospital stay (29). Gastric emptying begins as soon as two days postoperatively and colonic function generally begins within two to three days postoperatively. Providing a clear liquid diet as early as postoperative day one, and advancing to a regular diet after a patient has tolerated 500mLs of liquids, has been found beneficial in these patients (30). Gerardi et al (31) developed a clinical pathway that included rapid diet advancement, early discontinuance of nasogastric suction, criteria-based utilization of PN, selective laboratory testing, and deferring initiation of chemotherapy until after discharge in (primarily) women with advanced stage disease. Results found that early advancement of diet is feasible, safe, and associated with a significant reduction in length of hospital stay and hospital-related costs.

Unless otherwise indicated, the energy intake goal for malnourished ovarian cancer patients is estimated at 30-35 kcal/kg/day, reflecting the need for nutrition repletion in a predominantly malnourished population (32). Energy needs may be closer to 25-30 kcal/kg, among well-nourished ovarian cancer patients diagnosed at an early stage (32). Protein needs of cancer patients with normal renal function range from 1.0-1.5 g/kg, based on stress level (33). In cases of cancer cachexia, protein needs may increase to 1.5-2.5 g/kg, also depending on renal function and stress level (33). Micronutrient needs are consistent with Dietary Reference Intakes for the respective age group (34-36) or individualized as indicated by nutrition assessment.

Meal plans that emphasize small frequent meals; high energy, high protein foods; and texture modifications when mucositis is problematic are important for the goals of preserving weight and lean body mass in those experiencing nutrition impact symptoms. For more information on managing nutrition impact symptoms see chapter 12.

Medical Nutrition Therapy in Advanced Disease

Malignant bowel obstruction (MBO) is frequently seen in advanced cancer, may involve the small and/or large intestine, and can be related to the location of the tumor, radiation enteritis, or disease progression. From 20%-50% of patients with ovarian cancer may experience MBO (37). In some cases MBO may resolve spontaneously, but it is likely to recur. Conservative management measures include nasogastric (NG) suction, bowel rest, medication to control symptoms, and intravascular fluids (38). If conservative measures are ineffective, surgery is considered but may not be a viable option. At this point, when life expectancy may be less than four months and as short as four weeks (37,39), care transitions to palliative goals, i.e. non-surgical symptom management to improve quality of life. Carcinomatosis (metastatic disease throughout the abdominal region) can occur, and also may result in bowel obstruction. It can be temporarily treated with NG tube placement for suction, but is not comfortable for extended use, and therefore is usually replaced with a gastrostomy tube for drainage and decompression (37-41).

Few studies have examined potential benefits of PN on survival of patients with MBO. One study reported a mean survival rate of four to six months when PN was given. The complication rate was 13%. Results concluded that approximately 30% of patients with MBO who receive PN survive longer than three months; authors also stated that PN is not recommended in inoperable cases (37).

Energy needs also change in advanced cases. One study found that the Harris-Benedict equation is unreliable for determining needs in these patients as compared to indirect calorimetry (42). However, when goals transition to quality of life and comfort, it is not necessary to provide 100% of estimated energy needs, and diet as tolerated is provided. Certainly this is an area where clinical judgment and close patient monitoring are essential.

Research on the use of PN in advanced disease is conflicting. In one study terminally ill patients who received PN survived only four weeks longer than patients who did not receive PN (43). Survival was even shorter for patients who received chemotherapy as well as PN

(44). However, a study by Madhok et al. (45) found that patients who had an acceptable performance status and were able to provide self-care at home benefited from home PN. Performance status may be key when determining the appropriateness of home PN. In a small study, Soo and Gramlich (46) found that a higher performance status (i.e., Karnofsky score >50) was associated with a longer survival (i.e., median survival of six months) as compared with a Karnofsky score < 50 (i.e., median survival of three months). Larger studies are needed to confirm these findings. Poor prognosis has led researchers to call for inclusion of quality of life and symptom benefit to the list of primary endpoints in clinical trials investigating ovarian cancer treatment (5).

Studies examining use of PN in cases of advanced ovarian cancer have not yet provided clear and equivocal findings. Ripamonti (39) suggests that patients who may die of starvation rather than metastatic disease are appropriate for PN, but others are not convinced, given the potential discomfort and risks associated with PN. Other issues to consider are cost, quality of life, patient and family goals, and clinical judgment that includes feedback from the multidisciplinary team. Table 3 outlines medical nutrition therapy for phases of the ovarian cancer continuum.

Survivorship

Lifestyle changes after treatment for ovarian cancer can vary depending on the treatment, stage of disease, and future medical plans. For patients in remission, evidence-based cancer-prevention recommendations are appropriate (see Chapter 2), but may need to be modified per post-operative gastrointestinal anatomy and function. Symptom and function-based medical nutrition therapy should be provided when indicated. RDs are an essential resource for helping these patients decipher the many treatment and curative claims publicized. Providing evidence-based counseling on diets and dietary supplements proposed for cancer treatment can allay fears and help patients make confident decisions regarding a cancer-preventive lifestyle (see Chapter 8). Many long-term survivors who have undergone treatment for ovarian cancer will experience menopause and be at risk for developing heart disease and osteoporosis (47). It is important for RDs to emphasize medical nutrition therapy for preventing these diseases within a nutrition survivorship plan.

Conclusion

Ovarian cancer survivors may transition through many disease phases that pose unique and sometimes difficult nutrition challenges. Nutrition intervention provided by credentialed professionals (e.g., RDs and CSOs) will ensure that ovarian cancer patients receive the quality of nutrition care they deserve.

Table 3: Medical Nutrition Therapy for Ovarian Cancer

Continuum Phase or Complication	Potential Nutrition Impact	Medical Nutrition Therapy
Pre-Treatment	Early satiety, stomach pain, involuntary weight loss, abdominal swelling	Provide 5-6 small meals/day modified per nutrition impact symptoms (see chapter 12).
Chemotherapy	Anorexia, nausea, vomiting, constipation, diarrhea, abdominal pain, dysgeusia, stomatitis, esophagitis	After establishing nutrition needs and goals via nutrition assessment (32-33 and chapter 3), provide oral diet with 5-6 small meals/day. Provide energy & protein dense foods, utilize medical nutrition beverages and consider food sources of soluble fiber, probiotics or Metamucil® as indicated. Manage nutrition impact symptoms as suggested in chapter 12. Confirm use of supportive therapies such as anti-emetics as prescribed. Monitor efficacy of nutrition plan and modify as indicated.
Radiation Therapy	Diarrhea, fatigue	After establishing nutrition needs and goals via nutrition assessment (32-33 and chapter 3), provide oral diet with 5-6 small meals/day. Provide energy & protein dense foods, utilize medical nutrition beverages and consider food sources of soluble fiber, probiotics or Metamucil® as indicated. For diarrhea, confirm appropriate interventions per chapter 12 including use of soluble fibers. Consult with medical team on other interventions, include use of probiotics such as lactobacillus, bifidobacterium and streptococcus thermophiles, and use of 1-2 teaspoons of psyllium fiber (e.g. Metamucil ®) daily (19-20). Monitor efficacy of nutrition plan and modify as indicated.
Surgery	Abnormal bowel function (e.g. diarrhea), post-op nausea, anorexia, involuntary weight loss	Advance oral diet as tolerated; advise team on benefits of early postoperative feeding if appropriate (29-31); confirm adequate intake of nutrients (e.g., protein) needed for wound healing; manage nutrition impact symptoms per chapter 12.
Potential Complication: Bowel Obstruction	Nausea, vomiting including fecaloid vomiting, pain, absence of stools or gas, liquid stools	Complete obstruction: Bowel rest; PN as indicated (37-41 and chapter 13) Partial obstruction: low fiber diet; limit fatty/greasy foods and gas-forming foods; limit lactose if lactose intolerant; consume smaller, more frequent meals
Potential Complication: Malnutrition	Inadequate intake, possibly due to oral diet intolerance	As tolerated, maximize oral nutrition via high energy and protein foods (32-33). Consider 5-6 small meals and medical nutrition beverages. Consider need for nutrition support (27-28 and chapter 13)
Palliative and Hospice Care	Anorexia, nausea, vomiting, mucositis, stomatitis, diarrhea	Diet and fluids as tolerated and desired

References

1. American Cancer Society. Ovarian Cancer. http://www.cancer.org/acs/groups/cid/documents/webcontent/003130-pdf.pdf Last revised 03/21/2013. Accessed 05/01/2013.
2. Ovarian Cancer National Alliance. Statistics. http://www.ovariancancer.org/about-ovarian-cancer/statistics/
3. National Cancer Institute. What you need to know about ovarian cancer ™. http://www.cancer.gov/cancertopics/wyntk/ovary/page1/AllPages Posted 7/17/2006. Accessed 7/20/2013.
4. Howlader N, Noone AM, Krapcho M, et al. *SEER Cancer Statistics Review, 1975-2010*, National Cancer Institute. Bethesda, MD, http://seer.cancer.gov/csr/1975_2010/, based on November 2012 SEER data submission, posted to the SEER web site, 2013. http://seer.cancer.gov/statfacts/html/ovary.html
5. Vaughan S, Coward JI, Bast RC, Berchuck A, Berek JS, Brenton JC. Rethinking ovarian cancer: recommendations for improving outcomes. *Nat Rev Cancer*. 2011;11(10):719-725.
6. Burges A and Schmalfeldt B. Ovarian cancer: diagnosis and treatment. *Dtsch Arztebl Int*. 2011;108(38):635-641.
7. Collaborative Group on Epidemiological Studies of Ovarian Cancer (2012) Ovarian Cancer and Body Size: Individual Participant Meta-Analysis Including 25,157 Women with Ovarian Cancer from 47 Epidemiological Studies. *PLoS Med* 9(4): e1001200. doi:10.1371/journal.pmed.1001200
8. Jelovac D, Armstrong DK. Recent progress in the diagnosis and treatment of ovarian cancer. *CA: Cancer J Clin*. 2011;61(3):183-203.
9. Russo A, Calò V, Bruno L, Rizzo S, Bazan V, Di Fede G. Hereditary ovarian cancer. *Critical Reviews in Oncology/Hematology*. 2009;69(1):28-44.
10. South SA, Vance H, Farrell C, et al. Consideration of hereditary nonpolyposis colorectal cancer in BRCA mutation-negative familial ovarian cancers. *Cancer*. 2009;115(2):324-333.
11. Kotsopoulos J, Hecht JL, Marotti JD, Kelemen LE, Tworoger SS. Relationship between dietary and supplemental intake of folate, methionine, vitamin B6 and folate receptor α expression in ovarian tumors. *Int J Cancer*. 2010:126: 2191–2198. doi. 10.1002/ijc.24723
12. Kotsopoulos J, Baer H, Tworoger S. Anthropometric measures and risk of epithelial ovarian cancer: results from the Nurses' Health Study. *Obesity*. 2010:18(8):1625-1631.
13. Chandran U, Bandera E, Williams-King M, Paddock LE, Rodriguez-Rodriguez L, Lu S-E, et al. Healthy eating index and ovarian cancer risk. *Cancer Causes and Control*. 2011:22(4):563-571.
14. American Joint Committee on Cancer. Staging Resources. http://www.cancerstaging.org/staging/. Revised April 15, 2013.
15. Bragalone DL. *Drug Information Handbook for Oncology*. Ohio: Lexi-Comp, Inc., 2012.
16. Hess LM, Barakat R, Tian C, Ozols RF, Alberts DS. Weight change during chemotherapy as a potential prognostic factor for stage III epithelial ovarian carcinoma: a gynecologic oncology group study. *Gynecol Oncol*. 2007;107(2):260-265.

17. Dillon EL, Volpi E, Wolfe RR, et al. Amino acid metabolism and inflammatory burden in ovarian cancer patients undergoing intense oncological therapy. *Clin Nutr.* 2007;26(6):736-743.

18. McGough C, Baldwin C, Frost G, Andryev HJN. Role of nutritional intervention in patients treated with radiotherapy for pelvic malignancy. *Br J Cancer.* 2004;90(12): 2278-2287.

19. Murphy J, Stacey D, Crook J, Thompson B, Panetta D. Testing control of radiation-induced diarrhea with a psyllium bulking agent: A pilot study. *Canadian Oncology Nursing Journal.* 2000;(10)3:96-100.

20. Delia P, Sansotta G, Donato V, Frosina P, Messina G, De Renzis C, et al. Use of probiotics for prevention of radiation-induced diarrhea. *World J Gastroenterol.* 2007;13(6); 912-915.

21. Laky B, Janda M, Bauer J, Vavra C, Cleghorn G, Obermair A. Malnutrition among gynaecological cancer patients. *Eur J Clin Nutr.* 2007;61(5): 642-646.

22. Laky B, Janda M, Cleghorn G, Obermair A. Comparison of different nutritional assessments and body-composition measurements in detecting malnutrition among gynecologic cancer patients. *Am J Clin Nutr.* 2008;87(6):1678-1685.

23. Santoso JT, Cannada T, O'Farrel B, Alladi K, Coleman RL. Subjective versus objective nutritional assessment study in women with gynaecological cancer. *Int J Gynecol Cancer.* 2004;14(2):220-223.

24. Kathiresan AS, Brookfield KF, Schuman SI, Lucci JA 3rd. Malnutrition as a predictor of poor postoperative outcomes in gynecologic cancer patients. *Arch Gynecol Obstet.* 2011;284(2):445-451.

25. Asher V, Lee J, Bali A. Preoperative serum albumin is an independent prognostic predictor of survival in ovarian cancer. *Med Oncol.* 2012;29(3):2005-2009.

26. Geisler JP, Linnemeier GC, Thomas AJ, Manahan KJ. Nutritional assessment using prealbumin as an objective criterion to determine whom should not undergo primary radical cytoreductive surgery for ovarian cancer. *Gynecol Oncol.* 2007;106(1):128-131.

27. David AA, Huhmann MB. A.S.P.E.N. clinical guidelines: nutrition support therapy during adult anticancer treatment and in hematopoietic cell transplantation. *J Parent Enteral Nutr.* 2009;33(5):472-500.

28. Heyland DK, Cook DJ, Guyatt GH. Does the formulation of enteral feeding products influence infectious morbidity and mortality rates in the critically ill patients? A critical review of the evidence. *Crit Care Med.* 1994;22(7):1192-1202.

29. Keely DG, Stanhope CR. Postoperative enteral feeding: myth or fact? *Gynecol Oncol.*1997;67(3):235-240.

30. Schilder JM, Hurteau JA, Look KY, et al. A prospective controlled trial of early postoperative oral intake following major abdominal gynecologic surgery. *Gynecol Oncol.* 1997;67(3):235-240.

31. Gerardi MA, Santillan A, Meisner B, Zahurak ML, Diaz Montes TP, Gluntoll RL 2nd, et al. A clinical pathway for patients undergoing primary cytoreductive surgery with rectosigmoid colectomy for advanced ovarian and primary peritoneal cancers. *Gynecol Oncol.* 2008;108(2): 282-6.

32. Hurst JD and Gallagher AL. Energy, macronutrient, micronutrient, and fluid requirements In *The Clinical Guide to Oncology Nutrition, 2nd edition.* Editors: Elliott L, Molseed LL, McCallum PD. American Dietetic Association, p54-71.

33. Russell M, Malone AM. Nutrient Requirements in Charney P, Malone AM, ed. *ADA Pocket Guide to Nutrition Assessment,* Second Edition. Chicago IL: American Dietetic Association Publications; 2009: 167-191.

34. Dietary Reference Intakes for Vitamin A, Vitamin K, Arsenic, Boron, Chromium, Copper, Iodine, Iron, Manganese, Molybdenum, Nickel, Silicon, Vanadium and Zinc. Institute of Medicine of the National Academies, The National Academies Press, Washington DC 2001. Available at www.nap.edu Accessed July 2013.

35. Dietary Reference Intakes for Thiamin, Riboflavin, Niacin, Vitamin B6, Folate, Vitamin B12, Pantothenic acid, Biotin and Choline. Institute of Medicine of the National Academies, The National Academies Press, Washington DC 1998. Available at www.nap.edu Accessed July 2013.

36. Dietary Reference Intakes for Calcium and Vitamin D. Institute of Medicine of the National Academies, The National Academies Press, Washington DC 2011. Available at www.nap.edu Accessed July 2013.

37. Tuca A, Guell E, Martiniz-Losada E, Codorniu. Malignant bowel obstruction in advanced cancer patients: epidemiology, management, and factors influencing spontaneous resolution. *Cancer Manag Res.* 2012;4:159-169.

38. Tsahalina E, Woolas RP, Carter PG, Chan R, Gore ME, Blake PM, et al. Gastrostomy tubes in patients with recurrent gynaecological cancer and intestinal obstruction. *BJOG: Intl J Obstetr Gynaecol.* 1999;106(9):964-968.

39. Ripamonti C, Bruera E. Palliative management of malignant bowel obstruction. *Intl J Gynecol Cancer.* 2002;12(2):135-143.

40. Pothuri B, Meyer L, Gerardi M, Barakat RR, Chi DS. Reoperation for palliation of recurrent malignant bowel obstruction in ovarian carcinoma. *Gynecol Oncol.* 2004;95(1):193-195.

41. Pothuri B, Montenarano M, Gerardi M, Shike M, Ben-Porat L, Sabbatini P, et al. Percutaneous endoscopic gastrostomy tube placement in patients with malignant bowel obstruction due to ovarian carcinoma. *Gynecol Oncol.* 2005;96(2):330-334.

42. Dickerson RN, White KG, Curcillo PG 2nd, King SA, Mullen JL. Resting energy expenditure of patients with gynecologic malignancies. *J Am Coll Nutr.* 1995;14(5):448-454.

43. Brard L, Weitzen S, Strubel-Lagan SL, Swarmy N, Gordinier ME, Moore RG, et al. The effect of total parenteral nutrition on the survival of terminally ill ovarian cancer patients. *Gynecol Oncol.* 2006;103(1):176-80.

44. Abu-Rustum NR, Barakat RR, Venkatraman E, Spriggs D. Chemotherapy and total parenteral nutrition for advanced ovarian cancer with bowel obstruction. *Gynecol Oncol.* 1997;64(3):493-495.

45. Madhok BM, Yeluri S, Haigh K, Burton A, Broadhead T, Jayne DG. Parenteral nutrition for patients with advanced ovarian malignancy. *J Hum Nutr Diet.* 2011;24(2):187-91.

46. Soo I and Gramlich L. Use of parenteral nutrition in patients with advanced cancer. *Appl Physiol Nutr Metab.* 2008;33(1):102-106.

47. Schulz E, Arfai K, Liu X, Sayre J, Gilsanz V. Aortic calcification and the risk of osteoporosis and fractures. *J Clin Endocrinol Metab.* 2004:89(9):4246-4253.

Medical Nutrition Therapy for Pancreatic and Bile Duct Cancer

Maria Q. B. Petzel, RD, CSO, LD, CNSC

Overview

Due to the anatomical location of the cancer and its potential effects on exocrine, endocrine, and biliary function, patients with pancreatic and bile duct cancers are at an especially high risk for nutrition problems (1). Malnutrition is more common in patients with pancreatic and biliary cancers than in many other types of cancer (2).

The pancreas is located in the abdomen behind the stomach (see Figure 1). It is comprised of the head, body, and tail, and functions as part of both the endocrine and exocrine systems. Endocrine cells of the pancreas produce hormones such as insulin and glucagon, which are released directly into the blood and help regulate blood glucose. Exocrine cells produce pancreatic secretions, which contain bicarbonate and digestive enzymes (i.e., lipase, amylase and protease) that help neutralize stomach acid and digest fats, carbohydrates and proteins in foods. Pancreatic secretions are released into side ducts, which merge to form the main pancreatic duct. Bile, which promotes digestion and absorption of dietary fat, passes from the liver and gallbladder to the small intestine via the common bile duct. The common bile duct merges with the main pancreatic duct, emptying secretions into the small intestine (duodenum) at the ampulla of Vater. The superior mesenteric artery and superior mesenteric vein cross behind the pancreas; tumor involvement with these vessels may determine if the tumor is resectable or not (3-7).

Pancreatic tumors can form from either exocrine or endocrine cells. Exocrine tumors are most common, representing about 95% of pancreatic tumors with 90% being ductal cell carcinoma (adenocarcinoma). Less common malignant exocrine tumors include acinar cell carcinoma, adenosquamous carcinoma, squamous cell carcinoma and giant cell carcinomas. There is no tumor specific marker that exists specifically for pancreatic exocrine tumors, but carbohydrate antigen 19-9 (CA 19-9) is elevated in most patients with pancreatic cancer. CA 19-9 may be followed during or after treatment as a potential indicator of tumor response (3,5).

Pancreatic endocrine tumors are rare and make up 3%-5% of all pancreatic cancers diagnosed in the United States (U.S.); there are about 1000 cases per year (3,5,8). All endocrine tumors may be grouped together and called pancreatic neuroendocrine tumors or islet cell tumors. Pancreatic neuroendocrine tumors include: carcinoid tumors, insulinomas, glucagonomas, gastrinomas, somatostatinomas, VIPomas and PPomas (5).

Figure 1: Normal Anatomy

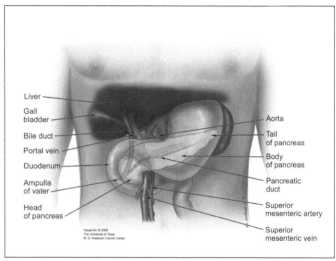

Reprinted with permission from the University of Texas M.D. Anderson Cancer Center

Other rare forms of periampullary cancer can arise in the region of the pancreas. These include ampullary cancer and distal bile duct cancer. Because of their anatomical location, many of the side effects and surgeries described in this chapter are also relevant to these types of cancer (4-5).

Incidence and Survival

In the U.S. in 2013, an estimated 45,220 people (22,740 men and 22,480 women) will likely be diagnosed with pancreatic cancer and about 38,460 people (19,480 men and 18,980 women) will die of this disease. The lifetime risk of developing pancreatic cancer is about 1 in 78 (3,5-6). It is the fourth leading cause of cancer death in this country. The overall survival rate for exocrine pancreatic cancer is 4% (5-6). However in 5%-10% of cases, the disease is caught early enough that complete surgical resection is achieved; in this group five-year survival is significantly better at 18%-24% (5-6). In patients with advanced pancreatic cancers, overall survival rate is less than 1% at 5 years, and most patients die within 1 year of diagnosis (5-6). Long-term success rates for pancreatic neuroendocrine tumors are often much better; these tumors are more likely to be cured with surgery (3). The five-year survival rate of resected localized endocrine tumor is about 55%, and is 15% in non-resectable tumors. Overall, five-year survival rate is 42% for all pancreatic neuroendocrine tumors (3,5-6).

Roughly 2,000 to 3,000 people in the U.S. develop bile duct cancer each year. Survival largely depends on the location of the tumor. Rarely can proximal bile duct tumors be resected, but in those arising in the distal bile duct, it is estimated that there is a 25% five-year survival (4). In many patients, ampullary cancer cannot be distinguished from pancreatic cancer until after surgery. Survival rate for ampullary cancer is about 30% to 50% at five years. More advanced ampullary cancers are treated like pancreatic cancer (5).

Treatment modalities and responses vary greatly between pancreatic exocrine tumors and neuroendocrine tumors. Surgical techniques and types are determined by anatomical location of the cancer rather than pathologic type. Because of the rarity of neuroendocrine tumors, the remainder of this chapter will focus on pancreatic exocrine tumors. However, clinicians should be aware that, in general, surgical considerations and side effects can be similarly managed. For more information regarding neuroendocrine tumors of the pancreas please refer to the resources listed in Box 1.

Box 1: Neuroendocrine Tumor Resources

NCI Pancreatic Neuroendocrine Tumors (Islet Cell Tumors) Treatment (PDQ®)
www.cancer.gov/cancertopics/pdq/treatment/ isletcell/HealthProfessional

Caring For Carcinoid Foundation
www.caringforcarcinoid.org

Nutrition Risk Factors for Diagnosis

Pancreatic cancer risk is associated with obesity and abdominal obesity (9-10). Lack of physical activity is also thought to increase risk of pancreatic cancer. Diabetes is more common in patients with pancreatic cancer, though it is difficult to ascertain which condition occurred first (3). Some studies suggest diets high in fat or high in red or processed meat increase the risk of pancreatic cancer but the mass of evidence so far remains inconclusive (3,5,11).

Nutrition Symptoms Associated with Diagnosis

Location of the tumor, type of tumor, and stage of disease may affect symptoms that trigger a diagnostic workup for pancreatic cancer. At early stages of the disease, symptoms are rarely present, but as disease progresses patients may experience one or more of the symptoms presented in Table 1 (3-5,7,12).

Nutrition Needs

The caloric needs of patients with pancreatic and biliary cancers may vary depending on stage of disease or treatment. Sasaki et al. found in a small study that those patients who presented for surgery had normal metabolic needs (about 25 kcal/kg/day) preoperatively. Those patients who underwent pancreaticoduodenectomy then had elevated needs during postoperative recovery, requiring about 30 kcal/kg/day (or resting energy expenditure per Harris-Benedict equation x1.2-1.3 activity/stress factor) (13). Conversely, studies have

Table 1: Symptoms Associated with Diagnosis (3-5,7,12)

Symptom	Etiology
Jaundice	Blocked bile duct
Abdominal Pain	Tumor involving or invading nerves Blocked digestive tract
Weight loss	Cancer cachexia Malabsorption
Poor appetite	Cancer cachexia
Malabsorption	Blockage of the pancreatic duct Reduced pancreatic enzyme production Blockage of the bile duct
Delayed gastric emptying Gastric outlet obstruction	Blockage or partial blockage of the duodenum
Diabetes	Reduced insulin production
Ascites	Cancer spread to peritoneum Portal vein hypertension Hepatic insufficiency Blockage of lymph system

found both newly diagnosed and those with cancer cachexia may be hypermetabolic (14-15). Because of the high incidence of advanced stage disease at presentation, one may infer that those patients found to be hypermetabolic at presentation may have had more advanced, unresectable tumors. Therefore needs may be estimated at 25 kcal/kg/day for resectable preoperative patients and higher for those with advanced disease. Ultimately nutrition needs should be estimated on an individual basis.

Patients with pancreatic exocrine insufficiency or who have had pancreatic surgery (see Table 2) are at risk for several micronutrient deficiencies. Medical nutrition therapy strategies for management of malabsorption will be discussed below. Additionally, patients may sometimes need special vitamin supplementation. To maximize absorption of dietary sources of vitamins, it is important for pancreatic enzyme replacement to be adequate. Patients who do not utilize adequate pancreatic enzyme replacement may become deficient in Vitamin B12 due to an inadequate amount of protease to cleave B12 from its carrier protein. It may be necessary to replace vitamin B12 in this group of patients using B12 via injection, nasal inhalation, or sublingual supplementation (16). Fat intolerance may require water miscible forms of fat soluble vitamins, including VITAMAX® and AquaDEKs® (17-18).

Pancreatic cancer and its treatments may require unique interventions for nutrition impact symptoms. Energy dense and high fat foods as well as medical nutrition beverages are often used to boost energy intake, but patients with pancreatic cancer may not tolerate high fat food or most supplemental drinks. Lower sugar "diabetic" supplement drinks may be better tolerated. General strategies for managing nutrition impact symptoms of cancer

Table 2: Common Surgeries for Pancreatic or Biliary Cancer and Associated Nutrition Impact Symptoms (3-4,6,21)

Surgical Procedure	Anatomic Changes	Nutrition Impact Symptoms				
		Exocrine Insufficiency (Figure 3)	Dumping Syndrome	Delayed Gastric Emptying	Lactose Intolerance	Diabetes/ Glucose Intolerance
Pancreaticoduodenectomy (PD); also known as Whipple Procedure (Figures 2 and 3)	Head of pancreas, duodenum, gallbladder, distal stomach, and part of common bile duct are removed.	3	3	3	3	3
Pylorus preserving pancreaticoduodenectomy (PPPD), also known as Pylorus preserving Whipple	Head of pancreas, duodenum, gallbladder, and part of common bile duct are removed; the stomach and pylorus are kept intact.	3		3	3	3
Total pancreatectomy (TP)	Removes the entire pancreas and sometimes the spleen. The additional structures removed with a PD are removed with a TP as well, and reconstruction is the same except there is no remnant pancreas.	v	3	3	3	v
Distal pancreatectomy	Removes only the tail of the pancreas or the tail and a portion of the body of the pancreas. The spleen may be removed as well.	3				3

3 *Indicates possible occurrence*
v *Indicates definite occurrence*

Table 3: Medical Nutrition Therapy Strategies for Impact Symptoms of Surgeries (3-4,6,21)

Nutrition Impact Symptoms	Exocrine Insufficiency (Figure 3)	Dumping Syndrome	Delayed Gastric Emptying	Lactose Intolerance	Diabetes/ Glucose Intolerance
Medical Nutrition Therapy Strategies	See recommendations for pancreatic enzyme replacement (table 4).	Anti-Dumping Diet (see Appendix 4)	Low-fiber, low-fat diet; 6-8 small meals/day; avoid eating 2-3 hours before bedtime; keep head of bed (HOB) elevated (22). Consider prokinetic meds (1,12,21,23)	Limit lactose containing foods and/or use lactase supplements with foods containing lactose.	Limit refined carbohydrate foods; consume meals and snacks at regular intervals; consume carbohydrate with protein and fat as tolerated (24-27). May need more aggressive insulin or medication management to allow more liberal diet due to side effects (27).

treatments are found in Chapter 12. Table 3 lists common recommendations for managing nutrition impact symptoms seen in the pancreatic cancer population; some special nutrition considerations are discussed later in this chapter and provide additional management tips.

Common Treatments and Impact on Nutrition Status

The most common treatments for pancreatic and bile duct cancers are surgery, chemotherapy, radiation therapy, and targeted therapy. In pancreatic and bile duct cancers that are resectable, the most common first line therapy is surgery (3-4,6,19). However, the use of preoperative (neoadjuvant) chemotherapy and/or chemoradiation for resectable and borderline resectable pancreatic tumors are being investigated, and are considered first line therapy at some institutions (19-20).

Surgery

There are three typical surgeries that may be performed to resect pancreatic and periampullary tumors: pancreaticoduodenectomy, total pancreatectomy and distal pancreatectomy. Figure 2 shows

Figure 2: Resected Anatomy

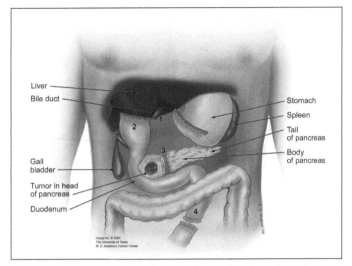

Reprinted with permission from the University of Texas M.D. Anderson Cancer Center

Figure 3: Reconstruction of Pancreaticoduodenectomy

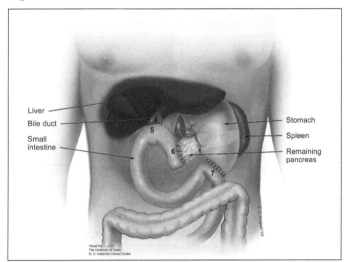

Reprinted with permission from the University of Texas M.D. Anderson Cancer Center

changes to the anatomy of the pancreas after the head of the pancreas is resected from the body of the pancreas. Figure 3 shows how organs are reconnected in pancreaticoduodenectomy. Pancreaticoduodenectomy and total pancreatectomy have greater nutritional implications than distal pancreatectomy. Regardless of the type of surgery, individuals who are malnourished at the time of surgery are at higher morbidity and mortality risk (21).

Surgical Reconstruction and Short-Term Postoperative Nutrition Considerations

For pancreaticoduodenectomy the GI tract is reconstructed by attaching a loop of the jejunum to the liver (hepaticojejunostomy), to the pancreatic remnant (pancreaticojejunostomy), and to the stomach (gastrojejunostomy) in PD or to the duodenum (duodenojejunostomy) in PPPD (3,4,6,21). Variations of surgery or reconstruction may include leaving the gallbladder, and connecting the jejunum to the gallbladder (choledocojejunostomy). Though it has been suggested that PPPD results in less dumping/diarrhea, better weight recovery, better quality of life and improved postoperative nutrition parameters, the literature does not support significant advantages of PPPD versus traditional PD (28-32). Studies also show no difference in delayed gastric emptying (DGE) with PPPD versus traditional PD (12,31,33-35). Some surgeons prefer to attach the pancreatic remnant to the stomach (pancreaticogastrostomy) instead of the small intestine to reduce the risk of developing a pancreatic fistula (6,20). Pancreaticogastrostomy does not appear to reduce incidence of pancreatic fistula and may lead to increased need for supplemental enzymes as exposure of pancreatic secretions directly to gastric acid will inactivate endogenous pancreatic enzymes (36-37).

In the short-term postoperative period after pancreaticoduodenectomy or total pancreatectomy, diet will often be started as clear liquids and transitioned to a soft, low-fiber, low-fat diet. The Anti-Dumping

Diet (Appendix 4) generally meets these requirements. The Anti-Dumping diet is recommended for at least six weeks after surgery. Enteral nutrition support also may be used in the post-operative setting to aid with recovery and prevent nutrient deficiency; a semi-elemental formula should be selected due to high likelihood of pancreatic exocrine insufficiency (38). After about six weeks, in the absence of dumping syndrome, the diet may then be liberized as tolerated. For many patients, symptoms may best be managed by avoiding high fat foods long term (such as fried foods, cream sauces, and full fat dairy products) and limiting the diet to 75 grams of fat per day (24).

Chemotherapy

Chemotherapy is standard first line therapy for pancreatic cancers that are locally advanced or metastatic. Gemcitabine is most often used, as it has been shown to extend survival and improve quality of life (3). It may be used alone or in combination with another drug. Chemotherapy is often given at the same time as radiation therapy to enhance radiosensitization of the tumor (19). Table 4 outlines nutrition impact symptoms associated with common chemotherapy agents and targeted therapies used to treat EC. Please see chapter 11 for a full discussion of types of cancer therapies and their full range of side effects and chapter 12 for strategies to manage nutrition impact symptoms. The Nutrition Needs section above provides for strategies unique to the pancreatic cancer population.

Radiation Therapy

Radiation therapy can be helpful in treating exocrine pancreatic cancer, however it is not commonly used for treatment of bile duct or pancreatic neuroendocrine tumors. External beam radiation therapy is most typically used (3-4,6,19). Common symptoms of radiation to the pancreas include anorexia, diarrhea, fatigue, nausea/vomiting, and weight loss (6).

Integrative Therapy

Given the poor prognosis of pancreatic cancer, many patients are interested in integrative therapies. In a survey of patients with cancer, 80% of respondents reported using such therapies (39). Tumeric/curcumin, fish oil, and the Gonzalez regimen have gained the attention of patients with pancreatic cancer. Curcumin is found in turmeric, a spice used in Asian and East Indian cooking as well as a traditional Asian medicine treatment for gastrointestinal "upset" (40). Some studies examining its use in pancreatic cancer show promise (41-43), but the body of research conducted is small and therefore inadequate for reaching a conclusion. It should be used with caution in patients with gastroesophageal reflux disease and by those with biliary obstructions and gallstones (40). Although early studies showed promise that high doses of eicosapentaenoic acid (EPA) may mitigate cancer cachexia syndrome, other studies have found no benefit (44-47). EPA and DHA are further addressed in chapters 7 and 8. The Gonzalez regimen (48-50) is addressed in chapter 8.

Special Considerations

Malabsorption, Pancreatic Exocrine Insufficiency, and Enzyme Supplementation

Pancreatic exocrine insufficiency (PEI) may be observed in patients upon diagnosis, during nonsurgical treatment and/or following surgery for pancreatic and periampullary cancer (1). It is often recognized because patients have frequent or loose bowel movements. However, due to narcotic pain medications required for many patients, gut motility is slowed and characteristic loose or frequent bowel movements may not be present. Tests exist to diagnose PEI but can be cumbersome, difficult to conduct in clinical practice and expensive. Tests include a fecal fat test, stool elastase sampling, 13C-triglyceride (13C-MTG) breath test and direct measures of secretin-cerulein or secretin-pancreozymin (51-53).

In clinical practice, directed questioning is usually used to determine if patients have frequent, loose stools or other symptoms of PEI (See Box 2) (1,54). Symptoms of malabsorption are generally observed in patients who have endogenous pancreatic enzyme output below 10% of normal (12). Recent studies indicate 80%-90% of patients with pancreatic cancer may have PEI and malabsorption (55-56). It is important to instill realistic expectations in patients with severe PEI; while it may be impossible to eliminate steatorrhea completely, treatment can reduce symptoms by 60%–70% (24,52). Malabsorption also can be attributed to inadequate bile salts in the GI tract; therefore biliary obstruction can lead to weight loss even if exocrine activity is sufficient (57). Following a low-fat diet and avoiding gas-producing foods may reduce symptoms of biliary obstruction until the obstruction is corrected (58).

Traverso and colleagues examined the effect of distal pancreatectomy or pancreaticoduodenectomy on PEI (59-60). Stool

Table 4: Nutrition Impact Symptoms for Treatments Used for Pancreatic Cancer and Bile Duct Cancer* (3-4,6-7,13)

Agent Generic Name (Brand Name)	Anorexia	Nausea / Vomiting	Diarrhea	Mucositis	Altered Taste	Myelo-suppression
Chemotherapy:						
Capecitabine (Xeloda®)		3	3			3
Cisplatin (Platinol AQ®)		3	3		3	3
Docetaxel (Taxotere®)		3	3	3		3
Doxorubicin * (Adriamycin®)	3	3	3	3		3
Fluorouracil (5-FU)**		3	3	3	3	3
Gemcitabine *** (Gemzar®)		3				3
Irinotecan (Camptosar®, CPT-11)	3	3	3			3
Mitomycin C* (Mutamycin ®)	3	3	3	3		3
Oxaliplatin (Eloxitan®)****		3	3			3
Paclitaxel (Taxol®, Abraxane ®)		3	3	3		3
Targeted Therapy:	Diarrhea, fatigue and anorexia					
Erlotinib (Tarceva ®)	Eriotinib is currently approved for use in advanced pancreatic cancers. It is provided in a pill and is generally used in combination with gemcitabine (3,6,19).					

* Chemotherapy agents used for treatment of bile cancer

** Suck on ice chips pre/post IV bolus to reduce mucositis

*** Gemcitabine may be used alone or in combination with Fluorouracil, Capecitabine, Cisplatin, Oxaliplatin, Erlotinib and Paclitaxel. It also may be used in combination with Docetaxel and Capecitabine (called GTX) or with 5-FU, Leucovorin, Irinotecan, and Oxaliplatin (called FOLFIRINOX). In addition to side effects above, Gemcitabine may cause clay colored stool.

**** Avoid cold foods when receiving this drug.

Note: For Docetaxel and Paclitaxel, nausea may be more limited than in other drugs associated with nausea. Nausea often occurs on the day the drug is given and the first few days after the drug is given; anti-nausea medications are often provided prophylactically.

Box 2: Signs and Symptoms of Pancreatic Exocrine Insufficiency (1,51-53,57)

• Abdominal Bloating
• Cramping after meals
• Excessive gas (burping or flatulence)
• Fatty stools
• Frequent stools
• Foul smelling stools or gas
• Floating stools
• Indigestion
• Loose stools
• Unexplained weight loss

elastase was evaluated in patients with normal pancreatic function preoperatively and then reevaluated at 3, 12, and 24 months after surgery. In patients who had extended distal pancreatectomy, 12% had PEI at three months post surgery but by 24 months postoperatively all of these patients had normal stool elastase levels (60). In those patients who had undergone a pancreaticoduodenectomy, Matsumoto and Traverso (59) found that 50% of patients who had normal exocrine function before Whipple surgery experienced PEI as a long-term side effect of surgery. It should also be noted that patients may still have adequate enzyme production (normal fecal elastase) after surgery but that surgery may lead to asynchrony within the gastrointestinal tract, and therefore symptoms of malabsorption, because enzymes are not meeting food at the appropriate point in the digestive system (52).

The primary strategy for management of malabsorption is the use of supplemental pancreatic enzymes. With adequate enzyme supplementation patients may not need to restrict the fat content of their diet (1,12,52). However, fat restriction may benefit some patients with severe steatorrhea. Sarner suggests consuming less than 75 grams of fat per day (24). For patients having trouble consuming adequate calories due to limited tolerance of fat, medium-chain triglyceride (MCT) oil may be substituted for other fats because MCTs do not require enzymatic action or bile salts for digestion or absorption (24,61). MCT oil is commercially available over the counter, though side effects can include diarrhea, vomiting, nausea, stomach discomfort, and intestinal gas. MCT oil should not be used as a patient's only source of fat because it does not provide essential fatty acids and can therefore lead to essential fatty acid deficiency (24). Patient compliance may also be an issue as it is not very palatable, however recipes are provided in Appendix 6 and are available from some manufacturers. Although coconut oil does not provide MCTs exclusively, it is very high in MCTs and may be substituted for other fat sources in the regular diet.

When PEI is present, pancreatic enzymes (pancrelipase) should be prescribed. See Table 5 for a list of FDA approved pancreatic enzyme products. Dosing recommendations vary, but generally suggest starting at 10,000–40,000 lipase units per meal and 5,000–25,000 lipase units per snack (1,24,52-54,57). Enzyme doses should start low and be titrated up every several days as needed based on the characteristics of stools and symptoms of each individual patient (53). Supplemental pancreatic enzyme dosages should not exceed 10,000 lipase units per kilogram per day or 2,500 lipase units per kilogram per meal up to 4 times a day (53). For optimal replacement, the enzyme dose should be divided and administered throughout the meal. Starting enzymes with the first bite of food and consuming them throughout the meal and at the end of the meal will ensure that enzyme is delivered with the food (24,53).

When pancreatic exocrine function is compromised, it is suggested that an H_2-receptor antagonist (e.g., ranitidine, famotidine, etc.) or proton-pump inhibitor (e.g., pantoprazole, omeprazole, etc.) should be used because bicarbonate production and transport to the small intestine could be impaired. A physiologically basic environment is needed for both enzyme function and bile acids to transport fatty acids into the blood (24,52). The following recommendations are advised should a patient continue to display symptoms of malabsorption after an enzyme dose has been titrated (51-53):

- Evaluate compliance with dose and timing
- Adjust dose and timing
- Change brand of enzyme and consider change in dosage form (Table 5)
- Add H_2-receptor antagonist or proton-pump inhibitor (if not already prescribed)
- Assess for bacterial overgrowth or other malabsorptive disorder

Those patients with diarrhea may need to consider use of medicinal fiber (e.g., one teaspoon fiber powder or dose providing 3.4 grams psyllium or methylcellulose blended with 2 ounces water). Fiber should be taken once a day after a meal and gradually increased as needed up to four times per day (68-69). The most effective symptom management for malabsorptive diarrhea may be to restrict high-fat foods (such as fried foods, cream sauces, full fat dairy products) and to limit dietary fat intake to 75 grams/day (24). Patients with altered taste who have a recent history of severe diarrhea or steatorrhea should consider short-term zinc replacement of 25–100 mg of elemental zinc daily (70-72).

Diabetes

The role of nutrition in management of diabetes varies depending on the side effects or symptoms a patient is experiencing and their stage of disease. It is appropriate to be more liberal with the diet and use more aggressive medication or insulin management due to side effects or symptoms that reduce or limit oral intake (24,27). Diet also should be liberalized with advanced disease (27). In those patients who have completed treatment and have no evidence of disease, carbohydrate counting is appropriate to aid with glycemic control (24). In general efforts may be made to minimize the use of refined carbohydrates, consume meals and snacks at regular intervals, and to consume a mix of protein, complex carbohydrates, and fat (as tolerated) at each meal/snack.

Table 5: FDA Approved Pancreatic Enzyme Replacement Products (Pancrelipase) (62-67)

Brand	Lipase Units	Dosage form	Marketer
Creon®	3000	Delayed-release capsule, enteric coated spheres/beads/microtablets	Abbvie
	6000		
	12000		
	24000		
	36000		
Pancreaze®	4,200	Delayed-release capsule, enteric coated spheres/beads/microtablets	Janssen Pharmaceuticals
	10,500		
	16,800		
	21,000		
Pertzye®	8000	Delayed-release capsule, bicarbonate-buffered enteric coated spheres/beads/microtablets	Digestive Care, Inc.
	16,000		
Ultresa™	13,800	Delayed-release capsule, enteric coated spheres/beads/microtablets	Aptalis
	20,700		
	23,000		
Viokace™	10,440	Tablet- no enteric coating	Aptalis
	20,880		
Zenpep®	3000	Delayed-release capsule, enteric coated spheres/beads/microtablets	Aptalis
	5000		
	10000		
	15000		
	20000		
	25000		

Ascites

Ascites may be present in advanced disease. It can generally be managed using the recommendations for delayed gastric emptying discussed in Table 3 with the addition of a sodium restriction (2 g per day) and a high protein intake (1.5 g/kg/day) (58).

Small Bowel Obstruction

Patients with advanced pancreatic cancer are at risk of developing a small bowel obstruction. A study by McCallum, Walsh, and Nelson (73) evaluated the use of prophylactic diet education regarding a soft, low-fiber diet with bowel management strategies for prevention of obstruction. Patients were also instructed to chew food thoroughly and to use laxatives (authors did not provide details of bowel management recommendations in the publication). Of the 17 patients given preemptive education none experienced obstruction versus 12 of the 17 patients not educated experienced obstruction (73). This study suggests that all patients at high risk for bowel obstruction (characterized by abdominal carcinomatosis, enlarged retroperitoneal nodes, or pelvic masses) should be educated regarding diet and bowel management strategies to prevent obstruction. An example of a bowel management regimen is provided in Appendix 9.

Gastric Outlet or Duodenal Obstruction

Gastric outlet or duodenal obstruction may affect 15%-20% of patients, though it is typically a late onset side effect of the cancer (12,74). Symptoms of obstruction are nausea, vomiting (often retained food), abdominal distention, and pain. It can cause dehydration and weight loss and lead to poor quality of life. Treatment for outlet obstruction may be surgical or endoscopic. Surgery, when indicated, typically involves gastrojejunostomy (gastric bypass) where a loop of jejunum is connected to a new opening in the stomach that allows food to pass out of the stomach and bypass the blocked portion of the small bowel. If endoscopic treatment is chosen, a metallic stent is placed into the duodenum to hold the obstructed area open (74). Sometimes stenting or gastric bypass is not possible; in these cases a gastrostomy tube (g-tube) is inserted for drainage and a jejunostomy tube (j-tube) for feeding (6).

Little information is published regarding appropriate diet after duodenal stent or drainage gastrostomy. Practice may vary, but diet in both circumstances is generally the same. Literature suggests that after a duodenal stent is placed, patients should first establish tolerance of liquids before transitioning to a soft, low fiber diet as tolerated a few days later. Patients should be instructed to chew all foods well and to drink plenty of liquids with meals to ensure a liquid food bolus (75-77). Patients with drainage gastrostomy tubes are advised to follow the same parameters as those for duodenal stents but at some institutions may be instructed to utilize blended foods before progressing to a diet of soft solids (78-79). Others may be allowed to progress to a regular diet as tolerated (79-81). Episodes of blockage may often be managed by flushing the tube and avoiding that specific food in the future (81).

Summary

It is important for the oncology RD to help patients cope with nutrition issues throughout the course of treatment and survivorship. Though disease prognosis is generally poor, medical nutrition therapy can improve treatment outcomes and empower patients and families to play an active role in their care for pancreatic and biliary cancers. For those patients who survive long term, the nutrition implications of the disease and treatments are likely to endure for the rest of their lives.

References

1. Ottery F. Supportive nutritional management of the patient with pancreatic cancer. *Oncology (Williston Park).* 1996;10(9 Suppl):26-32.
2. Bruera E. ABC of palliative care. Anorexia, cachexia, and nutrition. *BMJ.* 1997;315(7117):1219-1222.
3. American Cancer Society. Pancreatic Cancer Detailed Guide. 2013; http://www.cancer.org/Cancer/PancreaticCancer/DetailedGuide/index. Accessed February 3, 2013.
4. National Cancer Institute. PDQ(R) Extrahepatic Bile Duct Cancer Treatment. 2013; http://www.cancer.gov/cancertopics/pdq/treatment/bileduct/HealthProfessional. Accessed February 3, 2013.
5. National Cancer Institute. What You Need to Know(TM) About Cancer of the Pancreas. 2010; http://www.cancer.gov/cancertopics/wyntk/pancreas. Accessed February 3, 2013.
6. National Cancer Institute. PDQ(R) Pancreatic Cancer Treatment. 2012; http://www.cancer.gov/cancertopics/pdq/treatment/pancreatic/HealthProfessional. Accessed February 3, 2013.
7. The Pancreatic Cancer Action Network. Learn About Pancreatic Cancer. 2013; http://www.pancan.org/section_facing_pancreatic_cancer/learn_about_pan_cancer/index.php. Accessed February 3, 2013.
8. Halfdanarson TR, Rabe KG, Rubin J, Petersen GM. Pancreatic neuroendocrine tumors (PNETs): incidence, prognosis and recent trend toward improved survival. *Ann Oncol.* 2008;19(10):1727-1733.
9. World Cancer Research Fund / American Institute for Cancer Research. *Food, nutrition, physical activity, and the prevention of cancer: a global perspective.* Washington DC: AICR; 2007.
10. Aune D, Greenwood DC, Chan DS, et al. Body mass index, abdominal fatness and pancreatic cancer risk: a systematic review and non-linear dose-response meta-analysis of prospective studies. *Ann Oncol.* 2012;23(4):843-852.
11. Rohrmann S, Linseisen J, Nothlings U, et al. Meat and fish consumption and risk of pancreatic cancer: Results from the European Prospective Investigation into Cancer and Nutrition. *Int J Cancer.* 2013;132(3):617-724.
12. DiMagno EP, Reber HA, Tempero MA. AGA technical review on the epidemiology, diagnosis, and treatment of pancreatic ductal adenocarcinoma. American Gastroenterological Association. *Gastroenterology.* 1999;117(6):1464-1484.
13. Sasaki M, Okamoto H, Johtatsu T, et al. Resting energy expenditure in patients undergoing pylorus preserving pancreatoduodenectomies for bile duct cancer or pancreatic tumors. *J Clin Biochem Nutr.* 2011;48(3):183-186.
14. Cao DX, Wu GH, Zhang B, et al. Resting energy expenditure and body composition in patients with newly detected cancer. *Clin Nutr.* 2010;29(1):72-77.

15. Falconer JS, Fearon KC, Plester CE, Ross JA, Carter DC. Cytokines, the acute-phase response, and resting energy expenditure in cachectic patients with pancreatic cancer. *Ann Surg.* 1994;219(4):325-331.
16. Thomas S. Nutritional Implications of Surgical Oncology. In: Elliott L, Molseed LL, McCallum PD, Grant B, eds. *The clinical guide to oncology nutrition.* 2nd ed. Chicago, Ill.: American Dietetic Association; 2006: 94-109.
17. Cystic Fibrosis Services. Cystic Fibrosis Services Pharmacy Products and Prices. 2013; https://www.cfservicespharmacy.com/ProductsandPrices/. Accessed June 9, 2013.
18. Escott-Stump S. Cancer: Pancreatic Cancer. *Nutrition and Diagnosis-Related Care* 7th ed. Baltimore, MD: Lippincott Williams & Wilkins; 2012: 777-779.
19. American Society of Clinical Oncology. Pancreatic Cancer. 2012; http://www.cancer.net/patient/Cancer+Types/Pancreatic+Cancer?sectionTitle=Treatment. Accessed February 3, 2013.
20. Wray CJ, Ahmad SA, Matthews JB, Lowy AM. Surgery for pancreatic cancer: recent controversies and current practice. *Gastroenterology.* 2005;128(6):1626-1641.
21. Pappas S, Krzywda E, McDowell N. Nutrition and pancreaticoduodenectomy. *Nutr Clin Pract.* 2010;25(3):234-243.
22. Academy of Nutrition and Dietetics. Gastroparesis. *Nutrition Care Manual* 2012; http://nutritioncaremanual.org/topic.cfm?ncm_toc_id=255563&highlight=gastroparesis. Accessed February 3, 2013.
23. Leung J, Silverman W. Diagnostic and therapeutic approach to pancreatic cancer-associated gastroparesis: literature review and our experience. *Dig Dis Sci.* 2009;54(2):401-405.
24. Sarner M. Treatment of pancreatic exocrine deficiency. *World J Surg.* 2003;27(11):1192-1195
25. Barone BB, Yeh HC, Snyder CF, et al. Postoperative mortality in cancer patients with preexisting diabetes: systematic review and meta-analysis. *Diabetes Care.* 2010;33(4):931-939.
26. Irizarry L, Li QE, Duncan I, et al. Effects of Cancer Comorbidity on Disease Management: Making the Case for Diabetes Education (A Report from the SOAR Program). *Popul Health Manag.* 2013;16(1):53-57.
27. Poulson J. The management of diabetes in patients with advanced cancer. *J Pain Symptom Manage.* Jun 1997;13(6):339-346.
28. Takada T, Yasuda H, Amano H, Yoshida M, Ando H. Results of a pylorus-preserving pancreatoduodenectomy for pancreatic cancer: a comparison with results of the Whipple procedure. *Hepatogastroenterology.* 1997; 44(18):1536-1540.
29. Schniewind B, Bestmann B, Henne-Bruns D, Faendrich F, Kremer B, Kuechler T. Quality of life after pancreaticoduodenectomy for ductal adenocarcinoma of the pancreatic head. *Br J Surg.* 2006;93(9):1099-1107.
30. Di Carlo V, Zerbi A, Balzano G, Corso V. Pylorus-preserving pancreaticoduodenectomy versus conventional whipple operation. *World J Surg.* 1999;23(9):920-925.
31. Diener MK, Fitzmaurice C, Schwarzer G, et al. Pylorus-preserving pancreaticoduodenectomy (pp Whipple) versus pancreaticoduodenectomy (classic Whipple) for surgical treatment of periampullary and pancreatic carcinoma. *Cochrane Database Syst Rev.* 2011(5):CD006053.
32. Ohtsuka T, Yamaguchi K, Ohuchida J, et al. Comparison of quality of life after pylorus-preserving pancreatoduodenectomy and Whipple resection. *Hepatogastroenterology.* 2003;50(51):846-850.
33. Kawai M, Yamaue H. Pancreaticoduodenectomy versus pylorus-preserving pancreaticoduodenectomy: the clinical impact of a new surgical procedure; pylorus-resecting pancreaticoduodenectomy. *J Hepatobiliary Pancreat Sci.* 2011;18:755-761.
34. Wente MN, Bassi C, Dervenis C, et al. Delayed gastric emptying (DGE) after pancreatic surgery: a suggested definition by the International Study Group of Pancreatic Surgery (ISGPS). *Surgery.* 2007;142(5):761-768.
35. Kunstman JW, Fonseca AL, Ciarleglio MM, Cong X, Hochberg A, Salem RR. Comprehensive analysis of variables affecting delayed gastric emptying following pancreaticoduodenectomy. *J Gastrointest Surg.* Jul 2012; 16(7):1354-1361.
36. Ma JP, Peng L, Qin T, et al. Meta-analysis of pancreaticoduodenectomy prospective controlled trials: pancreaticogastrostomy versus pancreaticojejunostomy reconstruction. *Chin Med J (Engl).* 2012; 125(21):3891-3897.

37. Makni A, Bedioui H, Jouini M, et al. Pancreaticojejunostomy vs. pancreaticogastrostomy following pancreaticoduodenectomy: results of comparative study. *Minerva Chir*. 2011;66(4):295-302.

38. Zaloga GP. Intact proteins, peptides, and amino acid formulas. *Nutrition in Critical Care*: Mosby-Year Book; 1994:59-80.

39. Richardson MA, Sanders T, Palmer JL, Greisinger A, Singletary SE. Complementary/alternative medicine use in a comprehensive cancer center and the implications for oncology. *J Clin*. 2000;18(13):2505-2514.

40. Natural Medicines Comprehensive Database. Turmeric. 2012; http://naturaldatabase.therapeuticresearch.com/nd/Search.aspx?cs=&s=ND&pt=100&id=662&ds=&name=TURMERIC&lang=0&searchid=35371890. Accessed February 3, 2013.

41. Dhillon N, Aggarwal BB, Newman RA, et al. Phase II trial of curcumin in patients with advanced pancreatic cancer. *Clin Cancer Research*. 2008;14(14):4491-4499.

42. Bar-Sela G, Epelbaum R, Schaffer M. Curcumin as an anti-cancer agent: review of the gap between basic and clinical applications. *Curr Med Chem*. Jan 2010;17(3):190-197.

43. Epelbaum R, Schaffer M, Vizel B, Badmaev V, Bar-Sela G. Curcumin and gemcitabine in patients with advanced pancreatic cancer. *Nutr Cancer*. 2010;62(8):1137-1141.

44. Dewey A, Baughan C, Dean T, Higgins B, Johnson I. Eicosapentaenoic acid (EPA, an omega-3 fatty acid from fish oils) for the treatment of cancer cachexia. *Cochrane Database Syst Rev*. 2007(1):CD004597.

45. Natural Medicines Comprehensive Database. Fish Oil. 2012; http://naturaldatabase.therapeuticresearch.com/nd/Search.aspx?cs=&s=ND&pt=100&id=993&ds=&lang=0. Accessed February 3, 2013.

46. Moses AW, Slater C, Preston T, Barber MD, Fearon KC. Reduced total energy expenditure and physical activity in cachectic patients with pancreatic cancer can be modulated by an energy and protein dense oral supplement enriched with n-3 fatty acids. *Br J Cancer*. 2004; 90(5):996-1002.

47. Jatoi A, Rowland K, Loprinzi CL, et al. An eicosapentaenoic acid supplement versus megestrol acetate versus both for patients with cancer-associated wasting: a North Central Cancer Treatment Group and National Cancer Institute of Canada collaborative effort. *J Clin Oncology*. 2004; 22(12):2469-2476.

48. Gonzalez NJ, Isaacs LL. Evaluation of pancreatic proteolytic enzyme treatment of adenocarcinoma of the pancreas, with nutrition and detoxification support. *Nutr Cancer*. 1999;33(2):117-124.

49. National Cancer Institute. PDQ(R) Gonzalez Regimen. 2012; http://www.cancer.gov/cancertopics/pdq/cam/gonzalez/healthprofessional. Accessed February 3, 2013.

50. Chabot JA, Tsai WY, Fine RL, et al. Pancreatic proteolytic enzyme therapy compared with gemcitabine-based chemotherapy for the treatment of pancreatic cancer. *J Clin Oncol*. 2010;28(12):2058-2063.

51. Dominguez-Munoz JE. Pancreatic enzyme therapy for pancreatic exocrine insufficiency. *Gastroenterology Hepatol*. 2011;7(6):401-403.

52. Dominguez-Munoz JE. Pancreatic exocrine insufficiency: diagnosis and treatment. *J Gastroenterol Hepatol*. 2011;26 Suppl 2:12-16.

53. Fieker A, Philpott J, Armand M. Enzyme replacement therapy for pancreatic insufficiency: present and future. *Clin Exp Gastroenterol*. 2011;4:55-73.

54. Ellison NM, Chevlen E, Still CD, Dubagunta S. Supportive care for patients with pancreatic adenocarcinoma: symptom control and nutrition. *Hematol Oncol Clin North Am*. 2002;16(1):105-121.

55. Imrie CW, Connett G, Hall RI, Charnley RM. Review article: enzyme supplementation in cystic fibrosis, chronic pancreatitis, pancreatic and periampullary cancer. *Aliment Pharmacol Ther*. 2010;32 Suppl 1:1-25.

56. Wakasugi H, Hara Y, Abe M. A study of malabsorption in pancreatic cancer. *J Gastroenterol*. 1996;31(1):81-85.

57. Layer P, Keller J, Lankisch PG. Pancreatic enzyme replacement therapy. *Curr Gastroenterol Rep*. 2001;3(2):101-108.

58. Escott-Stump S. Hepatic, Pancreatic, and Biliary Disorders. In: *Nutrition and Diagnosis-Related Care*. 7th ed. Baltimore, MD: Lippincott Williams & Wilkins; 2012:471-518.

59. Matsumoto J, Traverso LW. Exocrine function following the whipple operation as assessed by stool elastase. *J Gastrointestinal Surgery*. 2006;10(9):1225-1229.

60. Speicher JE, Traverso LW. Pancreatic Exocrine Function Is Preserved After Distal Pancreatectomy. *J Gastroint Surg*. 2010;14(6):1006-1011.

61. Babayan VK. Medium chain triglycerides and structured lipids. *Lipids*. 1987;22(6):417-420.

62. Creon(R) [package insert]. North Chicago, IL: AbbVie Inc; 2013.

63. Pancreaze (R) [package insert]. Titusville, NJ: Janssen Pharmaceuticals, Inc; 2011.

64. Pertzye (R) [package insert]. Bethlehem, PA: Digestive Care, Inc.; 2012.

65. Ultresa(TM) [package insert]. Birmingham, AL: Aptalis Pharma US, Inc; 2012.

66. Viokace(TM) [package insert]. Birmingham, AL: Aptalis Pharma US, Inc; 2012.

67. Zenpep(R) [package insert]. Yardley, PA: Eurand Pharmaceuticals, Inc; 2011.

68. Murphy J, Stacey D, Crook J, Thompson B, Panetta D. Testing control of radiation-induced diarrhea with a psyllium bulking agent: a pilot study. *Can Oncol Nurs J*. Summer 2000;10(3):96-100.

69. Singh B. Psyllium as therapeutic and drug delivery agent. *Int J Pharm*. Apr 4 2007;334(1-2):1-14.

70. Takaoka T, Sarukura N, Ueda C, et al. Effects of zinc supplementation on serum zinc concentration and ratio of apo/holo-activities of angiotensin converting enzyme in patients with taste impairment. *Auris Nasus Larynx*. 2010;37(2):190-194.

71. Prasad AS. Clinical manifestations of zinc deficiency. *Annu Rev Nutr*. 1985;5:341-363.

72. Heyneman CA. Zinc deficiency and taste disorders. *Ann Pharmacother*. 1996;30(2):186-187.

73. McCallum P, Walsh D, Nelson KA. Can a soft diet prevent bowel obstruction in advanced pancreatic cancer? *Support Care Cancer*. 2002;10(2):174-175.

74. Gaidos JK, Draganov PV. Treatment of malignant gastric outlet obstruction with endoscopically placed self-expandable metal stents. *World J Gastroenterol*. 2009;15(35):4365-4371.

75. Adler DG, Baron TH. Endoscopic palliation of malignant gastric outlet obstruction using self-expanding metal stents: experience in 36 patients. *Am J Gastroenterol*. 2002;97(1):72-78.

76. Dormann A, Meisner S, Verin N, Wenk Lang A. Self-expanding metal stents for gastroduodenal malignancies: systematic review of their clinical effectiveness. *Endoscopy*. 2004;36(6):543-550.

77. Ly J, O'Grady G, Mittal A, Plank L, Windsor JA. A systematic review of methods to palliate malignant gastric outlet obstruction. *Surg Endosc*. 2009;24(2):290-297.

78. Meyer L, Pothuri B. Decompressive percutaneous gastrostomy tube use in gynecologic malignancies. *Curr Treat Options*. 2006;7(2):111-120.

79. Pothuri B, Montemarano M, Gerardi M, et al. Percutaneous endoscopic gastrostomy tube placement in patients with malignant bowel obstruction due to ovarian carcinoma. *Gynecol Oncol*. 2005;96(2): 330-334.

80. Teriaky A, Gregor J, Chande N. Percutaneous endoscopic gastrostomy tube placement for end-stage palliation of malignant gastrointestinal obstructions. *Saudi J Gastroenterology: official journal of the Saudi Gastroenterology Association*. 2012;18(2):95-98.

81. Brooksbank MA, Game PA, Ashby MA. Palliative venting gastrostomy in malignant intestinal obstruction. *Palliat Med*. 2002;16(6):520-526.

Medical Nutrition Therapy for Prostate Cancer

Greta Macaire, MA, RD, CSO

Overview:

The prostate, a walnut sized gland in men that surrounds the top of the urethra, produces seminal fluid. Prostate cancer is the most common cancer and the second most common cause of cancer deaths in men. Most prostate cancers are slow growing, although a small percentage of cases are aggressive. The National Cancer Institute has predicted that 238,590 men will be diagnosed with prostate cancer and 29,720 men will die of this disease in 2013 (1). The five-year relative survival rate for all stages combined is almost 100%. Metastatic prostate cancer is incurable with current therapies; the median survival is one to three years (2-3).

Screening/Diagnosis/Stages:

The American Cancer Society (ACS) recommends annual prostate-specific antigen testing (PSA) and digital rectal examination (DRE) starting at age 50 for men with at least a 10-year life expectancy (2). Screening at age 45 is recommended for men at high risk. However, PSA screening has become controversial. The U.S. Preventive Services Task Force recommends against PSA-based screening for healthy men because of the risk of overdiagnosis and adverse effects associated with overtreatment (4). The American Urological Association takes a third position, recommending that decisions regarding PSA-based screening and early treatment for prostate cancer be individualized (5). PSA screening cut-off points are among issues being debated with some questioning which PSA value to measure (e.g., levels circulating freely versus levels bound to protein) and the ideal cut-off points for various ages and status of general risk factors (6).

Symptoms of prostate cancer may include changes in urinary or sexual function and back or pelvic pain; early stage disease is asymptomatic. When suspected, a biopsy is used to make a prostate cancer diagnosis. The American Joint Committee on Cancer's TNM system is most often used to stage prostate cancer (7) and the Gleason score defines the histologic grade of the tumor (2-3).

Risk Factors:

Known risk factors for prostate cancer are age, race, nationality, family history, genetics and diet. About 60% of prostate cancers are diagnosed in men 65 years of age and older. African American men have the highest prostate cancer rates in the United States (U.S.). Having a first-degree relative with prostate cancer nearly doubles a man's risk, and 5%-10% of cases are believed to be genetic. Risk

Figure 1: The Prostate Gland

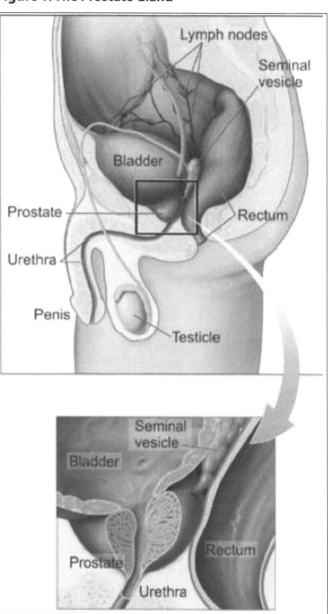

Reprinted with permission
The website of the National Cancer Institute (http://www.cancer.gov).

factors under investigation include obesity, infections, and vasectomy (2-3).

Metabolically, prostate cancer has been linked to androgen hormones, which stimulate prostate cancer growth. Increased levels of insulin-like growth factor-1 (IGF-1), over expression of cyclooxygenase (COX-2) and chronic inflammation also have been implicated in prostate cancer development (2-3). Research in this area is ongoing and dietary patterns likely influence these factors.

Medical Treatment

Treatment depends on the cancer stage, the patient's life expectancy and overall health. Early stage disease is treated with surgery, radiation therapy or active surveillance. For older men or men with less aggressive tumors, active surveillance may be the most appropriate option (2-3). Prostate cancer surgery removes the cancer, the prostate gland and some of the surrounding tissue. Various types of radiation therapy are used to treat prostate cancer. Hormone therapy, chemotherapy, radiation and combinations of these treatments are used to treat advanced prostate cancer (2-3).

Common side effects of surgery and radiation for prostate cancer are infertility and urinary, bowel, and erectile dysfunction (2-3). Hormone therapy, or androgen deprivation therapy (ADT), slows the growth of prostate cancer by reducing serum levels of androgens or interfering with the androgen receptor. Side effects of ADT include fatigue, hot flashes, sexual changes, mood changes, anemia, weight gain and body composition changes (2,8-10). ADT puts men at high risk for osteoporosis (3) and may raise the risk of cardiovascular disease and diabetes (2,5,8-10). Common chemotherapy agents used to treat prostate cancer include Carbazitaxel, Carboplatin, Docetaxel, Doxorubicin, Etoposide, Pacitaxel, Vinorelbine and Vinblastine (11). Chapter 11 provides information about the mechanisms of action and side effects of these and other cancer agents used to treat prostate cancer.

Nutrition and Prostate Cancer Risk

Observational data suggests that differences in diet and lifestyle play a role in the variability of prostate cancer rates worldwide (12). Preliminary evidence suggests that diet and lifestyle modifications may slow the progression of prostate cancer and lower the risk of recurrence (13-16).

A plant-based diet is associated with a lower risk of prostate cancer and its recurrence. Observational studies suggest that phytonutrients found in allium and cruciferous vegetables; diets high in lycopene; flaxseed; green tea; pomegranate and soyfoods may reduce prostate cancer risk (14,17-18). Plant foods provide vitamins, minerals, fiber and phytochemicals, which in experimental studies exhibit a variety of anticancer actions (11,16). Cruciferous vegetables have been consistently linked with a reduced risk of prostate cancer as well as its recurrence and metastasis (19-20); isothiocyanates and indoles in these foods have been shown to inhibit growth of prostate cancer cells (19). Allium vegetables such

as garlic provide organosulfur compounds that reduce prostate cancer risk by inducing cell cycle arrest and apoptosis of prostate cancer cells (21). Cell studies suggest that genistein, a cancer-fighting isoflavone in soy, may inhibit synthesis of prostaglandins that promote inflammation while genistein combined with daidzin and glycitin (also found in soy) may induce cell cycle arrest and apoptosis in prostate cancer cells (22-23). Lycopene may convey particular benefit against prostate cancer. The antioxidant activity of this carotenoid as well as its effects on cell cycles are believed to help protect against prostate cancer risk (24). Both the Health Professionals Follow-Up Study (25) and a study examining a large cohort of Seventh Day Adventist men (26) suggest that greater intakes of lycopene may reduce prostate cancer risk. These compounds help prevent DNA mutations that may initiate cancers; promote apoptosis of cancer cells; help limit inflammation; inhibit angiogenesis and regulate cell cycles to allow time for cellular repair of mutations (27).

Scientific evidence suggests that obtaining these compounds from whole foods (versus supplements) is most beneficial; to date studies examining anticancer benefits of single nutrient supplementation have been negative. Researchers speculate that bioactive compounds in fruits and vegetables work synergistically and on multiple biochemical pathways, and those benefits are difficult to capture in single-nutrient trials.

Research also suggests that the increased prostate cancer risk observed in developed countries may, in part, be due to the fact that a high-fat diet stimulates increased testosterone levels. Limited evidence shows that a low fat diet may be beneficial, though the types of fatty acids consumed may be more important than the amount of fat (11,18,28-29). Generally, studies have observed a positive association between prostate cancer and intake of saturated fat from meat and dairy foods (29-31). In addition, dairy foods may promote higher IGF-1 levels. Mutagens in meat cooked at high temperatures also contribute to prostate cancer risk (11,30-37).

While trans-fatty acid intake has been correlated with greater prostate cancer risk (38-39), omega-9 fatty acids appear to convey a neutral or a slightly inverse association (29,40). Higher blood levels of eicosapentaenoic and docosahexaenoic acid (EPA and DHA), the omega-3 fatty acids found in cold-water fish, have been associated with both greater and lower rates of prostate cancer (41-42). Greater fish consumption, however, has been associated with lower risk of prostate cancer and recurrence. Omega-6 fatty acids, linoleic acid (LA) and arachidonic acid (AA) may stimulate prostate cancer cell growth (29,34,40). Studies also suggest a benefit from diets containing a low omega-6 to omega-3 ratio, which may occur through the inhibition of AA-derived eicosanoids (28-31,40).

Calcium & Vitamin D

A number of epidemiologic studies have examined associations between calcium intake and total and/or fatal prostate cancer (43-44). In a large study, subjects who consumed more than 933 mg of dietary calcium had a 1.36 (but nonsignificant) increased risk of experiencing fatal prostate cancer when compared with those in the lowest quartile of intake; those who consumed more than 400 mg of supplemental calcium daily had a 50% greater (and statistically significant) risk of dying from prostate cancer than those who did not consume calcium supplements (43). Other studies have not found significant associations between prostate cancer and calcium intake (44) or found that whole milk (versus other types of milk or dairy intake) increased prostate cancer progression (45).

Biologic plausibility suggests that a higher calcium intake might suppress circulating levels of 1,25 dihydroxy vitamin D (25-26,43, 46-48). However, most studies examining relationships between vitamin D (intake or circulating levels) and prostate cancer have produced null results (41-43). Studies are underway to better understand the role of vitamin D in patients with prostate cancer (11,30-31,33,36).

Selenium & Vitamin E
Based on research suggesting an inverse association between selenium level and prostate cancer risk (49), the SELECT trial was initiated to examine effects of supplemental selenium, vitamin E or their combination on prostate cancer prevention (50). Results were

disappointing, showing a slightly increased risk of prostate cancer among those taking vitamin E supplements. Several hypotheses regarding the conflicting findings are under investigation (3,30,42,48).

Other food
Greater egg intake has been associated with increased risk of prostate cancer fatality (51). Choline, which is found in egg yolk, is highly concentrated in prostate cancer cells, leading researchers to question whether choline or a different dietary factor in egg yolk may be responsible for the observation.

Body Weight & Physical Activity
Evidence associating obesity with prostate cancer risk is inconsistent, however, gaining more than 2.2 kg after a prostatectomy has been associated with doubling the risk of disease recurrence (52). A meta-analysis suggested that a higher BMI increased mortality from prostate cancer (53). Obtaining three or more hours per week of vigorous activity is associated with lower mortality in prostate cancer survivors. Additionally, exercise appears to mitigate the side effects of ADT (54-57).

Table 1: Medical Nutrition Therapy Matrix for Prostate Cancer (14, 17-18, 21-26, 29-31, 38-39, 41-42)

Treatments and Nutrition Impact Symptoms	MNT During Treatment	MNT Post-treatment
Active Surveillance	n/a	Long Term: See nutrition recommendations in Table 2
Surgery: Radical Prostatectomy	Consume adequate energy, protein, and micronutrients required for healing	Following recovery, adopt nutrition recommendations in Table 2
Radiation Therapy: Directed at the entire prostate, caudal portion of seminal vesicles and in advanced cases the pelvic lymph nodes, which exposes the bladder, rectum, sigmoid colon and small bowel to radiation.	Modify fiber and fat intake for rectal urgency, loose stools, and/or diarrhea (e.g., emphasize soluble fibers and lower fat foods; reduce intake of insoluble fibers and higher fat foods). See chapter 12 for additional suggestions. Confirm use of anti-diarrheal medications recommended by the medical team, possibly including Imodium®, Metamucil® and probiotics.	Same as MNT during treatment; gradually relax dietary restrictions as symptoms resolve.
Androgen (ADT) Hormone Therapy decreases serum testosterone levels >95% and increases estrogen levels >80%	Long-term side effects of ADT (58): **Osteoporosis:** Total calcium intake should meet Dietary Reference Intakes with predominant calcium sources being low fat dairy and vegan sources. It is important to maintain an adequate vitamin D status (> 20 ng/mL) and a daily vitamin D supplement (e.g., 400 IU) daily may be indicated to achieve this goal. **Preserve Lean Body Mass:** To preserve lean body mass, intentional weight loss (when indicated) should be gradual and combined with physical activity. **Elevated Lipids:** Weight management interventions combined with NCEP ATP III guidelines and engaging in 30 minutes of physical activity daily will promote desired lipid levels. As part of a heart-healthy diet, survivors should consider consuming 25 grams soy protein daily. **Decreased insulin sensitivity:** Weight management combined with NCEP ATP III guidelines is advised; monitor for need to regulate carbohydrate intake. **Normochromic, normocytic Anemia:** Provide education on maximizing iron absorption and consuming adequate iron if indicated.	
Hot Flashes	Avoid hot beverages, spicy foods, alcohol, caffeine and smoking. Consume one serving of soyfood daily (see Table 2 for options).	Avoid hot beverages, spicy foods, alcohol, caffeine and smoking. Consume one serving of soyfood daily (see Table 2 for options).

Table 2: Nutrition Recommendations for Prostate Cancer Survivors

Food or Nutrient	Recommended Intake	Comments
Vegetables & Fruits	Consume 8-10 servings per day including ≥ 5 servings vegetables and ≥ 3 servings fruits daily. Select a variety of colors of vegetables and fruits. Emphasize regular intake of cruciferous vegetables.	One serving = ½ cup fruit or vegetable; 1 cup leafy green vegetables; ¼ cup dried fruit or vegetable; 6 ounces vegetable or fruit juice
Lycopene	30 mg daily	Tomato paste (6½ Tbsp); tomato sauce (3/4 cup); raw tomatoes (8 medium); Guava (3½ cups) and watermelon (4¼ cups) each provide approximately 30 mg of lycopene.
Dietary Fiber	30-45 grams daily	Include vegetables, fruits, beans/legumes, nuts, seeds and whole grains in the diet.
Refined Grains & Added Sugars	Limit intake of refined grains and added sugars	Limit intake of refined grains and foods with added sugars including white rice, foods made with enriched white flour, sugary drinks, desserts and pastries.
Red & Processed Meat	Reduce red meat; avoid processed meats and grilled or fried meats	Limit intake of beef, lamb and pork. Limit intake of hot dogs, bacon, salami and other processed meats.
Dairy Products	Select reduced fat or nonfat dairy foods; moderate dairy food intake (2 servings daily); combine vegetarian sources of calcium with limited dairy selections	Select reduced fat or nonfat cheese, milk, yogurt and similar dairy products. Select leafy green vegetables and soyfoods are non-dairy sources of calcium while cold water fish is an acceptable non-dairy source of vitamin D.
Saturated Fat	Limit to <7% of energy intake	Limit whole milk dairy foods, red meats, processed meats (unless formulated to be low in saturated fat), poultry skin and baked goods (unless formulated to be low in saturated fat and trans fat).
Trans Fats	Avoid food sources of trans fat	Limit margarines and baked foods unless label states the product contains no trans fat. Limit or avoid fried foods.
Eggs	Limit egg yolk intake to 2 per week	Egg whites are acceptable; consume a maximum of 2 egg yolks per week.
Omega-6 Fats: Arachodonic Acid (AA) and Linoleic Acid (LA)	Limit intake of meat, butter, egg yolks and whole milk Limit vegetable oil sources of LA to 1 Tablespoon daily	AA: Limit meat, butter, egg yolks, whole milk dairy foods. LA: Limit intake of vegetable oils such as corn oil, safflower oil, sunflower oil, cottonseed oil and processed foods made with these oils to 1 Tablespoon daily.
Omega-3 Fats EPA & DHA Alpha Linolenic Acid (ALA)	Consume cold water fish twice weekly, or fish oil supplements providing an equivalent amount of EPA and DHA	Include sources of EPA and DHA in the diet such as: salmon, sardines, black cod, trout, herring and DHA enriched eggs (within the egg allowance). Include sources of ALA such as: flaxseed, chia seeds, walnuts, hemp seeds and pumpkin seeds.
Omega-9 Fats	A handful of peanuts or sunflower seeds per day is acceptable.	Humans can synthesize omega-9 fats, so they are not considered essential. Oleic acid is a primary source of omega-9 fat, and is found in olive oil, canola oil, peanut oil and sunflower oil (which is also a source of omega-6 fat). Limit intake of these fats to 2 tablespoons daily.
Flaxseed	2 Tablespoons ground flaxseed daily	Ground flaxseed and flax seed oil (whole flaxseeds may not be absorbed) are acceptable at intakes up to 2 Tablespoons daily.
Soy	Include 1 or more servings of soyfood daily (1 serving = 1 cup soy milk, 4 ounces tofu, ½ cup edamame, ¼ cup soy nuts); 2-3 servings of natural soyfoods such as tofu and tempeh are considered safe and acceptable.	Acceptable sources of soyfoods are: edamame, tempeh, tofu, soymilk and miso. Soy supplements are not recommended.
Green Tea	Drink 1 or more cups daily	
Calcium	RDA: 1000-1200 mg daily from diet Do not consume > 1500 mg calcium daily	Preferred sources of calcium include reduced fat or nonfat dairy products, canned fish with soft bones, beans, leafy greens, tofu, almonds, calcium fortified soy and almond beverages and other calcium fortified foods.
Vitamin D	RDA: 600-800 IU daily UL: 4000 IU daily *High dose may be recommended if serum 25 (OH) D is <36 ng/mL(57)	Sources of vitamin D include sunlight, fish and vitamin D fortified foods.
Vitamin E	RDA: 15 mg daily UL: 1000 mg daily	Vegetable oils, wheat germ, nuts, seeds, avocado are sources of vitamin E; consume within recommended limits.
Alcohol	≤ 2 drinks daily	1 serving of alcohol = 1 ounce liquor, 5 ounces wine, 12 ounces beer.

To help achieve or maintain a healthy body weight, prostate cancer survivors are also encouraged to engage in ≥ 30 minutes of physical activity on most days.

Nutrition Screening and Assessment for Prostate Cancer

Few men diagnosed with early stage prostate cancer are underweight or present with recent weight loss or eating difficulty. Most of these patients complete their cancer treatment without major complications, though it is important for RDs to counsel patients on strategies to manage nutrition impact symptoms (NIS) that may occur, as outlined in Chapter 12. Otherwise, in this group interventions should focus on optimizing health and quality of life, including strategies to prevent long-term effects of some prostate cancer therapies such as osteoporosis and cardiovascular disease.

Patients with advanced disease are more likely to present with weight loss and decreased intake, which increases the risk of incomplete chemotherapy treatment and/or treatment breaks and poorer outcomes. These men also are at greater risk of experiencing NIS from systemic therapy and additional weight loss during treatment. Diarrhea is a particular risk as it commonly occurs after full pelvic radiation, which some patients with advanced prostate cancer receive. Nutrition interventions include an increased intake of soluble fiber, decreased intake of insoluble fiber and other interventions as suggested in chapter 12. In this population a comprehensive nutrition care plan for the treatment phase most often needs to address weight maintenance (to promote full treatment and preserve muscle mass) and diarrhea management (to prevent excess nutrient and fluid losses and promote weight maintenance).

With emerging research suggesting that weight gain and overweight/obesity may increase the risk of disease recurrence, post-treatment nutrition intervention should address weight maintenance when weight is within the normal range and a gradual weight loss that also preserves lean body mass for overweight and obese survivors. Recommendations from the National Cholesterol Education Program Adult Treatment Panel III are appropriate for achieving healthy lipid levels. Nutrition intervention post ADT treatment also should address calcium needs and sources (e.g. reduced fat or nonfat dairy and non-dairy sources) for maintaining bone density. All survivors would benefit from nutrition education targeting foods and dietary intake patterns believed to help prevent disease recurrence. Medical nutrition therapy for the treatment phase is summarized in Table 1. Table 2 provides nutrition recommendations for survivors who have completed treatment for prostate cancer.

References

1. National Cancer Institute. Surveillance Epidemiology and End Results. SEER Stat Fact Sheets: Prostate. http://seer.cancer.gov/statfacts/html/prost.html. 2013 data. Accessed 9/15/2013.
2. American Cancer Society. Detailed guide: Prostate Cancer. http://www.cancer.org/Cancer/ProstateCancer/DetailedGuide/index. Accessed 7/9/2012.
3. National Cancer Institute. Prostate Cancer Treatment (PDQ®). Stage Information for Prostate Cancer. http://www.cancer.gov/cancertopics/pdq/treatment/prostate/HealthProfessional/page3. Last modified 8/13/2013. Accessed 9/20/2012.
4. U.S. Preventive Services Task Force. Screening for Prostate Cancer. http://www.uspreventiveservicestaskforce.org/prostatecancerscreening.htm. Release date May 2012. Accessed 9/1/2013.
5. American Urological Association. Early detection of prostate cancer; AUA Guideline. http://www.auanet.org/education/guidelines/prostate-cancer-detection.cfm. Approved April 2013. Accessed 9/04/2013.
6. National Cancer Institute. Prostate-Specific Antigen (PSA) Test. http://www.cancer.gov/cancertopics/factsheet/detection/PSA. Reviewed 7/24/2012. Accessed 09/04/2013.
7. American Joint Committee on Cancer. AJCC Cancer Staging Manual. 6th ed. New York, NY: Springer; 2002.
8. Guise TA, Oefelein MG, Eastham JA, et al. Estrogenic side effects of androgen deprivation therapy. Rev Urol. 2007;9(4):163-180.
9. Storer TW, Miciek R, Travison TG. Muscle function, physical performance and body composition changes in men with prostate cancer undergoing androgen deprivation therapy. Asian J Androl. 2012;14(2):204-221.
10. Levine GN, D'Amico AV, Berger P, et al. Androgen-deprivation therapy in prostate cancer and cardiovascular risk: a science advisory from the American Heart Association, American Cancer Society, and American Urological Association: endorsed by the American Society for Radiation Oncology. Circulation. 2010;21(6):833-840.
11. American Cancer Society. Chemotherapy for Prostate Cancer. http://www.cancer.org/cancer/prostatecancer/detailedguide/prostate-cancer-treating-chemotherapy Last Revised 8/26/2013. Accessed 9/26/2013.
12. World Cancer Research Fund/American Institute for Cancer Research. Food, Nutrition, Physical Activity, and the Prevention of Cancer: a Global Perspective. Washington DC: AICR (2007)
13. Ornish D, Weidner G, Fair WR, et al. Intensive lifestyle changes may affect the progression of prostate cancer. J Urology. 2005:174(3):1065-1070.
14. Frattaroli J, et al. Clinical events in prostate cancer lifestyle trial: results from two years of follow-up. Urology. 2008;72(6):1319-1323.
15. Nguyen JY, Major JM, Knott CJ, et al. Adoption of a plant-based diet by patients with recurrent prostate cancer. Integr Cancer Ther. 2006;5(3):214-223.
16. Dubenmier JJ, Weidner G, Marlin R, et al. Lifestyle and health-related quality of life of men with prostate cancer managed with active surveillance. Urology. 2006;67(1):125-130.
17. Salem S, Salahi M, Mohseni M, et al. Major dietary factors and prostate cancer risk: a prospective multicenter case-control study. Nutr Cancer. 2011;63(1):21-27.
18. Hardin J, Cheng I, Witte JS. Impact of consumption of vegetable, fruit, grain, and high glycemic index foods on aggressive prostate cancer risk. Nutr Cancer. 2011;63(6):860-872.
19. Higdon JV, Delage B, Williams DE, Dashwood RH. Cruciferous vegetables and human cancer risk: epidemiologic evidence and mechanistic basis. Pharmacol Res. 2007;55(3):224-236.
20. National Cancer Institute Fact Sheet. Cruciferous Vegetables and Cancer Prevention. http://www.cancer.gov/cancertopics/factsheet/diet/cruciferous-vegetables. Reviewed 07/07/2012. Accessed 09/01/2013.
21. Hsing AW, Chokkalingam AP, Gao YT, et al. Allium vegetables and risk of prostate cancer: A population-based study. J Natl Cancer Inst. 2002;94(21):1648-1651.
22. Yan L and Spitznagel EL. Soy consumption and prostate cancer risk in men: a revisit of a meta-analysis. Am J Clin Nutr. 2009.89(4):1155-1163.
23. National Cancer Institute: PDQ® Prostate Cancer, Nutrition, and Dietary Supplements. Bethesda, MD: National Cancer Institute. http://cancer.gov/cancertopics/pdq/cam/prostatesupplements/healthprofessional. Date last modified 8/06/2013. Accessed 9/10/2013.
24. Campbell JK, Canene-Adams K, Lindshield BL, Boileau TW, Clinton SK, Erdman JW. Tomato phytochemicals and prostate cancer risk. J Nutr. 2004;134(12Suppl):3486S-3492S.
25. Giovannucci E. Tomatoes, tomato-based products, lycopene, and cancer: review of the epidemiologic literature. J Natl Cancer Inst. 1999;91:317-331.
26. Giovannucci E, Rimm EB Liu Y, Stampfer MJ, Willett WC. A prospective study of tomato products, lycopene, and prostate cancer risk. J Natl Cancer Inst. 2002;94(5):391-398.
27. Pan MH, Ghai G, Ho CT. Food bioactives, apoptosis, and cancer. Molecular Nutrition & Food Research. 2008;52(1):43-52.

28. Hsu A, Bray TM, Helferich WG, Doerge DR. Differential effects of whole soy extract and soy isoflavones on apoptosis in prostate cancer cells. *Exp Biol Med.* 2010;235(1):90-97.

29. Suburu J. & Chen Y.Q. Lipids and prostate cancer. *Prostaglandins Other Lipid Mediat.* 2012;98(1-2):1-10.

30. Kushi LH, Doyle C, McCullough M., et al.; American Cancer Society 2010 Nutrition and Physical Activity Guidelines Advisory Committee. American Cancer Society Guidelines on nutrition and physical activity for cancer prevention: reducing the risk of cancer with healthy food choices and physical activity. *CA Cancer J Clin.* 2010;62(1):30-67.

31. Rock CL, Doyle C, Demark-Wahnefried W, et al. Nutrition and physical activity guidelines for cancer survivors. *CA: A Cancer Journal for Clinicians.* 2012;62:242–274.

32. Richman EL, Carroll PR, Chan JM. Vegetable and fruit intake after diagnosis and risk of prostate cancer progression. *Int J Cancer.* 2012; 131(1): 201-210.

33. Kurahashi N, Inoue M, Iwasaki M, et al. Japan Public Health Center Based Prospective Study Group.Collaborators (102). Dairy product, saturated fatty acid, and calcium intake and prostate cancer in a prospective cohort of Japanese men. *Ca Epidemiol Biomarkers Prev.* 2008;17(4): 930-937.

34. Hu J, La Vecchia C, Gibbons L, Negri E, Mery L. Nutrients and risk of prostate cancer. *Nutr Cancer.* 2010;62(6):710-718.

35. McGreevy KM, Hoel BD, Lipsitz SR, Hoel DG. Impact of nutrients on insulin-like growth factor-I, insulin like growth factor binding protein-3 and their ratio in African American and white males. *Public Health Nutrition.* 2007;10(1):97-105.

36. Ahn J, Albanes D, Peters U, et al. Prostate, Lung, Colorectal, and Ovarian Trial Project Team. Dairy products, calcium intake, and risk of prostate cancer in the prostate, lung, colorectal, and ovarian cancer screening trial. *Ca Epidemiol Biomarkers Prev.* 2007;16(12):2623-2630.

37. Koutros S, Cross AJ, Sandler DP, et al. Meat and meat mutagens and risk of prostate cancer in the Agricultural Health Study. *Cancer Epidemiology and Biomarkers Prevention.* 2008;17(1):80-87.

38. Lu QY, Arteaga JR, Zhang Q, et al. Inhibition of prostate cancer cell growth by an avocado extract: role of lipid-soluble bioactive substances. *J Nutr Biochem.* 2006;16(1):23-30.

39. Gonzalez CA, Salas-Salvado J. The potential of nuts in the prevention of cancer. *Br J Nutr.* 2006;96(suppl 2):S87-S94.

40. Szymanski KM, Wheeler DC, Mucci LA. Fish consumption and prostate cancer risk: a review and meta-analysis. *Am J Clin Nutr.* 2010;92(5): 1223-1233.

41. Brasky TM, Till C, White E, et al. Serum phospholipid fatty acids and prostate cancer risk: results from the Prostate Cancer Prevention Trial. *Am J Epidemiol.* 2011;173(21):1429-1439.

42. Torfadottir JE, Valdimarsdottir UA, Mucci LA, et al. Consumption of fish products across the lifespan and prostate cancer risk. PLoS One. 2013 Apr 17;8(4):e59799. doi: 10.1371/journal.pone.0059799.

43. Giovannucci E, Liu Y, Stampfer MJ, Willett WC. A prospective study of calcium intake and incident and fatal prostate cancer. *Cancer Epidemiol Biomarkers Prev.* 2006;15(2):203-210.

44. Park SY, Murphy SP, Wilkens LR, Stram DP, Henderson BE, Kolonel LN. Calcium, vitamin D, and dairy product intake and prostate cancer risk: the Multiethnic Cohort Study. *Am J Epidemiol.* 2007;166(11):1259-1269.

45. Pettersson A, Kasperzyk JL, Kenfield SA, et al. Milk and dairy consumption among men with prostate cancer and risk of metastases and prostate cancer death. *Cancer Epidemiol Biomarkers Prev.* 2012;21(3):428-436.

46. Chan JM, Giovannucci EL. Dairy products, calcium, and vitamin D and risk of prostate cancer (Sweden). *Epidemiol Rev* 2001;23(1):87-92.

47. Kristal AR, Arnold KB, Neuhouser ML. Diet, supplement use, and prostate cancer risk: results from the Prostate Cancer Prevention Trial. *Am J Epidemiol.* 2010;172(5):566-577.

48. Chan JM, Stampfer MJ, Ma J, Gann PH, Gaziano JM, Giovannucci EL. Dairy products, calcium, and prostate cancer risk in the Physicians' Health Study. *Am J Clin Nutr.* 2001;74(4):549-554.

49. Hurst R, Hooper L, Norat T, et al. Selenium and prostate cancer: systematic review and meta-analysis. *Am J Clin Nutr.* 2012;96(1):111-122.

50. Klein EA, Thompson IM, Tangen CM, et al. Vitamin E and the risk of prostate cancer the selenium and vitamin e cancer prevention trial (select). *JAMA.* 2011;306(14):1549-1556.

51. Richman EL, Stampfer MJ, Paciorek A, Broering JM, Carroll PR, Chan JM. Intakes of meat, fish, poultry, and eggs and risk of prostate cancer progression. *Am J Clin Nutr.* 2010;91(3):712-721.

52. Joshu CE, Mondul AM, Menke A. Weight gain is associated with an increased risk of prostate cancer recurrence after prostatectomhy in the PSA era. *Cancer Prev Res.* 2011;4(4):544-551.

53. Cao Y, Ma J. Body-mass index prostate cancer-specific mortality and biochemical recurrence: A systematic review and meta-analysis. *Cancer Prev Res.* 2011;4(4):486-501.

54. Hernandez BY, Park SY, Wilkens LR, et al. Relationship of body mass, height, and weight gain to prostate cancer risk in the multiethnic cohort. *Cancer Epidemiol Biomarkers Prev.* 2009;18(9):2413-2421.

55. Liu Y, Hu F, Li D, et al. Does physical activity reduce the risk of prostate cancer? A systematic review and meta-analysis. *Eur Urol,* 2011;60(5): 1029-1044.

56. Kenfield SA, Stampfer MJ, Giovanucci E, Chan J.M. Physical activity and survival after prostate cancer diagnosis in the health professionals follow-up study. *J Clin Oncol.* 2011;29(6):726-32

57. Keogh JW, MacLeod RD. Body composition, physical fitness, functional performance, quality of life, and fatigue benefits of exercise for prostate cancer patients: a systematic review. *J Pain Symptom Manag.* 2012;43(1):96-110.

58. Michaelson MD, Cotter SE, Gargollo PC, Zietman AL, Dahi DM, Smith MR. Management of complications of prostate cancer treatment. *CA Cancer J Clin.* 2008;58(4):196-213.

Medical Nutrition Therapy for Thyroid Cancer

Shanna Bernstein, MPH, RD

Background

The thyroid is a small gland located in the front part of the neck. It makes thyroid hormone, which helps regulate heart rate, body temperature and weight, and also calcitonin, a hormone that helps maintain normal calcium levels. It is estimated that in the United States (U.S.) in 2013, 60,220 cases of thyroid cancer are expected while 1,850 people are expected to die from this disease (1). The lifetime risk of developing thyroid cancer is 1.03% (1). Since the mid-1970s, the incidence of thyroid cancer has increased significantly, though this trend is widely attributed to new technology allowing earlier diagnosis and identification of smaller carcinomas (2). Most thyroid cancers are relatively indolent, and five-year relative survival is 97.7% (1).

Thyroid cancers are a heterogeneous group of diseases, often distinguished by cellular classification and categorized by clinical features and management. Early thyroid cancer is often asymptomatic, but as the cancer grows, symptoms may develop. While symptoms vary by type of thyroid cancer, they may include cough, difficulty swallowing or breathing, enlargement of or lump on the thyroid gland, neck pain, and hoarseness or change in voice (3).

For purposes of clinical management, thyroid cancer is divided into differentiated or undifferentiated cancers. Table 1 summarizes types of thyroid cancer.

Diagnosis of thyroid cancer usually involves blood tests for abnormal levels of thyroid stimulating hormone (TSH) or calcitonin, thyroid ultrasounds, radioactive scans, and biopsies (3). Staging of thyroid cancer is based on primary tumor assessment, regional lymph node metastasis and distant metastasis. Stages range from I-IV for all thyroid cancer types except for anaplastic carcinoma, which is always stage IV (3).

Risk Factors

Various risk factors for thyroid cancer have been identified while many others remain under investigation. One of the most-established risk factors is exposure to high levels of radiation, particularly during infancy or early childhood. Multiple genetic mutations have been associated with thyroid cancer, with genetic factors being responsible for up to 20%-25% of medullary carcinoma (7). Additionally, increased risk is associated with being over 45 years of age and being female (4). Family and personal history of benign

Figure 1: Thyroid Gland

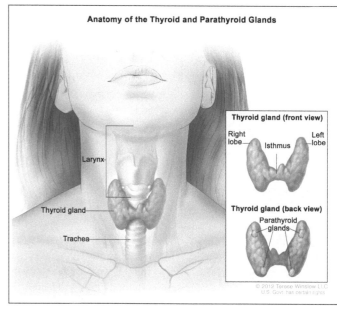

© 2012 Terese Winslow, U.S. Govt. has certain rights

thyroid conditions, such as goiters, also are considered risk factors for thyroid cancer.

New evidence suggests that a higher BMI is weakly associated with an elevated risk of thyroid cancer with risk estimates ranging from 1.1-2.3 in males and 1-7.4 in females (8). Though it has been hypothesized that this finding may be due to detection bias, it is an important factor to consider, as it could potentially contribute to the increasing incidence of thyroid cancer.

Perhaps the most widely accepted dietary factor related to thyroid cancer is iodine intake. Research has consistently shown that chronic iodine deficiency is associated with an increased risk of follicular carcinoma, while high iodine intake, such as in iodine supplementation programs, is associated with an increased incidence of papillary carcinoma (7). Given that seafood is a major natural source of dietary iodine, associations between fish intake and thyroid cancer have been examined. Findings have been inconsistent with risk estimates ranging from 0.6-2.2, but overall the effect of fish consumption on thyroid cancer risk seems negligible (7-8). Epidemiological studies

Table 1: Types of Thyroid Cancers (4-6)

Type	Prevalence	Comments
Papillary (differentiated)	80%	Slow-growing; curable when diagnosed early; best prognosis of all thyroid cancers
Follicular (differentiated)	10-15%	Originates in follicular cells; outcome is generally good but is more likely to recur than papillary
Medullary (Cancer of the C cells)	2%	Raises calcitonin levels
Anaplastic (undifferentiated)	2%	Aggressive; usually fatal; usual survival is 3-6 months

provide limited support for an association between thyroid cancer and intake of cruciferous vegetables, which contain goitrogens that can induce thyroid cancer in animals. Inverse associations have been found between thyroid cancer risk and non-cruciferous vegetable intake. It is hypothesized that any unfavorable effect of goitrogenic substances is outweighed by the protective effect of other vegetable constituents that inhibit carcinogenesis (7). Single studies have suggested potential associations between thyroid cancer risk and soy (7), nitrate (9), alcohol (10) and green tea (11) intake, but further studies are needed to clarify these associations. It should be noted that much of the research exploring dietary factors and thyroid cancer risk are limited by the difficulties inherent in measuring diet, which is a multi-dimensional exposure. Issues specific to assessment of iodine intake also must be acknowledged, as iodine content of foods varies enormously based on local factors and therefore limits the accuracy of generalized food composition tables for this nutrient (7).

Dysphagia

Patients with thyroid cancer may experience dysphagia, usually occurring when an enlarged thyroid compresses on structures involved in swallowing (12). Conventional strategies used to manage this symptom include small frequent feedings of moist food. For additional recommendations, please see chapter 12. A Speech-Language Pathologist consult should be considered when there is concern for safe swallowing function.

Treatment

In many cases of thyroid cancer, surgery is the therapy of choice. Often a total or near-total thyroidectomy is indicated, though in low-risk cases, a lobectomy may be performed. In cases of metastases to lymph nodes, removal of lymph nodes and neck dissection is recommended. For anaplastic cancer, surgery is rarely indicated due to advanced disease (2-3). In all instances of total thyroidectomy, postoperative thyroid hormone replacement should be provided, sometimes at doses sufficient to suppress TSH (4). Also, damage to the recurrent laryngeal nerve can occur after thyroid surgery, which may compromise swallowing function (13).

In high-risk cases of differentiated thyroid cancer (DTC), radioactive iodine (RAI) therapy is indicated postoperatively. RAI can be used to detect residual or recurrent disease as well as to treat persistent disease, as RAI is concentrated by thyroid cancer cells, leading to their destruction (4). Nutrition impact symptoms (NIS) of RAI include transient nausea, dry mouth, change in taste, a low risk of late-onset damage of salivary glands and dental caries. Secondary malignancies are an additional risk of RAI (2).

RAI has no role in the treatment of medullary or anaplastic thyroid cancers. In cases of advanced medullary cancer and DTC in which further surgery or RAI is ineffective, radiation therapy should be considered. Radiation therapy is also used with chemotherapy in combined modality treatment for anaplastic cancer. While there is no supportive evidence for use of chemotherapy in DTC, it may be used for palliative purposes in medullary cancer. Unfortunately, there are limited randomized, controlled trials examining treatment of medullary and anaplastic cancers because of their low incidence, and as a result there is limited consensus regarding management. Potential alternative options for treatment, including immunotherapy, vaccine-based therapies, and gene therapies, are being explored (5-6).

Presenting symptoms of thyroid cancer do not commonly include weight loss, and energy, macronutrient and micronutrient needs are consistent with age and gender specific Dietary Reference Intakes (DRIs) unless otherwise indicated by a nutrition assessment. However, thyroid cancer treatments, including chemotherapy, radiation therapy, and RAI, can result in a range of NIS that may compromise the ability to eat. RDs identify NIS when conducting a nutrition assessment, and provide appropriate education and counseling; Chapter 12 provides effective strategies for managing NIS. The RD will also educate and counsel patients receiving RAI on the low iodine diet.

Thyroid Cancer Treatment and The Low-Iodine Diet

Low iodine diets (LID) are used in conjunction with RAI scans and therapy. The rationale for utilization of LID is to deplete whole-body iodine stores and thereby optimize RAI uptake in thyroid cells (14). Studies of urinary iodine concentration, which are used to assess iodine status, support the use of LID. In comparison to non-restricted diets, LID have been repeatedly shown to reduce urinary iodine, with significantly lower values after two weeks, as compared with one week, of iodine restriction (14). Research also shows that following LID will increase tumor uptake, lengthen the half-life of RAI and improve ablation rates. It is not known whether LID improves long-term outcomes, and though the usual dietary goal is ≤ 50 μg iodine/day, the superiority of this intake to less restrictive diets has not been adequately studied (14). In general, research on LID is hindered by limited numbers and the retrospective nature of studies. Nonetheless, the American Thyroid Association Management Guidelines, endorsed by nine international professional organizations, recommends LID "… for 1-2 weeks for patients undergoing RAI remnant ablation, particularly for those patients with high iodine intakes (Recommendation rating: B)" (2).

Few risks are associated with LID, though there are case reports of symptomatic hyponatremia while following LID. This is likely due to the unnecessary restriction of all, including non-iodized, salt. Patient feedback has indicated that the diet is boring, unpalatable, "overwhelming while adapting to a new diagnosis" and difficult to understand (15). Confusion regarding LID is largely related to limited and inconsistent data on the iodine content of foods worldwide. Growing conditions, food production practices related to the use of iodized salt, and iodine-fortification and food-labeling laws vary throughout the world; thus LID guidelines developed for one country may not be valid in another country. In the U.S., the FDA does not require Nutrition Facts labels to list iodine content unless the food item is fortified with this nutrient (16). Iodine content of many common foods varies greatly, with one study showing iodine content of bread ranging from 2.2-587.4 µg/slice. This degree of variation is attributed to inconsistent use of iodate conditioners (17). However, even iodine content of less processed foods, such as fresh produce, varies according to soil, fertilizer and irrigation practices. This in turn affects iodine content of meat and animal products, as produce may be used for animal feed (14). Use of iodine-based sanitizing solutions on dairy equipment also contributes to variable iodine content in dairy products, and the variability of iodine in salt water affects iodine content of seafood (18).

Iodine content of foods in the average U.S. diet was most recently examined as part of the 2006-2008 U.S. Food and Drug Administration Total Diet Study (TDS). Results showed that dairy and grain products contributed >65% of total daily iodine intake in adults (19). Data also showed high iodine content in eggs and a variety of seafood and baked good products (19). Though not examined in TDS, iodized salt is recognized as a major dietary source of iodine. While a voluntary practice, most salt manufacturers in the U.S. add iodine to table salt, leading to iodized salt that contains approximately 400 µg iodine/ tsp. salt (16,20).

The variability in iodine content of foods as well as the use of outdated and misinterpreted data has led to inconsistencies in LID guidelines published by various organizations (20-21). However, key features of most LID include avoidance of the following:
- Iodized salt
- Seafood and all sea products
- Dairy products
- Egg yolks
- Red-dye #3/erythrosine
- Iodate dough conditioners
- Any foods containing significant amounts of these products as ingredients (20-22)

When following LID, it is necessary to check ingredient lists on package labels. See Table 2 for a detailed list of foods allowed and not allowed on the LID (22-26). Unless otherwise indicated, these recommendations reflect the most current U.S. data on iodine content of foods. Note that these lists may not be appropriate for use outside the U.S. due to differences in iodine content of foods in other countries.

Though iodized salt should be avoided on LID, non-iodized salts are acceptable for use. Due to presence of iodine in seawater, avoidance of sea salt is often recommended, however actual analysis of sea salt shows only trace levels of iodine (27). Therefore, evidence does not support the restriction of sea salt. Most processed or prepared foods made by large food manufacturers in the U.S. use non-iodized salt; if iodized or sea salt is used, it should be specified on the ingredient list (16). Table 3 lists names of manufacturers and associated brands that have confirmed use of non-iodized salt in their U.S. food production as of 2012. It is important to periodically review manufacturers' websites for the most current information on products made with non-iodized salt because processing techniques can change over time. Fresh foods are most reliable on LID. It is not usually possible to determine the type of salt used for food preparation in restaurants and thus, it is most prudent to avoid eating out while on LID.

Other products to be avoided while on LID include multi-vitamins that contain iodine and any supplements, including selenium or fish oil, made from sea-based products such as oyster shells, kelp or fish. While on LID, iodine tablets should not be used for water purification and creams or lotions made from seaweed should be avoided. Topical products and antiseptics that contain iodine, such as Betadine® (Purdue Products, Stamford), should not be used (22,27).

Though rare, it is possible that LID may be required for those dependent on tube-feedings (TF) or parenteral nutrition (PN). Most PN formulations and trace element products do not contain iodine and supplementation for those receiving PN is not routinely recommended. Thus, for purposes of LID, it is crucial to avoid iodine containing medications and antiseptics, which are the primary source of iodine in this population (28). In cases of TF dependence there is a recognized lack of low-iodine commercial formulas. Therefore, it is recommended that a low-iodine TF formula be prepared by pureeing food products that are acceptable for LID (29). Table 2 outlines the low iodine diet and Table 3 lists foods processed with non-iodized salt. It is essential for patients undergoing RAI to adhere to the low iodine diet for the timeframe recommended. RDs should be consulted regarding any questions about this diet.

Conclusion

While the survival rate is high, thyroid cancer is now recognized as one of the most frequently diagnosed cancers in the U.S. Therefore, it is essential that RDs and other health practitioners be aware of the elements involved in care and management of those with thyroid cancer. Though still being studied, it has become clear that diet plays a role in the risk of development of thyroid cancer. Additionally, it is necessary to consider the application of the LID as a component of therapy and the NIS of thyroid cancer treatment.

Table 2: Low Iodine Diet Food Chart

Food Category	Foods Allowed	Foods Not Allowed
Milk and Milk Products	• Possible milk substitutes include almond milk, rice milk, coconut milk and hemp milk • Non-dairy cream substitutes	• All milk including whole, low-fat, skim, buttermilk and powdered milk • Cream • Lattes and cappuccinos • Cream and milk-based soups or sauces • Yogurt and kefir • Cheese, cottage cheese • Ice cream, sherbet
Eggs	• Egg whites and egg substitutes made from egg whites	• Whole eggs • Egg yolks
Seafood	• None	• All fish including canned tuna and sardines • All shellfish including lobster, crab, shrimp, and oysters • Imitation crab meat • Fish sauces, pastes, and spreads • Sushi, nori, seaweed or any sea vegetables, such as kelp and algae
Animal Proteins	• All fresh red meats–beef, pork, lamb, veal • All fresh poultry including turkey and chicken • Wild or game meats including venison and bison • Luncheon meats including ham, turkey and chicken • Frankfurters and sausages • Bacon	• Bologna • Cured meats including pepperoni and salami
Vegetable Proteins and Soy	• Protein powders made from wheat or nuts and allowed ingredients • Meal replacement bars made from wheat or nuts and allowed ingredients • Tofu* • Soybeans*	• Protein powders made from soy or whey • Meal replacement bars and drinks made from soy or whey • Veggie burgers and other meat imitation products* • Soymilk*
Nuts and Seeds	• Any unsalted nuts and seeds • Nuts and seeds salted or roasted by large food producers • Peanut butter in limited amounts (less than 2 Tbsp. per day)	• Nuts and seeds salted or roasted by local or small producers • Trail mixes that contain any chocolate, yogurt or other *not allowed* ingredients
Fruits	• All fresh, canned, dried, or frozen fruits and fruit juices	• Maraschino cherries containing red dye #3/erythrosine
Vegetables	• Most fresh, frozen and canned vegetables including potato, peas, lentils, squash, most beans and corn	• Nori, seaweed or any sea vegetables, such as kelp and algae • Cowpeas, navy and red beans
Breads, Grains and Cereals	• Home-made breads prepared with only allowed ingredients • Commercial breads, including tortillas, that do not contain iodate conditioners • Pasta (white and wheat), noodles, rice, bulgur, couscous, oats, quinoa, polenta, cornmeal and other grain • Cold and hot cereals (without milk)	• Breads containing iodate conditioners (i.e. calcium iodate, potassium iodate) or other *not allowed* ingredients • Any grain or cereal prepared with or containing *not allowed* ingredients
Baked goods	• Home-made cakes, cookies and fruit desserts only if prepared with allowed ingredients	• Cakes, muffins, cookies, or pastries prepared with *not allowed* ingredients
Snack foods	• Commercially prepared plain crackers, pretzels, chips (potato and tortilla) and popcorn • Fruit ice and popsicles • Gelatin dessert • Dark chocolate • Most nuts and seeds	• Snacks made with *not allowed* ingredients. • Milk chocolate and any chocolate products that contain milk • Puddings or custards • Cocoa or hot chocolate mix
Mixed dishes and Soups	• Home-made or canned soups, stews, and casseroles prepared with only allowed ingredients • Hamburger or meatloaf if prepared with only allowed ingredients	• Lasagna, pizza, burritos and other dishes made with cheese • Hamburgers or meatloaf if prepared with egg yolk or other *not allowed* ingredients *(Continued)*

Table 2: Low Iodine Diet Food Chart *(continued)*

Food Category	Foods Allowed	Foods Not Allowed
Condiments	• Margarine • Sugar and sugar substitutes • Jelly • Catsup and mustard • Gravy made without milk • Oil and non-creamy salad dressings • Vinegar • Mayonnaise, soy sauce and butter in limited amounts (less than 2 Tbsp. per day)	• Blackstrap molasses • Creamy or cream-based sauces and salad dressings • Sour cream • Fish sauce or anchovy paste
Beverages	• Water, coffee, tea, carbonated beverages, fruit juices and drinks • Beer, wine and alcohol if permitted by physician	• Milk or cream • Any beverages containing *not allowed* ingredients
Miscellaneous	• Non-iodized salt • Fresh and dried herbs and spices	• Iodized salt • Red dye #3/ erythrosine • Alginate, agar-agar, carrageenan and algae (check labels for these additives)

*U.S data on iodine content of these foods is lacking and therefore guidelines are based on food composition data from other countries. However, it may be safest to avoid all soy and tofu foods unless you follow a vegetarian or vegan diet with limited protein sources.

References

1. National Cancer Institute, Surveillance Epidemiology and End Results, Fact Sheets: Thyroid. Available at: http://seer.cancer.gov/statfacts/html/thyro.html. Accessed May 2013.
2. Cooper DS, Doherty GM, Haugen BR, et al. Revised American Thyroid Association Management Guidelines for Patients with Thyroid Nodules and Differentiated Thyroid Cancer. *Thyroid.* 2009;19(11):1167-1214.
3. PubMed Health, Thyroid Cancer. Available at: http://www.ncbi.nlm.nih.gov/pubmedhealth/PMH0002193/. Accessed July 2012.
4. National Cancer Institute, What you need to know about thyroid cancer. Available at: http://www.cancer.gov/cancertopics/wyntk/thyroid/page1. Accessed July 2012.
5. Pudney D, Lau H, Ruether JD, Falck V. Clinical experience of the multimodality management of anaplastic thyroid cancer and literature review. *Thyroid.* 2007;17(12):1243-1249.
6. Wu LS, Roman SA, Sosa JA. Medullary thyroid cancer: an update of new guidelines and recent developments. *Curr Opin Oncol.* 2011;23(1):22-27.
7. Dal Maso L, Bosetti C, Vecchia CL, Franceschi S. Risk factors for thyroid cancer: an epidemiological review focused on nutritional factors. *Cancer Causes Control.* 2009;20(1):75-86.
8. Peterson E, Prithwish D, Nuttall R. BMI, diet and female reproductive factors as risks for thyroid cancer: a systematic review. *PLoS One.* 2012;7(1): e29177.
9. Ward MH, Kilfoy BA, Weyer PJ, Anderson KE, Folsom AR, Cerhan JR. Nitrate intake and the risk of thyroid cancer and thyroid disease. *Epidemiology.* 2010;21(3):389-395.
10. Meinhold CL, Park Y, Stolzenberg-Solomon RZ, Hollenbeck AR, Schatzkin A, Berrington de Gonzalez A. Alcohol intake and risk of thyroid cancer in the NIH-AARP diet and health study. *Br J Cancer.* 2009;101(9):1630-1634.
11. Michikawa T, Inoue M, Shimazu T, et al. Green tea and coffee consumption and its association with thyroid cancer risk: a population-based cohort study in Japan. *Cancer Causes Control.* 2011;22(7):985-993.
12. Lindgren S, Janzon L. Prevalence of swallowing complaint and clinical findings among 50-79 year old men and women in an urban population. *World J Surg.* 2009;33(2):255-260.
13. Zabrodsky M, Boucek J, Kastner J, Kuchar M, Chovanec M, Betka J. *Acta Otorhinolaryngol Ital.* 2012;32(4):222-228.
14. Sawka AM, Ibrahim-Zada I, Galacgac P, et al. Dietary iodine restriction in preparation for radioactive iodine treatment or scanning in well-differentiated thyroid cancer: a systematic review. *Thyroid.* 2010; 20(10):1129-1138.
15. Morris LF, wilder MS, Waxman AD, Braunstein GD. Reevaluation of the impact of a stringent low-iodine diet on ablation rates in radioiodine treatment of thyroid carcinoma. *Thyroid.* 2001;11(8):749-755.
16. Pearce EN, Pino S, He X, Bazrafshan HR, Lee SL, Braverman LE. Sources of dietary iodine: bread, cows' milk, and infant formula in the Boston area. *J Clin Endocrinol Metab.* 2004;89(7):3421-3424.
17. Office of Dietary Supplements, Dietary supplements fact sheet: iodine. Available at: http://ods.od.nih.gov/factsheets/Iodine-HealthProfessional/ . Accessed 7/2012.
18. Pennington JA, Schoen SA, Salmon GD, Young B, Johnson RD, Marts RW. Composition of core foods of the U.S. food supply, 1982-1991. *J Food of Compost Analysis.* 1995;8(2):171-217.
19. Murray CW, Egan SK, Kim H, Beru N, Bolger PM. US Food and Drug Administration's total diet study: dietary intake of perchlorate and iodine. *J Expo Sci Environ Epidemiol.* 2008;18(6):571-580.
20. Thyroid Cancer Survivors' Association, Inc. Available at: http://thyca.org/rai.htm . Accessed July 2012.
21. Thyroid Cancer Canada, Low Iodine Diet. Available at: http://www.thyroidcancercanada.org/low-iodine-diet.php?lang=en . Accessed July 2012.
22. National Institutes of Health, Clinical Center, Low iodine diet Available at: http://www.cc.nih.gov/ccc/patient_education/conditions_diseases.html. Accessed 7/2012
23. *Total diet Study Statistics on Element Results- 2006-2008.* College Park, MD: US Food and Drug Administration, Center for Food Safety and Applied Nutrition; 2010.
24. Technical University of Denmark, National Food Institute, Danish Food Composition Database Version 7.01. Available at: http://www.foodcomp.dk/v7/fcdb_default.asp . Accessed 7/2012.
25. Food Standards Australia New Zealand, NUTTAB 2010 Online Searchable Database. Available at: http://www.foodstandards.gov.au/consumerinformation/nuttab2010/nuttab2010onlinesearchabledatabase/onlineversion.cfm?&action=nutrientFoods&category=Minerals&nutrientID=I . Accessed 7/2012.
26. Haldimann M, Alt A, Blanc A, Blondeau K. Iodine content of food groups. *J Food Compost Analysis.* 2005;18:461-471.
27. Preedy VR, Burrow GN, Watson RR. *Comprehensive Handbook of Iodine: Nutritional, Biochemical, Pathological and Therapeutic Aspects.* Burlington, MA: Elsevier Inc; 2009.
28. Zimmerman MB, Crill CM. Iodine in enteral and parenteral nutrition. *Best Pract Res Clin Endocrinol Metab.* 2010;24(1):143-158.
29. Ain KB, Dewitt PA, Gardner TG, Berryman SW. Low-iodine tube-feeding diet for iodine-131 scanning and therapy. *Clin Nucl Med.* 1994;19(6): 504-507.

Table 3: Food manufacturers and brands using non-iodized salt

The following list of food manufacturers and product brands using non-iodized salt in their food products sold in the U.S. is based on written inquiry in 2012. This list does not include all manufacturers or brands and inclusion on this list does not suggest endorsement of any particulars brands or products. Remember to check labels for *non-allowed* ingredients. It is also important to consider that manufacturing processes can periodically change, which can potentially alter iodine content of these products.

Conagra Foods®	**FritoLay®**	**Kraft Foods®**
http://www.conagrafoods.com/	http://www.fritolay.com/index.html	http://www.kraftrecipes.com/Products/
Banquet®	Cheetos®	ProductMain.aspx
Chef Boyardee®	Cracker Jacks®	A1®
Egg Beaters®	Doritos®	Boca®
Fleischmann's®	Funyuns®	Breakstone's®
Healthy Choice®	Grandma's®	Capri Sun®
Hebrew National®	Lays®	Chips Ahoy®
Hunt's®	Nut Harvest®	Cool Whip®
La Choy®	Rold Gold®	Cracker Barrel®
Marie Callender's®	Ruffles®	Crystal Light®
Orville Redenbacher's®	Sabra®	Honey Maid®
PAM®	Sabritones®	Jell-o®
Peter Pan®	Simply Natural®	Kool-Aid®
Slim Jim®	Stacy's®	Maxwell House®
	Sun Chips®	Miracle Whip®
		Nabisco®
		Nilla®
		Oreo®
		Oscar Mayer®
		Planters®
		Ritz®
		Snackwell's®
		Stove Top®
		Triscuit®
		Wheat Thins®
General Mills®	**Hormel Foods®**	**PepsiCo®**
http://www.generalmills.com/Betty Crocker®	http://www.hormelfoods.com/brands/default.aspx	http://www.pepsico.com/Brands.html
Big G cereals®	Chi-chi's®	(owns FritoLay® and Quaker®, previously listed)
Bisquick®	Dinty Moore®	Aquafina®
Cascadian Farm®	Farmer John®	Brisk®
Cheerios®	HerbOx®	Dole®
Chex®	Jennie-O®	Frappuccino®
Fiber One®	Spam®	Gatorade®
Green Giant®	Stagg Chili®	IZZE®
Haagen- Dazs®	World Food®	Lipton®
Hamburger Helper®		Mountain Dew®
Nature Valley®		No Fear®
Old El Paso®		Ocean Spray®
Pillsbury®		Pepsi®
Progresso®		Propel®
Total®		Sierra Mist®
		Sobe®
		Tropicana®
Campbell's® US	**Heinz®**	**Quaker®**
http://www.campbellsoupcompany.com/	http://www.heinz.com/our-food/products.aspx	http://www.quakeroats.com/home.aspx
Default.aspx	Bagel Bites®	Aunt Jemima®
Pace®	Classico®	Chewy®
Pepperidge Farm®	Jack Daniels Sauces®	Cap'n Crunch®
Prego®	Ore-Ida®	Life®
Swanson®	Smart Ones®	Mother's®
V8®	T.G.I.Friday's ®	Near East®
		Pasta Roni®
		Rice-A-Roni®
Kashi®		
http://www.kashi.com/products		
GOLEAN®		
Heart to Heart®		

Nutrition Management of Oncology Patients in Palliative and Hospice Settings

Kelay Trentham, MS, RD, CSO, CD

Introduction

Palliative care and hospice are forms of specialized care that are distinct from curative care. Simply defined, "to palliate" is to lessen or ease symptoms of disease independently of curative efforts (1). The World Health Organization (WHO) defines palliative care as "an approach that improves quality of life of patients and their families facing problems associated with life-threatening illness, through the prevention and relief of suffering by means of early identification and impeccable assessment and treatment of pain and other problems, physical, psychosocial and spiritual" (2). Additionally, palliative care activities are characterized as those which, through a team approach, affirm life; neither hasten nor postpone dying; incorporate psychological and spiritual aspects of care; provide a support system such that patients may actively live until death; help families cope with a loved one's illness and their grief; enhance quality of life; and, possibly, have a positive impact on the course of the illness (3). Palliative care for oncology patients should be considered as essential to patients' care as curative therapy itself. Provision of palliative care is appropriate in all care settings, including hospitals, extended care facilities, home healthcare, assisted living facilities, outpatient clinics, and emergency departments (3).

The Hospice Foundation of America defines hospice as "a special concept of care designed to provide comfort and support to patients and their families when a life-limiting illness no longer responds to cure-oriented treatments" (4). Goals of hospice care include improving quality of life (QoL), preserving dignity, providing comfort and controlling pain (4). Like palliative care, hospice care is provided by a multidisciplinary team, and includes emotional, psychological and spiritual components (4). In addition, bereavement and counseling services are offered to families prior to and for up to one year following a patient's death (4). Hospice care also may be provided in a variety of settings, including the patient's home, hospitals, skilled nursing facilities and freestanding hospice care facilities. In the United States (U.S.) patients must have a life expectancy of six months or less for hospice to be covered by most insurance plans, including Medicare and Medicaid (5). An estimated 1.65 million people received hospice services in 2011 (6).

Philosophies of hospice and palliative care have many similarities. Both seek to palliate symptoms, improve quality of life and incorporate physical, psychological, spiritual and emotional care for both patients and families. As symptom palliation is a primary goal of hospice, hospice and palliative care services have often been linked within healthcare systems. Though long considered equivalent to hospice, palliative care is now emerging as a distinct system of care that is appropriately delivered any time between diagnosis and end-stages of chronic disease (7). In March of 2012, the American Society of Clinical Oncology issued a Provisional Clinical Opinion recommending that a combination of palliative and standard oncology care be considered in the early stage of illness for cancer patients with metastatic disease or high symptom burden (8).

Malnutrition is a prevalent and significant issue for advanced cancer patients. Nutrition impact symptoms and the nutritional decline experienced by oncology patients negatively impact QoL (9-11). Many medical nutrition therapy interventions that address these issues, such as those designed to manage digestive and oral symptoms in order to improve the enjoyment and tolerance of food intake, are indeed palliative in nature. Depending on the clinical circumstances, enteral and parenteral nutrition also may be considered palliative therapies, though they may be deemed aggressive or contraindicated interventions as patients near the end of life. Nutrition care is an integral element of palliative and hospice care. In these settings, the Registered Dietitian's (RD's) role is to provide medical nutrition therapy interventions to improve symptom management; educate patients, family members and the medical team on evidence-based nutrition interventions; and assist with decision-making regarding the use of artificial nutrition and hydration.

Nutritional Impact Symptoms and Quality of Life

Patients with advanced cancer experience a variety of symptoms that impact nutritional status and QoL. Cancer-induced malnutrition can impair mental and physical health, reduce performance status and diminish social well-being (11-13). A study of head and neck, esophageal, stomach and colorectal cancer patients found that QoL function scores were significantly lower in patients with weight loss and decreased dietary intake (9). For hospice patients with advanced cancer, nutrition screening scores significantly correlated with QoL, functional well-being and social-spiritual well-being scores (12). Malnourished patients with advanced colorectal cancer, as assessed by the Subjective Global Assessment (SGA), had diminished physical, role and cognitive functionality as well as diminished QoL (14). These same patients also experienced more fatigue and appetite loss.

Table 1: Prevalence of Some Nutrition Related Symptoms in Cancer Patients

	Study Population Characteristics				
	Advanced Cancer, Inpatients and Outpatients (26)	Palliative Treatment, Outpatients (27)	Advanced Cancer (72% of patients), Inpatients (28)	After 12 months of treatment, Outpatients (29)	Advanced Cancer (82% of patients), Inpatients (30)
Symptom	N = 218	N=571	N = 100*	N = 159	N = 45
Appetite Loss	61%*	18%	69%	16%	67%
Constipation	40%	15%	44%	14%	40%
Diarrhea	10%	6%	29%	22%	7%
Dysgeusia	33%	-	44%	13%	11%
Dysphagia	13%	-	15%	6%	7%
Early Satiety	50%	-	60%	-	31%
Nausea	28%	14%	65%	21%	22%
Sore Mouth	13%	-	22%	5%	13%
Vomiting	12%	6%	32%	4%	18%
Weight loss	56%	-	57%	-	49%
Xerostomia	66%	28%	59%	34%	27%

Estimates of the prevalence of malnutrition in advanced cancer patients vary depending on setting, screening methods used, diagnosis and severity of disease. Incidence of malnutrition in cancer patients with stage III and IV disease is significantly greater than in those with stage I or II disease (15). A study of Spanish patients in a variety of settings (e.g., hospital, outpatient, home care) indicated that 52% were moderately or severely malnourished (16). Malnutrition prevalence among hospitalized cancer patients ranges from 31% to 69%, depending on screening method and cancer type (17-19). Studies of non-hospitalized advanced cancer patients suggest that 33% to 68% were considered to be at nutrition risk or malnourished, while 13% to 63% were severely malnourished (12,20-21). In general, patients with stomach, esophageal, pancreatic, liver, lung and head and neck cancers are at greatest risk for malnutrition with pancreatic and gastric cancer patients experiencing the greatest weight loss (11,19,22). Diagnoses most commonly associated with weight loss and malnutrition in advanced cancer patients include gastrointestinal, larynx, gynecological, lung, hematological, and prostate cancers (16,20).

In addition to disease processes, factors that impact symptom burden, malnutrition and QoL include physiologic and psychosocial conditions, treatment modality and medications (11). In patients undergoing cancer treatment, typical physiologic symptoms with nutritional impact include oral issues (e.g., dysgeusia and parageusia, odynophagia, sore mouth, xerostomia), gastrointestinal issues (e.g., nausea, constipation, diarrhea), anorexia and pain (23). In a study of patients newly starting chemotherapy, a screening tool used to identify those with palliative care needs found that 26% of patients were referred to palliative care services for appetite loss, nausea and constipation (24). A 2007 review of symptom prevalence in advanced cancer patients showed that between 31% and 53% of patients studied experienced nausea, constipation, xerostomia, weight loss and anorexia, while 11% to 23% experienced diarrhea,

dysphagia, vomiting, sore mouth, dysgeusia and early satiety (25). Symptom prevalence rates from studies of advanced cancer patients, patients receiving palliative treatment and medical oncology patients at 1 year of treatment are shown in Table 1. In the studies of advanced cancer patients, prevalent symptoms include appetite loss, constipation, early satiety, weight loss and xerostomia (26-30).

Other causes of distress, including functional and psychosocial factors and pain, also may significantly influence nutritional status, intake and QoL (11,13). The reported prevalence of pain in advanced cancer patients varies widely. In one study of 505 newly diagnosed stage IV ambulatory patients, 33% reported some degree of pain, while pain was reported by 82% of hospitalized patients in a Kuwaiti cancer center (30-31). Pain and its treatment with opioids can result in decreased appetite, constipation and distress (32-33). Common psychosocial and functional symptoms include anxiety or nervousness, depressed mood, and confusion (25-26,34). Fatigue (also termed tiredness or weakness) is seen in 45% to 96% of patients (10,34) and is associated with weight loss, anorexia, and poor performance status (25).

Nutritional Screening and Assessment for Palliative and Hospice Care

Patients in all settings who receive palliative and hospice care should be screened to determine the need for nutrition intervention. The Patient-Generated Subjective Global Assessment (PG-SGA) is a modified version of the Subjective Global Assessment (SGA) that has been validated for use in the oncology population (35). The PG-SGA has long been considered a standard for the nutrition screening of cancer patients (36-37). Several other screening tools, discussed in Chapter 3, have been found to be appropriate for the oncology patient and are reviewed in the Evidence Analysis Library of the Academy of Nutrition and Dietetics. However, because of their unique needs, specific screening tools, in addition to the SGA and PG-SGA, have been evaluated for use with advanced cancer patients. These include the Malnutrition Universal Screening Tool (MUST), the Mini-Nutritional Assessment (MNA), and a modified version of Nutrition Risk Screening (NRS-2002) (38-41). Studies comparing the predictive value of the SGA and PG-SGA to anthropometric indicators in advanced cancer patients found that they correlate well with such measurements as Mid Upper Arm Circumference, Mid Upper Arm Muscle Circumference, Triceps Skin Fold and weight loss (38,42). The MNA has been found to correlate with baseline history of weight loss but not weight change (40). BMI appears to have limited usefulness as an indicator of nutritional status in advanced cancer patients. In one study, although BMI was correlated with the SGA, malnutrition was not established until values dropped below 20 kg/m^2 (38). In other studies, there was no consistent correlation between BMI and subjective screening methods, and patients with BMIs indicative of obesity were screened as malnourished or at risk of malnutrition (40,42).

Malnutrition is prevalent, significantly more likely to occur in patients with poorer performance status (43) and is thought to significantly contribute to functional decline (44). Patients in a home care hospice setting found to have poor nutritional status (using the PG-SGA) also scored lower for psychophysiological, functional and social/spiritual well-being as well as total QoL (45). The French Nutrition Oncology Study Group suggested that nutritional status be used to define cancer patients' clinical condition as it may more accurately reflect tolerance to treatment than performance status (44). Thus, functional and QoL assessments performed in palliative and hospice care settings may serve as an additional tool to identify patients who would benefit from nutritional intervention.

Nutrition care and goals for palliative care patients differ depending on whether palliative care is initiated early in the disease process, concurrent with curative treatment, versus later, when treatment options are limited or cure is no longer a goal. Thus, early palliative care nutrition may be as aggressive as early cancer treatment with an eye towards improving treatment outcome, body composition and physical function as well as symptom palliation. As the focus of care shifts from curative treatment to end of life or hospice care, nutrition goals appropriately become less aggressive, focusing primarily on comfort.

Accurate and unbiased patient assessment may be challenging, but is essential. Studies have shown poor agreement between palliative care patients and their providers regarding symptoms and QoL (46-47). In one such study, providers were found to have underestimated physical symptoms including anorexia, constipation, nausea, vomiting and diarrhea (47). Differences in symptom estimates were influenced by such factors as cancer diagnosis and previous history of drug abuse (47). In another study, patient and provider assessment of QoL were significantly different for all physical and functional domains assessed (46). In a qualitative exploration of patients' experience with cancer cachexia, a dominant theme was that of "lack of response from healthcare

professionals" regarding their weight loss (48). Patients wanted their weight loss acknowledged, desired information about its cause and were interested in interventions to manage weight change (48). A similar study sought to evaluate emotional distress experienced by family members and the need for improved communication when terminally ill cancer patients are no longer able to take oral nourishment (49). Of those who experienced a loved one becoming unable to take daily oral nourishment, 71% reported being distressed or very distressed, and 46% indicated the need for at least some improvement in professional practice (49). Given these examples, it is clear that assessing the needs and goals of patients and families is of primary importance if one is to provide high quality care for the advanced cancer patient receiving palliative or hospice care services.

Artificial Nutrition and Hydration

Patients, caregivers and healthcare professionals alike often consider the provision of food and fluids to be basic care at the end of life. The use of artificial nutrition and hydration (ANH) for this purpose has long been a complex and controversial topic. Factors which may influence the desire of patients and caregivers to employ ANH at the end of life include cultural and religious practices; perceived benefit versus burden; belief that it may prolong life or reduce suffering; and attitudes or advice of healthcare providers. For some patients, financial cost, insurance coverage and increased care needs play a large role in the decision. For others, religion or culture may play the greatest role in decision-making. Religious and cultural traditions vary as regards to the use of ANH at the end of life; some may hold that it is obligatory while others consider withholding or withdrawing it an acceptable practice (50). Given the prevailing principle of autonomy in the American bioethics culture as well as the increasing diversity of our population, the views of patients and families regarding ANH use at end of life may conflict with those of healthcare providers (51). For those less compelled by religious or cultural factors, lack of knowledge about all nutrition care options during the dying process may lead to unrealistic expectations of medical interventions. Here exists an important role for the RD: to provide objective and evidence-based education for patients, families and healthcare providers regarding the benefits and burdens of ANH at the end of life. Select resources for patient education are listed at the end of this chapter.

Artificial Nutrition

From 3% to 53% of end-stage cancer patients receive artificial nutrition in the last week of life (52). It is most commonly used when bowel obstruction precludes tolerance of an oral diet and in ovarian cancer patients (53). Perceived benefits of AN include its potential ability to prolong life, improve quality of life, reduce suffering, maintain weight or body composition and improve energy levels (54). In studies of advanced cancer patients undergoing palliative cancer treatments (e.g., chemotherapy, radiation therapy or both), those receiving parenteral nutrition (PN) had significantly more stable Body Mass Index (BMI), improved QoL, increased survival time and decreased gastrointestinal symptoms compared with patients only receiving intensive oral and enteral nutrition therapy

(55-56). In advanced head and neck cancer patients undergoing chemoradiotherapy, early initiation of enteral nutrition (EN) reduced weight loss, but when used long-term also was correlated with poorer performance status and QoL (57-58). Ovarian cancer patients with intestinal obstruction receiving PN had a median increased survival time of 4 weeks, but this was reduced in those patients receiving concurrent chemotherapy (59). For patients admitted to an inpatient hospice and palliative care unit in Taiwan, the use of ANH from either time of admission or two days before death had no significant influence on survival (60). Studies have indicated that both performance status and albumin are predictors of survival for advanced cancer patients using PN (61,53). In contrast with non-cancer patients, reviews of home AN use have suggested that use of PN in the setting of advanced cancer often has a positive impact on QoL (61-62). In a qualitative interview regarding the experience of home PN, patients and their families reported a sense of relief that nutritional needs were met and that this positively affected QoL, weight, energy and activity levels. Perceived negative effects included interference with sleep and restrictions on family activities and social contacts (63). In summary, the advantage of using AN in the advanced cancer population differs depending on diagnosis, whether treatment continues, prognosis, performance scores and patient and family perceptions. Table 2 illustrates various published recommendations for the use of AN in this stage of care.

Artificial Hydration
As with AN, a variety of factors influence the perspectives of patients, caregivers and healthcare providers (HCPs) regarding the use of AH during palliative and end-of-life care. The provision of fluids is often viewed as meeting a "basic human need" (69). Patients and families commonly believe that the use of AH will improve quality and length of life, reduce discomfort, and promote a sense of well being (70,53). Studies of Japanese community members found that 38% to 43% of those surveyed believed that AH and AN should continue until death, while 52% to 62% indicated they would want AH for the purpose of prolonging life (53). In a review of advanced directives of elderly Swiss cancer patients, 78% indicated a desire for AH (71). Views of HCPs on including AH in end-of-life care vary considerably. A review of several studies suggested that from 22% to 100% of HCPs recommend using AH, while up to 75% recommend against it (53). Persons influencing their support for AH at the end of life included attending physicians (or superiors) (45%) and patients (38%).

Terminal dehydration is thought to cause or contribute to symptoms of confusion, opioid toxicity, constipation, dry mouth, and thirst (71). It has been argued that provision of hydration would assist in preventing or relieving these problems while allowing providers a means to maintain the patient relationship and continue attempts to improve QoL (69). In contrast, opponents of AH argue that it may cause pain, is intrusive and may increase symptoms such as vomiting, ascites, edema, and pulmonary congestion (69). Studies of the use of AH at the end of life have focused on evaluating whether it improves or worsens symptoms, discomfort and overall QoL. A 2008 Cochrane Review evaluated two randomized

controlled trials and three prospective controlled trials of AH in adult palliative care patients with advanced cancer (72). In these studies, one found improvements in sedation and myoclonus as well as in the total score for target symptoms (e.g., sedation, fatigue, hallucinations, myoclonus). Authors questioned the reported result of improvement of chronic nausea in another study, and found no significant differences in other outcomes evaluated in the remainder of the studies. Of three studies not included in this review, one found fewer clinical signs of dehydration but more ascites in the AH group, another found increased intestinal drainage but no difference in ascites and pleural drainage, and a third found no differences in delirium and agitation (53). A study presented at the ASCO 2012 Annual Meeting evaluated the effect of AH on hospice patients with advanced cancer and found no differences between hydration and placebo groups in dehydration and other symptoms including delirium, QoL and survival (73). Though poorly or not at all evidenced, the following are suggested detriments to the use of AH at the end of life: that it creates a barrier between patient and family; promotes false hope or denial of the terminal nature of disease; increases urine output with subsequent difficulties managing same; and increases risk of infections (71).

When palliative care accompanies chemotherapy and/or radiation therapy, addressing hydration needs is crucial for a variety of reasons. First, these treatments can cause a variety of side effects that may lead to dehydration and subsequently impact patients' overall well-being. Nausea, vomiting, dysgeusia, diarrhea, dysphagia and the presence of an ostomy are all factors that can increase risk for dehydration. Certain chemotherapies are nephrotoxic, and adequate hydration is imperative if patients wish to continue receiving treatment (74). Dehydration also contributes to morbidity and carries a financial cost to patients continuing with curative or palliative therapy, as it is often associated with unplanned clinic and emergency room visits (74). In this case, palliation involves managing dehydration as best as possible to allow patients to continue treatment and to alleviate symptoms. When the focus of care shifts to comfort, treatment of dehydration should be focused solely on palliation of symptoms resulting from it.

Whether or not to use ANH is a complex topic in the setting of palliative and hospice care. Its use may evoke a sense of hope and comfort for patients and caregivers. HCPs may be hesitant to recommend it due to concern about its potential complications. Differing views of its use, whether between patients and their families or HCPs, can lead to challenging discussions about end-of-life care. Recommendations regarding the use of ANH should be individualized for each patient, carefully considering the patient's disease and current physical condition, symptoms, care setting, religious- and cultural-based preferences and the benefit versus burden of this treatment modality.

Summary
Palliative care, though once considered the same as hospice care, is emerging as a distinct care process for persons with life-threatening illnesses such as cancer. Patients with advanced cancer often have a

Table 2: Guidelines for the Use of Nutritional Support in Advanced Cancer Patients

Guideline	Description	Summary of Recommendations	Source
Enteral/Parenteral Nutrition: Palliative or terminal nutrition in adults with progressive cancer	Enteral Nutrition Palliative care, Head/Neck CA: Terminal stage CA: Parenteral Nutrition Malignant bowel obstruction, Other food intolerances Karnofsky < 50%, or performance status > 2	May slow nutritional deficiency, prevent dehydration, improve QoL Gastrostomy is not recommended due to risk of complications May slow nutritional deficiency, prevent dehydration, improve QoL Use not justified	French National Federation of Cancer Centers, 2001 (64)

Parenteral Nutrition: Advanced cancer	Enteral nutrition not feasible; Intestinal obstruction, short bowel syndrome, malabsorption	Trial of PN offered if:
		1) Death expected from starvation/malnutrition before disease progression
		2) Expected survival of months, PN to be at least 6 weeks
		3) High QoL
		4) Adequate functional status, home environment to support home PN:
		    a) Problems manageable at home or with out-patient services
		    b) Karnofsky > 50%
		    c) Caregiver available to assist
		    d) Clinical, laboratory follow up are easily accessed
		    e) Patient/caregiver cognitively, psychologically capable of home administration
		    f) Home environment clean, safe, free of hazards
			Capital Health Home Parenteral Nutrition Program – Edmonton, 2005 (65)

Enteral/Parenteral Nutrition: Adults during anti-cancer treatment, HSCT	During palliative care	Use is rarely indicated	ASPEN, 2009 (66)
Parenteral Nutrition: Non-surgical Oncology	Patients with weight loss, decreased nutrient intake: Patients with intestinal failure:	Probable benefit for use of "supplemental" PN PN should be offered if: 1) Enteral nutrition is inadequate to maintain nutrition status 2) Expected survival is > 2-3 months 3) PN expected to stabilize or improve QoL, performance status 4) Patient desires PN for nutrition support	ESPEN, 2009 (67)
Parenteral Nutrition: Non-surgical oncology	Incurable patients with severely impaired intestinal absorption:	PN should be initiated if: 1) Enteral nutrition inadequate to maintain nutritional status 2) Expected survival is > 4 weeks 3) PN expected to stabilize or improve QoL 4) Patient desires PN for nutrition support	German Association for Nutritional Medicine, Working Group for Developing Guidelines for parenteral nutrition, 2009 (68)

significant symptom burden that impacts well-being and QoL. More and more often, palliative care services are being initiated soon after cancer diagnosis and concurrently with curative treatment to assist patients with maintaining an optimum QoL. As the focus of care shifts from curative intent to the provision of comfort at the end of life, palliative care continues as hospice care. Throughout this continuum of care, there exists a role for the RD to provide medical nutrition therapy that aims to manage symptoms and improve QoL. As part of the palliative and hospice care teams, the RD can be instrumental in educating patients, caregivers and HCPs and in facilitating discussion about nutrition care options, including the use of ANH.

Patient Education Resources

http://www.caringinfo.org/files/public/brochures/ArtificialNutritionAndHydration.pdf

http://www.cancer.gov/cancertopics/cancerlibrary/epeco/selfstudy/module-11-pdf pp.20-21

http://www.caregiver.org/caregiver/jsp/content_node.jsp?nodeid=399

http://www.americanhospice.org/articles-mainmenu-8/caregiving-mainmenu-10/48-artificial-nutrition-and-hydration-beneficial-or-harmful

References

1. Definition: palliate, in Merriam Webster's online dictionary. Available at: http://www.merriam-webster.com/dictionary/palliate. Accessed May 29, 2012.

2. World Health Organization. WHO definition of palliative care. Available at: http://www.who.int/cancer/palliative/en/. Accessed May 6, 2012.

3. National Consensus Project for Quality Palliative Care (2009). *Clinical Practice Guidelines for Quality Palliative Care, Second Edition.* http://www.nationalconsensusproject.org. Accessed May 6, 2012

4. Hospice Foundation of America. About hospice: What is hospice? Available at: http://www.hospicefoundation.org/whatishospice. Accessed May 29,2012.

5. National Cancer Institute. Coping with cancer: Preparing for the end of life – Hospice. Available at: http://www.cancer.gov/cancertopics/factsheet/Support/hospice. Accessed May 29,2012.

6. National Hospice and Palliative Care Association. NHPCO Facts and Figures: Hospice Care in America. 2012 Edition. Available at: http://www.nhpco.org/sites/default/files/public/Statistics_Research/2012_Facts_Figures.pdf Released November 2012. Accessed January 20, 2013.

7. Reville B, Axelrod D, Maury R. Palliative care for the cancer patient. *Prim Care.* 2009;36(4):781-810.

8. Smith TJ, Temin S, Alesi ER, et al. American Society of Clinical Oncology Provisional Clinical Opinion: The Integration of palliative care into standard oncology care. *J Clin Onc.* 2012; 30(8):880-887.

9. Ravasco P, Monteiro-Grillo I, Vidal PM, Camilo ME. Cancer: disease and nutrition are key determinants of patients' quality of life. *Support Care Cancer.* 2004;12(4):246-252.

10. van den Beuken-van Everdingen MHJ, de Rijke JM, Kessels AG, Schouten HC, van Kleef M, Patijin J. Quality of life and non-pain symptoms in patients with cancer. *J Pain Symptom Manage.* 2009;38(2)216-233.

11. Van Cutsem E, Arends J. The causes and consequences of cancer associated malnutrition. *Eur J Oncol Nurs.* 2005;9(Suppl2):S51-S63

12. Shahmoradi N, Kandiah M, Peng LS. Impact of nutritional status on quality of life of advanced cancer patients in hospice home care. *Asian Pac J Cancer Prev.* 2009;10(6):1003-1010.

13. Caro MMM, Laviano A, Pichard C. Impact of nutrition on quality of life during cancer. *Curr Opin Clin Nutr Metab Care.* 2007;10(4):480-487.

14. Thoresen L. Nutrition care in cancer patients. Nutrition assessment: diagnostic criteria and the association to survival and health-related quality of life in patients with advanced colorectal carcinoma. Doctoral theses at NTNU, 2012:82. ISBN 978-82-471-3438-2 (electronic version).

15. Ravasco P, Monteiro-Grillo I, Vidal PM, Camilo ME. Nutritional deterioration in cancer: the role of disease and diet. *Clin Onc.* 2003;15(8):433-450.

16. Segura A, Pardo J, Jara C, et al. An epidemiological evaluation of the prevalence of malnutrition in Spanish patients with locally advanced or metastatic cancer. *Clin Nutr.* 2005;24(5):801-814.

17. Pirlich M, Schutz T, Norman K, et al. The German hospital malnutrition study. *Clin Nutr.* 2006;25(4):563-572.

18. Kwang AY, Kandiah M. Objective and subjective nutritional assessment of patients with cancer in palliative care. *Amer J Hosp Pall Care.* 2010;27(2):117-126.

19. Wie G-A, Cho Y-A, Kim S-Y, Kim S-M, Bae J-M, Joung H. Prevalence and risk factors of malnutrition among cancer patients according to tumor location and stage in the National Cancer Center in Korea. *Nutr.* 2010;26(3):263-268.

20. Orrevall Y, Tishelman C, Permert T, Cederholm T. Nutritional support and risk status among cancer patients in palliative home care services. *Supp Care Cancer.* 2009;17(2):153-161.

21. Slaviero K, Read J, Clarke S, Rivory L. A baseline nutrition assessment in advanced cancer patients receiving palliative chemotherapy. *Nutr Cancer.* 2003; 46(2):148-157.

22. von Meyenfeldt M. Cancer-associated malnutrition: an introduction. *Eur J Onc Nurs.* 2005;9(Suppl2):S35-S38.

23. Tong H, Isenring E, Yates P. The prevalence of nutrition impact symptoms and their relationship to quality of life and clinical outcomes in medical oncology patients. *Support Care Cancer.* 2009;17(1):83-90.

24. Morita T, Fujimoto K, Namba M, et al. Palliative care needs of cancer outpatients receiving chemotherapy: an audit of a clinical screening project. *Support Care Cancer.* 2008;16(1):101-107.

25. Teunissen SC, Wesker W, Kruitwagen C, de Haes HC, Voest EE, de Graeff A. Symptom prevalence in patients with incurable cancer: a systematic review. *J Pain Symptom Manage.* 2007;34(1):94-104.

26. Kirkova J, Walsh D, Rybicki L, et al. Symptom severity and distress in advanced cancer. *Palliat Med.* 2010; 24(3):330-339.

27. van den Beuken-van Everdingen MH, de Rijke JM, Kessels AG, Schouten HC, van Kleep M, Patijn J. Quality of life and non-pain symptoms in patients with cancer. *J Pain Symptom Manage.* 2009;38(2)216-233.

28. Halawi R, Aldin ES, Baydoun A, et al. Physical symptom profile for adult cancer inpatients at a Lebanese cancer unit. *Eur J Intern.* 2012;23(8):e185-e189. doi: 10.1016/j.ejim.2012.08.018.

29. Tong H, Isenring E, Yates P. The prevalence of nutrition impact symptoms and their relationship to quality of life and clinical outcomes in medical oncology patients. *Support Care Cancer.* 2009;17(1):83-90.

30. Alshemmari S, Ezzat H, Samir Z, Sajnani K, Alsirafy S. Symptom burden in hospitalized patients with cancer in Kuwait and the need for palliative care. *Am J Hosp Palliat Care.* 2010; 27(7):446-449.

31. Isaac T, O Stuver S, Davis RB, et al. Incidence of severe pain in newly diagnosed ambulatory patients with stage IV cancer. *Pain Research & Management.* 2012;17(5):347-352.

32. Dhingra L, Shuk E, Grossman B, et al. A qualitative study to explore psychological distress and illness burden associated with opioid-induced constipation in cancer patients with advanced disease. *Palliat Med.* 2013; 27(5):447-456.

33. Rodriguez RF, Bravo LE, Castro F, et al. Incidence of weak opioids adverse events in the management of cancer pain: a double-blind comparative trial. *J Palliat Med.* 2007;10(1):56-60.

34. Cheung WY, Le LW, Zimmermann C. Symptom clusters in patients with advanced cancers. *Support Care Cancer.* 2009;17(9):1223-1230.

35. Ottery F. Definition of standardized nutritional assessment and interventional pathways in oncology. Nutrition.1996;12(1 Suppl):S15-19.

36. Wojtaszek CA, Kochis LM, Cunningham RS. Nutritional screening and assessment: an overview. In: Integrating nutrition into your cancer program. *Oncology Issues.* 2002;17(2):S11-12.

37. Bauer J, Capra S, Ferguson F. Use of the Patient-generated subjective global assessment (PG-SGA) as a nutrition assessment tool in patients with cancer. *Eur J Clin Nutr.* 2002;56(8):779-785.

38. Thoresen L, Fjeldstad I, Krogstad K, Kaasa S, Falkmer UG. Nutritional status of patients with advanced cancer: the value of using the subjective global assessment of nutritional status as a screening tool. *Palliat Med.* 2002;16(1):33-42.

39. Isenring E, Cross G, Daniels L, Kellett E, Koczwara B. Validity of the malnutrition screening tool as an effective predictor of nutritional risk in oncology patients receiving chemotherapy. *Support Care Cancer.* 2006;14(11):1152-1156.

40. Slaviero KA, Read JA, Clarke SJ, Rivory LP. Baseline nutritional assessment in advanced cancer patients receiving palliative chemotherapy. *Nutr Cancer.* 2003;46(2):148-157.

41. Orrevall Y, Tishelman C, Permert J, Cederholm T. The use of artificial nutrition among cancer patients enrolled in palliative home care services. *Palliative Medicine.* 2009;23(6):556-564.

42. Kwang AY, Kandiah M. Objective and subjective nutritional assessment of patients with cancer in palliative care. *Am J Hospice & Palliative Medicine.* 2010;27(2):117-126.

43. Mateus C, Cacheux W, Lemarie E. Relationship between performance status and malnutrition in non-selected cancer patients: A nation-wide one-day survey. *J Clin Oncol.* 2007; ASCO Annual Meeting Proceedings Part 1. 25(18S):9126.

44. Cessot A, Hebuterne X, Coriat R. Defining the clinical condition of cancer patients: it is time to switch from performance status to nutritional status. *Support Care Cancer.* 2011;19(7):869-870.

45. Shahmoradi N, Kandiah M, Peng LS. Impact of nutritional status on the quality of life of advanced cancer patients in hospice home care. *Asian Pac J Cancer Prev.* 2009;10(6):1003-1009.

46. Petersen MA, Larsen H, Pedersen L, Sonne N, Groenvold M. Assessing health-related quality of life in palliative care: comparing patient and physician assessments. *Eur J Cancer*. 2006;42(8)1159-1166.

47. Laugsand EA, Sprangers MAG, Bjordal K, Skorpen F, Kaasa S, Klepstad P. Health care providers underestimate symptom intensities of cancer patients: a multicenter European study. *Health QOL Outcomes*. 2010;8:104-117. doi:10.1186/1477-7525-8-104

48. Reid J, Mckenna HP, Fitzsimmons D, McCance TV. An exploration of the experience of cancer cachexia: what patients and their families want from healthcare professionals. *Eur J Cancer Care*. 2010;19(5):682-689.

49. Yamagishi A, Morita T, Miyashita M, Sato K, Tsuneto S, Shima Y. The care strategy for families of terminally ill cancer patients who become unable to take nourishment orally: recommendations from a nationwide survey of bereaved family members' experiences. *J Pain Symptom Manage*. 2010;40(5):671-683.

50. Geppert CMA, Andrews MR, Druyan ME. Ethical issues in artificial nutrition and hydration: a review. *J Parenter Enteral Nutr*. 2010;34(1):79-88.

51. Maillet JO, Potter RL, Heller L. Position of the American Dietetic Association: Ethical and legal issues in nutrition, hydration, and feeding. *J Am Diet Assoc*. 2002;102(5)716-726.

52. Raijmakers NJH, Fradsham S, van Zuylen L, Mayland C, Ellershaw JE, van der Heide A. Variation in attitudes towards artificial hydration at the end of life: a systematic literature review. *Curr Opin Support Palliat Care*. 2011;5(3):265-272.

53. Soo I and Gramlich L. Use of parenteral nutrition in patients with advanced cancer. *Appl Physiol Nutr Metab*. 2008;33(1):102-106.

54. Suter PM, Rogers J, Strack C. Artificial nutrition and hydration for the terminally ill. *Home Healthc Nurse*. 2008;26(1):23-29.

55. Shang E, Weiss C, Post S, Kaehler G. The influence of early parenteral nutrition on quality of life and body composition in patients with advanced cancer. *J Parenter Enteral Nutr*. 2006;30(3):222-230.

56. Hasenberg T, Essenbreis M, Herold A, Post S, Shang E. Early supplementation of parenteral nutrition is capable of improving quality of life, chemotherapy-related toxicity and body composition in patients with advanced colorectal carcinoma undergoing palliative treatment: results from a prospective, randomized clinical trial. *Colorectal Dis*. 2010 ct;12(10 Online):e190-9. doi: 10.1111/j.1463-1318.2009.02111.x.

57. Morton RP, Crowder VL, Mawdsley R, Ong E, Izzard M. Elective gastrostomy, nutritional status and quality of life in advanced head and neck cancer patients receiving chemoradiotherapy. *ANZ J Surg*. 2009;79(10):713-718.

58. Wiggenraad RGJ, Flierman L, Goosens A, et al. Prophylactic gastrostomy placement and early tube feeding may limit loss of weight during chemoradiotherapy for advanced head and neck cancer, a preliminary study. *Clin Otolaryngol*. 2007;32(5):384-390.

59. Brard L, Weitzen S, Strubel-Lagan SL, et al. The effect of total parenteral nutrition on the survival of terminally ill ovarian cancer patients. *Gynecol Oncol*. 2006;103(1):176-180.

60. Chiu T-Y, Hu W-Y, Chuang R-B, Chen C-Y. Nutrition and hydration for terminal cancer patients in Taiwan. *Support Care Cancer*. 2002;10(8):630-636.

61. Dy SM. Enteral and parenteral nutrition in terminally ill cancer patients: a review of the literature. *Am J Hosp Palliat Care*. 2006;23(5):369-377.

62. Winkler MF. Quality of life in adult home parenteral nutrition patients. *J Parenter Enteral Nutr*. 2005;29(3)162-170.

63. Orrevall Y, Tishelman C, Permert J. Home parenteral nutrition: a qualitative interview study of the experiences of advanced cancer patients and their families. *Clin Nutr*. 2005;24(6):961-970.

64. Bachmann P, Marti-Massoud M, Blanc-Vincent MP, et al. Summary version of the standards, opinions, options and recommendations for palliative or terminal nutrition in adults with progressive cancer (2001). *Br J Cancer*. 2003;89(Supp1):S107-S110.

65. Mirhosseini N, Fainsinger RL, Baracos V. Pareneral nutrition in advanced cancer: indications and clinical practice guidelines. *J Palliat Med*. 2005;8(5):914-918.

66. August DA, Huhmann MB, American Society for Parenteral and Enteral Nutrition (A.S.P.E.N.) Board of Directors. A.S.P.E.N. clinical guidelines: nutrition support therapy during adult anticancer treatment and in hematopoietic cell transplantation. *J Parent Enteral Nutr*. 2009;33(5):472-500.

67. Bozetti F, Arends J, Lundholm K, Micklewright A, Zurcher G, Muscaritoli M. ESPEN guidelines on parenteral nutrition: non-surgical oncology. *Clin Nutr*. 2009;28(4):445-454.

68. Arends J, Zuercher G, Dossett A, et al. Non-surgical oncology – guidelines on parenteral nutrition, Chapter 19. *GMS Med Sci*. 2009;7:1612-1625

69. Dev R, Dalal S, Bruera E. Is there a role for parenteral nutrition or hydration at the end of life? *Curr Opin Support Palliat Care*. 2012; 6(3):365-370.

70. Cohen MZ, Torres-Vigil I, Burbach BE, de la Rosa A, Bruera E. The meaning of parenteral hydration to family caregivers and patients with advanced cancer receiving hospice care. *J Pain Symptom Manage*. 2012;43(5):855-865.

71. Bavin L. Artificial rehydration in the last days of life: is it beneficial? *Int J Palliat Nurs*. 2007;13(9):445-449.

72. Good P, Cavenagh J, Mather M, Ravenscroft P. Medically assisted hydration for adult palliative care patients. Cochrane Database of Systematic Reviews. 2008; Issue 2. Art no: CD006273. DOI: 10.1002/14651858.CD006274.pub2.

73. Dalal S, Hui D, Torres-Vigil I, et al. Parenteral hydration (PH) in advanced cancer patients: a multicenter, double-blind, placebo-controlled randomized trial. ASCO 2012; *J Clin Oncol* 30, 2012 (suppl; abstr 9025).

74. Price KAR. Hydration in cancer patients. *Curr Opin in Support Palliat Care*. 2010;4(4):276-280.

APPENDIX 1: Public Health Guidelines for Cancer Prevention and Survivorship

	Cancer Prevention		Cancer Survivorship	
	American Institute for Cancer Research[1]	World Health Organization[2,3]	American Cancer Society[4]	National Comprehensive Cancer Network[5]
BODY WEIGHT	Be as lean as possible within the normal range of body weight. Maintain body weight within the normal range from age 21. Avoid weight gain and increases in waist circumference throughout adulthood.	Achieve energy balance and a healthy weight. Maintain weight such that BMI is in the range of 18.5- 25 kg/m2 and avoid weight gain during adulthood.	Achieve and maintain a healthy weight (BMI between 18.5-25 kg/m2). After cancer treatment, weight gain or loss should be managed with a combination of diet, physical activity and behavioral strategies.	Maintain a healthy weight. Weight gain and being overweight during cancer treatment and survivorship may increase risk of recurrence and lower odds for survival.
PLANT-BASED DIET	Choose a plant-based diet rich in a variety of vegetables and fruits, pulses (legumes) and minimally processed starchy staple foods.	Increase consumption of fruits and vegetables, legumes and whole grains and nuts.	Achieve a dietary pattern that is high in vegetables, fruits, and whole grains.	Eat a variety of foods. Create a plate that is ½ cooked or raw vegetables, ¼ lean protein, and ¼ whole grains.
VEGETABLE & FRUIT	Eat five or more portions (14 oz or 400 grams) of a variety of non-starchy vegetables and of fruits daily.	Increase consumption of fruits and vegetables, legumes and whole grains and nuts. Consume at least 400g of total fruits and vegetables per day.	Achieve a dietary pattern that is high in vegetables and fruits. Eat at least 2.5 cups of vegetables and fruits each day.	Eat a minimum of 5 servings of fruits and vegetables per day. Use plant-based seasonings such as herbs and spices.
BREADS, GRAINS & CEREALS	Eat relatively unprocessed cereals (grains) and/or pulses (legumes) with every meal.	Increase consumption of fruits and vegetables, legumes and whole grains and nuts.	Choose whole grains instead of refined grain products. Eat plenty of high-fiber foods.	Go for whole grains. Opt for high-fiber breads and cereals. Avoid refined foods and those high in sugar.
ANIMAL PRODUCTS	People who eat red meat should limit intake to less than 18 oz per week, very little, if any, to be processed.	Moderate consumption of preserved meat (sausage, salami, bacon, ham) and red meat (beef, pork, lamb). Poultry and fish are preferable.	Limit intake of processed and red meats. Avoid cooking these and other high-fat sources of protein at high temperatures.	Choose lean protein such as fish, poultry and tofu. Limit red meat and processed meats. Consume fatty fish at least twice a week. Keep dairy low-fat. Select skim milk, low fat yogurt and reduced fat cheeses.
DIETARY FAT	Consume energy-dense foods sparingly. Certain plant oils, nuts, and seeds are important sources of fat and nutrients and should not be avoided.	Limit energy intake from fat and shift fat consumption away from saturated fats to unsaturated fats. Eliminate trans-fat consumption.	Limit the intake of foods and beverages high in fat and with added sugar to promote healthy weight control.	Eat fatty fish, such as salmon, sardines and canned tuna at least twice a week. Walnuts, canola oil, and flaxseeds are additional sources of healthy dietary fat.
PROCESSED FOODS & REFINED SUGAR	Eat relatively unprocessed cereals (grains) and/or pulses (legumes) with every meal. Limit refined starchy foods. Avoid sugary drinks.	Limit the intake of free sugars.	Limit the intake of foods and beverages high in fat and with added sugar to promote healthy weight control.	Avoid refined foods and those high in sugar.
SALT & SODIUM	Limit consumption of processed foods with added salt to ensure an intake of less than 6 g (2.4 g sodium) per day.	Limit salt (sodium) consumption from all sources and ensure that salt is iodized.	No recommendations provided.	No recommendations provided.
ALCOHOL	If consumed at all, limit alcoholic drinks to no more than two drinks a day for men and one for women.	Consumption of alcoholic beverages is not recommended. If consumed, do not exceed 20g per day.	Alcoholic drinks up to one or two drinks per day (for women and men, respectively) can lower the risk of heart disease, but higher levels may increase the risk of specific cancers. It is important for the health care provider to tailor advice on alcohol consumption to the individual survivor.	Limit alcohol consumption. Men should have no more than two drinks per day and women no more than one drink per day.
SUPPLEMENTS	For those who follow the above recommendations, dietary supplements are not recommended for reducing cancer risk. Aim to meet nutrient needs through diet alone. Talk with your health care team about supplements for other specific health reasons.	No recommendations provided.	Before supplements are prescribed or taken, all attempts should be made to obtain needed nutrients through dietary sources. Supplements should be considered only if a nutrient deficiency is biochemically or clinically demonstrated.	Food, not supplements, is the best source of vitamins and minerals. There is no evidence that dietary supplements provide the same anti-cancer benefits as fruits and vegetables and some high-dose supplements may actually increase cancer risk.
PHYSICAL ACTIVITY	Be moderately physically active for at least 30 minutes every day. As fitness improves, aim for 60 minutes or more of moderate, or 30 minutes or more of vigorous physical activity every day. Limit sedentary habits like watching television.	Engage in regular physical activity. Adults aged 18 to 64 should accumulate at least 150 minutes of moderate-intensity aerobic activity or at least 75 minutes of vigorous aerobic activity throughout the week. Strength training should be done at least 2 days per week.	Engage in regular physical activity. Avoid inactivity and return to normal daily activities as soon as possible following diagnosis. Aim to exercise at least 150 minutes per week. Include strength training at least 2 days per week.	Engage in at least 30 minutes of moderate-intensity activity on 5 days per week or more, or at least 20 minutes of vigorous-intensity activity on 3 days or more. In addition, perform strength training at least 2 days per week.

(Continued) |

"Public Health Guidelines for Cancer Prevention and Survivorship" was developed by Colleen K. Spees, PhD, MEd, RD and Elizabeth Grainger, PhD, RD, with thanks to Anna Maria Bittoni

References

1. World Cancer Research Fund/American Institute for Cancer Research. *Food, Nutrition, Physical Activity and the Prevention of Cancer: a Global Perspective.* Washington DC: AICR;2007.

2. Key TJ, Schatzkin A, Willett WC, Allen NE, Spencer EA, Travis RC. Diet, nutrition and the prevention of cancer. *Public Health Nutr.* 2004 Feb;7(1A):187-200.

3. World Health Organization. Global Strategy on Diet, Physical Activity and Health. Available at: http://www.who.int/dietphysicalactivity/diet/en/index.html. Accessed September 3, 2013.

4. Rock, CL, Doyle C, Demark-Wahnefried W, et al. Nutrition and physical activity guidelines for cancer survivors. *CA Cancer J Clin.* 2012;62(4):243-74.

5. National Comprehensive Cancer Network. Patient and Caregiver Resources. http://www.nccn.com/index.php?option=com_content&view=article&id=129:nutrition-for-cancer-survivors&catid=66. Accessed September 16, 2013.

APPENDIX 2: Assessing Performance Status

The Karnofsky Performance Status Scale and the Eastern Cooperative Oncology Group (ECOG) grade are used to assess performance status. Developed in 1948 by David A Karnofsky (1914-1969), MD and medical oncologist, the Karnofsky Performance Status Scale assigns a percent rating (from 0 to 100%) that estimates functional status of activity, work and self-care. In 1982 the Eastern Cooperative Oncology Group (ECOG) developed a performance status tool for the assessment of ways cancer may impact the daily living abilities of each patient. Each grade of this tool represents a different reference for describing performance status.

Table 1: Karnofsky Performance Status Scale

KARNOFSKY PERFORMANCE STATUS SCALE: percent ratings		
	Percent	
Able to independently carry on normal activity and work	100	No functional complaints and no evidence of disease
	90	Able to carry on normal activity; minor signs or symptoms of disease
	80	Normal activity with increased effort; some signs or symptoms of disease
Unable to work outside of the home (may be able to work from home); able to live at home with some assistance; able to independently provide personal needs	70	Provides self-care but unable to complete normal activity or be active
	60	Provides self-care but requires assistance on occasion
	50	Requires considerable assistance and frequent medical care
Unable to provide self-care; requires institutional or hospice care (at home or in a hospice center); disease may be progressing rapidly and prognosis for recovery is poor	40	Disabled; requires special care and assistance
	30	Severaly disabled; hospital admission or hospice care (at home or in a hospice center) is indicated but death is not imminent
	20	Very sick; active supportive treatment is necessary, whether in a hospital, hospice center, or via in-home hospice care
	10	Moribund; fatal processes progressing rapidly
	0	Dead

Source: Karnofsky D, Abelmann W, Craver L, Burchenal J. The use of nitrogen mustard in the palliative treatment of cancer. *Cancer.* 1948;1:634-656.

Table 2: ECOG Reference Status

ECOG Grade	Reference Status
0	Fully active, able to carry on all pre-disease activities without restrictions (KS 90-100)
1	Restricted in physically strenuous activity but ambulatory and able to carry out work of a light and sedentary nature (KS 70-80)
2	Ambulatory and capable of all self-care but unable to carry out any work activities. Out of bed over 50% of the time (KS 50-60)
3	Capable of only limited self-care, confined to bed or chair >50% of waking hours (KS 30-40)
4	Completely disabled, cannot carry on any self-care, totally confined to bed or chair (KS 10-20)
5	Dead

Source: Oken MM, Creech RH, Tormey DC, et al. Toxicity and response criteria of the Eastern Cooperative Oncology Group. *Am J Clin Oncol.* 1982;5:649-655. http://ecog.dfci.harvard.edu/general/perf_stat.html Accessed November 3, 2012.

APPENDIX 3: Diet and Nutrition Guidelines after Intestinal Surgery

After your surgery, your body will need time to adapt to a regular diet. By adjusting your food choices, you can help your body heal and prevent problems such as nausea, abdominal cramping, and diarrhea. These problems are most common in the first few weeks after surgery.

Most people are able to resume a normal diet after the first 4 to 6 weeks. This handout will provide specific diet guidelines as well as examples of meals to choose in the first 4 to 6 weeks. It will also discuss how to transition to a regular diet.

General diet recommendations for the first 4 to 6 weeks

1. **Eat small, frequent meals.** Aim for 5 to 6 small meals per day. See the sample menus for examples of meals.
2. **Chew foods well.** Chewing foods well will help you better absorb the nutrients. It will also prevent foods from causing a blockage or obstruction as they pass through your intestine.
3. **Choose a high protein food at each meal or snack.** Protein helps your body heal after surgery. Examples of high protein foods are tender meat, poultry, fish, eggs, tofu, cheese, milk, soy milk, yogurt, and smooth peanut butter.

4. **Avoid high fiber foods.** Dietary fiber refers to the part of plant foods that cannot be digested by your intestines. It is important to avoid both types of fiber, insoluble fiber and soluble fiber.
    a. **<u>Avoid</u> foods high in insoluble fiber.** Insoluble fiber makes the intestines contract and may move food through your intestines too quickly, which may interfere with wound healing. Foods high in insoluble fiber include skins of fruits, stringy fibers from raw vegetables, seeds, and whole grain breads or cereals.
    b. **<u>Limit</u> foods high in soluble fiber.** Soluble fiber absorbs fluid in your digestive tract and thickens the stool. Thicker output will increase the pressure in your intestine and may interfere with wound healing. Limit food sources of soluble fiber including rice, applesauce, and bananas.
    c. **<u>Limit</u> total fiber intake to less than 20 grams of fiber per day.** Here are some examples of fiber content of well-tolerated foods:
       • 1 banana = 3 grams fiber
       • ½ cup applesauce = 2 grams fiber
       • ½ cup rice = 0-2 grams fiber
5. **See the table below for specific examples of foods to choose.**

Foods to choose and foods to avoid after intestinal surgery

The following table lists foods that are best tolerated after intestinal surgery. Use this table to guide your food choices.

Food Categories	Well-tolerated foods	Poorly tolerated foods (avoid for the first 4 to 6 weeks) *Note: Reintroduce these foods slowly. You may have difficulty tolerating some of these foods long-term.*
Fruits	Bananas	All raw, fresh fruits except bananas
	Canned fruit such as applesauce, peaches, pears, and other canned fruit without skins	All canned fruits with skins, seeds, or membranes
	All canned fruit should be packed in juice or water (not heavy syrup)	All dried fruits (raisins, prunes, apricots, etc.)
Vegetables	Tender cooked and canned vegetables without seeds or skins such as carrots, spinach, or winter squash Peeled potatoes	All raw vegetables Cooked vegetables with large seeds such as tomato, zucchini, or cucumber Corn Potato skins
Starches	**Hot Cereals** Products with <u>less than 3 grams of fiber</u> such as plain cream of rice, cream of wheat, grits, or instant oatmeal **Cold Cereals** Products with <u>less than 3 grams of fiber</u> per serving such as Cheerios®, Corn Flakes®, or Rice Krispies® **Breads, pastas, and potatoes** Bread with less than 2 grams of fiber per slice (white bread, potato bread, seedless Italian, corn tortilla, etc) Plain bagels or dinner rolls (no seeds) Pasta: plain macaroni, spaghetti, egg noodles Potatoes (no skin), baked or mashed Rice, white Saltines or other low fiber cracker	**Hot Cereals** Cereals with raisins, nuts, seeds, coconut, or other dried fruits **Cold Cereals** Whole wheat or wheat bran cereals; Cereals with raisins, nuts, seeds, coconut, or other dried fruits **Breads, pastas, and potatoes** Whole grain or multigrain breads Breads and cereals with raisins, nuts, seeds, coconut, or other dried fruits Whole grain pastas, crackers, or other starch *(Continued)*

Foods to choose and foods to avoid after intestinal surgery (continued)

Food Categories	Well-tolerated foods	Poorly tolerated foods (avoid for the first 4 to 6 weeks) *Note: Reintroduce these foods slowly. You may have difficulty tolerating some of these foods long-term.*
High Protein Sources	Well cooked, plainly prepared, lean fish, meat, poultry, or tofu (broiled, steamed, poached, or baked) Creamy peanut butter Eggs	All fried meats (poultry, fish, tofu or other meat), meat with casing (sausage, hot dogs) Nuts and seeds; crunchy peanut butter; beans, lentils, legumes
Dairy Products	Low-fat milk (skim or 1%) Low-fat lactose-free milk or soy milk Low-fat plain or light flavored yogurt Low-fat cottage or cream cheese Low-fat, unflavored mild cheeses	Whole milk Fruited yogurt with seeds, such as strawberry or raspberry High fat cheeses Strongly flavored cheeses
Fluids	**Soups** Broth (beef, chicken, or vegetable) Chicken noodle or rice or puréed soups made with allowed ingredients **Beverages** Tea or coffee: hot or iced (limit caffeinated items to 2 cups per day) Sports drinks, such as Gatorade® Sugar-free drinks, such as Crystal Lite® **Juices** All fruit juices except for prune juice, tomato juice, or juice with pulp	**Beverages** All carbonated beverages, including soda, pop, and carbonated waters **Juices** Prune juice, tomato juice, or juice with pulp
Desserts	Angel food cake Plain baked goods without nuts, raisins, or seeds Frozen yogurt, pudding, or fruit ice Jell-O®	Desserts with nuts or seeds
Other	Sugar, 1 packet or teaspoon per meal Artificial sweetener Salt, as desired Margarine, butter, oil, mayonnaise – limit to 1-2 teaspoons per meal	Chewing gum Catsup and mustard; Pickles Large spices such as oregano Strongly flavored spices or herbs such as chili, curry, and pepper

Sample meals

Below are conservative dietary recommendations. Remember to aim for 5 or 6 small meals per day and to chew your foods well.

Sample meals for breakfast

¾ cup Rice Krispies®
½ banana
½ cup low-fat milk
1 cup tea

* * * *

1 hard boiled egg
1 slice white toast
1 teaspoon butter or margarine
1 teaspoon grape jelly
1 cup orange juice

Sample meals for lunch

Turkey sandwich on white bread with light mayonnaise
2 canned peach halves
12 ounces sports drink

* * * *

½ cup plain tuna salad
(prepared with light mayonnaise and without celery)
6 saltine-type crackers
½ cup mandarin oranges
12 ounces iced tea with lemon

Sample meals for dinner

3-4 ounces grilled, skinless chicken
½ cup mashed potatoes (without skins)
½ cup tender cooked green beans
1 teaspoon butter or margarine
12 ounces water

* * * *

3-4 ounces grilled tender steak (visible fat removed)
1 baked potato (do not eat the skin)
1 tablespoon light sour cream
½ cup cooked spinach
12 ounces iced tea

Transitioning to a regular diet

After you have recovered, you should be able to resume your usual diet slowly. Here is a list of recommendations to help you transition to your usual diet:

1. Add new foods back to your diet one at a time to make sure that you can digest each new food correctly.
2. If you notice any discomfort or new symptom, use a food diary to keep track of the foods and fluids you are eating and drinking. Record the type of food/fluid, the amount, and any symptoms you experience after eating/drinking.
3. Bring your food diary to follow-up appointments. Your doctor, dietitian, and/or nurse will be able to help you identify foods and/or patterns that are causing any symptoms.

Adapted with permission from the Clinical Nutrition Service, National Institutes of Health Clinical Research Center, Bethesda, MD

APPENDIX 4: Anti-Dumping Diet

Dumping Syndrome occurs when large amounts of food pass too quickly through the digestive tract and fills the small intestine with undigested food that is not ready for absorption. Usually, the pyloric valve located at the base of the stomach helps to release only small amounts of food at a time into the duodenum. If your pyloric valve was removed or manipulated during your surgery, you are at risk for dumping syndrome.

Symptoms associated with dumping syndrome have been classified as **early dumping syndrome** and **late dumping syndrome.**

- **Early dumping syndrome** usually occurs within 15 to 60 minutes of eating. One possible explanation for the early symptoms is that they are caused by the body's response to concentrated sugar entering into the small intestine too quickly. Your body tries to dilute the sugar by pulling fluid from your bloodstream and tissues into your intestine. This can cause cramping, bloating, nausea, and diarrhea. Also, the loss of water from your blood can cause your blood pressure to go down, which can make you feel weak and faint. Increased release of gut hormones may also play a role in the symptoms associated with early dumping syndrome.
- **Late dumping syndrome** usually occurs 2 to 3 hours after eating. When sugar from the intestine is absorbed into the bloodstream quickly, your blood sugar levels rise so your body produces more insulin. When more insulin is released, your blood sugar levels can suddenly drop below normal, causing "hypoglycemia" or low blood sugar. Low blood sugar can cause weakness, a faster heart rate, dizziness, shakiness, sweating, fainting, and mental confusion.

Not everyone experiences these symptoms. Others may experience one or both sets of symptoms. Usually these symptoms decrease as your body adjusts and you learn what types and amounts of foods your body can handle.

If you do not see improvement in these symptoms, report this to your doctor. Ask about medications that can help slow the movement of food through your digestive tract or medications that can help manage the symptoms you are experiencing.

Need for Extra Vitamins and Minerals

Without the production of the digestive enzymes and acids usually present in the stomach, digestion of protein, vitamin B-12, folate, calcium, and iron may be affected. You may also have difficulty absorbing Vitamin D. In addition, when you have dumping syndrome, the food may pass too quickly through the gut and your body may not absorb all of the nutrients from the food you eat. For these reasons, you may be at risk for vitamin and mineral deficiencies.

If you are not absorbing enough nutrients, you may need to take a daily multivitamin with minerals and/or additional vitamin supplements. You may also need injections of vitamin B-12. Ask your doctor or your dietitian what is right for you.

How can I minimize unwanted side effects?

By choosing the right foods and following some basic diet guidelines, you can minimize these unwanted side effects. In this handout you will find diet guidelines about meal planning and food choices.

Immediately after surgery you will be given only clear liquids such as broth, Jell-O, tea or juices. Beverages that have too much sugar, even "natural" fruit sugar, may pull fluid into your intestines, which could cause or worsen diarrhea. Diluting juices and other drinks can reduce the chance that you will have diarrhea from it. Also, limit the portions to ½ cup at a time until you can tolerate the food without discomfort. For example, try the following liquids first: ½ cup broth (vegetable, beef, chicken) OR ½ cup Gatorade or similar Sport drink OR ½ cup diluted grape or cranberry juice (½ water, ½ juice). Your dietitian is available to provide additional suggestions.

When your body is ready, your diet will be advanced to a Phase 1 diet and then to a Phase 2 diet. Phase 1 should be followed during the first 6 – 8 weeks while your body is still recovering and adjusting to the change. After this time period, you may be able to move onto Phase 2 of the diet, which involves slowly adding foods back into your diet. Your dietitian will help you learn when and which foods and drinks are right for you.

A sample meal plan is included to help you plan the timing and sizes of your meals, snacks, and drinks.

Keep in mind that it is important that you focus not only on **which** foods you choose, but also on **how much** of those foods you eat and when you are eating them. By following these guidelines and working with your dietitian, you will be able to minimize unwanted symptoms and increase your comfort level.

See the final section of this handout for ways to minimize nausea, vomiting, diarrhea, early dumping syndrome, and late dumping syndrome through your food choices.

Phase 1: Recovery Period Following Surgery (usually 6 – 8 weeks)

General Guidelines

- Eat at least 6 **small** meals each day.
- Eat slowly and relax while eating.
- **Chew foods completely** so that food becomes liquid before swallowing because your stomach may not be able to grind food like it used to do.
- Do not drink liquids or have soup with your meals. Instead, consume these fluids 45 minutes **before** eating or 1 hour **after** eating.
- Try lying down for 15 minutes after eating. This may help slow the movement of food through your intestine.
- Choose foods low in fiber. Avoid whole grains, fruit and vegetable skins, nuts, seeds, peas and beans.
- Choose soft, well-cooked foods. Avoid raw fruits and vegetables.
- Have a good source of protein with each meal and snack.

○ **High protein foods:** Tender meat, poultry, fish, eggs, tofu, cheese, milk, soy milk, yogurt, and smooth peanut butter.
• Avoid high-sugar foods.
○ **Foods to avoid:** Fruit juice, sugar-sweetened beverages, added sugar, syrup, honey, candy, jam, jelly, molasses, marshmallows, chocolate, ice cream, pudding, pastries, pies, cakes, frosting, cookies, fruit ice, sherbet, gelatin.
○ **Ingredients to avoid (if listed in the first 3 ingredients on the food label):** Sugar, honey, corn syrup, fructose, lactose, dextrose, maltose, sorbitol, xylitol, or mannitol.

○ You **may use** artificial sweeteners that come in yellow, blue, or pink packets. These sweeteners contain sucralose, aspartame, or saccharin respectively.
○ **Limit fruit** to ½ cup cooked or canned at a time.
• Avoid tough or doughy foods like chewy meats and bagels.
• If you find that high fat foods cause discomfort, use low-fat cooking methods and avoid greasy or fried foods. Prepare meat and other foods by broiling, baking, or grilling rather than frying.
• Avoid foods listed in the "Avoid these Foods" column below.

Phase 1: Foods to choose and foods to avoid

Food Group	Choose These Foods	Avoid these Foods
Breads/ Starches/ Grains	Bread, soft rolls, crackers, pasta, white rice Hot and cold cereals with less than 5 grams of sugar and no more than 2 grams of fiber per serving Examples: Corn Chex, Rice Chex, Rice Krispies, Corn Flakes, Cream of Wheat, Special K and Product 19	Sugar-sweetened breads such as sweet rolls, coffeecake, muffins, breakfast bars, donuts, sugar-sweetened cereals, breads with syrup or sweetened sauces Doughy, tough foods like bagels High fiber foods with 3 or more grams of fiber per serving
Protein Sources	Tender, well-cooked meats, poultry, fish, eggs, or soy foods prepared without added fat Smooth nut butters Milk, mild cheese	Sweetened yogurt and flavored milk, nuts, seeds, dried beans and peas If you find that foods high in fat cause discomfort, avoid fried meat, poultry, or fish; high-fat deli meats, such as bologna and salami; and nuts and nut butters
	Note: If you find that milk and dairy products cause discomfort, try lactose-free products or soy milk instead of regular milk and milk products.	
Vegetables	Well-cooked vegetables like carrots without tough skin or seeds Potatoes without skin Strained vegetable juice	All raw vegetables Beets, broccoli, brussel sprouts, cabbage, cauliflower, corn, potato skins, and collard, mustard, or turnip greens Vegetables served with tough skin or seeds
Fruits	Canned, soft fruits without added sugar or syrup like unsweetened applesauce	All raw fruits, dried fruits, fruit juice, and fruits canned in sugar or syrup
Fats & Oils	Oils, butter, margarine, cream, cream cheese, mayonnaise	Sweetened cream cheese, honey butter, salad dressings made with honey
Beverages and Soups **(taken 45 minutes before or 1 hour after meals and snacks)**	Decaffeinated coffee, caffeine-free tea, and caffeine- and sugar-free (diet) soft drinks—(let diet sodas sit until flat) Sweeten with artificial sweeteners Soup - mildly flavored	Caffeinated coffee or tea Alcoholic beverages Beverages containing sugar, corn syrup, or honey Fruit juices and fruit drinks
Other	Artificial sweetener in yellow, blue, or pink packets (sucralose, aspartame, and saccharin)	Sugar, honey, syrup Sorbitol, xylitol Foods that list sugar, honey, syrup, high fructose corn syrup, xylitol, or sorbitol as one of the first three ingredients on the food label

Phase 1: Sample Meal Plan with Timing Schedule

This example has 2200 calories and 85 grams of protein. Your dietitian can help design a meal plan to meet your specific calorie and protein needs.

Time	Food	Fluids
Breakfast		
8:00 am		1 cup decaf tea with sugar substitute ¾ cup milk
8:45 am	1 boiled egg ½ cup cream of wheat with margarine or butter	
Snack		
10:00 am	1 oz. mild cheese 6 crackers ½ cup canned fruit in water	
11:00 am		1 cup water
Lunch		
Noon	3 oz. turkey on white bread with mayonnaise	
1:00 pm		¾ cup milk
Snack		
2:00 pm	½ cup unsweetened apple sauce ¾ cup plain yogurt 6 crackers	
3:00 pm		1 cup soup, like chicken noodle
Dinner		
6:00 pm	3 oz. baked chicken ½ cup cooked carrots ½ cup rice with margarine or butter	
7:00 pm		1 cup water
Snack		
8:15 pm		1½ cup decaf tea with sugar substitute
9:00 pm	4 graham cracker squares with 2 tablespoons smooth peanut butter	

Diet Strategies for Specific Symptoms
NOTE: Some of the suggestions may not be appropriate for the diet phase you are currently following

Symptom	Strategy
Nausea	• Drink small amounts of liquids throughout the day, between meals and snacks. • Eat many (6 – 8) small meals or snacks throughout the day. • Choose light, low-fat, cold foods, such as cold cereal with milk, or a cold turkey sandwich. • Avoid hot temperature foods and foods with strong odors or flavors.
Vomiting	• Chew food completely before swallowing. Eat very slowly. • Contact your doctor if you experience persistent vomiting and discomfort when swallowing. This could indicate that scar tissue is causing part of the gut to be too narrow to allow food to pass easily.
Diarrhea	Drink plenty of allowed fluids between meals and snacks to replace the fluids lost from diarrhea. Consume plenty of allowed foods high in potassium, such as bananas, avocados, cantaloupes, tomatoes, and skinless potatoes. Eat many (6 – 8) small meals or snacks throughout the day. After the first 6-8 weeks, try foods with soluble fiber such as oats, barley, peeled fruit, and cooked vegetables. Products such as Metamucil™ or Benefiber™ can also serve as a source of soluble fiber. Soluble fiber helps to solidify stool. Avoid insoluble fiber such as wheat bran, stringy fibers, seeds, and thick skins. Insoluble fiber can speed up the flow of food through the gut. Limit milk and milk products if not tolerated. They contain a natural sugar called "lactose" that can be hard to breakdown and can worsen diarrhea for some people. You may need to be tested for malabsorption. Avoid sugar alcohols like sorbitol.
Early Dumping Syndrome	Avoid high-sugar foods (including "natural sugars") such as sweetened beverages, fruit juice, cookies, cakes, pies, and other sweets. High-sugar foods pull more water into the intestine to dilute the sugars, causing dumping.
Late Dumping Syndrome	With each meal and snack, eat a source of protein, fat, and/or soluble fiber that you tolerate well. Examples may be meat, cheese, oats, barley, peeled fruit, and cooked vegetables. These foods may slow the rate that sugars are absorbed into the blood. Avoid high-sugar foods and large portions of carbohydrate (i.e., Do not eat more than 3 servings of grains, juice and/or fruit in one meal) Limit fluids with meals.

Phase 2: When you are no longer experiencing symptoms after eating
General Guidelines
Continue to:
- Eat at least 6 **small** meals each day.
- Eat slowly and relax while eating.
- **Chew foods completely** before swallowing.
- **Limit liquids or soup with meals to ½ cup.** Consume additional liquids and soups 45 minutes **before** eating or 1 hour **after** eating.
- Have a good source of protein with each meal or snack.
- **Limit** high-sugar foods.
- If high-fat foods cause you discomfort, use **low-fat** cooking methods and **avoid** greasy or fried foods.
- Add new foods back to your diet one at a time to make sure that you can digest each new food correctly.
- If you notice any discomfort or new symptom, use a food diary to keep track of the foods and fluids you are eating and drinking. Record the type of food/fluid, the amount, and any symptoms you experience after eating/drinking.

- Bring your food diary to follow-up appointments. Your doctor, dietitian, and/or nurse will be able to help you identify foods and/or patterns that are causing any symptoms.

Conclusion
You CAN do this! While all of this may seem overwhelming at first, keep in mind that it is really all about listening to your body. There is no doubt that stomach surgery may change the way your body handles food. By following the diet guidelines provided in this handout you will be able to minimize unwanted symptoms and discomfort. Also, by *slowly* adding foods back into your diet you will learn which foods, and in what amounts, your body is able to handle. Your dietitian is available to answer any questions and to help you with any problems you come across every step of the way.

Adapted with permission from the Clinical Nutrition Service, National Institutes of Health Clinical Research Center, Bethesda, MD

APPENDIX 5: Diet and Nutrition Guidelines after Ileostomy Placement

After your ileostomy is placed, your body will need time to adapt to a regular diet. By adjusting your food choices, you can prevent problems such as excess gas production, dehydration, diarrhea, and constipation. These problems are most common in the first few weeks after surgery.

Most people are able to resume a near-normal diet after the first 6 to 8 weeks. This handout will provide specific diet guidelines for the first 6 to 8 weeks after surgery, as well as discuss how to transition to a regular diet. Finally, this handout will provide useful tips on how to manage symptoms that are likely to continue for as long as you have the ileostomy.

General diet recommendations for the first 6 to 8 weeks

1. **Eat small, frequent meals.** Aim for 5 to 6 small meals per day. Do not skip meals. Skipping meals may increase gas production. See the sample menu for examples of meals.
2. **Chew foods well.** Chewing foods well will help you better absorb the nutrients. It will also prevent foods from causing a blockage or obstruction as stool exits the ileostomy.
3. **Stay hydrated.** Drink <u>at least</u> 8 to 10 cups of liquid per day. See the list of fluids to choose (in the table).
   If you experience diarrhea or have a lot of liquid output from your ileostomy, you may need to drink more to prevent dehydration. <u>Do not try to control diarrhea or high ileostomy output by restricting fluids.</u> Call your health care provider if you have signs of dehydration, which include the following:
   • Feeling thirsty
   • Dry skin and mouth
   • Feeling lightheaded
   • Decreased amount of urine or very dark urine
   • Feeling tired

4. **Avoid foods high in dietary fiber.** Dietary fiber refers to the part of plant foods that cannot be digested by your intestines. It is important to avoid both types of fiber, insoluble fiber and soluble fiber.
   • **Avoids foods high in insoluble fiber.** Insoluble fiber stimulates intestinal contractions and may move food through your intestines too quickly, which may interfere with wound healing. Foods high in insoluble fiber include skins of fruits, stringy fibers from raw vegetables, seeds and whole grain breads or cereals.
   • **Avoid foods high in soluble fiber.** Soluble fiber absorbs fluid in your digestive tract and may help thicken ileostomy output. However, the thicker output will increase the pressure in your intestine and may interfere with wound healing. <u>Therefore, you should avoid foods high in soluble fiber until your doctor reports that your intestine has healed. After you have healed from the surgery, you will need to eat more soluble fiber to make your stools more formed.</u> Examples of foods high in soluble fiber are rice, oats, applesauce, and bananas.
5. **Choose low-fat foods.** Low-fat foods are easier to digest than high-fat foods. Examples of low-fat foods include low-fat dairy products such as skim or 1% milk, lean meats (visible fat and/or skin removed), and reduced-fat or fat-free sauces, gravies, and/or salad dressings.
6. **Limit simple sugars.** Foods such as desserts and sugar-sweetened beverages may cause diarrhea. Avoid these foods for the first 6 to 8 weeks after surgery, or until you are tolerating a regular diet without difficulty. You can gradually reintroduce sweetened foods once your ileostomy output is well managed.

Foods to choose and foods to avoid for the first 6 to 8 weeks

The following table tells you which specific foods are best tolerated in the first 6 to 8 weeks after surgery. Also make sure to read the nutrition facts label on food products and limit foods to those with 2 grams of fiber or less per serving during the first 6 to 8 weeks after surgery.

Food Categories	Well-tolerated foods	Poorly tolerated foods (avoid for the first 6 to 8 weeks) *Note: Reintroduce these foods slowly. You may have difficulty tolerating some of these foods long-term.*
Fruits	Bananas (limit portion to ½)	All raw, fresh fruits except bananas
	Canned fruit such as applesauce, peaches, pears, and other canned fruit without skins	All canned fruits with skins, seeds, or membranes
	All canned fruit should be packed in juice or water (not heavy syrup).	All dried fruits (raisins, prunes, apricots, etc.)
Vegetables	Tender cooked and canned vegetables	All raw vegetables, all gas forming vegetables
	Begin with soft, cooked green beans, wax beans, carrots and beets	Cooked vegetables with large seeds such as zucchini or squash
	Peeled potatoes	Potato skins
Starches	**Hot Cereals** Plain cream of rice, cream of wheat, grits, or oatmeal	**Hot Cereals** Cereals with raisins, nuts, seeds, coconut or other dried fruits
	Cold Cereals Cheerios®, Corn Flakes®, Rice Krispies®, Puffed Rice or other low fiber cereal	**Cold Cereals** Whole wheat or wheat bran cereals; Cereals with raisins, nuts, seeds, coconut, or other dried fruits
	Breads, pastas, and potatoes White bread or toast Plain bagels English muffins Plain dinner rolls Pasta: plain macaroni, spaghetti, egg noodles Potatoes (no skin), baked or mashed Rice, white Saltines	**Breads, pastas, and potatoes** Whole grain or multigrain breads Breads and cereals with raisins, nuts, seeds, coconut, or other dried fruits
High Protein Sources	Well cooked, plainly prepared, lean fish, meat, poultry, or tofu (broiled, steamed, poached, or baked)	All fried meats (poultry, fish, tofu or other meat), meat with casing (sausage, hot dogs)
	Creamy peanut butter (1 Tablespoon)	Nuts and seeds; crunchy peanut butter
	Eggs (cooked until the yolk is firm)	Beans, lentils, legumes
Dairy Products	Low-fat milk (skim or 1%) Low-fat Lactaid® milk or soy milk Low-fat plain or light flavored yogurt Low-fat cottage cheese Low-fat, unflavored and/or mild cheeses	Whole milk Fruited yogurt (with seeds, such as strawberry or raspberry) High fat cheeses Strongly flavored cheeses
Fluids	**Soups** Broth (beef, chicken, or vegetable) Chicken noodle, chicken rice, or pureed soups	**Soups** Soups made with ingredients that are poorly tolerated, such as gas forming vegetables, corn, heavy cream or whole milk
	Beverages Tea or coffee: hot or iced (limit caffeinated items to 2 cups per day) Sports drinks, such as Gatorade® Sugar-free drinks, such as Crystal Lite® **Juices** Dilute all juices to ½ juice, ½ water	**Beverages** All carbonated beverages, including soda, pop and carbonated waters
Desserts	Angel food cake Plain baked goods without nuts, raisins, or seeds Frozen yogurt, pudding, fruit ice Jell-O®	All other desserts
Other	Sugar, 1 packet or teaspoon per meal Artificial sweetener except sugar alcohols Salt, as desired Margarine, butter, oil, mayonnaise – limit to 1-2 teaspoons per meal	Sugar alcohols Chewing gum Chocolate Catsup and mustard; pickles Strongly flavored spices or herbs such as chili powder, curry powder, horseradish, and pepper

Sample menu for the first 6 to 8 weeks

Below are conservative dietary recommendations. Remember to aim for 5 or 6 small meals per day and to chew your foods well.

Sample breakfast

¾ cup Rice Krispies®
½ banana
½ cup Lactaid®, soy, or low-fat milk
1 cup tea

Sample lunch

Turkey sandwich on white bread with light mayonnaise
2 canned peach halves (in water or juice)
12 ounces Gatorade®

Sample dinner

3-4 ounces grilled, skinless chicken
½ cup mashed potatoes (without skins, prepared without
added fat such as butter, margarine or cream)
½ cup tender cooked green beans
1 teaspoon butter or margarine
12 ounces water

Recommendations for snack foods and desserts

Angel food cake with or without canned peaches
and light whipped topping
Plain cookies such as vanilla wafers or animal crackers
Hot or cold cereal with low-fat milk
Baked chips or pretzels
Jell-O® or Fruited Jell-O®
Pudding (if you tolerate milk products)
Small slice pound cake
Reduced-fat ice cream
Canned fruit

Transitioning to a regular diet

After you have recovered, you should be able to resume your usual diet slowly.

1. Add new foods back to your diet one at a time to make sure that you can digest each new food correctly.
2. If you notice any discomfort or new symptom, use a food diary to keep track of the foods and fluids you are eating and drinking.
   Record the type of food/fluid, the amount, and any symptoms you experience after eating/drinking.
3. Bring your food diary to follow-up appointments. Your doctor, dietitian and/or nurse will be able to help you identify foods and/or patterns that are causing any symptoms.

Adapted with permission from the Clinical Nutrition Service, National Institutes of Health Clinical Research Center, Bethesda, MD

MCT oil may be appropriate when conventional fats are not tolerated. Patients using MCT oil should begin with a daily intake of 15mL; should not consume more than 20mL at one time; and should not consume more than 100 mL in one day (http://www.nestlehealthscience.us/products/mct-oil%C2%AE), Accessed September 25, 2013. Those using MCT oil should only do so under the direction of an MD and with the support of an RD. Sample recipes provide ideas for incorporating MCT oil in a diet.

Recipe #1: MCT Margarine
Reprinted with permission from Diana Pantalos, MS, RDN, LD, Metabolic Nutritionist, University of Louisville

Ingredients
4 T fat free cream cheese
4 T non-fat liquid margarine
½ cup MCT oil
1/8 t salt

Use as a margarine spread.
Not recommended for cooking or baking.

Combine cream cheese and liquid margarine with hand blender, food processor or mixer. Add salt. Slowly add MCT oil, mixing until combined. Whip if desire.

Yield: 1 cup
1 t margarine = 2.5 mL MCT oil
1 T margarine = 7.5 mL MCT oil

Recipe #2: MCT Vinaigrette Dressing
Reprinted with permission from Diana Pantalos, MS, RDN, LD, Metabolic Nutritionist, University of Louisville

Ingredients
½ cup MCT oil
½ cup cider vinegar
1 Tablespoon sugar
¾ teaspoon salt
¾ teaspoon dry mustard
1/8 teaspoon pepper

Shake all ingredients together vigorously in a covered jar.
Dressing will separate, but shake just before using.
Yield: ½ cup dressing
1 Tablespoon – 1½ teaspoons (7.5 mL) MCT oil

APPENDIX 7: Overview of a Ketogenic Diet

In recent years the ketogenic diet has gained attention as a potential cancer treatment. To induce ketosis, the diet provides no more than 5% to 10% of daily calories from carbohydrate, or < 50 grams of carbohydrate daily (1). After metabolic adaptation, fatty acids provide approximately 70% of energy needs, ketone bodies 20% and glucose 10% (from the metabolism of dietary protein and fat) (1). Evidence suggests that the ketogenic diet may blunt the appetite, but the weight goal is usually maintenance.

The carbohydrate content of diets providing 5%-10% of carbohydrate for various calorie levels:

Calories	Grams of Carbohydrate Equal to 5% of Calories	Grams of Carbohydrate Equal to 10% of Calories
1200	15	30
1500	19	37.5
1600	20	40
1800	22.5	45
2000	25	50

Foods that contain significant amounts of carbohydrate are eliminated or severely restricted:

Fruits and juices
"Starchy" vegetables such as peas
Many dairy foods (e.g., milk, yogurt)
Grains (e.g. breads, pasta, rice, potatoes, noodles, cereals, crackers)
Sugar-sweetened desserts and sweets (e.g. cakes, pies, cookies, ice cream, caney, sugars, honey, karo syrup and other sweeteners)

Foods that contain minimal amounts of carbohydrate are often included in limited amounts:

Non-starch vegetables (e.g. leafy greens, asparagus, zucchini, tomatoes, celery)

Foods that contain small amounts of carbohydrate may be included in limited amounts:

Nuts and seeds

Foods that do not contain carbohydrate are recommended:

Meats, poultry, fish, eggs, fats

Adhering to a ketogenic diet is challenging and the diet must be individualzed for each patient. Meal plans should meet each patient's unique needs and incorporate as wide a range of foods as possible. These diets are deficient in many nutrients; vitamin/ mineral, calcium, and vitamin D supplementation is usually required.

Constipation is a common problem. It is essential to drink recommended amounts of fluid. The diet should be as high in fiber as possible, though this is challenging. Use of stool softeners and laxatives may be indicated.

The Charlie Foundation serves the community of children who have seizure disorders and follow a ketogenic diet. This foundation provides a range of resources that can assist children and adults who follow this diet http://www.charliefoundation.org/.

A full discussion of ketogenic diets is beyond the scope of this document, but this overview provides a general review of important points and considerations.

1. Westman EC, Feinman RD, Mavropoulos JC. Low-carbohydrate nutrition and metabolism. *Am J Clin Nutr.* 2007;86(2):276-284.

While interest in the Ketogenic Diet is increasing, there is still much to learn about its metabolic effects. Cancer patients should follow this diet only under the direction of an MD and with careful monitoring by an RD.

APPENDIX 8: Drug, Nutrient, Food, and Dietary Supplement Interactions with Cancer Medications

Chemotherapy, Biotherapy and Hormonal Agents, Trade Names and Route of Administration	Possible Drug, Nutrient, Food, and Dietary Supplement Interactions
Axitinib Inlyta® Oral Directions: Take 2 times a day, 12 hours apart.	• CYP3A4 inducers may decrease drug activity (e.g., St. John's Wort, Phenobarbital). • Avoid CYP3A4 inhibitors which may increase drug activity (e.g., grapefruit juice, ketoconazole, erythromycin).
Bexarotene Targretin® Oral Directions: Take as a single dose with food.	• Grapefruit juice may increase concentration and toxicities. • Limit Vitamin A intake to ≤ 1,500 IU/day to avoid possible additive toxicity with drug.
Bortezomib Velcade® Intravenous or subcutaneous	• Green tea should be avoided while taking this drug, especially in liquid and capsule forms. • CYP3A4 inhibitors or inducers may alter drug activity, monitor closely.
Busulfan Myleran® Oral Directions: Take on an empty stomach.	• Aspirin-containing OTC medications should be avoided while taking this drug.
Capecitabine Xeloda® Oral Directions: Take as directed within 30 minutes of a meal with a full glass of water.	• Altered coagulation when taken with Warfarin, monitor closely. • Vitamin B6 (dose of 50 to 100 mg two to three times a day) may help to prevent/reduce the incidence and severity of hand-foot syndrome.
Cetuximab Erbitux® Intravenous	• Monitor serum magnesium and calcium levels closely. At risk populations: elderly, hypomagnesemia at baseline, patients who have received prior treatment with oxaliplatin (Eloxatin®).
Chlorambucil Leukeran® Oral Directions: Take on empty stomach, either 1 hour before meals or 2 hours after meals.	• Risk of toxicity increases if barbiturates have been taken.
Cisplatin Platinol® Intravenous	• Rigorous hydration is necessary to prevent nephrotoxicity (e.g., oral hydration and in some instances patients may benefit from intravenous infusions of fluid). • Carefully monitor renal function (BUN and Creatinine) and serum electrolytes (magnesium, calcium, sodium, potassium) levels closely. At risk populations: elderly, hypomagnesemia or those with impaired renal function at baseline.
Cyclophosphamide Cytoxan® Intravenous or Oral Oral Directions: take preferably earlier in the day and with vigorous hydration throughout the day.	• Advise vigorous oral hydration (3 liters of fluid per day) throughout the day. Instruct patients to empty bladder every 2 to 3 hours during waking hours, as well as at night if getting up or awake. • Of note, Mesna is given with high-dose cyclophosphamide to prevent hemorrhagic cystitis. • Increases the effect of anticoagulants, so dose of anticoagulants may need to be decreased.
Dasatinib Sprycel® Oral Directions: Take with or without food.	• Avoid CYP3A4 inducers which may decrease drug activity (e.g., St. John's Wort, Phenobarbital). • Avoid CYP3A4 inhibitors which may increase drug activity (e.g., grapefruit juice, ketoconazole, and erythromycin). • Do not crush or cut drug.
Deferasiox Exjade® Directions: Dissolve tablets completely in water before taking.	• If drug is not fully dissolved it can cause diarrhea. • Drug contains lactose. May cause diarrhea in lactose intolerant patients. Recommend lactase enzyme supplement with dosing.
Erlotinib Tarceva® Oral Directions: Take on empty stomach, either 1 hour before meals or 2 hours after meals. Take at the same time every day with a full glass of water.	• Avoid CYP3A4 inducers which may decrease drug activity (e.g., St. John's Wort, Phenobarbital). • Avoid CYP3A4 inhibitors which may increase drug activity (e.g., grapefruit juice, ketoconazole, and erythromycin).

(Continued)

APPENDIX 8: Drug, Nutrient, Food, and Dietary Supplement Interactions with Cancer Medications *(cont.)*

Chemotherapy, Biotherapy and Hormonal Agents, Trade Names and Route of Administration	Possible Drug, Nutrient, Food, and Dietary Supplement Interactions
Everolimus Afinitor® Oral Directions: Take once a day at the same time, with or without food. Swallow whole with a glass of water.	• Avoid CYP3A4 inducers which may decrease drug activity (e.g., St. John's Wort, Phenobarbital). • Avoid CYP3A4 inhibitors which may increase drug activity (e.g., grapefruit juice, ketoconazole, and erythromycin). • Do not chew or crush drug.
Exemestane Aromasin® Oral Directions: Take daily after a meal.	• Avoid CYP3A4 inducers which may decrease drug activity.
Fluorouracil 5-FU or Adrucil® Intravenous	• For IV bolus infusions only – Have patient melt ice chips in the mouth 10 to 15 minutes pre- and post- IV bolus infusion to reduce incidence of oral mucositis. • Vitamin B6 (dose of 50 to 100 mg two to three times a day) may help to prevent/reduce the incidence and severity of hand-foot syndrome.
Gefitinib Iressa® Oral Directions: Dissolve tablets in half glass of water and stir until dissolved. Drink immediately and follow with another full glass of water.	• Drug toxicity may be increased if barbiturates have been used.
Imatinib mesylate Gleevec® Oral Directions: Take with a meal and a full glass of water.	• If tablets are difficult to swallow, drug may be dissolved in a glass of water or apple juice. Drink immediately and follow with another full glass of water. • CYP3A4 inducers may decrease drug activity (e.g., St. John's Wort, Phenobarbital, and dexamethasone). • CYP3A4 inhibitors may increase drug activity (e.g., grapefruit juice, ketoconazole, and erythromycin).
Lapatinib Tykerb® Oral Directions: Take on an empty stomach, either 1 hour before meals or 2 hours after meals. Take with a full glass of water.	• CYP3A4 inhibitors may increase drug activity (e.g., grapefruit juice, ketoconazole, and erythromycin). • Do not crush or chew drug.
Melphalan Alkeran® Intravenous or oral Oral Directions: Take on an empty stomach, either 1 hour before meals or 2 hours after meals.	• Premedicate with antiemetic one hour before oral dose. • Encourage small, frequent meals and snacks.
Mercaptopurine 6-MP or Purinethol® Oral Directions: Take on empty stomach, 1 hour before meals or 2 hours after meals.	• Avoid consuming dairy-containing foods around the time of taking this drug.
Methotrexate Folex® or Rheumatrex® Intravenous, Intrathecal or Oral Oral Directions: Take on an empty stomach, either 1 hour before meals or 2 hours after meals.	• Avoid folic acid and its derivatives during methotrexate drug therapy. • Avoid alcohol as it may increase hepatotoxicity.
Nilotinib Tasigna® Oral Directions: Take on an empty stomach with a full glass of water.	• CYP3A4 inhibitors may increase drug activity (e.g., grapefruit juice, ketoconazole, and erythromycin). • Contains lactose. May cause diarrhea in lactose intolerant patients. Recommend lactase enzyme supplement with dosing.
Oxaliplatin Eloxatin® Intravenous	• To prevent pharyngolaryngeal dysesthesia minimize exposure to cold for up to five days after the infusion by avoiding eating and drinking cold or frozen foods. Sensitivity to cold may persist for longer periods of times with subsequent dosing. • Use care when handling cold or frozen foods from the refrigerator or freezer. • Vitamin B6 (dose of 50 to 100 mg two to three times a day) may help to prevent/reduce the incidence and severity of hand-foot syndrome. *(Continued)*

APPENDIX 8: Drug, Nutrient, Food, and Dietary Supplement Interactions with Cancer Medications *(cont.)*

Chemotherapy, Biotherapy and Hormonal Agents, Trade Names and Route of Administration	Possible Drug, Nutrient, Food, and Dietary Supplement Interactions
Panitumumab Vectibix®. Intravenous	• Monitor serum magnesium levels closely. At risk populations: elderly, patients with hypomagensemia at baseline.
Pemetrexed Alimta® Intravenous	• To prevent possibly severe anemia ensure the following dietary supplementation prior to and during drug therapy: – Folic acid (350 to 1000 µg) po beginning 1 week prior to first treatment continuing daily throughout treatment and post treatment – Vitamin B-12 (1000 µg) IM injections given every 3 cycles, beginning 1 week prior first treatment, and continuing throughout treatment.
Procarbazine Hydrochloride Matulane® Oral	• Exhibits weak MAO (monoamine oxidase) inhibitor activity. • Foods containing tyramine should be avoided while taking this drug and for 2 weeks after. Tyramine-containing foods include: beer, red wine, sherry, distilled spirits, brewer's yeast, fava beans, raspberries, figs, dried fruits (raisins and prunes), avocados, bananas, miso soup, soy sauce, sauerkraut, aged and strong cheeses, anchovies, caviar, beef and chicken livers, meat extracts, meats such as sausage, bologna, pepperoni, and salami. Avoid caffeine. Consuming these foods may lead to hypertensive crisis or intracranial hemorrhage. • Patients should be advised to avoid all alcoholic beverages for possible Antabuse®-like reaction.
Regorafenib Stivarga® Oral Directions: Take in the morning with a low fat meal that contains ≤ 8 grams of fat	• High fat meals can alter the absorption of the drug. • One study (with 24 healthy men) found that this medicine was better absorbed when taken with a meal providing 8.2 grams of fat and 319 calories as compared with a meal providing 54.6 grams of fat and 945 calories.
Sipuleucel-T Provenge® Intravenous Directions: leukapheresis is performed 3 days prior to each of the 3 planned treatment infusions.	• Patients should be advised to avoid caffeinated beverages on the day of their leukapheresis. • Patients should be instructed to drink more water than usual 2 to 3 days prior to their treatments and to consume a calcium-rich breakfast prior to receiving their treatment infusions.
Streptozocin Zanosar® Intravenous	• Alters glucose metabolism (hypoglycemia) in some patients.
Sorafenib Nexavar® Oral Directions: Take on an empty stomach, either 1 hour before meals or 2 hours after meals. Take with a full glass of water.	• CYP3A4 inducers may decrease drug activity (e.g., St. John's Wort, Phenobarbital, and dexamethasone).
Sunitinib Sutent® Oral Directions: Take with or without food.	• Avoid CYP3A4 inducers which may decrease drug activity (e.g., St. John's Wort, Phenobarbital). • Avoid CYP3A4 inhibitors which may increase drug activity (e.g., grapefruit juice, ketoconazole, and erythromycin).
Tamoxifen Nolvadex® Oral Directions: Take with or without food. Take at the same time each day.	• Avoid antacids within 2 hours of taking the drug. • Avoid CYP3A4 inducers which may decrease drug activity (e.g., St. John's Wort, Phenobarbital). • Avoid CYP3A4 inhibitors which may increase drug activity (e.g., grapefruit juice, ketoconazole, and erythromycin).
Temsirolimus Torisel® Intravenous	• Alters glucose metabolism (hyperglycemia) and cause hypercholesterolemia in some patients.
Temozolomide Temodar® Oral Directions: Take at bedtime or on an empty stomach with a full glass of water.	• Do not crush or dissolve drug.

(Continued)

APPENDIX 8: Drug, Nutrient, Food, and Dietary Supplement Interactions with Cancer Medications *(cont.)*

Chemotherapy, Biotherapy and Hormonal Agents, Trade Names and Route of Administration	Possible Drug, Nutrient, Food, and Dietary Supplement Interactions
Thalidomide Thalomid® Oral Directions: Take at bedtime, at least 1 hour after evening meal.	• Drug interactions with barbiturates, chlorpromazine, reserpine, and alcohol.
Vinblastine Velban® Intravenous	• CYP3A4 inducers may decrease drug activity (e.g. St. John's Wort, Phenobarbital, and dexamethasone). • CYP3A4 inhibitors may increase drug activity (e.g. grapefruit juice, ketoconazole, and erythromycin). • Stool softeners and/or stimulant laxative may help to prevent severe constipation.
Vincristine Oncovin® Intravenous	• CYP3A4 inducers may decrease drug activity (e.g. St. John's Wort, Phenobarbital, and dexamethasone). • CYP3A4 inhibitors may increase drug activity (e.g. grapefruit juice, ketoconazole, and erythromycin). • Stool softeners and/or stimulant laxative may help to prevent severe constipation.
Zoledronic Acid Zometa® Intravenous	• Patients should take an oral supplement of 500 mg calcium and 400 IU of Vitamin D daily

Sources:
- Wilkes GM and Barton-Burke, 2012; Wilkes GM, 2011; Chu and DeVita, 2012; Polovich et al, 2009; Golden et al, 2009; Saif, 2008; Chemocare, 2013.
- Chemocare. Available at: http://chemocare.com/chemotherapy/drug-info/default.aspx. Accessed June 2, 2013.
- Chu E, DeVita VT. Physicians' Cancer Chemotherapy Drug Manual: 2012. Burlington, MA: Jones and Bartlett Learning; 2012.
- Golden EG, Lam PY, Kardos A, et al. Green tea polyphenols block the anticancer effects of bortezomib and other boronic-acid based porteasome inhibitors. Blood. Epub: February 3, 2009.
- Polovich M, Whitford JM, Olsen M. Chemotherapy and Biotherapy Guidelines: Recommendations for Practice. Pittsburgh, PA: Oncology Nursing Society; 2009.
- Saif MW. Management of hypomagnesemia in cancer patients receiving chemotherapy. *J Support Oncology.* 2008;6:243-248.
- Wilkes GM. Target Cancer Therapy: A Handbook for Nurses. Burlington, MA: Jones and Bartlett; 2011.
- Wilkes GM, Barton-Burke M. Oncology Nursing Handbook: 2012. Burlington, MA: Jones and Bartlett Learning; 2012.

APPENDIX 9: Bowel Regimen

For healthy people, the keys to bowel regularity are an adequate and varied fiber intake, an adequate fluid intake, and regular physical activity. However, these habits may not be sufficient, appropriate or even possible for some cancer patients and survivors. Pain medication requirements slow gastrointestinal (GI) functions; surgeries may re-route usual GI pathways; and advanced cancer can be associated with intestinal blockages that prevent normal stool passage.

Bowel regimens are used to improve bowel function and passage of stool when a cancer and its treatments limit, prevent and/or impede normal GI function. They often combine bulk-forming agents with osmotic laxatives; may incorporate stool softeners; and may utilize enemas. Agents may be used in a step-wise pattern. It is important to use as few agents as possible and indicated for the setting. While there is concern that frequent laxative use can create dependence in healthy individuals, this may not be a concern in an advanced cancer setting when palliation may be the primary goal.

Bowel regimens can significantly improve quality of life and prevent serious GI complications. When a bowel regimen is indicated, it is important to consult with the multidisciplinary team as many institutions have developed preferred bowel regimens. It also is important to consider the following points:
- Advise the patient on the type(s) and amounts of dietary fiber indicated, if any.
- Advise the patient on the importance of consuming small, frequent meals and chewing food well to improve digestion and absorption.
- Confirm the preferred bowel regimen with the multidisciplinary team so that all team members are reinforcing the same message.

Baseline doses of stool softeners and laxatives are often initially ordered. Doses are increased slowly as needed, with the goal of providing the lowest and most effective doses for the combination of medications prescribed.

Products considered for bowel regimens may include bulk forming agents such as Metamucil® and Benefiber®; oral osmotic laxatives such as Phillips' Milk of Magnesia® and Miralax®; oral stool softeners such as Colace® and Kaopectate®; oral stimulants such as Senokot®, and rectal stimulants such as Bisacodyl® and Dulcolax®. Bowel regimens also may include products used for pre-operative bowel cleanses such as Magnesium Citrate® and may consider enemas such as sodium phosphate enema.

Patients on a bowel regimen will receive specific instructions on the prescribed combination of agents (with specific doses for each), and time when agents should be used. Patient communication is essential to monitor outcomes and assess need for changes in the bowel regimen.